# Sustainable Development Goals Series

The **Sustainable Development Goals Series** is Springer Nature's inaugural cross-imprint book series that addresses and supports the United Nations' seventeen Sustainable Development Goals. The series fosters comprehensive research focused on these global targets and endeavours to address some of society's greatest grand challenges. The SDGs are inherently multidisciplinary, and they bring people working across different fields together and working towards a common goal. In this spirit, the Sustainable Development Goals series is the first at Springer Nature to publish books under both the Springer and Palgrave Macmillan imprints, bringing the strengths of our imprints together.

The Sustainable Development Goals Series is organized into eighteen subseries: one subseries based around each of the seventeen respective Sustainable Development Goals, and an eighteenth subseries, "Connecting the Goals", which serves as a home for volumes addressing multiple goals or studying the SDGs as a whole. Each subseries is guided by an expert Subseries Advisor with years or decades of experience studying and addressing core components of their respective Goal.

The SDG Series has a remit as broad as the SDGs themselves, and contributions are welcome from scientists, academics, policymakers, and researchers working in fields related to any of the seventeen goals. If you are interested in contributing a monograph or curated volume to the series, please contact the Publishers: Zachary Romano [Springer; zachary.romano@ springer.com] and Rachael Ballard [Palgrave Macmillan; rachael.ballard@ palgrave.com].

Anna Stewart Ibarra
A. Desiree LaBeaud
Editors

# Transforming Global Health Partnerships

Critical Reflections and Visions of Equity at the Research-Practice Interface

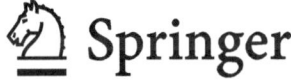 Springer

*Editors*
Anna Stewart Ibarra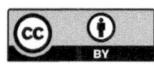
Inter-American Institute for Global
Change Research (IAI)
Panama City, Panama

A. Desiree LaBeaud
Department of Pediatrics
Division of Infectious Diseases
Stanford University
Stanford, CA, USA

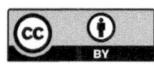

ISSN 2523-3084          ISSN 2523-3092   (electronic)
Sustainable Development Goals Series
ISBN 978-3-031-53792-9          ISBN 978-3-031-53793-6   (eBook)
https://doi.org/10.1007/978-3-031-53793-6

Color wheel and icons: From https://www.un.org/sustainabledevelopment/, Copyright © 2020
United Nations. Used with the permission of the United Nations.
The content of this publication has not been approved by the United Nations and does not
reflect the views of the United Nations or its officials or Member States.

This Springer imprint is published by the registered company Springer Nature Switzerland AG
The registered company address is: Gewerbestrasse 11, 6330 Cham, Switzerland

If disposing of this product, please recycle the paper.

# Preface

## Introduction

If you are reading this book, you may be a scientist, clinician, or public health practitioner engaged in global health partnerships, a student considering a career in global health, or someone who wants to learn about creating equitable and transformative partnerships at the intersection of research and practice. If you're like us, you may wear multiple hats as a clinician, researcher, international civil servant, leader, learner, teacher, mentor, activist, advocate, healer, and diplomat. Such is the nature of global health partnerships and those of us who work in this dynamic, evolving space.

This is a book about the human experience of conducting global health research linked to operational responses to the control and prevention of diseases worldwide. Rather than a manual or "how to" guide, we propose a roadmap and vision of equitable, sustainable, and impactful partnerships shared through a rich interweaving of voices—North and South, academics and community practitioners, senior mentors and trainees/students, multiple generations, and multiple disciplines. We focus on the stories that need to be told, the successes and the failures, and visions for a healthier and more compassionate future for humanity.

This book was written by 90 authors from 26 countries, bringing diverse perspectives on global health partnerships' past, present, and future. Although many of the chapters use examples related to infectious diseases, the ideas in this book are relevant to the broader field of global health research and practice.

## How This Book Is Organized

This book is organized into three sections, broadly related to foundational concepts, present experiences (case studies), and future visions.

The first section focuses on the historical colonial legacy of global health and the foundations needed for equitable partnerships, introducing key themes explored throughout the book. These include concepts related to decolonization, ethics, gender, systems approaches and transdisciplinary science, Planetary Health, One Health, team science, and communication. Authors explore the power inequities, biases, and stigmas that shape and distort partnerships. They emphasize a holistic systems approach to infectious disease and global health work and discuss the science of teams, including the nature of conflicts in the context of multicultural and transdisciplinary teams and their resolution as opportunities for growth. Lastly, the authors emphasize the critical role of communication strategies in driving change in global health work.

The book's second section draws on case studies of global health partnerships to understand where we are today in global health. Authors share their experiences responding to global health threats, including disease outbreaks, refugee health, stigma, and sexually transmitted diseases, and post-disaster community recovery. Through these stories, they impart lessons learned from building partnerships to improve the health of the world's people. This section highlights the need for a team culture of continual learning, especially learning from our mistakes and missteps. Authors explore how to reshape partnership models to respond to ongoing and future global health threats, such as the COVID-19 pandemic.

The book's third section articulates a new vision for global health partnerships to co-create a more peaceful, equitable, and loving world. This vision is urgently needed to address the challenges that have emerged in the context of global climate change, the COVID-19 pandemic, and other human threats. Authors emphasize the critical role of Indigenous People in articulating a future narrative focused on the inherent interconnectedness of all life. Other authors envision transformative research funding and educational systems that support the equitable sharing of resources and power, with examples of action driven by social movements, students, and women from the Global South. Finally, the authors share a vision of a new paradigm of science that values other ways of knowing, which may contest or complement Western systems of global health work.

## Why This Book Now?

Our motivation for convening these stories is to place human partnership as the foundation of global health work. How we engage as humans (with who, when, where, and by whose rules) is critical yet often overlooked in formal university education and scientific discourse, leading to planetary and civilatory crises resulting from a blatant disregard for our relationship with other people and all other life forms, waters, air, and soils. This book is an opportunity to be explicit about *relationships* and to center them in global health discourse, to be honest, and introspective, and to examine the field of global health in a way that is constructive and critical. The authors name the collective wounds of colonization and other inequitable and extractive relationships to reveal their ties to the origins of global health and the unbalanced structures and power dynamics of current global health practice. We do so to heal, transform, and transcend these violent ways of relating and to create an alternative vision of the future. We are compelled to work to improve human health and well-being—the foundation of global health—but know that it needs to be done differently.

Our hope is that this book can plant many seeds that contribute to a new global conversation about how we, as humanity, work together and with other life forms, to understand better our role, our responsibility, and our deep interconnectedness. This requires humility and courage to self-reflect, to see the damage that has been done to us or that we have done, to be willing to repair and make amends, to forgive, and to transform our relationships purposefully. We hope this book demonstrates the agency and opportunity within partnerships that can propel global health to thrive. Authors worldwide have shared examples from their work that make lessons learned and best practices in global health partnerships more accessible. We hope this book will inspire all readers beyond the field of global health to put relationships first.

## Cross-cutting Themes

We recognize our responsibility to serve a global community, to address historical and present-day injustices, and to humbly listen and learn from our colleagues and friends whose writings are in this book. Through weaving together this book, the following themes emerged and re-emerged in the stories of global health partnerships, including the need to:

- Acknowledge the origins of global health and apply decolonization, gender, and intersectional frameworks to redress historical injustices and disrupt the status quo that reinforces inequalities.
- Center trust, communication, and ethical principles as the foundation of partnerships. Actively level power imbalances and elevate vulnerable voices and their needs. Respect, dignify, and empower women, girls, and the feminine.
- Educate ourselves on the history of the place and the people with whom we partner, and how they intersect with our history. Recognize that local communities are central to the co-creation process in this work, and seek mechanisms to empower and support local leaders and communities.
- Transform funding schemes, educational systems, and research incentives to increase equitable recognition in science, equitable benefits, and improved resource sharing.
- Expand the boundaries of what is accepted as legitimate science, particularly Indigenous and other non-Western science and ways of understanding the world. Value and work to repair our interconnectedness with beings of all life systems.
- Embrace the diverse, often challenging roles of global health work: we are scientists, practitioners, leaders, mentors, learners, advocates, activists, and champions for those who are the most vulnerable and impacted by disease. Nurture this diversity of perspectives through adaptive teamwork, flexibility, and the purposeful creation of a shared vision.
- Work within imperfect systems to drive change, while maintaining our humanity and sensitivity. Experience the joy and power of basic human

connections to catalyze and sustain the work. This is instrumental to the fulfillment and long-term commitment of individuals and teams.

- Stay open and humble to learn, practice respectful listening, use authentic storytelling, lay aside biases, self-reflect, learn from our failures, and grow with the process. Exercise these habits to bring our whole selves in service.
- Persist in hopefulness! Despite many challenges, we have agency and we can use our partnerships to foster needed change. It is not just *what* we do or *who* does it, but also *how* we work together in global health that matters.

Many of these themes align, explicitly or implicitly, with the UN Sustainable Development Goals (SDGs). Most centrally, SDG 17: Partnerships for the Goals and SDG 3: Good Health and well-being, but in the spirit of interconnectedness and partnership emphasized throughout this book, there are links to SDG 1: No Poverty, SDG 4: Quality Education, SDG 5: Gender Equality, SDG 6: Clean Water and Sanitation, SDG 8: Decent Work and Economic Growth, SDG 10: Reduced Inequalities, SDG 11: Sustainable Cities and Communities, SDG 12: Responsible Consumption and Production, SDG 13: Climate Action, SDG 15: Life on Land, and SDG 16: Peace, Justice, and Strong Institutions. The SDG framework is intended to galvanize the global community, from individuals to nations, to partner for progress and sustainability now and in the future. It highlights the interconnectedness of all life on this planet, humanity's responsibility to sustain and nurture it, and to leave a healthier planet for the generations to come. To accomplish this, we must critically examine our past and present, our successes and failures, and how these create and inform opportunities for the future. This book endeavors to do exactly that through the lens of global health and partnerships.

## What This Book Is Not

This book is not a systematic review of scientific literature on global health partnerships. We recognize that this book is biased towards the Americas, given our experience and network of contacts, and we recognize our positions of privilege in the realm of global health. It is impossible to include every voice and nation in this book. We recognize regional gaps in authorship, most notably from Asia and Eastern Europe, and in content, for example, participatory community research. We do not intend to be the "experts" or to capture and represent all realities in this text; we recognize this with humility. We are limited by our own framing/background/training/country of origin, as are all authors in this book. Global crises like COVID-19 will continue to shape the landscape of global health partnerships. We need to remain attentive and flexible to respond to the ever-changing needs of the communities that we serve.

## Conclusion

We hope this book can contribute to the rich discussion by colleagues world-wide about the need to radically transform global health partnerships, research systems, and funding structures. We also hope that this book contributes toward a new vision of the future and that the authors of this book can inspire others to think critically, be courageous agents of change, and work for the health of people and the planet. Ultimately, the transformation of global health partnerships will require a transformation of consciousness through deep introspection and personal contemplation. This is what we have asked of the authors of this book. We have asked them to bring their whole selves, uniting hearts and minds. This is unconventional, even scorned or ridiculed in academic circles as insufficiently technical. The authors of this book are courageous in their willingness to be vulnerable and share their stories. The authors of this book humble us, as this is an act of great service and a tremendous opportunity to teach and learn from the human experience, and we thank them sincerely.

*This book is dedicated to the next seven generations of humanity. May your world be more loving, peaceful, and healthy than today. May it be so.*

Panama City, Panama                                             Anna Stewart Ibarra
Stanford, CA, USA                                              A. Desiree LaBeaud

### Editor Perspective

We are self-identified women leaders in science and beyond. As scientists, we have investigated arboviral epidemiology and links to climate, environment, and social/structural forces, with public health partners in different countries. We have worked at universities, nonprofit organizations, and intergovernmental organizations, where we have weaved communities of practice across cultures and disciplines. We are descendants of European colonizers of the Americas, Indigenous Peoples of the Andes, and enslaved people from Western and Central Africa. We are women, mothers, friends, and colleagues. We met in 2018 when we shared a project in Ecuador, and we came together to co-create this book in March 2020 in the first weeks of the COVID-19 pandemic. We recognize our privilege and biases as citizens of the United States, having received higher education and employment at U.S. universities. Anna is also an Ecuadorian citizen and has lived in Latin America for over a decade. At the time of writing, we respectfully acknowledge that we live on the ancestral and seized territory of the Charua and Guarani people in Uruguay (Anna) and the Ramaytush Ohlone people in the United States (Desiree).

# Prologue: Global Health Partnerships Must Evolve from Saviorism to Solidarity

*If you have come here to help me, you are wasting your time. But if you have come because your liberation is bound up with mine, then let us work together*
—Lilla Watson, Indigenous elder.

Global health, in the past, and even today is a Global North-dominated, "white-savior industrial complex," to borrow a phrase from Teju Cole (2012). And we are all a part of this complex, nested within a "chaotic landscape of geopolitical chess" (Wenham 2023) wherein rich nations, lobbied by big corporates, maximize their power, influence, and benefits.

There is no aspect of global health that is not dominated by the most powerful and privileged individuals and institutions (Abimbola et al. 2021; Abimbola and Pai 2020). Leadership of organizations (Global Health 50/50 2020), inclusion on boards (Global Health 50/50 2022), access to funding (Charani et al. 2022), key authorship positions on publications (Hedt-Gauthier et al. 2019), editorial roles (Nafade et al. 2019), speaking roles in conferences (Velin et al. 2021), passport privilege that allows easy travel (Pai 2022), awards and prizes (MacLean et al. 2021), access to degrees in global health (Svadzian et al. 2020), every single aspect is tipped in favor of Global North entities.

Needless to say, global health partnerships are often designed to benefit the same, dominant groups (Hodson et al. 2023). It is remarkable and rather sad that even recommendations to promote more ethical and equitable global health partnerships are dominated by Global North teams (Hodson et al. 2023).

Since colonial times, global health has always been more about charity, goodwill, and saviorism, rather than justice, rights, and equity (Khan et al. 2023). The hierarchical terms we use to categorize people and countries reflect this (Khan et al. 2022). Even the images we use reflect this (Charani et al. 2023).

This saviorism or charity model of global health is antiquated, unjust, and unfit for purpose, as we saw, firsthand, during the COVID-19 pandemic. During a global crisis, we saw that rich nations talk a lot about global solidarity, partnerships, and equity. But when it was time to act, they chose to hoard life-saving products and actively block measures that would have enabled Global South nations to make their own products and become self-sufficient (Pai and Olatunbosun-Alakija 2021).

Global South nations learned a hard lesson: relying on the generosity of rich countries is a bad idea. They also learned that buzzwords like global solidarity mean very little, unless words are translated into concrete actions. Mere pledges and slogans are worthless.

The North-South power asymmetry has serious consequences, especially when life and death decisions about the health of people in the Global South are made in countries far away, by elite, privileged people. Very often, because they lack lived experience, contextual understanding, and genuine community engagement, people in the Global North will just get things wrong, even if they are well-intentioned. They did, as we saw during the pandemic.

Indeed, the COVID-19 pandemic taught us a lot about the deeply entrenched structural inequities and power asymmetries that pervade all of global health (Svadzian et al. 2020). Global health and development are current versions of old, colonial systems, and hence deeply rooted in white supremacy and white saviorism (Khan et al. 2023; Binagwaho et al. 2022; Khan 2021). Anti-Blackness and de-prioritization of Black, Brown, and Indigenous lives is a consequence, as described by Kyobutungi and colleagues (Kyobutungi et al. 2023). From HIV to Ebola, and COVID-19 to mpox, the de-prioritization of Black and Brown lives by the rest of the world has had devastating consequences (Kyobutungi et al. 2023).

Given these repeated and egregious failures of solidarity and equity in global health, is there any hope for equity and genuine solidarity? Can we possibly shift power to create equitable, fair, reciprocal partnerships? Can we pivot from saviorism and charity to authentic allyship and solidarity? These are urgent and important questions, even as the world is negotiating a pandemic accord, and trying to mitigate the consequences of climate change.

In this context, *Transforming Global Health Partnerships*, a timely and well-written book by 90 authors from 26 countries, brings diverse perspectives on global health partnerships, and offers many concrete suggestions on how we can do better with collaboration, partnerships, and solidarity.

The book begins with historical and foundational concepts, as it is critical to understand how and why global health partnerships came to be dominated by the elites, and why a better understanding of coloniality, power, and privilege are critical to not repeat the mistakes of the past. This section also offers helpful frameworks to guide the work—e.g., transdisciplinary science, systems approaches, One Health, Planetary Health, team science, and best practices in communication.

The second section, the heart of the book, includes 12 case studies of partnerships and offer insights from people on the ground, their learnings, and their efforts to make partnerships work better. These case studies cover a diverse array of partnerships, including local community-based NGOs, academic research models, mentorship and leadership partnerships, and government to government partnerships.

In the third section, the authors articulate a new vision for global health partnerships to co-create a just, equitable world.

It is important to acknowledge that global health partnerships do not automatically imply North-South collaborations. In fact, many things need no involvement of the Global North. But since North-South power dynamics are so dominant and powerful, it is particularly important to confront this issue and fight for equity.

As I see it, North-South partnerships will achieve equity only when we stop centering global health on people and countries in the Global North. It is time for people in the Global South to claim the seat they have historically been denied at the global health decision-making table (Gitahi 2022). It is time to abandon the charity, saviorism model of global health, and fight for a model that is rooted in justice, equity, human rights, and self-determination. As Sewankambo and colleagues put it, "the narrative of global health needs to be reoriented from saving, helping, and educating vulnerable others, towards working in solidarity and building transformative change" (Sewankambo et al. 2023).

This will require Global South colleagues and institutions to push back against unfair and unjust practices in global health. This is already happening and will increasingly happen (Kyobutungi et al. 2023; Gitahi 2022; Ssennyonjo et al. 2023). It will also require genuine South-South solidarity among stakeholders within low and middle-income countries (Gitahi 2022; Ssennyonjo et al. 2023). Global South nations must work together in solidarity and realize the agenda of self-determination and self-reliance.

Within every nation, it is critical to center on people with lived experience and communities that are most oppressed or disadvantaged. As Abimbola put it, "people understand their own lives better than we could ever do, that they and only they can truly improve their own circumstances and that those of us who work in global health are only, at best, enablers" (Abimbola 2018).

Where does that leave Global North people and organizations? Can they still contribute to global health? Do they still have a role? The answer is yes, but their role shifts from being leaders and saviors, to that of being good allies and co-conspirators (Pai 2023). People that typically hold power and privilege must practice allyship, where they see their primary role as allies or enablers or co-liberators rather than leaders (Pai 2023). Allyship is vastly different from saviorism (Figure).

| Saviorism | Allyship |
|---|---|
| A savior is a person who saves, rescues, or delivers. Not about dismantling oppression. | An ally works in solidarity with an oppressed group, to *dismantle* systemic oppression. |
| Often without consent. | With consent. |
| Elevates whiteness. | Elevates the oppressed groups. |
| Work on behalf of. | Works alongside. |
| Centers the saviors & validates their privilege. | Centers the needs of others. |
| Undermines agency. | Assumes & respects agency. |

Allyship is "an active, consistent, and arduous practice of unlearning and re-evaluating, in which a person in a position of privilege and power seeks to operate in solidarity with a marginalized group" (The Anti-Oppression

Network 2023; Nixon 2019). Allyship is not an identity. It is a lifelong practice (The Anti-Oppression Network 2023). The goal of allyship is to dismantle systemic oppression, so there is no need for allies. It rests on the idea of collective liberation—"none of us is free until all of us is free" (Nixon 2019).

Allies always work alongside oppressed groups and elevate them. Allies deeply respect the agency of the groups they work with and act with consent, when invited. Most importantly, allies do not center themselves. It is never about them. Good allies cede power, resources, space, and privileges. And they expect no medals or awards for doing the work. In the end, allies work toward a world where there is no need for allies anymore.

Saviors, on the other hand, often act without consent, and their goal is not to dismantle oppression. Saviors center themselves and work on behalf of others who they think need to be saved and cannot save themselves. "The White Savior Industrial Complex is not about justice. It is about having a big emotional experience that validates privilege," wrote Teju Cole (2012).

"White saviorism is simultaneously a state of mind and a concrete unequal power structure between the Global North and the Global South," wrote Themrise Khan and colleagues in their book "White Saviorism in Global Development" (Khan et al. 2023). "White saviorism not only strips the agency of racialized people but also falsely implies that White agents need to save them from their positions as victims. While it ends up alleviating poverty on the margins, it undermines the struggles of Global South people to emancipate themselves from economic, social, and political oppression, and often reinforces the capitalist-heteropatriarchal system," Khan and colleagues wrote.

What can allyship look like in global health? As I have written elsewhere (Pai 2023), people in the Global North must be allies to people in the Global South. White people in global health must be allies to Black, Indigenous and people of color people. Men in global health must be allies to women. Able-bodied and cis-hetero people must be allies to people with disabilities and LGBTQ+. The list goes on, as we all have intersectional identities (Nixon 2019).

This then is the defining challenge for global health professionals in the Global North: can they meaningfully shift power and pivot from saviorism and charity to genuine solidarity and allyship? The authors of this book tackle this question, among others, and offer valuable suggestions on how to transform and reimagine partnerships.

As we deal with massive, transnational challenges that threaten our very existence (namely, widening economic inequities, conflicts, pandemics, and climate change), our ability to act as global citizens, forge genuine partnerships and demonstrate authentic solidarity and allyship may well determine our shared future. In the end, we sink or swim as humankind. To paraphrase Archbishop Desmond Tutu, our humanity is caught up in the humanity of others. For we can only be human together.

**Author Perspective**

I was once called a "double agent" because I grew up and trained in India, but now do global health research and teaching in North America. As I have written elsewhere, like all double agents, I worry about being complicit in maintaining the power asymmetries inherent in global health. As an established, male academic in the Global North, I see myself as being very privileged, and I am looking for ways to spend my power and privilege and walk the path of allyship in global health.

Madhukar Pai
School of Population and Global Health
McGill University
Montreal, QC, Canada

## References

Abimbola S (2018) On the meaning of global health and the role of global health journals. Int Health 10(2):63–65. https://doi.org/10.1093/inthealth/ihy010. PubMed PMID: 29528402

Abimbola S, Pai M (2020) Will global health survive its decolonisation? Lancet 396(10263):1627–8. https://doi.org/10.1016/S0140-6736(20)32417-X. PubMed PMID: 33220735

Abimbola S, Asthana S, Montenegro C, Guinto RR, Jumbam DT, Louskieter L, et al (2021) Addressing power asymmetries in global health: imperatives in the wake of the COVID-19 pandemic. PLoS Med 18(4):e1003604. https://doi.org/10.1371/journal.pmed.1003604. PubMed PMID: 33886540

Binagwaho A, Ngarambe B, Mathewos K (2022) Eliminating the white supremacy mindset from global health education. Ann Glob Health 88(1):32. Epub 20220517. https://doi.org/10.5334/aogh.3578. PubMed PMID: 35646611; PubMed Central PMCID: PMCPMC9122008

Charani E, Abimbola S, Pai M, Adeyi O, Mendelson M, Laxminarayan R, et al (2022) Funders: the missing link in equitable global health research? PLOS Glob Public Health 2(6):e0000583. Epub 20220603. https://doi.org/10.1371/journal.pgph.0000583. PubMed PMID: 36962429; PubMed Central PMCID: PMCPMC10021882

Charani E, Shariq S, Cardoso Pinto AM, Farooqi R, Nambatya W, Mbamalu O, et al (2023) The use of imagery in global health: an analysis of infectious disease documents and a framework to guide practice. Lancet Global Health 11(1):e155–e164. Epub 20221201. https://doi.org/10.1016/S2214-109X(22)00465-X. PubMed PMID: 36463917

Cole T (2012) The White-Savior Industrial Complex. URL: https://www.theatlantic.com/international/archive/2012/03/the-white-savior-industrial-complex/254843/. Date accessed 4 Apr 2023. The Atlantic

Gitahi G (2022) Africa, it's time to take charge of our health agenda. URL: https://www.devex.com/news/opinion-africa-it-s-time-to-take-charge-of-our-health-agenda-103800. Date accessed 8 Jan 2023

Global Health 50/50 (2020) The Global Health 50/50 report 2020: power, privilege and priorities. URL: https://globalhealth5050.org/2020report/. Date accessed 13 Mar 2021. London

Global Health 50/50 (2022) The Global Health 50/50 report 2022: boards for all? URL: https://globalhealth5050.org/2022-Report/. Date accessed 9 Jan 2023. London

Hedt-Gauthier BL, Jeufack HM, Neufeld NH, Alem A, Sauer S, Odhiambo J, et al (2019) Stuck in the middle: a systematic review of authorship in collaborative health research in Africa, 2014–2016. BMJ Glob Health 4(5):e001853. https://doi.org/10.1136/bmjgh-2019-001853. PubMed PMID: 31750000; PubMed Central PMCID: PMCPMC6830050

Hodson DZ, Etoundi YM, Parikh S, Boum Y, 2nd (2023) Striving towards true equity in global health: a checklist for bilateral research partnerships. PLOS Glob Public Health 3(1):e0001418. Epub 20230118. https://doi.org/10.1371/journal.pgph.0001418. PubMed PMID: 36963065; PubMed Central PMCID: PMCPMC10021183

Khan T (2021) Racism doesn't just exist within aid. It's the structure the sector is built on. URL: https://www.theguardian.com/global-development/2021/aug/31/racism-doesnt-just-exist-within-aid-its-the-structure-the-sector-is-built-on. Date accessed: 12 May 2022. Guardian

Khan T, Abimbola S, Kyobutungi C, Pai M (2022) How we classify countries and people-and why it matters. BMJ Glob Health 7(6). https://doi.org/10.1136/bmjgh-2022-009704. PubMed PMID: 35672117; PubMed Central PMCID: PMCPMC9185389

Khan T, Dixon K, Sonderjee M (2023) White saviorism in international development. URL: https://darajapress.com/publication/the-white-savior-complex-in-international-development-theory-practice-and-lived-experiences. Date accessed 4 Apr 2023. Daraja Press

Kyobutungi C, Gitahi G, Wangari M-C, Siema P, Gitau E, Sipalla F, et al (2023) From vaccine to visa apartheid, how anti-Blackness persists in global health. PLOS Global Public Health 3(2):e0001663.

MacLean E, Bigio J, Singh U, Klinton J, Pai M (2021) Global tuberculosis awards must do better with equity, diversity, and inclusion. Lancet 397(10270):192–193

Nafade V, Sen P, Pai M (2019) Global health journals need to address equity, diversity and inclusion. BMJ Glob Health 4(5):e002018. https://doi.org/10.1136/bmjgh-2019-002018. PubMed PMID: 31750004; PubMed Central PMCID: PMCPMC6830051

Nixon SA (2019) The coin model of privilege and critical allyship: implications for health. BMC Public Health 19(1):1637. Epub 2019/12/07. https://doi.org/10.1186/s12889-019-7884-9. PubMed PMID: 31805907; PubMed Central PMCID: PMCPMC6896777

Pai M (2022) Passport and visa privileges in global health. Forbes. URL: https://www.forbes.com/sites/madhukarpai/2022/06/06/passport-and-visa-privileges-in-global-health/. Date accessed 9 Jan 2023

Pai M (2023) Disrupting global health: from allyship to collective liberation. URL: https://www.forbes.com/sites/madhukarpai/2022/03/15/disrupting-global-health-from-allyship-to-collective-liberation/. Date accessed 4 Apr 2023

Pai M, Olatunbosun-Alakija A (2021) Vax the world. Science 374(6571):1031. Epub 2021/11/26. https://doi.org/10.1126/science.abn3081. PubMed PMID: 34822275

Sewankambo NK, Wallengren E, De Angeles KJC, Tomson G, Weerasuriya K (2023) Envisioning the futures of global health: three positive disruptions. Lancet 401(10384):1247–1249. Epub 20230316. https://doi.org/10.1016/S0140-6736(23)00513-5. PubMed PMID: 36934734

Ssennyonjo A, Wanduru P, Omoluabi E, Waiswa P (2023) The 'decolonization of global health' agenda in Africa: harnessing synergies with the continent's strategic aspirations. Eur J Public Health 33(3):358–359. https://doi.org/10.1093/eurpub/ckad056. PubMed PMID: 37263014; PubMed Central PMCID: PMCPMC10234636

Svadzian A, Vasquez NA, Abimbola S, Pai M (2020) Global health degrees: at what cost? BMJ Glob Health 5(8). Epub 2020/08/08. https://doi.org/10.1136/bmjgh-2020-003310. PubMed PMID: 32759185; PubMed Central PMCID: PMCPMC7410003

The Anti-Oppression Network (2023) Allyship. URL: https://theantioppressionnetwork.com/allyship/. Date accessed 4 June 2023

Velin L, Lartigue JW, Johnson SA, Zorigtbaatar A, Kanmounye US, Truche P, et al (2021) Conference equity in global health: a systematic review of factors impacting LMIC representation at global health conferences. BMJ Glob Health 6(1). https://doi.org/10.1136/bmjgh-2020-003455. PubMed PMID: 33472838; PubMed Central PMCID: PMCPMC7818815

Wenham C (2023) Creating more and more new institutions may not make the world safer from pandemics. PLOS Glob Public Health 3(5):e0001921. Epub 20230517. https://doi.org/10.1371/journal.pgph.0001921. PubMed PMID: 37195920; PubMed Central PMCID: PMCPMC10191324

# Acknowledgments

We thank our families for their support, love, and patience as we devoted our time and energy to this book for over four years. We also thank our ancestors who taught us lessons about humanity, perseverance, generosity, and the strength of the human spirit that guided us through the book's inception and creation.

We thank our mentors and global health research collaborators and participants, who have trusted us, learned with us, and allowed us to make mistakes to move forward in global health amidst our human imperfections.

We thank the authors who were brave and generous, sharing their stories and lessons in pursuit of the greater good for all. Their dedication to this book throughout the COVID pandemic, given that many of them were actively involved in the pandemic response, was unparalleled. We also thank those authors who hoped to contribute to the book but could not do so-- many were frontline COVID workers.

We thank the team at Springer, notably our phenomenal editor Alison Ball, who supported us every step of the journey.

We thank those authors who were able to donate funding to allow open-access publication for this book so that it will be available for everyone.

We thank the artists who contributed to this book: Mira Cheng (Laying roots, Seeking sun, and What is yet to be), Orion Lavery (elephant), Everest Lavery (cheetah), and Phoenix Lavery (rhinoceros).

We thank the makers of technology, specifically ZOOM, for allowing us to pull together a global book during a global pandemic. We became even better friends during and through this journey, despite the distance between Uruguay and California.

We thank all of our teachers who have shined a light on our paths, providing the tools and courage to be agents of change, speak up, and meet our true selves. In particular, we thank our spiritual teachers, teachings, and communities that support our work.

We thank our planet for the abundant air, water, soil, food, medicine, animals, plants, and shelter provided and for the daily reminders of beauty that inspired this collaborative effort and sustained our dreams and visions for a better future for and on our sacred planet.

We respectfully acknowledge that during the writing of this book we live on the ancestral and seized territory of the Charua and Guarani people in Uruguay (Anna) and the Ramaytush Ohlone people in the United States (Desiree).

Finally, we thank each other for all the gifts of time, wisdom, and story over these last four years together and we look hopefully to a more peaceful, equitable, and healthy future for all life through transformed global health partnerships.

# Contents

# Contributors

**Maya Adam** Department of Pediatrics, Stanford School of Medicine, Stanford University, Stanford, CA, USA

**Cristina Alonso** La Colaborativa, Chelsea, MA, USA

Harvard T.H. Chan School of Public Health, Boston, MA, USA

**Marc Altshuler** Department of Family and Community Medicine, Thomas Jefferson University Hospital, Philadelphia, PA, USA

**Sonia Alvarez** Stanford School of Medicine, Stanford University, Stanford, CA, USA

**Till Bärnighausen** Heidelberg University, Heidelberg Institute of Global Health (HIGH), Heidelberg, Germany

Department of Global Health and Population, Harvard T. H Chan School of Public Health, Africa Health Research Institute (AHRI), Somkhele, KwaZulu-Natal, South Africa

**Daniel G. Bausch** London School of Hygiene and Tropical Medicine, London, UK

**Anil S. Bilimale** School of Public Health, JSS Medical College, Mysuru, Karnataka, India

**Mercy Borbor-Cordova** Faculty of Maritime Engineering and Sea Sciences, Escuela Superior Politécnica del Litoral (ESPOL), Guayaquil, Ecuador

Pacific International Center for Disaster Risk Reduction (PIC-DRR, ESPOL), Guayaquil, Ecuador

**Aude Bouagnon** School of Medicine, University of California San Francisco, San Francisco, CA, USA

**Amaya L. Bustinduy** Clinical Research Department, London School of Hygiene & Tropical Medicine, London, UK

**David Cedeño Rodriguez** Walking Palms Global Health, Bahía de Caráquez, Manabí, Ecuador

**Ismelda Cedeño** Walking Palms Global Health, Bahía de Caráquez, Manabí, Ecuador

**Namakau Chola** Zambart, Lusaka, Zambia

**Kareem Coomansingh** Office of Research, Windward Islands Research & Education Foundation (WINDREF), St. George's University, Grenada, West Indies

**Yves Coppieters** Health Systems and Policies – International Health Research Centre, School of Public Health, Université libre de Bruxelles (ULB), Brussels, Belgium

**Ibrahim Daud** CRC Laboratory at United States Army Medical Research Directorate-Africa (MRD-A/K)| Kenya Medical Research Institute, Kericho, Kenya

**Jessica Deffler** Department of Family and Community Medicine, Thomas Jefferson University Hospital, Philadelphia, PA, USA

**Avriel Diaz** Walking Palms Global Health, Bahía de Caráquez, Manabí, Ecuador

**Annie Dori** PATH, Port Moresby, Papua New Guinea

**Willy Dunbar** Health Systems and Policies – International Health Research Centre, School of Public Health, Université libre de Bruxelles (ULB), Brussels, Belgium

**Jonathan H. Epstein** EcoHealth Alliance, New York, NY, USA

**Rachael Farquhar** Burnet Institute, Melbourne, VIC, Australia

**Jennifer Gates** Icahn School of Medicine at Mt. Sinai, Mt. Sinai, NY, USA

**Jenna Gosnay** Department of Family and Community Medicine, Thomas Jefferson University Hospital, Philadelphia, PA, USA

**Rebecca F. Grais** Epicentre, Paris, France

**Manisha Gupte** Mahila Sarvangeen Utkarsh Mandal (MASUM), Pune, Maharashtra, India

**Anita Hargrave** Department of Internal Medicine, University of California, San Francisco, San Francisco, CA, USA

**Nusrat Homaira** University of New South Wales (UNSW), Sydney, NSW, Australia

**Nathalie Imbault** The Coalition for Epidemic Preparedness Innovations, Oslo, Norway

**Gloria Jaramillo** Walking Palms Global Health, Bahía de Caráquez, Manabí, Ecuador

**Andrew Jeffery** Walking Palms Global Health, Bahía de Caráquez, Manabí, Ecuador

**Krisada Jongsakul** Contractor, Royal Thai Army, based at US Armed Forces Research Institute of Medical Sciences (AFRIMS), Bangkok, Thailand

**Robert Kanwagi** World Vision, Dublin, Ireland

**Hugo Kavunga-Membo** National Institute for Biomedical Research, Kinshasa, Democratic Republic of the Congo

**Trevor Kelebi** West Sepik Provincial Health Authority, Vanimo, Sandaun, Papua New Guinea

**Zebedee Kerry** PNG Institute of Medical Research, Goroka, Papua New Guinea

**Lydiah W. Kibe** Kenya Medical Research Institute, Eastern Southern Africa Centre of International Parasite Control, Nairobi, Kenya

**Jacqueline Kitulu** Kenya Medical Association, Hospital Holdings B.V., PATH, Nairobi, Kenya

**A. Desiree LaBeaud** Department of Pediatrics, Division of Infectious Diseases, Stanford University, Stanford, CA, USA

**Moses Laman** PNG Institute of Medical Research, Goroka, Papua New Guinea

**Rachel Lowe** Barcelona Supercomputing Center (BSC), Barcelona, Spain

Catalan Institution for Research and Advanced Studies (ICREA), Barcelona, Spain

Centre for Climate Change and Planetary Health and Centre for Mathematical Modelling of Infectious Diseases, London School of Hygiene & Tropical Medicine, London, UK

**Stephen P. Luby** Infectious Diseases and Geographic Medicine, Stanford University, Stanford, CA, USA

**Valerie A. Luzadis** State University of New York College of Environmental Science and Forestry and Heart Forward Science, Syracuse, NY, USA

**Cheryl Macpherson** Department of Clinical Skills, Windward Islands Research & Education Foundation (WINDREF), St. George's University, Grenada, West Indies

**Leo Makita** National Malaria Control Program, NDoH, Port Moresby, Papua New Guinea

**Nokwanele Mbewu** The DG Murray Trust, Cape Town, South Africa

**Samuel McEwen** Burnet Institute, Melbourne, VIC, Australia

**Kelly Menzel** Gnibi College of Indigenous Australian Peoples, Southern Cross University, Lismore, Australia

**Blas Mera Rodriguez** Walking Palms Global Health, Bahía de Caráquez, Manabí, Ecuador

**Miriam Mutebi** Department of Surgery, Aga Khan University, Nairobi, Kenya

**Meggie Mwoka** Rockefeller Foundation-Boston University 3D Commission, Nairobi, Kenya

**Angela Nalwoga** Department of Immunology and Microbiology, University of Colorado Anschutz Medical Campus, Aurora, CO, USA

**Kesavan Rajsekharan Nayar** Global Institute of Public Health, Trivandrum, India

**Christine Ngaruiya** Department of Emergency Medicine, Stanford School of Medicine, Stanford University, Stanford, CA, USA

**Sia Nowrojee** United Nations Foundation, Washington, DC, USA

**Denisse Vega Ocasio** Rollins School of Public Health, Emory University, Atlanta, GA, USA

**Yessenia Pallaroso** Walking Palms Global Health, Bahía de Caráquez, Manabí, Ecuador

**Anjana Penugondla** Independent Public Health Professional, Bhubaneshwar, India

**Comfort R. Phiri** Zambart, Lusaka, Zambia

**Barbara Profeta** Independent consultant, Bern, Switzerland

**P. Arathi Rao** Prasanna School of Public Health, Manipal, India

**Mahmudur Rahman** Global Health Development/EMPHNET, Dhaka, Bangladesh

**Nicole Redvers** Schulich School of Medicine & Dentistry, University of Western Ontario, London, ON, Canada

Arctic Indigenous Wellness Foundation, Yellowknife, NT, Canada

**Nadia Ali Rimi** icddr,b, Dhaka, Bangladesh

**Natalie Roberts** MSF-France, Paris, France

**Leanne Robinson** Burnet Institute, Melbourne, VIC, Australia

Walter and Eliza Hall Institute, Parkville, VIC, Australia

**Rosemary Rochford** Department of Immunology and Microbiology, University of Colorado Anschutz Medical Campus, Aurora, CO, USA

**Shazia Ruybal-Pesántez** Burnet Institute, Melbourne, VIC, Australia

Walter and Eliza Hall Institute, Parkville, VIC, Australia

**Sadie Ryan** Department of Geography and the Emerging Pathogens Institute, University of Florida, Gainesville, FL, USA

College of Life Sciences, University of KwaZulu Natal, Pietermaritzburg, South Africa

**Chelsea Salas-Tam** Department of Family and Community Medicine, Thomas Jefferson University Hospital, Philadelphia, PA, USA

**Maritza Salazar** UCI Paul Merage School of Business, University of California Irvine, Irvine, CA, USA

**Gabriela Samayoa-Reyes** Department of Immunology and Microbiology, University of Colorado Anschutz Medical Campus, Aurora, CO, USA

**Sameera Sarma** School of Medicine, St. George's University, Grenada, West Indies

**Krish Seetah** Stanford Doerr School of Sustainability, Departments of Environmental Social Sciences, and Oceans, Stanford, CA, USA
Center for Innovation in Global Health, Stanford, CA, USA
Woods Institute for the Environment, Stanford, CA, USA

**Meena Som** Independent Public Health Professional, Bhubaneshwar, India

**Michele Spring** Department of Microbiology and Immunology, State University of New York (SUNY) Upstate Medical University, Syracuse, NY, USA
Formerly, based at Armed Forces Research Institute of Medical Sciences (AFRIMS), Bangkok, Thailand

**Anna Stewart Ibarra** Inter-American Institute for Global Change Research (IAI), Panama City, Panama

**Harold Agusto Suazo Laguna** Department of Community Projects and Entomology, Sustainable Sciences Institute, Managua, Nicaragua

**Rebeca Sultana** icddr,b, Dhaka, Bangladesh
University of Copenhagen, Copenhagen, Denmark
Institute of Health Economics, University of Dhaka, Dhaka, Bangladesh

**Jean-Jacques Muyembe Tamfum** National Institute for Biomedical Research, Kinshasa, Democratic Republic of the Congo

**Diana Timbi** PNG Institute of Medical Research, Goroka, Papua New Guinea

**Irene Torres** Inter-American Institute for Global Change Research, Montevideo, Uruguay
Uruguay and Fundación Octaedro, Quito, Ecuador

**Amie Tyler** Higher Love Healing, Burlingame, CA, USA

**Rosa von Borries** World Meteorological Organization, Geneva, Switzerland
Charité Universitätsmedizin Berlin, Berlin, Germany

**Randall Waechter** Caribbean Center for Child Neurodevelopment (CCCN) at Windward Islands Research & Education Foundation (WINDREF), Grenada, West Indies

**Enoch Waipeli** West Sepik Provincial Health Authority, Vanimo, Sandaun, Papua New Guinea

**Deborah Watson-Jones** London School of Hygiene and Tropical Medicine, London, UK

**Breana Wonsey** Walking Palms Global Health, Bahía de Caráquez, Manabí, Ecuador

**Ashok Gladston Xavier** Loyola College, Chennai, Tamil Nadu, India

**Margarita Zambrano** Walking Palms Global Health, Bahía de Caráquez, Manabí, Ecuador

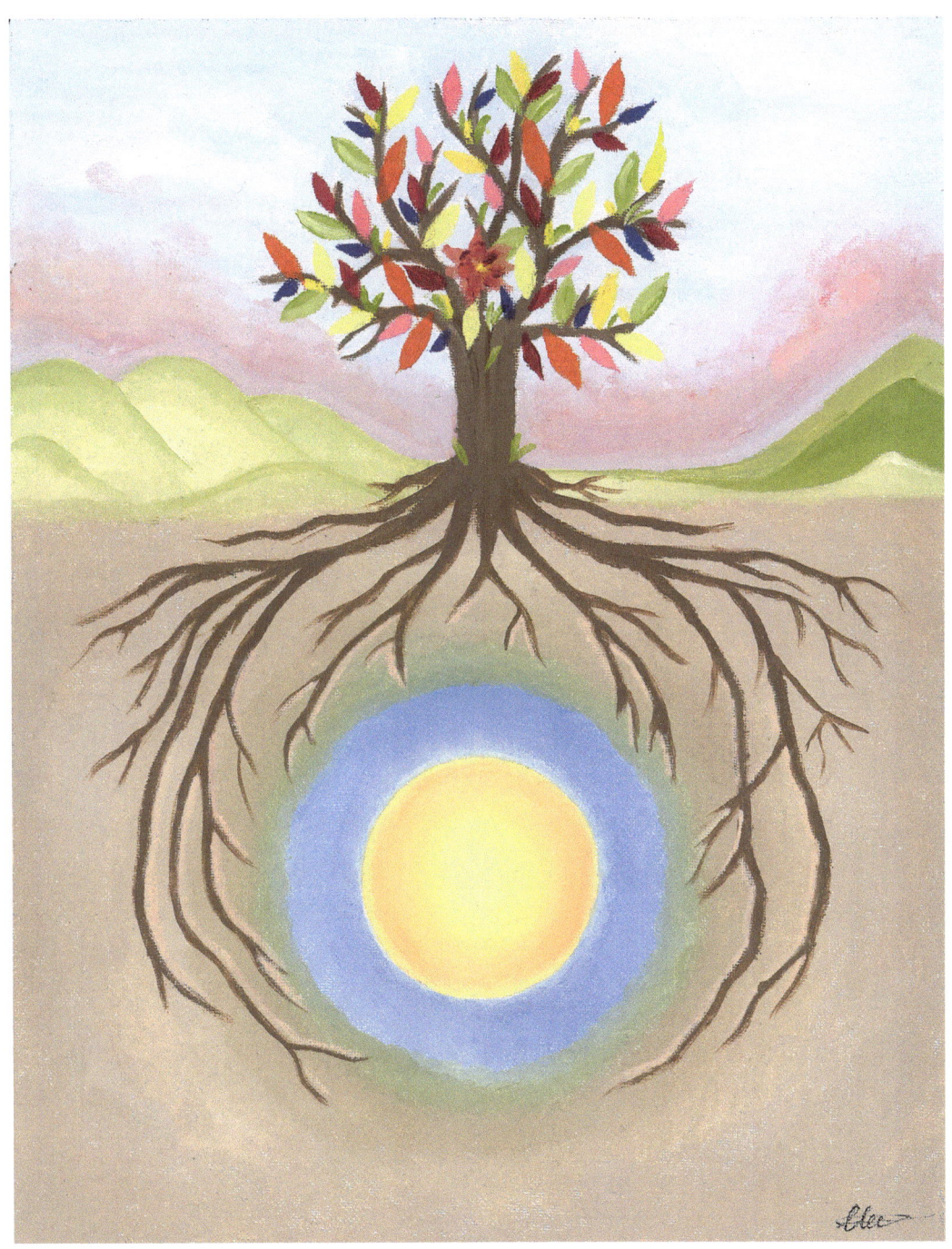

"Laying roots" by Mira Cheng

# Colonialism, Decolonization, and Global Health

Krish Seetah

## Abstract

This chapter serves as a bridge between the social sciences and humanities, and clinical research. It identifies the utility of anthropological and historical perspectives for the purposes of decolonizing global health, demonstrating the relevance of multidisciplinary approaches for the discipline. The chapter illuminates the historical trajectory of global health from its roots in colonial medicine, tracing the negative legacies that now impact former-colonial nations, and the modern discipline of global health. Using the case of Mauritius, the chapter presents how the processes of colonialism led to poor health in the past, disenfranchisement, and high mortality in laboring peoples. Lines are then drawn between the historical and modern context, urging the reader to consider how the heterogenous nature of colonialism must now be accounted for during the ongoing process of decolonization, particularly regarding global health partnership.

K. Seetah (✉)
Stanford Doerr School of Sustainability, Departments of Environmental Social Sciences, and Oceans, Stanford, CA, USA

Center for Innovation in Global Health, Stanford, CA, USA

Woods Institute for the Environment, Stanford, CA, USA
e-mail: kseetah@stanford.edu

## Keywords

Global health · Colonialism · Decolonization · Legacies · Enslavement · Indenture

**Author Perspective**

In this chapter I draw on both academic and personal backgrounds. I am a first-generation college graduate, educated in biology, ecology, health studies, and archaeology. Born in Mauritius of indentured ancestry, I was educated in the British system. This included the instruction I received in Mauritius (a former British colony), and throughout my formal schooling to doctoral level. I have worked in the USA for the last decade, primarily focused on how longitudinal and social evidence can help us better understand the relationships between society and disease. This chapter is written for junior scholars new to global health, and combines anthropological, socio-ecological, and longitudinal perspectives on disease and health. This work is biased in favor of English-speaking academic traditions.

*Colonialism is an economic, social, and political system that relies on the principles of cultural hierarchy and supremacy as justification for the multifaceted domination of the 'other'. The power structures of colonialism both relies on and perpetuates ideas of racial difference and superiority as tools for economic exploitation and cultural*

A. Stewart Ibarra, A. D. LaBeaud (eds.), *Transforming Global Health Partnerships*, Sustainable Development Goals Series, https://doi.org/10.1007/978-3-031-53793-6_1

*sovereignty – infantilizing colonized populations and situating them as incapable of self-governance – using evolutionary and essentialist rationalizations. In doing so, beyond its fundamental economic function, colonialism formalizes, institutionalizes, and structures racism.*

(Daffé et al. 2021, p. 557)

# 1 Introduction

## 1.1 Colonialism and Its Impacts on the World

Colonialism is an ancient concept, with distinct forms practiced by the Greeks and Romans for example (Van Dommelen 2012), which has become more closely associated with European expansion from the fifteenth century. The main impacts were as a consequence of hegemonic control of territorial lands and subjugation of local populations. By the 1800s, 35% of the globe had fallen under European colonialism; by the time of industrialization, circa 1900, this figure had reached over 80% (Hoffman 2015) (Fig. 1). The Portuguese effectively began the period of Europeanization when they established African outposts from 1445, and the Spanish expanded European interests into the New World from 1492. Nations as varied as America, Japan, Sweden, Austria, and Oman, all held colonies. However, by 1914, three nations had emerged as the main imperial forces. At the height of colonialism, just before the outbreak of the First World War, approximately 560 million people were under colonial rule: 70% of those where under the British, 10% under the French, and nine percent under the Dutch (US Tariff Commission 1922).

Colonialism was exploitative, and extractive. Huge profits were made by establishing plantations of sugar, tea, and tobacco, none of which were native to Europe. The period of colonialism witnessed the expansion of mercantilism, capitalism, and commodification, creating economies of material consumption on a massive scale, which initiated many of the challenges we now associate with climate change.

**Key Tenets**

1. Reducing disparity in partnerships requires acknowledging that global health is founded on colonial ideology.
2. Partners across socio-economic and geographic boundaries may knowingly and unknowingly perpetuate negative ideologies that originated during colonialism.
3. Partnerships that actively work to decolonize global health practice ultimately benefit all, practitioner and patient alike.
4. This chapter addresses the following SDGS: #3 good health & well-being, #4 quality education, and #10 reduction of inequalities.

While the economic ramifications of colonialism are well studied, the conceptual and social consequences have received less attention but were no less profound. Colonial ideology, driven by millennia of European thought on social hierarchy, elevated the written over the spoken word, and thus, vast tracks of knowledge gained over centuries on ecology, disease, and food by Indigenous Peoples were discarded as invalid (Box 2). Gender roles were radically reorganized. In many colonized nations, women had traditionally held power and prestige. This notion was undermined through European, but also for example, Japanese, patriarchy leading to the disenfranchisement of women in local governance (Ferguson and Beouch In press). Throughout the nineteenth century, opium produced in India and traded with China by the British helped offset the balance of deficit owed to China, a nation that had little need for European goods (Richards 2002). However, this led to an unprecedented epidemic of dependency—and attendant social crisis—for the Chinese, with 13–14 million addicts by 1906 (Lu et al. 2008).

Conversely, the British tried to restrict opium use in India and promote alcohol consumption,

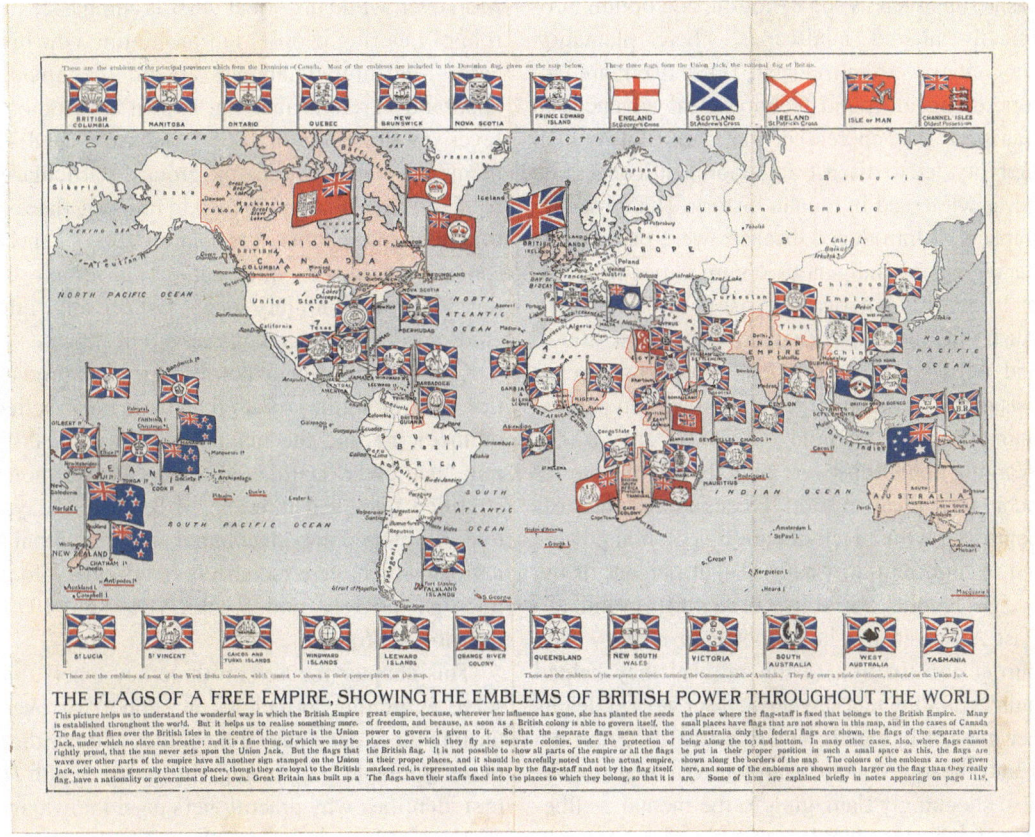

**Fig. 1** Map of the world circa 1910 showing colonial British territories. (Arthur Mees 'Flags of A Free Empire 1910', Cornell, CUL.PJM.1167.01)

which it could monopolise. The socio-political backlash in Britain to the opium trade in China, and the burgeoning addiction to opium and marijuana in European and American cities by the early twentieth century, led to draconian regulation on drug use in 1928. These regulations were based on colonial attitudes to laboring and migrant communities and continue to structure drug control and policing, as well as medicinal studies of plant-based intoxicants, to the present day.

In combination, the factors summarized above have drastically reconfigured the planet's ecology, geography, and demography. Unsurprisingly, our ideas around medicine, health, and health care, have also been fundamentally shaped by colonialism. Practices that favoured European elites and their interests have become institutionalized, with debilitating consequences for

formerly-colonized populations today. Decolonization of global health has become of primary interest to the modern discipline. However, as Bump and Aneibo indicate, '*a major obstacle for advocates of decolonization in global health is the field's very weak connections to history and the rich tradition of anti-colonial scholarship*' (Bump and Aneibo 2022, p. 2).

## 1.2 Hard Truths: The Colonial Foundation of Global Health

Global Health is rooted in colonial science and attitudes (Farmer et al. 2013; Richardson 2020). The movement of colonists, enslaved, indentured, and convict labor radically transformed populations in colonized geographies (Allen 1999, 2015). Concomitantly, the drive to produce cash crops such as sugar, cotton, and opium, profoundly altered landscapes where plantation economies were introduced. These two main factors, alongside rapid technological advances in transport that increased the speed of human mobility, led to disease and poor health on a scale never witnessed in human history. The devasting impacts of introduced diseases were particularly damaging for indigenous communities in North and South America (Crosby 1976, 2003), Australia and New Zealand (Anderson 2007), and Africa (Dawson 1979). Infectious disease was part of a much larger and broader impact on human health (Arnold 1993; Crosby 2003). Working conditions were directly responsible for poor individual health. Occupational hazards combined with a lack of care by colonial powers led to high mortality rates. Eight percent of the 31,983 'coolie' workforce brought from India to East Africa in the late nineteenth century died during construction of the railway they helped build, equating to a staggering four worker deaths per mile of line laid (Nowrojee 2014). From the scant statistics that are available, colonialism was also shockingly damaging to the mental wellbeing of laboring peoples, resulting in extremely high relative rates of suicide (Parahoo 1986).

In response, colonial elites sought to insulate Europe from diseases of the 'primitive-uncivilized' world (Aginam 2003), protect the health of Europeans in overseas territories (King 2002), and maintain the output, not necessarily the health, of the labor force. The study of 'diseases of warm climates' emphasized the then-dominant etiology of health as connected to geography and climate (Bashford 2000). This led to the establishment of iterative institutions of Public Health, International Health, and ultimately, Global Health. Schools of 'tropical medicine and hygiene' were established to tackle the rising scourge of infectious disease in colonized nations from the 1700s and early 1800s (Arnold 1993, pp. 24–25). The naming of these institutions as 'tropical' represents an enduring misnomer that can only be described as hypocrisy. Many diseases these institutions wrestled with were or had been endemic and epidemic in Europe.

Moreover, while historical records emphasize the role of laboring peoples in transmitting new diseases—indentured laborers aboard the *Spunky* apparently brought malaria, known as 'Bombay fever' to Mauritius in 1865 (Anderson 1918)—members of the colonizing groups, particularly soldiers, were also implicated in bringing disease to colonized nations (Toussaint 1966). These schools, alongside interventions governed by missionary and military ideals, collectively 'othered', evangelized, and militarized healthcare.

Consequently, many non-European communities were infantilized with regards to the practice of medicine and the maintenance of a healthy mind and body (Daffé et al. 2021). Furthermore, stratified two- and three-tiered health care systems developed in both colonial and non-colonial nations which were racialized and divided along lines of poverty and wealth (Dawson 1979; Parahoo 1986).

This chapter focuses on three key tenets that serve as guiding principles in support of overturning these deep-seated inequities and building more equitable partnerships in global health. It first identifies why practitioners need knowledge of colonial legacies; secondly, using the case of Mauritius, a small Indian Ocean island colonized from 1638, it highlights how colonial practice now negatively impacts modern populations. Finally, the chapter identifies several conceptual and practical routes to support the process of decolonizing global health, focusing on authorship, education, research frameworks, and the participant experience. These four categories form critical components of global health partnerships, and all are heavily influenced by colonial legacies.

## 1.3 Why Do Global Health Practitioners Need an Understanding of Colonial Fingerprints?

Tenet 1: Reducing disparity in partnerships requires acknowledging that global health is founded on colonial ideology.

This tenet seeks to situate the fact that colonial relationships established on extractive and exploitative practices have now evolved into seemingly benevolent modern relationships. For example, donor support, the intervention of foreign policy from Western nations in the global south, the global pharmaceutical industry, and the negative socio-political response in times of epidemics, as seen with both Ebola and COVID-19 (Adida et al. 2020; Büyüm et al. 2020), all trace their roots to power inequalities stemming from colonialism.

The legacy of colonialism on modern global health is a well-established phenomenon (Amrith 2006; Smith 2013). Similarly, the lack of historical contextualization has also been long recognized (Navarro 1977; Parahoo 1986), as has the fact that healthcare in former colonial states was largely evaluated as ahistorical and natural, rather than historical and social (Djurfeldt and Lindberg 1975). However, the use of history and anthropology in these earlier studies was directed at providing context. More recent work has illustrated how a lack of historical and social contextualization has undermined major global health efforts, such as the malaria eradication programs of the 1950s and 60s (Greene et al. 2013, p. 33). We are now at an unprecedented moment whereby the social sciences and humanities can meaningfully support the process of decolonization of global health in fundamental ways.

The roots of global health do not have to define nor characterize the discipline. However, legacies of colonialism persist in both the practice and partnerships of global health. These legacies are pervasive, often concealed, nuanced, and institutionalized. Negative legacies can only be resolved once they are recognized and acted upon. Colonialism has shaped our education, systems of governance, human-environmental relationships, and socio-economic interactions. Thus, decolonization is a far-reaching endeavor encompassing many disciplines, and itself part of a wave of social justice activity sweeping our world. Decolonization of global health specifically would benefit by engaging and learning from area studies that have not traditionally formed an alliance with clinical and disease research.

Alongside helping to establish where negative legacies stem, anthro-historical perspectives also reveal the underlying human cosmologies that shape how partners interact and how historical actions resonate socially today. For example, within the context of the participant experience, which is at the core of transnational research partnerships (TRPs), colonial histories have led to mistrust of health providers and systems, which ultimately influence clinical studies and outcomes. These legacies are observed explicitly in several ways. Through a long history of valorizing European medical practice at the expense of local healthcare, individuals may have less trust in traditional healers and, conversely feel incapable of questioning foreign practitioners. Missionary efforts during colonialism transformed from providing spiritual solace to health advice and medication. Similarly, efforts to support the health of military personnel facing the onslaught of infectious disease were merged with practices to cure troops sourced from local populations, as well as those individuals who came under the hegemony of the colonial state after conflicts ended (Greene et al. 2013). For research participants in former colonial states, the lines between past and present may remain blurred. Medical practitioners may present in a medico-spiritual guise to sick individuals, even when this is unintentional on the part of the foreign professional. Moreover, doctors may have to be accompanied by the military in zones of conflict, again replicating a model that has historical resonance passed on through oral accounts. In the absence of ethnographic research, these relevant facets of modern health care may remain invisible to clinicians. Indeed, as of 2020, no clinical studies on the participant experience in Lower-Middle Income Countries (LMIC) have been conducted (Lawrence and Hirsch 2020).

## 2 Case study: Colonialism, Health, and Disease in Mauritius

The following case illustrates how colonialism shaped the historical disease context in Mauritius (Fig. 2), and how the legacies of colonialism

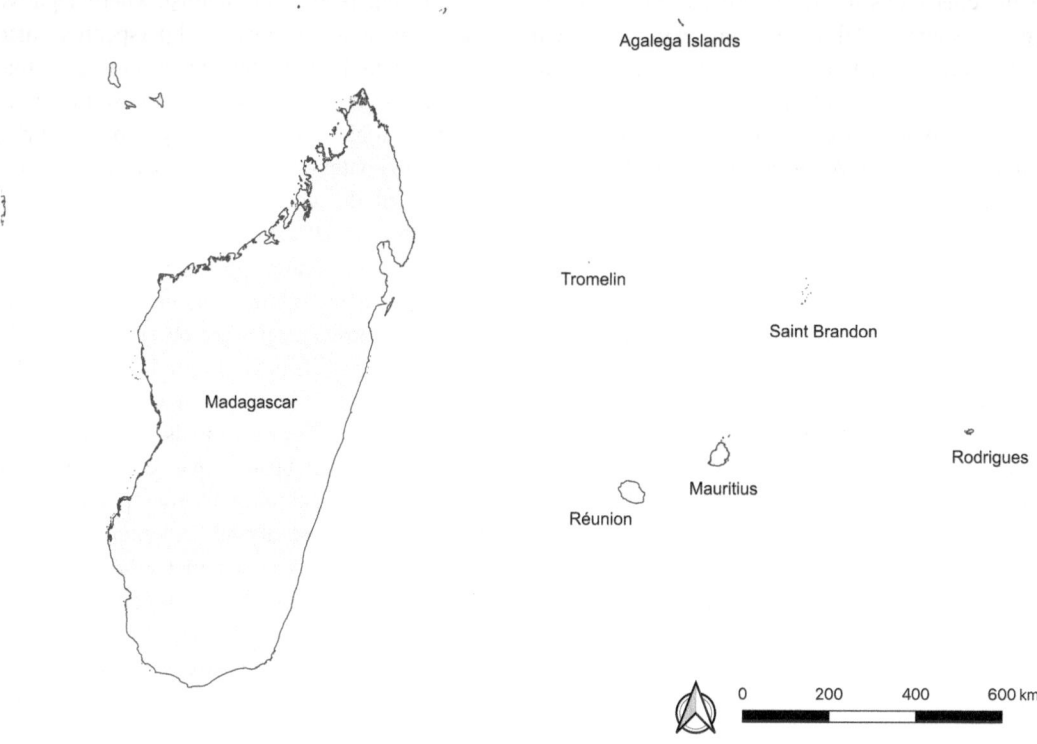

**Fig. 2** Map of Mauritius, situated regionally

continue to perpetuate colonial ideology, inequity in access to healthcare, and ecological degradation.

## 2.1 Demographic and Ecological Impacts of Labor Diaspora

Mauritius had no indigenous population. Peoples of mainly European, African, Indian, and Chinese origins now form the island's populace of some 1.3M individuals on a surface area of only 1865 km², the highest population density in Africa. The island underwent three phases of European colonialism, Dutch from 1568, French from 1710, and finally British from 1810. Throughout these successive waves of colonial hegemony, enslaved, indentured, convict, and merchant diasporas rapidly enlarged the island's population. The Slavery Abolition Act, 1833, enacted by Britain, led to a major demographic flux. From 1835, Mauritius became the location for the 'Great Experiment', used by the British to replace enslaved with indentured labor. This trial led to a rapid demographic transformation. In a few decades, the island went from around 90,000 mainly African peoples, to over 400,000 mainly Indian individuals. Each colonial administration was galvanized to transform the island's ecology. Mauritius has no customary systems of ecological governance and knowledge from pre-colonial times. All the island's peoples were engaged in the transformation of the landscape for agricultural purposes. Thus, the local ecology is now unrecognizable, retaining only two percent of its native forest, down from 98% at the onset of colonialism. More problematic, efforts to redress past ecological damage, which could have major benefits for human and environmental health (WHO 2019c), are hampered by a lack of cohesive strategies or shared values built from deep-seated, indigenous knowledge (Seetah et al. 2022).

## 2.2 History of Infectious Disease Transmission in Mauritius

These rapid demographic and ecological changes were mediated via ship transport, bringing people and goods, but also, cattle and other commensals that accelerated ecological damage and simultaneously served as vectors of disease (Box 1). The socio-economic dimensions of disease reveal the convoluted long-term impacts of colonialism on

**Box 1**

The introduction of infectious disease began with the French (Fig. 4). The first epidemic in 1754 of smallpox served as a harbinger of disease that would characterize the island for decades. French troops from India brought subsequent smallpox outbreaks in 1772 and 1782; rabies was introduced in 1813; in 1819, cholera was brought from the Philippines via *La Topaz* (Parahoo 1986). With the advent of indenture under British rule, which coincided with a concerted and large-scale drive for sugar production (from the 1850s, Mauritius produced 7% of the world's sugar (Allen 2008, p. 152)), the situation escalated exponentially. The need for labor overshadowed health concerns. Indentured laborers were transported in increasing numbers. Measures to control disease were circumvented, and ships suspected of carrying disease were permitted to dock rather than being held in quarantine (Toussaint 1966, p. 107). This led to new epidemics of cholera in the capital of Port Louis in 1854, 1856, 1859, and 1861 (Parahoo 1986). From 1866-68, malaria killed 41000 people, 10% of the entire Mauritian population at the time (Pike 1873). It was not until this massive epidemic that measures for quarantine and improved sanitation were implemented and adhered to, although these were criticized and undermined as they reduced profits (Parahoo 1986).

human well-being. With the abolition of enslavement, the advent of indenture, and a booming sugar industry, one might have expected the former enslaved to have had an improved situation. As with the Americas, this was far from the case. The small population constituting the landowning French plantocracy prospered. The former enslaved fell increasingly into poverty. They suffered from malnutrition and incidence of infectious diseases (Parahoo 1986). Archaeological research from the Le Morne 'Old Cemetery', a burial ground of emancipated peoples, provides scientific evidence of prolonged osteological infection and dental disease that likely debilitated many former enslaved peoples (Fig. 3). Part of the reason for this spiral into poverty, exposure to infectious disease, and malnutrition, was due to the influx of indentured laborers. This 'cheap' labor force effectively pauperized the former enslaved by removing opportunities to work on the plantation (Parahoo 1986).

## 2.3 Occupational Hazards for Indentured Laborers

The laborers appear to have suffered even greater levels of ill health than the former enslaved. A report from the Civil Hospital in the capital conducted by Beaugeard in 1870, paints a horrific picture. The immensely arduous work, combined with minimal food rations and repeated bouts of malaria, meant that when laborers presented with illness at the hospital, they were debilitated to the point that they were unlikely to recover (Parahoo 1986). Laborers were docked a day's pay if they were sick, effectively creating a debt trap when any time was taken off from work, even for illness. As such, laborer's avoided treatment. Thus, while mortality per thousand amongst Europeans was 18.4, and 66.6 for former enslaved peoples, for laborers the rate was 158.6. The defining issue was ideological, not clinical. Colonial Europeans effectively saw laborers within the same mental framework as enslaved peoples (Parahoo 1986). However, they were not responsible for the well-being of laborers in the same way as they had

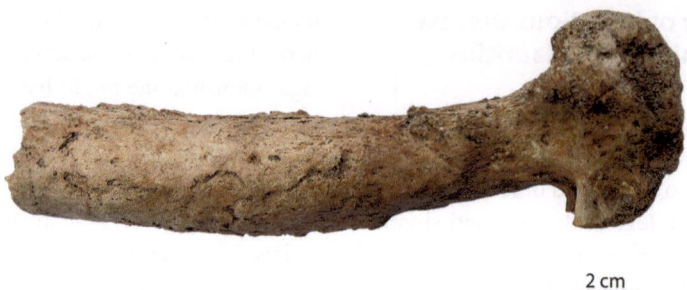

2 cm

**Fig. 3** This is an image of osteomyelitis, an infection of the bone caused by a bacterial or fungal infection in the humerus, from Le Morne 'Old Cemetery', a burial ground of emancipated peoples in Mauritius. Such infections may be caused by traumatic injury, allowing infectious agents to penetrate the body. The image suggests a debilitating working environment and lack of access to healthcare. From the extensive state of infection, it is evident that treatment was not administered in time for healing to occur before death.

## Major disease introductions and outbreaks

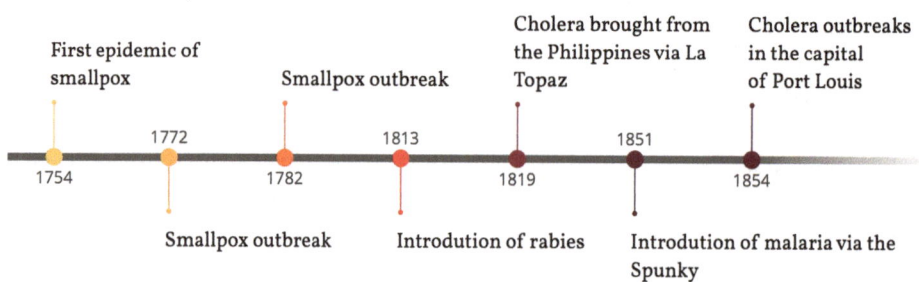

**Fig. 4** A timeline of the introduction and outbreaks of the major diseases affecting Mauritius during colonialism

been under the guidelines to manage the enslaved, such as those established in the *Code Noir*.[1] Laborers were expected to maintain their own health. Legislation to support the health of laborers was flouted; the unbearable working conditions were not factored into the likely causes for poor health, rather the blame was apportioned to poor sanitation in the laboring camps. The impacts of disproportionate gender balance (~90% of laborers were male) and fractured family lives were ignored. Alcoholism was rife and the use of marijuana was initially permitted to alleviate the boredom of monotonous work, with smoking complexes developing that also included opium (Seetah et al. in prep). Unsurprisingly, the psychological health of laborers suffered alongside their physical deterioration.

Parahoo states '...*neither the alcohol or Gandia [marijuana] could prevent the psychological or physical suffering of the Indians. Tragically, for too many of them, suicide was the only way out of their miseries*' (Parahoo 1986, p. 417).

---

[1] The *Code Noir* (Black code) was established in 1685 in order to provide conditions and a legal structure under which enslavement was to be practiced within the French Empire. The edict required that enslaved peoples were baptized into the Roman Catholic Church, restricted their movement, and defined the boundaries of punishment, amongst other conditions.

Beaugeard's 1870 report compared local suicide rates with those from England and paints an extremely bleak picture. For every million individuals in England, 70 committed suicide. In Mauritius, for the general population, 67 suicides were recorded per million; among laborers, that figure was four-fold higher at a staggering 280 per million.

## 2.4 Colonial Legacies on Health and Well-Being Post-independence

The lasting legacies of these inequalities remain, as do other socioeconomic factors that affect human and ecological well-being. Some of these legacies are direct. Like many former colonies, the healthcare system in Mauritius was established during the colonial period, with the post-independence government either unwilling or incapable of changing the underlying inequalities (Parahoo 1986). Health provision was tiered in favor of European elites, with plantation 'pharmacies' serving the needs of laboring peoples. While modern hospitals now exist, local pharmacies still serve the needs of a large portion of the population. A pharmacist, not a doctor, diagnoses and administers medication, mimicking the historical setting. The best locally available medical equipment, methods, and best-trained doctors are in private clinics. Costs to access these clinics are prohibitive for the majority of the population. Thus, class, ethnic, and regional availability of healthcare and access to medical care remains modeled on a colonial approach.

Other legacies are more subtle but no less problematic. With the advent of indenture, British capitalists saw an opportunity for financial gain. The British (who governed the island) encouraged the sale of rice and flour, alongside ghee, and dhal, all staples of Indian cuisine, by French landowners to the workforce. However, even today, the local government has not been able to convince the plantocracy to diversify the products grown to reduce the island's dependency on imported goods. Mauritians remain reliant on food—the core element of a healthy lifestyle— with inflated costs because of a legacy of import-export/production-consumption practices. The poorest individuals are the most affected.

## 2.5 Health Care Systems Today

The island's modern health system constitutes an infrastructure with 124 public health care facilities, mainly comprising of health posts (88.7%), alongside regional, district, and provincial hospitals (9.76%) (Musango et al. 2020; WHO 2015). Health care workers constitute some 2550 physicians, alongside 4261 nursing, 380 dentistry, and 497 pharmaceutical personnel, supported by 2700 technical, administrative, managerial, and community staff (WHO 2019a). For the year 2016, healthcare spending amounted to US$553 per capita, US$552 of which was derived from domestic general governmental and private sectors and only US$1 from external sources (WHO 2019b).

As the above summary suggests, Mauritius has achieved a status of general self-reliance, and indeed, the health of the nation has a positive outlook, with an average life expectancy of 74.4 years; mortality from infectious, parasitic, and waterborne disease has decreased from seven percent in 1976 to 2.8% in 2019 (HSSP 2020, pg. xiv). However, non-communicable disease (NCD), and the needs of an aging population pose significant healthcare challenges. Tackling these and other health challenges is complicated by the fact that Mauritius has gradually received less and less overseas development assistance (ODA) as gross national income has increased. ODA amounted to US$65.2M from 2005 to 2006, described as 'meagre' by the WHO Country Corporation Strategy report (WHO 2009). While development partnerships such as the World Diabetes Foundation, UNFPA, the World Bank, UNAIDS and the French Corporation Agency all contribute to the development of the health sector, UNICEF and UNFPA have both closed their respective offices in Mauritius as socio-economic and health indicators improved. Partnerships have also generally been limited, the main efforts focusing on diabetes with the World Diabetes

Foundation; multilateral partnerships have been developed with the World Bank, and bilateral partnerships exist with the French government. The local government, recognizing the need to build stronger partnerships, outlined a 5-year Health Sector Strategic Plan (HSSP) covering the period from 2020 to 2024, with Strategic Goal 24 focused specifically on "*developing a charter for NGOs and other private partners, strengthening of partnership with both local and foreign private health institutions for capacity building and the strengthening of outsourcing services to the private sector*" (HSSP 2020, pg. xxi).

## 3    Conceptual Pathways to Decolonize Global Health

Tenet 2: Partners across socio-economic and geographic boundaries may knowingly and unknowingly perpetuate negative ideologies that originated during colonialism.

Institutions must acknowledge their past and make clear statements on the unacceptability of racial and systemic inequality, as the London School of Hygiene and Tropical Medicine has recently done (Erondu et al. 2020). Institutional leadership must also take bold steps in stating lucidly and emphatically that inequality, specifically around education for example, causes damage in the very contexts we seek to support (Barry 2021). These high-level actions must be combined with ways of educating the next generation of global health scholars to recognize, learn from, and dismantle the historical and social imbalances that affect the discipline.

The Mauritian case study has two main purposes. Firstly, it illustrates the relationships between human and ecological health over time and identifies how specific attitudes and actions now impact modern populations. Effectively, this example identifies why we need to add time depth to contemporary 'One Health' approaches (see Chapter "Team Science and Infectious Disease Work: Exploring Challenges and Opportunities"); contemporary planetary and human health have been negatively affected by

the period of colonialism. Secondly, the case demonstrates that colonialism was heterogeneous; differential colonial groups had various impacts on the peoples under imperial rule, as seen with introduced infectious disease. The interactions between different colonial administrations, languages and cultures, geographies, temporalities, local elites, and lay communities, to name a few, led to the creation of distinct disease and health ecologies and subsequently, medical responses. The dimensionality and relationships between these dynamic factors form complex networks that cannot be disentangled through clinical-type efforts alone. Thus, models and approaches for the decolonization of global health will need to be both adaptive and reflexive. Decolonization is and will be a complex and enduring process requiring multivocality.

How we learn from and utilize these perspectives will be critical to the success or failure of the process of decolonization of global health. Academic relationships have been identified as a critical area in need of change if the decolonization process is to be successful. Power imbalances need to be redressed to improve partnerships between academic peers and enhance the relationship between researchers and communities (Lawrence and Hirsch 2020). To that end, this section will focus on four key areas of academic relationships: authorship (Abimbola 2019; Abimbola and Pai 2020), curriculum development (Erondu et al. 2020), equitability across research frameworks, and the participant experience (Lawrence and Hirsch 2020).

### 1. *Authorship*

Coming back to the Mauritian case and its illustration of heterogeneity in colonialism, consider first: the generations of educational institutionalization that favored foreign knowledge, ways of learning, and systems of thought around western medicine and research. To this, consider how each colonial context enacted the same principle, valorizing European knowledge, but in different ways. Conversely, consider the generational history of refining written academic English, grant writing, and proposal development, which high-income country (HIC) scholars take for granted and may even reduce resources in low- and middle-income countries (LMIC) (Barry 2021). These factors emphasize the importance of authorship, academic publications, and research funding within the decolonization process.

Numerous articles have pointed to the need for more equitable authorship to recognize the contribution of scholars from LMIC versus HIC (Eichbaum et al. 2021; Erondu et al. 2020). Many factors are involved. These include a lack of funding to facilitate LMIC-led research, and institutional inequity (See Chapter "Funding for Equitable Infectious Disease Research and Development"). The simple answer would be to avoid the practices of parachute science (Bockarie et al. 2018), and fairly attribute authors' work based on their contribution. Equally, improved inclusion is suggested for sharing responsibilities in research and grant writing. However, we need to consider several points. Who has defined the areas that need improvement? They may appear obvious and merit-worthy, but how will we enact these changes? Discussing authorship, Abimbola observes that local scholars often feel the 'foreign gaze…', writing for audiences which are not their own (Abimbola 2019). Now that HIC academics are waking to the realities of white supremacy, racism, and colonial legacies in global health, there is a pressing emphasis on action. Abimbola points to but one example of a failure to acknowledge local contexts. Juxtaposing these points, what role do we anticipate local LMIC colleagues to have in the face of numerous obstacles within their own country, and few if any of the opportunities enjoyed by HIC scholars? Do we risk setting up LMIC scholars for failure? This is a pitfall we must avoid as it will only promote future asymmetry. Authorship is central to our recognition of scholars' intellectual contributions to knowledge. Balanced authorship provides a way to overturn not only the immediate inequity between those involved in research and those who gain recognition, but also, how we recognize the contributions of Black, Indigenous, and Peoples of Color scholars. Decolonization in

global health will thus have a ripple effect beyond the boundaries of the discipline.

## 2. *Curricula development*

Epistemic violence against non-European ways of thought and institutions of knowledge characterized colonialism. How do global health practitioners work against and resolve heterogeneous legacies, and overturn the coloniality of knowledge (Daffé et al. 2021), when global health has been developed to enact broad change from a distance; distance that is ideological as well as physical? Curricula development that includes historical knowledge of colonialism, and anthropological perspectives, will go part of the way to creating a balanced understanding of lasting inequalities (see Chapters "Educational Perspectives from the Field: Pathways to the Future" and "Learning from the Past to Inform the Future: Perspectives on Future Directions in International Health and Research"). On the research front, greater involvement of social sciences (see Chapter "Partnership-Based Approach to Infectious Disease Research in Papua New Guinea"), and integration of approaches that reveal the social dimensions of disease transmission (Gerken et al. 2023; Seetah et al. 2020), will illustrate to global health students how cross-disciplinary research leads to improved knowledge of disease transmission, but also, modern health disparities. The moment is ripe for new forms of collaborations across schools, departments, and centers. For example, institutions of global health and global ethnography could fruitfully develop collaborations to formalize how clinical and ethnographic research can be mutually supportive. Overall, we will have to acknowledge the place of the humanities and social sciences not only in helping us to think about modern legacies, but also in building knowledge for descendant communities. We have precious little scientific knowledge of the disease context of laboring peoples. Our knowledge of disease in the colonial period is overwhelmingly historical, which itself is biased towards the colonial elite. New knowledge of past disease could be instrumental both to better understanding modern disease (Seetah 2018), and to help descendant communities reckon with their own legacies of colonialism. Thus, the process of increasing our understanding of colonialism, and learning how to decolonize global health, are unified.

### 3. Building equitable research frameworks

While the preceding two examples emphasize deep and encompassing root-and-branch changes to overturn colonial legacies within academic institutions, to promote better partnerships specifically change is also needed within the context of clinical trials (see Chapter "Community-Based Approaches to Respond to Epidemics and Natural Disasters in Coastal Ecuador"). Such trials are often undertaken as part of transnational research partnerships (TRPs). Trials, particularly to tackle global disease challenges such as those posed by HIV, are invariably conceptualized, designed, funded, and directed by institutions and partners in HIC locations. In-country partners are then identified, recruited, and trained to work on the trial. In such examples, essential aspects of the inception, development, oversight, and data organization routinely occur in the HIC. Thus, while the LMIC partner(s) implement the trial and serve as the direct interface with the study participants, they are effectively excluded from core development stages and lose the opportunity to gain critical skills that could support their local trials if they so choose to pursue that route (Lawrence and Hirsch 2020).

To create more equitable research frameworks, several developments are needed. Establishing new and improving existing clinical laboratories in LMIC would serve as a locus for funded research, support the transition from research outcomes to policy within the local context, and provide the necessary infrastructure for local teams to develop the training and experience they gain into expertise and capacity. Ultimately, this leads to increased competency and competitiveness in LMICs (Crane 2013).

Change is also needed in the HIC context. Using research funding and publication output as the overarching quantitative metric for measuring performance and success in academia and global health does not recognize or value efforts to promote local capacity. Thus, despite the benefits of promoting local capacity, HIC partners who do make an effort to support local researchers receive little incentive or recognition for doing so. Emphasizing, evaluating, and acknowledging efforts at capacity and expertise building for local researchers, although subjective, could be integrated into performance assessment to promote and sustain these areas as part of a broader effort to decolonize the discipline.

**Box 2**

Within the context of building equitable research relationships, valuing indigenous and other oral cultures and orally transmitted knowledge should be emphasized, given the dependence on the written word, which is celebrated in Western academia. Writing from the perspective of ocean science, Johannes summarizes the existing situation succinctly: *"Natural scientists have routinely overlooked the practical knowledge possessed by artisans... It is one manifestation of the elitism and ethnocentrism that run deep in much of the Western scientific community. If unpublished notebooks containing the detailed observations of a long line of biologists and oceanographers were destroyed, we would be outraged. But when specialized knowledge won from the sea over centuries by formally unschooled but uniquely qualified observers – fishermen – is allowed to disappear as the westernization of their cultures proceeds, hardly anyone seems to care."* (Johannes 1981, ix). Valuing indigenous knowledge and perspectives, as opposed to viewing indigenous and formerly-colonized communities as in need of care, vulnerable, and requiring external resolutions, is integral to the paradigmatic shift needed to decolonize global health (see Chapter "Transforming the Planetary Health Crisis Through an Indigenous Land-

Based Meta-Narrative"). *"Intercultural dialogue recognises the validity and value of Indigenous standpoints, and participatory research promotes reciprocal respect for stakeholder input in knowledge creation."* (Sarmiento et al. 2020).

### 4. *Participant experience in research partnerships*

Inequitable relations extend beyond that of HIC-LMIC researchers, and building good partnerships needs to accommodate and consider those from whom we gather data. However, '*To date, there exists no published research that has specifically explored the perspective of participants in LMICs when it comes to the structure of global health research.*' (Lawrence and Hirsch 2020, p. 519). This absence of published work on the structure of research trials from participants' viewpoint reinforces the extent to which colonial mentalities permeate modern global health partnerships. Improving opportunities for locally-led clinical trials, as above, would also likely increase the integration of participant views. Considering that clinical trials depend on participants, it is fair and just to seek ways to include their perspectives into the development process, and not have those views inferred by external observation, often by researchers in HICs. Connecting this point to point 2, one way to improve the integration of participant viewpoints would be through ethnographic studies, such as 'The Lived Experience of Participants in an African Ramdomised Trial' (LEOPARD) currently underway by D.S. Lawrence and colleagues (see: https://clinicaltrials.gov/ct2/show/NCT04296292, accessed 07, Feb. 2022).

Broader developments are needed when it comes to valuing participants. These relate to international research standards, including ethical standards (see Chapter "Ethical Challenges in Global Health Research") which may not immediately align with local contexts, such as processes related to the informed consent of study participants (Lawrence and Hirsch 2020). Ethics and consent are two major pillars of clinical research, which are largely defined by researchers in the Global North. Increasing local involvement, developing more flexible interpretations of research standards, and redefining consent processes that respond to local perspectives, would support equitability in partnerships more broadly. Such developments would also respond to ethical concerns raised by cases of misconduct, especially in trials that involve genetic evidence (Stokstad 2019).

## 4 Conclusions

Tenet 3: Partnerships that actively work to decolonize global health practice ultimately benefit all, practitioner and patient alike.

Partnerships are at the of core of global health practice. This chapter has focused on education as one of several paths to building a better discipline in the future and features of global health partnerships that will need to change to develop more equitable practice. Other chapters of this book emphasize the way power and trust shape partnerships (see Chapter "Role of Social Science in Infectious Disease Research: a Case Study of Partnering with Communities in Vector Control in a Kenyan Village"), how the existing ethical standards we adhere to influence the practice of infectious disease research and partnerships therein (see Chapter "Ethical Challenges in Global Health Research"), and how diversity across many parameters is necessary to promote collaborative team science (see Chapter "Foundations and Future Directions of Global Health Communication").

In concluding this chapter, my aim has been to make clearer some of the contributions anthropological and historical perspectives can make to support the decolonization of global health. We should recognize that it is our underlying cosmologies and ideologies that need to change and that this can improve how we build partnerships. Changing cosmologies in HICs will be fundamentally different from changing cosmologies in LMICs. It seems unimaginable today to suggest that COVID-19 vaccines be 'tested in Africa'; yet French scientists expressed this idea in March of 2020 (Büyüm et al. 2020). Such sentiments make clear the extent to which colonialism remains rooted in western thought. This point also illustrates how significant education of new global health scholars, alongside reeducation, will help build a strong discipline for the future. However, the more important development will need to revolve around colleagues in LMIC. For decolonization to take place in global health, it will be necessary for well-intentioned professionals from HICs to step back and allow the time and space for equitable realignment between traditional and modern western health care practices and for the self-valorization of local scholars to flourish.

## Glossary

**Colonialism:** the policy or practice of acquiring full or partial political control over another country, occupying it with settlers, and exploiting it economically.

**Decolonization:** the action or process of a state withdrawing from a former colony, leaving it independent. In the contemporary context, also used to describe the process of removing attitudes and institutions of thought that have colonial legacies.

**Epistemic violence:** violence exerted against or through knowledge.

**Industrialization:** the development of industries in a country or region on a wide scale.

**Multivocality:** 'many voices'; encourages the articulation of numerous different narratives or parallel discourses.

**Parachute science:** practice whereby international scientists, typically from higher-income countries, conduct field studies in another country, typically of lower income, and then complete the research in their home country without any further effective communication and engagement with others from that nation.

**Plantocracy:** a population of planters regarded as the dominant class.

**Structural violence:** indicative of social forces that harm certain groups of people, produc-

ing and perpetuating inequality in health and well-being.

**Systemic violence:** refers to the harm people suffer from the social structure and the institutions sustaining and reproducing it.

## References

Abimbola S. The foreign gaze: authorship in academic global health. BMJ Global Health. 2019;4(5):e002068.

Abimbola S, Pai M. Will global health survive its decolonisation? Lancet (London, England). 2020;396(10263):1627–8.

Adida CL, Dionne KY, Platas MR. Ebola, elections, and immigration: how politicizing an epidemic can shape public attitudes. Polit Groups Identities. 2020;8(3):488–514.

Aginam O. The nineteenth century colonial fingerprints on public health diplomacy: a postcolonial view. Law Social Justice Global Dev J. 2003;1(6)

Allen RB. Slaves, freedmen and indentured laborers in colonial Mauritius. Cambridge University Press; 1999.

Allen RB. Capital, illegal slaves, indentured labourers and the creation of a sugar plantation economy in Mauritius, 1810–60. J Imp Commonw Hist. 2008;36(2):151–70.

Allen RB. European slave trading in the Indian Ocean, 1500–1850. Ohio University Press; 2015.

Amrith S. Decolonizing international health: India and Southeast Asia, 1930–65. Springer; 2006.

Anderson DE. The epidemics of Mauritius. HK Lewis & Company; 1918.

Anderson W. The colonial medicine of settler states: comparing histories of Indigenous health. Health History. 2007;9(2):144–54.

Arnold D. Colonizing the body: state medicine and epidemic disease in nineteenth-century India. University of California Press; 1993.

Barry M. COVID provides opportunity to rethink inequitable roles in global health partnerships. Global Health. 2021. https://globalhealth.stanford.edu/education/covid-provides-opportunity-to-rethink-inequitable-roles-in-global-health-partnerships.html/. Accessed 5 Dec 2021.

Bashford A. 'Is White Australia possible?' Race, colonialism and tropical medicine. Ethn Racial Stud. 2000;23(2):248–71.

Bockarie M, Machingaidze S, Nyirenda T, Olesen OF, Makanga M. Parasitic and parachute research in global health. Lancet Global Health. 2018;6(9):e964.

Bump, J. B., & Aniebo, I. Colonialism, malaria, and the decolonization of global health. PLOS Global Public Health. 2022;2(9):e0000936.

Büyüm AM, Kenney C, Koris A, Mkumba L, Raveendran Y. Decolonising global health: if not now, when? BMJ Global Health. 2020;5(8):e003394.

Crane JT. Scrambling for Africa: AIDS, expertise, and the rise of American global health science. Cornell University Press; 2013.

Crosby AW. Virgin soil epidemics as a factor in the aboriginal depopulation in America. William Mary Q. 1976;1:289–99.

Crosby AW. The Columbian exchange: biological and cultural consequences of 1492. Greenwood Publishing Group; 2003.

Daffé ZN, Guillaume Y, Ivers LC. Anti-racism and anti-colonialism praxis in global health—reflection and action for practitioners in US academic medical centers. Am J Trop Med Hyg. 2021 Sep;105(3):557.

Dawson MH. Smallpox in Kenya, 1880–1920. Social Sci Med Part B Med Anthropol. 1979;13(4):245–50.

Djurfeldt G, Lindberg S. Pills against poverty: a study of the introduction of western medicine in a Tamil village. Studentlitt; 1975.

Eichbaum QG, Adams LV, Evert J, Ho MJ, Semali IA, van Schalkwyk SC. Decolonizing global health education: rethinking institutional partnerships and approaches. Acad Med. 2021;96(3):329–35.

Erondu NA, Peprah D, Khan MS. Can schools of global public health dismantle colonial legacies? Nat Med. 2020;26(10):1504–5.

Ferguson C, Bells, S. Between the shore and the reef, there is a school. In, Seetah K, Leidwanger J. Across the shore. Integrating perspectives on heritage. Springer Science + Business Media: 'When the Land Meets the Sea' Series. In press.

Farmer P, Kim JY, Kleinman A, Basilico M. Reimagining global health: an introduction. University of California Press; 2013.

Gerken KN, Maluni J, Mutuku FM, Ndenga BA, Mwashee L, Ichura C, Shaita K, Mwaniki M, Orwa S, Seetah K, LaBeaud AD. Exploring potential risk pathways with high risk groups for urban Rift Valley fever virus introduction, transmission, and persistence in two urban centers of Kenya. PLOS Neglect Trop Dis. 2023;17(1):e0010460.

Greene J, Basilico MT, Kim H, & Farmer P. Colonial medicine and its legacies. In, Farmer P, Kim JY, Kleinman A, Basilico M. Reimagining global health: an introduction. University of California Press; 2013.

Health Sector Strategic Plan 2020–2024. Republic of Mauritius, Ministry of Health and Wellness. 2020. https://health.govmu.org/Communique/HSSP%20 Final%2015%20September%202020.pdf. Accessed 18 Aug 2022.

Hoffman PT. Why did Europe conquer the world? Princeton University Press; 2015.

Johannes RE. Words of the lagoon: fishing and marine lore in the Palau district of Micronesia. Univ of California Press; 1981.

King NB. Security, disease, commerce: ideologies of postcolonial global health. Social Stud Sci. 2002;32(5-6):763–89.

Lawrence DS, Hirsch LA. Decolonising global health: transnational research partnerships under the spotlight. Int Health. 2020;12(6):518–23.

Lu L, Fang Y, Wang X. Drug abuse in China: past, present and future. Cell Mol Neurobiol. 2008;28(4):479–90.

Navarro V. Social security and medicine in the USSR: a Marxist critique, 1977.

Nowrojee P. A Kenyan Journey. Transafrica Press; 2014.

Musango L, Timol M, Burhoo P, Shaikh F, Donnen P, Kirigia JM. Assessing health system challenges and opportunities for better noncommunicable disease outcomes: the case of Mauritius. BMC health services research. 2020 Dec;20(1):1–21.

Parahoo KA. Early colonial health developments in Mauritius. International journal of health services. 1986 Jul;16(3):409–23.

Pike N. Sub-tropical Rambles in the Land of Aphanapteryx: Personal Experiences, Adventures, and Wanderings in and Around the Island of Mauritius. 1873.

Richards JF. Opium and the British Indian Empire: the Royal Commission of 1895. Modern Asian Studies. 2002;36(2):375–420.

Richardson ET. Epidemic illusions: on the coloniality of global public health. MIT Press; 2020.

Sarmiento, I., Zuluaga, G., Paredes-Solís, S., Chomat, A. M., Loutfi, D., Cockcroft, A., & Andersson, N. Bridging Western and Indigenous knowledge through intercultural dialogue: lessons from participatory research in Mexico. BMJ Global Health, 2020;5(9): e002488.

Seetah K. Connecting continents: Archaeology and history in the Indian Ocean world. Ohio University Press; 2018.

Seetah K, LaBeaud D, Kumm J, Grossi-Soyster E, Anangwe A, Barry M. Archaeology and contemporary emerging zoonosis: A framework for predicting future Rift Valley fever virus outbreaks. International Journal of Osteoarchaeology. 2020;30(3):345–54.

Seetah K, Manfio S, Balbo A, Farr H, Florens FB. Colonization during colonialism: developing a framework to assess the rapid ecological transformation of Mauritius's pristine ecosystem. Front Ecol Evol. 2022:186. https://doi.org/10.3389/fevo.2022.791539.

Seetah K, Ricci G, Calaon D, Trazzi R, Zanaboni M, Balliana E, Izzo FC, Zendri E. In prep. Insights into the inception of modern drug use: Chemical analysis reveals the smoking complexes of labouring peoples in colonial Mauritius. In prep.

Smith LT. Decolonizing methodologies: research and indigenous peoples. Zed Books Ltd; 2013.

Stokstad E. Genetics lab accused of misusing African DNA. Science. 2019. https://www.science.org/content/article/major-uk-genetics-lab-accused-misusing-african-dna. Accessed 7 Feb 2022.

Toussaint A. Une cité tropicale: Port-Louis de l'île Maurice. Presses universitaires de France; 1966.

United States Tariff Commission. Colonial tariff policies. US Government Printing Office; 1922.

Van Dommelen P. Colonialism and migration in the ancient Mediterranean. Ann Rev Anthropol. 2012;(41):393–409.

WHO. Regional Office for Africa. WHO country cooperation strategy 2008-2013: Mauritius. World Health

Organization. Regional Office for Africa. 2009. https://apps.who.int/iris/handle/10665/136064

WHO. World health statistics 2015. Geneva: WHO; 2015.

WHO. Global health workforce statistics database. Geneva: WHO; 2019a. http://www.who.int/hrh/statistics/hwfstats/. Accessed 22 Aug 2022.

WHO. Global health expenditure database. Geneva: WHO; 2019b. http://apps.who.int/nha/database/ViewData/Indicators/en. Accessed 22 Aug 2022.

WHO. Health, environment and climate change; 2019c https://www.who.int/docs/defaultsource/climate-change/who-global-strategy-on-health-environment-and-climate-change-a72-15.pdf?sfvrsn=20e72548_2. Accessed 22 Aug 2022.

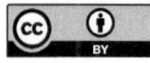

# Ethical Challenges in Global Health Research

Randall Waechter, Kareem Coomansingh,
Cheryl Macpherson, and Sameera Sarma

*The first step in the evolution of ethics is a sense of solidarity with other human beings.*

Albert Schweitzer.

## Abstract

Understanding global health ethics requires insight into factors that influence inequalities in global health such as economic disparities, extreme poverty, limits on human rights, political oppression, and unequal distribution of research funding. We review some ethical issues related to global health, focusing on global infectious disease research. Significant ethical concerns include inequities and disparities in national and institutional capacity to conduct global health research on infectious diseases because these can influence the extent to which low-resource countries benefit from the research. Research funding for global health or infectious disease often comes from the governments and institutions of developed countries. It is allocated based on their institutional priorities, which may not align with those of the developing country. When they do align, developing countries may lack the necessary research, manufacturing, and logistical capacity to discover, produce, and distribute medicines and/or vaccines for infectious diseases within their countries. Research ethics guidelines evolve iteratively to help global health practitioners and researchers navigate concerns involving global health and infectious disease. There is an ongoing need for legal and regulatory frameworks, support for research capacity building—including ethics capacity, and systems to audit the impacts of capacity-building programs. While partnerships are essential to carrying out global health research, inequities between high- and low-resource countries drive ethical challenges in global health and infectious disease work. Recognizing and mitigating these inequities is a core challenge in global health research ethics supported by wider efforts toward decolonization.

R. Waechter (✉)
Caribbean Center for Child Neurodevelopment
(CCCN) at Windward Islands Research & Education
Foundation (WINDREF), Grenada, West Indies
e-mail: randallwaechter@cccnd.org

K. Coomansingh
Office of Research, Windward Islands Research &
Education Foundation (WINDREF), St. George's
University, Grenada, West Indies

C. Macpherson
Department of Clinical Skills, Windward Islands
Research & Education Foundation (WINDREF), St.
George's University, Grenada, West Indies

S. Sarma
School of Medicine, St. George's University,
Grenada, West Indies

## Keywords

Research ethics · Bioethics · Global Health ·
Global infectious disease · Inequity

© The Author(s) 2024
A. Stewart Ibarra, A. D. LaBeaud (eds.), *Transforming Global Health Partnerships*, Sustainable
Development Goals Series, https://doi.org/10.1007/978-3-031-53793-6_2

**Author Perspective**

We are colleagues, mentors and students of a growing center of bioethics training and expertise in a low-resource tropical region. We strongly believe that curiosity about and responsiveness to inequities is at the core of bioethics and research ethics and something that every student of global health research, and health in general, should be aware of. Most of the authorship team have spent most of their career living in and carrying out global health research in developing countries. We hope that the diversity of author perspectives provides the reader with a comprehensive overview of the ethical issues in global health, including inequities that can be rectified only by the many stakeholders in research, including researchers themselves.

Key Tenets

1. Global health ethics is driven by inequality.
2. Global health research funding often comes from developed countries and is allocated based on their priorities, which may not align with those of developing countries
3. Health research and ethics capacity-building within developing countries should be a priority.
4. Clear, ongoing communication and partnership building is key to addressing some of the ongoing gaps and disparities.
5. This chapter addresses the following SDGs: #4 To ensure inclusive and equitable quality education and promote lifelong learning opportunities for all; #10 To reduce inequality within and among countries; #17 To strengthen the means of implementation and revitalize the Global Partnership for Sustainable Development.

# 1 Global Health and Global Infectious Disease

Global Health addresses the health of disadvantaged populations regardless of where they live while acknowledging the importance of equity for health and well-being. It has been defined as public health *everywhere* (Fischer et al. 2020). It has also been defined as health for all (driven by equity principles), health by all (influenced and improved by a broad scope of actors), and health in all (health in all policies) (Garay et al. 2013). Public health—the early diagnosis and/or prevention of disease, prolonging life, and promotion of physical health through sanitation of the environment, control of communicable infections, and the education of the individual (Winslow 1920)—is closely related to global health but differs in scope. Public health professionals are charged with the health of prescribed populations within a city, state, region, or nation. In contrast, global health professionals address healthcare challenges and policies across national borders. This is especially important in addressing infectious diseases because pathogens do not respect political borders. Infectious disease, which is caused by pathogenic microorganisms, such as bacteria, viruses, parasites, or fungi, and can be spread, directly or indirectly, from one person to another, is a central concern in global health.

# 2 Bioethics, Research Ethics, and Global Health Ethics

In this chapter, we review significant ethical issues related to global health, specifically focusing on global infectious disease work. Ethics are concerned with establishing rules and guidelines that distinguish between acceptable and unacceptable behavior when interacting with others, especially when inequity, or power differentials, between individuals and groups of people may be present. Laws are rules that direct behavior within a society. Ethical guidelines are less formal and more widely applicable than laws. Ethics also provides guidelines and principles for deciding how to analyze complex problems and issues and act thoughtfully and deliberately. When people think of ethics in medicine and health, or bioethics, they often think about research ethics guidelines such as the World Medical Association's (WMA) Declaration of Helsinki or the Council for International Organizations of Medical Sciences' (CIOMS) International Ethical Guidelines for Health-related Research involving Humans. These guidelines encompass perspectives from medicine and patient care as well as public health but fail to resolve conflicts between, for example, restricting an individual's freedom of movement to protect others from contact with an infectious pathogen. Institutional review boards (IRBs)—called research ethics committees (RECs) in much of the world—should not be the sole or primary focus of teaching about ethics in global health research because this minimizes other significant ethical concerns, including the need to make host country partners' perspectives and priorities central to global health and global health research (DeCamp et al. 2019).

Global health practitioners work with a "global state of mind about the world and our place in it" (Benatar et al. 2003), allowing for a consideration of the context in which ethical dilemmas emerge. Understanding global health ethics requires one to acknowledge factors that influence enormous inequalities in global health: Economic disparities, extreme poverty, limits on human rights, political oppression, and the 90/10 gap, wherein 90% of global research dollars are spent on health problems that affect only 10% of the world (Ostlin et al. 2004; Bhutta 2002; Neufeld et al. 2001). According to the World Bank, 8.4% or 644.6 million people, mostly in tropical developing regions worldwide, lived in poverty in 2019. They do not have access to the basic necessities of life: reliable shelter, clean water, nutritious food, and healthcare. Improving access to these necessities significantly impacts health and quality of life. This 'health in all poli-

cies' concept (Pan American Health Organization/World Health Organization 2021) acknowledges that addressing socio-economic disparities is an essential step in addressing health disparities (i.e., the social determinants of health) (Rowson et al. 2012). Global health requires an acknowledgment of and attempts to address socioeconomic inequities. Simultaneously, global health workers and researchers must understand that the inequitable factors underlying global health are also the drivers of ethical dilemmas (Pinto and Upshur 2009). For example, disparities can increase vulnerability among developing-world patients and research participants and developed-world clinicians and researchers (Edejer 1999). Patients in low-resource countries may lack the knowledge or empowerment to question their physician, seek clarification, or refuse consent to participate in research (Pinto and Upshur 2009). Neglect of the health and well-being of the poorest and most disadvantaged threatens the health of all (Benatar 2002).

## 3 Global Infectious Disease Work

Infectious disease control involves the prevention of transmission at individual and population levels and the effective management of infectious diseases within individuals. These are major areas of global infectious disease work. Before the turn of the twentieth century, infectious diseases were responsible for the greatest global burden of death and disability. Due to advances in public health, such as water source sanitation, vaccine development, pharmacological therapies such as antibiotics, and educational resources, that distinction has been passed to non-communicable diseases (Holmes et al. 2017). However, infectious diseases still account for a significant global burden, primarily in low- and middle-income countries (LMICs) (GBD 2019 Diseases and Injuries Collaborators 2020). There are many ways to measure the impact of infectious diseases on human health. One is to measure the number of people who die from a given infectious disease every year (i.e., mortality), and another is to measure the number of people who get infected and are living with an infectious disease each year (i.e., morbidity). Using these parameters, the most impactful global infectious diseases in 2019 included: (1) HIV/AIDS and other sexually transmitted infections (STIs); (2) influenza; (3) tuberculosis (TB); (4) malaria; and (5) neglected tropical diseases (NTDs)—a group of 18 diseases which affect over 1 billion of the most impoverished and marginalized people globally (World Health Organization 2021a). Morbidity and mortality from these infectious diseases have a significant socioeconomic impact on individuals, communities, and nations because of the cycle of poverty, disability, and misinformation surrounding the transmission of these diseases. There is a great need for multidisciplinary research efforts to address these preventable disease conditions (Mhalu 2006). There is also a great need for researchers and public health workers to continue collaborating across international borders—to take a global health perspective—when addressing these infectious diseases. Increasing world trade and international travel mean that infectious diseases do not respect political borders. The spread of viruses such as Chikungunya, Zika, Ebola, and most recently, SARS-CoV-2 demonstrate what awaits humanity in the future. By taking a global health perspective, infectious disease researchers, public health officials, governments, and private industry have united to address the SARS-CoV-2 pandemic unlike any other health threat in human history (Daszak 2021). This collaboration has been possible because of technological innovations in communication and the outcome of globalization itself—the interconnectedness of experts into specialized knowledge groups spread across the globe.

# 4 Ethical Considerations in Global Infectious Disease Work

We can now pull together the information presented in the first parts of this chapter to understand the types of ethical issues encountered in global infectious disease work. An overarching concern is the inequities and disparities in national and institutional capacity to conduct global health research on infectious disease, particularly between low and high-resource countries. These inequities influence the extent to which low-resource countries benefit from the research (Garay et al. 2013; The Council for International Organizations of Medical Sciences (CIOMS) 2016). Advancing ethical implementation of global infectious disease work will require an acknowledgment of this inequity by stakeholders and a dedication to addressing the inequity through the process of decolonization[1] (see chapter "Colonialism, Decolonization, and Global Health").

Creating and sustaining a successful research partnership to address global health issues involves showing mutual respect between partners, having trust, good communication and outlining the clear roles and expectations of those involved (John et al. 2016). Though these factors appear straightforward, many obstacles impede their implementation and success, such as a paternalistic view held by researchers from higher-income countries, a lack of transparency of research agendas, inequity in compensation, and an overall lack of proper communication (John et al. 2016). To decolonize research in global health, transnational research partnerships can be strengthened by focusing on participants' views of the research, ensuring that researchers from high-income countries not only prioritize their own needs but work towards transferring skills to research partners in low-income countries so that they may lead their own research in future, and allowing for fair authorship, so researchers from lower-income countries can receive more prestigious listings and fair recognition on publications (Lawrence and Hirsch 2020).

Addressing these key areas may strengthen new and long-standing global health research

---

[1]According to the United Nations, only 17 non-self-governing territories comprising fewer than 2 million inhabitants remain. Thus, when we use the term decolonization, we are referring to addressing the ongoing effects of colonization and related forms of exploitation and domination.

partnerships between lower- and higher-income countries (John et al. 2016). Open discussion regarding existing power imbalances between high- and low-income country researchers, at both the country and institutional level, is encouraged to progress with solutions that meet the needs of all partners and avoid international research groups putting their needs above those of their local partners due to the assumption that they are more knowledgeable, which can be an unfortunate spillover effect of colonization (Lawrence and Hirsch 2020).

## 4.1 Research Priorities and Capacity Building

At the turn of the twenty-first century, LMICs accounted for 85% of the world's population and 92% of the global disease burden. Still, only 10% of global health research funding was devoted to addressing these persistent challenges (Global Forum for Health Research 2004). Most global health research is carried out in high-income countries, which only sometimes consider the burden of specific diseases within LMICs when allocating funding. Recognition of this '90/10 gap' led to renewed calls for health research capacity development in LMICs and further investment (John et al. 2016). Whether individuals, including the vulnerable and disadvantaged around the globe, receive preventative care and treatment for their illnesses in part depends on what public health interventions and what medicines have been developed and whether health systems can deliver them efficiently and affordably. This, in turn, depends on what global health research has been prioritized and performed in the places where these individuals live. Much research fails to consider the most pressing health issues in low-resource countries or offers solutions that are too costly or depend on well-developed infrastructures (White 2004). Where global health research does not focus on health conditions (e.g., neglected tropical diseases), effective public health interventions and medicines will not be developed for them. Where global health research does not generate new

knowledge on strategies for implementing effective interventions in low-resource contexts, health systems will have limited capacity to promote population health and reduce health disparities.

Consequently, some individuals, especially in LMICs, will be more likely to acquire preventable illnesses and lack access to effective treatments (Pratt 2018). Despite the need for more research on health concerns within LMICs, these countries often possess limited capacity to conduct relevant health research, including the capacity for ethical review of research. This limits the accumulation of needed local evidence to inform policies designed to improve population health (Mansour et al. 2021). Research funding for global health or infectious disease comes primarily from pharmaceutical companies, academic institutions, North American and European governments, non-governmental organizations (e.g., Wellcome Trust, Bill and Melinda Gates Foundation), and the World Health Organization (WHO) (see chapter "Funding for Equitable Infectious Disease Research and Development"). Each funding body commissions research on topics that reflect institutional priority and the perceived needs of various stakeholders (Bowsher et al. 2019). Building research infrastructure and capacity in LMICs does not address immediate health challenges and has not been a focus of most funding agencies. The limited infrastructure and capacity in low-resource countries can make it challenging to obtain funding for research on their health priorities. This cycle of limited capacity leading to reliance on research being carried out by developed countries can trap LMICs in a perpetual loop of research dependency. Investment and funding from wealthy countries that extend beyond immediate research study needs is required to build research infrastructure and capacity in LMICs (Matthews and Ho 2008).

The primary focus on institutional review boards (IRBs) and research ethics committees (RECs) when teaching ethics in global health and global health research neglects significant concerns, particularly in global and international health research where the perspectives and priorities of host country governments, institutions, and researchers tend to receive little attention (DeCamp et al. 2019; Macpherson 2019). This inequity stems partly from reliance on the Western bioethics' principles of autonomy (more accurately stated as respect for persons), beneficence, nonmaleficence, and justice, which have different implications and significance in non-Western settings (Pinto and Upshur 2009). By including additional principles and the widely accepted fundamental requirements for ethical research (e.g., value, validity, fair subject selection, favorable risk-to-benefit ratio, independent review, informed consent, and respect for participants), global health researchers can help to ameliorate the reliance on Western bioethics principles. By including other principles in the discussion, host country governments, institutions, and researchers may find it easier to provide their perspectives. This opens the door to discussions about maximal resource allocation (e.g., would the implementation of existing knowledge be a better use of resources than a proposed research project?) and promotes the four concepts central to global health itself: humility, introspection, solidarity, and social justice (Pinto and Upshur 2009).

## 4.2    Access to Treatment and Benefits of Research

Despite a recent push towards equitable access, there remain large global disparities in the distribution of vaccines, diagnostics, and treatments for infectious diseases. LMICs have limited research, manufacturing, and logistical capacity (e.g., cold chain storage) to discover, produce, and distribute medicines and/or vaccines for infectious diseases within their countries (World Health Organization 2021b). Many rely on the charity of developed nations to provide knowledge and capacity to produce or supply medicines and vaccines. As the SARS-CoV-2 pandemic demonstrated, LMICs must often wait for wealthy countries' donations of vaccines, and many are still waiting for adequate supplies as of this writing (OECD 2021).

There is a longstanding consensus in research ethics that fair benefits to host countries, institutions, researchers, and research participants are requirements for ethical research conducted in low-resource countries (Macpherson 2019). The Fair Benefits Framework relies on three ethical conditions: (1) The research should address a significant health problem within the developing country population; (2) The research objectives should provide strong justification for carrying out the study in any given population; and (3) The benefits to the population must outweigh the risks (Participants in the 2001 Conference on Ethical Aspects of Research in Developing Countries 2002). Whether access to treatments that would otherwise be unavailable to a host country population constitutes a fair benefit, how and for how long researchers should provide this access, and how it should be paid for remain unresolved by this and subsequent frameworks. Box 1 presents a real-world example illustrating how these considerations can be addressed. Ethical answers will likely vary with each study and local context as to what is proportionally appropriate. Some guidance, founded in the partial-entrustment model of the researcher-participant relationship, has been provided regarding the ancillary-care responsibilities researchers owe study participants (Richardson and Belsky 2004).

Ethical concerns regarding early international HIV/AIDS research reflect those that persist today. For example, the use of placebo-controlled trials in developing countries when sufficient evidence exists in developed countries to justify an active-controlled trial remains a concern for HIV and other types of international research today (Lurie and Wolfe 1997). These concerns are compounded by advances in genetics and artificial intelligence (AI) that raise questions about privacy, confidentiality, and data ownership. Attempts to obtain informed consent from research participants involve researchers disclosing risks to participants and the opportunity to withdraw from the study at any time. Still, it is nearly impossible for participants to withdraw their demographic, digital, or biological specimens from a biobank or AI repository (Ashcroft

**Box 1**

One ethical challenge we as global health researchers who live and work in a developing country have encountered is the narrow focus of research aims prescribed by funding agencies. In one epidemiological surveillance study, the aim was to determine the impact of a viral infection in pregnant women on fetal and early child development. In considering the needs of the study population, our research team wanted to provide remedial intervention to address developmental delays identified in specific children as part of the research protocol. However, the funding agency, which was in a developed country, was not willing to provide funds for such interventions because it was beyond the core aims of the epidemiological study, and thus, beyond the scope of funding. This was an ethical dilemma for the research team because it was an area of need identified by the developing country research participants. To address this challenge, the research team developed a protocol to provide clear feedback to each study participant about the developmental status of her child and coordinated with the local Ministry of Health to provide follow-up assessment of any child that was determined by the research team to be experiencing developmental delay. This demonstrates the importance of local partnership building for successful implementation of Global health studies.

and Macpherson 2019). Participants in low-resource settings have even less ability to do so because their data is almost always exported to a wealthy country repository. Informed consent has other implications in medicine and public health because participants can be described as both victims and vectors of an infectious disease (Francis et al. 2005).

These implications may play out differently for individuals who are seen primarily as vectors and are stigmatized and marginalized in accessing care, for example, sexually transmitted diseases like HIV/AIDS (see chapter "Building Partnerships to Empower Women Through Home Self-Sampling for Sexual and Reproductive Tract Infections"), a highly lethal disease like Ebola (see chapter "Community-Based Approaches to Respond to Epidemics and Natural Disasters in Coastal Ecuador"), or a pandemic disease where they are blamed or feared for infecting others. Understanding individuals as vulnerable to disease transmission, who are unwilling vectors to others, may provide different analyses of informed consent and justice (Francis et al. 2005) in low- and high-resource countries. The COVID-19 pandemic has generated new and reconsidered old ethical questions in global health research, giving rise to new research ethics guidance and a wealth of literature in prominent Western medical and bioethics journals (e.g., International Development Research Center 2021; Pan American Health Organization 2020; Wolff et al. 2021).

## 4.3 Climate Change

Climate change is accelerating environmental degradation and increasing the frequency and intensity of extreme weather, among other impacts. The effects of both gradual environmental degradation and sudden shocks, such as hurricanes and floods, disproportionately affect vulnerable populations. Whether they impinge on infrastructure, livelihoods, resources, health, or even the loss of lives and homes, these impacts are in no way equal across countries or population groups with varying economic disparities (United Nations 2020). Those in high-income countries which have contributed the most to greenhouse gas emissions that accelerate climate change are more likely to have the needed resources to adapt to increasing environmental degradation. In contrast, those in LMICs which have contributed relatively little to greenhouse gas emissions, are at the greatest risk.

Equally important are the indirect effects involving, among others, infectious diseases which may be climate sensitive. The distribution of infectious diseases can be impacted by variables such as air and water temperature, rainfall, humidity, sun exposure, and water and food sources (Hall et al. 2021). Some of these variables impact the distribution of vectors, such as mosquitoes that spread infectious diseases, including malaria (Lafferty and Mordecai 2016). Rising temperatures are adversely affecting economic growth in some tropical countries, and these tend to be low-resource countries. The disparity between the income of the richest and poorest 10% of the global population is 25% larger than it would be without global warming (Diffenbaugh and Burke 2019).

Global health goes hand in hand with planetary health (see chapter "Team Science and Infectious Disease Work: Exploring Challenges and Opportunities") and health professionals, given their often trusted and respected position in the community. These professionals have taken an oath to provide ethical care to their patients and must mediate between science, policy, and practice in the face of global climate change. This makes them potential agents of individual and systemic efforts to increase climate change mitigation and resilience (Wabnitz et al. 2020). Bioethicists have responsibilities in communicating, educating, and sometimes advocating for justice and other concerns relevant to climate change (Solomon 2021; Scully 2019; Macpherson 2013). Research is needed on what makes for effective and ethical climate change communication and how individual beliefs affect related behaviors and policies (Valles 2015).

## 5    Ethical Guidelines for Global Health Research

The importance of and need for research on global infectious disease is clear, as is the need to conduct research following internationally accepted guidelines. Research ethics guidelines have evolved over 75 years and include the Nuremberg Code, Declaration of Helsinki, and Belmont Report, which were partly established because of the egregious Tuskegee experiments (The Tuskegee Timeline 2019). The Belmont

Report emphasizes respect for persons, beneficence, and justice, which guide the assessment of risks and benefits, selection of human research participants, and how informed consent is understood and obtained (National Commission for the Protection of Human Subjects of Biomedical and Behavioral Research 1978). The US National Institutes of Health (NIH) Clinical Center recently updated guidance for the ethical conduct of research, which builds on the U.S. Common Rule (1991). The new guidelines emphasize the social and clinical value of research, scientific validity, fair participant selection, favorable risk-benefit ratio, independent review, informed consent, and respect for potential and enrolled participants (National Commission for the Protection of Human Subjects of Biomedical and Behavioral Research 1978). Ethical guidelines for international research build on widely shared principles and add several caveats.

The Nuffield Council on Bioethics report on Research in Global Health Emergencies (NIH Clinical Center 2021) calls for research stakeholders to (1) ensure that research addresses the concerns of those most affected; (2) design studies with cultural sensitivity to host country and community needs; (3) modify approaches to informed consent when the situation warrants this; (4) treat researchers and research institutions in host countries as equal partners; (5) review and justify how data and biological materials will be collected and shared; and (6) provide support for researchers and others encountering ethical dilemmas during the conduct of research. Release of an ethical compass by the Nuffield Council on Bioethics (Nuffield Council on Bioethics 2020) emphasizes equal respect, fairness, and helping reduce suffering as values that researchers should consider if their research is to be sensitive to host culture, respectful of participants, equitably balance risks and benefits, be inclusive and transparent, and respond to host research needs. The Pan American Health Organization (PAHO) highlights ethical oversight as critical for research in public health emergencies when the rapid production of evidence impacts risk/benefit ratios and ethical acceptability. Results may call for modification, suspension, or cancelation of a given study, so REC analysis and oversight are essential (The Pan American Health Organization 2020).

World Health Organization (WHO) guidelines call for working closely with national governments in surveillance and preparedness, particularly for infectious disease outbreaks. This may require financial, technical, and scientific assistance from the international community, which it calls on to allocate resources equitably and with utility (i.e., to minimize burdens and maximize benefits). Importantly, the research itself should be designed and implemented, when feasible, in tandem with other public health interventions, and investigators should promote rapid sharing of data and findings to facilitate interventions and prevention (The World Health Organization 2016). The International Ethical Guidelines for Health-related Research Involving Humans from the Council for International Organizations of Medical Sciences (CIOMS) provides 25 succinct guidelines with detailed commentary to explain their intent (The Council for International Organizations of Medical Sciences (CIOMS) 2016). Other bodies and authors offer guidance designed for different stakeholders or to address specific areas of interest (Emanuel et al. 2004). These call on researchers and sponsors to partner with host country institutions and researchers in assessing what research priorities to pursue; what forms of benefit-sharing and capacity building to provide and how best to provide them; and share and deliver appropriate benefits to host institutions, researchers, and populations.

Existing guidelines aim, among other things, to prevent what is known as 'ethics dumping'—the exploitation of research participants or resources in low-resource host countries. Ethics dumping involves using research methods and practices in low-resource countries when those practices would be unethical and unacceptable in the country from which research is designed and funding obtained, which is usually a wealthy country. Factors contributing to ethics dumping include absent or ineffective laws and oversight for research ethics and limited understanding by institutions and researchers of what ethics dumping is, why it's wrong, and that they are engaging in it (Schroeder et al. 2018). Schroeder and colleagues (2018) provide numerous real-life case examples that demonstrate the severity of the problem.

The TRUST consortium offers useful guidance for funders to better ensure that the research they support is equitable and includes partnerships with host countries based on fairness, respect, care, and honesty (TRUST Consortium 2020). TRUST guidelines stress the importance of (1) establishing an understanding of all research stakeholders about their respective roles and responsibilities during the research; (2) including host country researchers equitably as partners unless there is sound justification not to; (3) sharing research data and analyses with host partners and participants; (4) providing support for research infrastructure including IRBs and their staff and members; (5) establishing a mechanism for receiving feedback and complaints from participants and partners; (6) creating measures to protect participants from stigmatization and discrimination; (7) determining what host resources may be depleted by the research and investing in replenishing or sustaining these; and (8) and protecting animal welfare and natural environments (TRUST Consortium 2020).

The common theme across current ethical guidelines for global health research is a focus on partnership building between high-income countries and LMIC researchers that actively engages the LMIC researchers to respond to the priorities of their own countries, as determined by the LMIC country itself. This requires an equal collaboration between partners that account for the unique circumstances and requirements within each LMIC and an understanding that those needs may evolve. Wealthy countries committed to attaining this ideal must invest in the capacity of LMIC host countries if they are to become equal partners.

## 6 Ongoing Challenges in Global Health Research

The guidelines discussed above reflect ethical standards and values that have endured and evolved since the mid-twentieth century. Access to and familiarity with these guidelines is necessary for those working in global health and research, as is the ability to apply these to real-world scenarios. It is important to note that the organizations listed above regularly review and update their guidelines as new issues and challenges in global health arise. In this way, ethics is ongoing—the work is never finished.

## 6.1 Need for Legal and Regulatory Frameworks in Low Resource Countries

There is no international convention or law binding countries to CIOMS or any other ethics guideline. Some countries have laws in place, for example, the Code of Federal Regulations (45CFR46) and the Common Rule in the United States. Countries with legal and regulatory frameworks can monitor compliance with their research ethics laws and regulations. Although many countries regulate some aspects of research, they fail to address other equally important topics (TRUST Consortium 2020). Many low- and high-resource countries rely on bureaucratic and uncoordinated systems that use varied standards for research ethics review (e.g., institutional, national, or international) and different types of committees to conduct reviews (e.g., IRBs, RECs, national ethics committees, hospital ethics committees). Many IRB or REC members in low-resource countries have little research ethics training and expertise and inadequate time allocated by their employers for IRB or REC work. To a lesser extent, these deficits exist in wealthy countries too.

Efforts in some countries to centralize and streamline timely research ethics reviews through national or institutional systems can effectively standardize the level of knowledge and expertise of reviewers and the quality of reviews while reducing the number of reviewers where these are limited. Efforts to partner with and delegate reviews for certain types of research to an IRB or REC in different jurisdictions may help balance heavy workloads or boost the capacity of IRBs with limited membership, expertise, or institutional resources. Such partnerships are some-

times called 'research ethics equivalency' but have had limited success. Helpful resources include the International Compilation of Human Research Standards enumerating over 1000 laws, regulations, and guidelines (collectively referred to as standards) governing human subjects research in 130 low- and high-resource countries (Office for Human Research Protections U.S, Department of Health and Human Services 2021). In addition to familiarity with international research ethics guidelines, those with a responsibility to be aware of relevant laws and regulations where they collect data include researchers, sponsors, and institutional officials. Problems involving ethics dumping have persisted and spread in the absence of such frameworks and given the limited research and research ethics capacity in low-resource countries.

Limited capacity can lead to the marginalization of low-resource country researchers and institutions in dialogues about research ethics. For example, what, in their country, constitutes a fair distribution of benefits and burdens, recruitment and selection of participants, adequate community engagement, collection and storage and use of data and biological materials, and the extent to which a study has both social and scientific validity. The resource needs, health priorities, and unique circumstances of a host country influence how their researchers, institutions, and government respond to invitations to host or partner with others in international research. Potential economic and educational benefits of such partnerships tempt some to accept any benefits and terms offered without negotiating for more equitable sharing and distribution. This challenges host country institutions and researchers in conducting research on host country health priorities and hinders their ability to obtain compensation for the use of their resources and infrastructure, fair distribution of benefits, and research funding and lead authorship on publications (Macpherson 2019).

With respect to financial payments, there is no consensus about how much to remunerate research participants or incentive to pay participants (what amount is too little or too much) and what post-trial benefits (medications, vaccines, others) should be provided to participants (or by who and for how long). Informed consent is challenging in all countries, and more so when wealthy country researchers ascertain that host country participants understand the purpose of a study or the risks and benefits of participating. Respect for participants is embodied in sensitivity to what information they want to know and how to disclose it effectively to a given participant and population.

## 6.2 Need for Research Ethics Capacity Building

Global health research in the twenty-first century is increasingly funded and conducted by commercial entities, sometimes in partnership with academic or research institutions or governments. Corporations and industries led by those from wealthy countries conduct research in low-resource countries, although doing so may harm host countries and participants and worsen inequities. With limited success, CIOMS (2016) and others such as the Council on Health Research and Development (COHRED https://www.cohred.org/home/) call for sponsors from wealthy countries to consult and engage host country researchers, communities, and other stakeholders about health challenges, research design, benefit sharing, and research ethics capacity. Research ethics capacity requires resources such as IRB or REC infrastructure, staffing, operational budgets, office space and equipment, training of members and administrators, and protected time for members to provide adequate review of research proposals. There is a widespread perception that being a health professional or 'good' person qualifies one to serve on an IRB. Still, those lacking education about research and research ethics have limited ability to review the subtle ethical and practical implications of proposed research objectively and insightfully for participants and their families and communities.

Continuing education in research ethics is needed to deepen reviewer knowledge and keep them updated about evolving ethical issues and guidance. Among the many helping to build

capacity through infrastructure and education are the WHO, PAHO, CIOMS, European Commission, Health Canada, International Society for Environmental Epidemiology (ISEE), Nuffield Council on Bioethics, Wellcome Trust, Drugs for Neglected Diseases initiative (DNDi), European & Developing Countries Clinical Trial Partnership (EDCTP), NIH-Fogarty International Center (FIC), Medical Education Partnership Initiative, African Malaria Network Trust, and the Training & Resources in Research Ethics Evaluation group.

Research ethics education and infrastructure development programs are generally required to report and disseminate outcomes, but tools for doing so are limited. It is difficult to assess their impact and value objectively. The African Bioethics Training Program (FABTP), supported by the NIH-FIC, developed a tool for evaluating institutional research ethics capacity that explores changes in individual knowledge, institutional commitment, and the research environment by looking at faculty training, ethics coursework, ethics policies, financing of research ethics oversight, and functionality of IRB infrastructure (Deutsch-Feldman et al. 2018).

## 7 Hope for Progress

Research ethics is always evolving. A Congressional hearing in the 1970s led to the Belmont Report and legal protection for human participants in the United States Code of Federal Regulations. Despite its wealthy, Western country origin and lens, the principles of the Belmont Report still ground international and national standards for research ethics. The United States Office of Human Research Protections (OHRP) provides oversight and educational resources. The NIH mandates research ethics training for all its researchers, including postdoctoral and other training fellows from other countries.

The NIH-FIC supports capacity building for research and ethics by funding awards to establish graduate-level research ethics training programs in low-resource countries. These awards build the capacity of researchers and institutions by developing the knowledge and skills essential to research ethics and IRB reviews. Research ethics knowledge and skills take years to hone and are vital to capacity building (Carracedo et al. 2021; Saenz et al. 2014). NIH-FIC supports such projects in the Caribbean, South America, the Middle East, Africa, Asia, and South Asia. Each is unique and tailors the educational approach to the needs of the country or region, but all are founded on the mentor-mentee model (see Box 2). The NIH-FIC award supports the Caribbean Research Ethics Education initiative (CREEi) in delivering a master's degree in bioethics (MScB) simultaneously to English- and Spanish-speaking fellows in low-resource countries of the Caribbean basin (www.creeii.org). The bilingual curriculum facilitates communication and nurtures trusting fellow-fellow and fellow-faculty relationships across language, culture, and distance. Trusting partnerships are essential to equitable international research partnerships. They can strengthen research ethics networks by enhancing the awareness of and access to resources and information among low resource country researchers and research ethicists. This strengthens their capacity to negotiate equitable partnerships with wealthy country researchers and sponsors, address local health issues, and deliver benefits to host country participants, researchers, institutions, and governments (Bowsher et al. 2019). Despite ongoing investment in research ethics education and capacity, wealthy country researchers and sponsors continue to harm participants and other stakeholders in low and high resource countries through ethics dumping and other ways (Schroeder et al. 2018; OHRP 2021; Pillar 2021).

**Box 2**

Another challenge we as global health researchers and ethicists who live and work in a developing country often encounter is poorly planned and written research proposals that do not take the peer-reviewed literature, regulatory frameworks, ethics guidelines, and cultural norms into consid-

eration. These limitations are exacerbated by imprecise research questions that cannot be meaningfully answered by any scientific method, and which therefore lack social value. This value is an important consideration in ethical review and is determined by whether a protocol will provide information that is useful to other researchers, healthcare professionals, health authorities, healthcare organizations, patients, or communities. Studies of questionable social value, like flawed research questions or methods, are often accompanied by other ethical weaknesses such as overlooking geographic, socioeconomic, and cultural circumstances that influence recruitment and confidentiality or seeking to collect demographic data that has no direct relevance to the research, and thus, unnecessarily violate privacy or confidentiality. To avoid these pitfalls, new researchers should collaborate with experienced researchers until they have the experience to design and lead ethical global health studies independently.

## 8    Conclusion

As social and environmental conditions continue to change, facilitating infectious disease transmission and contributing to other global health challenges, research is needed to prevent and mitigate harm. Global health research on infectious diseases and other areas relies on ethically conducted international research and equitable research partnerships. Often funded by commercial bodies, this research is mandated to provide equitable benefits to host countries. What constitutes an equitable benefit varies with a given study and country. Contributing to the capacity for host country research and research ethics may constitute a benefit of research for some studies and countries and is essential to increase the number of equitable research partnerships between high- and low-resource countries and better provide fair benefits to host country stakeholders. High income country sponsors must invest in host country research and research ethics partnerships and establish and maintain long-term trust between stakeholders and partners. New or enhanced legal and regulatory frameworks, and cultures of research integrity, must be developed in institutions and governments. With their research ethics expertise, bioethicists should be invited to contribute to their development and implementation.

As global health challenges are met, new ones will arise and often be accompanied by ethical questions. Bioethics, like science, medicine, and healthcare, evolves over time. Educating professionals in low- and high-resource countries about research ethics will deepen and broaden their capacity for identifying and resolving ethical challenges in global health research. This capacity may be generalizable to other fields and endeavors. The take-home message for global health professionals is that bioethics work is iterative and evolving in its applications to global health and other realms. The work of bioethics is never finished.

## Glossary of Key Terms in Research Ethics (Adapted from Resnik 2015)

**Autonomy:** The capacity for self-governance (ability to make reasonable decisions for and about oneself)

**Beneficence:** An ethical obligation to do good and avoid causing harm

**Bioethics:** The study of ethical, social, or legal issues in biomedicine and biomedical research

**Commercialization:** The process of developing and marketing commercial products such as drugs, devices, or other technologies from research

**Confidentiality:** The obligation to keep some types of information confidential or secret

**Disparity:** An outcome that is seen to a greater or lesser extent between individuals or populations

**Equity:** Social justice or fairness

**Ethics dumping:** Exportation of unethical research practices from a higher-income to lower-income setting

**Guideline:** A non-binding recommendation for conduct

**Informed consent:** The process of making an informed decision such as to participate in research (often a document giving permission to researchers to use one's data for various purposes and share them with other researchers)

**Institutional review board (IRB):** A committee responsible for reviewing and overseeing human subjects research (also be called a research ethics committee (REC) or research ethics board (REB) and usually include members from different backgrounds and disciplines)

**Justice:** An ethical principle that obligates one to treat people fairly

**Law:** A rule enforced by the coercive power of the government

**Nonmaleficence:** Avoiding harming others

**Privacy:** Being free from unwanted intrusion into one's personal space, private information, or personal affairs

**Research sponsor:** An organization, such as a government agency or private company, which funds research

**Research subject (also called research participant):** A living individual who is the subject of an experiment or study involving the collection of biological samples from or demographic or other information about that individual

**Right:** A legal or moral entitlement that generally implies duties or obligations

**Utilitarianism:** Basing ethical decisions on what will maximize benefits, happiness, and well-being for all affected individuals

**Vulnerability:** An elevated susceptibility to harm or exploitation due to circumstances that compromise one's ability to make decisions or advocate for their interests or independence (may derive from age, mental state, institutionalization, language barriers, socio-economic or other environmental conditions, or other factors)

# References

Ashcroft JW, Macpherson CC. The complex ethical landscape of biobanking. Lancet Public Health. 2019;4(6):e274–5.

Benatar SR. Reflections and recommendations on research ethics in developing countries. Soc Sci Med. 2002;54(7):1131–41. https://doi.org/10.1016/s0277-9536(01)00327-6.

Benatar SR, Daar AS, Singer PA. Global health ethics: the rationale for mutual caring. Int Aff (Royal Institute of International Affairs 1944-). 2003;79(1):107–38.

Bhutta ZA. Ethics in international health research: a perspective from the developing world. Bull World Health Organ. 2002;80:114–20.

Bowsher G, et al. A narrative review of health research capacity strengthening in low and middle-income countries: lessons for conflict-affected areas. Global Health [Internet]. 2019;15(23). Available from: https://globalizationandhealth.biomedcentral.com/articles/10.1186/s12992-019-0465-y

Carracedo S, Palmero A, Neil M, Hasan-Granier A, Saenz C, Reveiz L. El panorama de los ensayos clínicos sobre COVID-19 en América Latina y el Caribe: evaluación y desafíos. Rev Panam Salud Publica. 2021;45:e33.

Daszak P. Lessons from COVID-19 to help prevent future pandemics. China CDC Wkly. 2021;3(7):132–3. https://doi.org/10.46234/ccdcw2021.035.

DeCamp M, Kalbarczyk A, Manabe YC, Sewankambo NK. A new vision for bioethics training in global health. Lancet Glob Health. 2019;7(8):e1002–3.

Deutsch-Feldman M, Hamapumbu H, Lubinda J, Musonda M, Katowa B, Searle KM, et al. Efficiency of a malaria reactive test-and-treat program in southern Zambia: a prospective, observational study. Am J Trop Med Hyg. 2018;98(5):1382–8.

Diffenbaugh NS, Burke M. Global warming has increased global economic inequality. PNAS. 2019;116(20):9808–13.

Edejer TT. North-south research partnerships: the ethics of carrying out research in developing countries. BMJ. 1999;319:438–41.

Emanuel EJ, Wendler D, Killen J, Grady C. The benchmarks of ethical research. J Infect Dis. 2004;189(5):930–7.

Fischer S, Patil P, Zielinski C, Baxter L, Bonilla Escobar F, Hussain S, et al. Is it about the 'where' or the 'how'? Comment on defining global health as public health somewhere else. Br Med J Glob Health. 2020;5:e002567.

Francis LP, Battin MP, Jacobson JA, Smith CB, Botkin J. How infectious diseases got left out—and what this omission might have meant for bioethics. Bioethics. 2005;19(4):307–22.

Garay J, Harris L, Walsh J. Global health: evolution of the definition, use and misuse of the term. Face à face Regards sur la santé [Internet]. 2013 [cited 2021 Sep 19];12. Available from: https://journals.openedition.org/faceaface/745

GBD 2019 Diseases and Injuries Collaborators. Global burden of 369 diseases and injuries in 204 countries and territories, 1990–2019: a systematic analysis for the Global Burden of Disease Study 2019. Lancet. 2020;396(10258):1204–22.

Global Forum for Health Research & World Health Organization. The 10/90 (ten ninety) report on health research 2003-2004. World Health Organization. 2004. Available from: https://iris.who.int/handle/10665/44386

Hall NL, Barnes S, Canuto C, Nona F, Redmond AM. Climate change and infectious diseases in Australia's Torres Strait Islands. Aust N Z J Public Health. 2021;45(2):122–8. Available from: https://onlinelibrary.wiley.com/doi/full/10.1111/1753-6405.13073

Holmes KK, Bertozzi S, Bloom BR, Jha P, Gelband H, DeMaria LM, Horton S. Major infectious diseases: key messages from *disease control priorities*. In: Holmes KK, et al., editors. Major infectious diseases. 3rd ed. Washington, DC: The International Bank for Reconstruction and Development/The World Bank; 2017.

International Development Research Center. Research ethics practices during COVID-19. 2021. [cited 2021 Nov 10]. Available from: https://www.idrc.ca/en/research-ethics-practices-during-covid-19

John CC, Ayodo G, Musoke P. Successful Global Health research partnerships: what makes them work? Am J Trop Med Hyg. 2016;94(1):5–7. https://doi.org/10.4269/ajtmh.15-0611. https://www.ncbi.nlm.nih.gov/pmc/articles/PMC4710444/

Lafferty KD, Mordecai EA. The rise and fall of infectious disease in a warmer world. F1000Res 2016.;5:F1000 Faculty Rev-2040. Available from:https://www.ncbi.nlm.nih.gov/pmc/articles/PMC4995683/

Lawrence DS, Hirsch LA. Decolonising global health: transnational research partnerships under the spotlight. Int Health. 2020;12(6):518–23. https://doi.org/10.1093/inthealth/ihaa073. https://academic.oup.com/inthealth/article/12/6/518/5962065?login=true

Lurie P, Wolfe SM. Unethical trials of interventions to reduce perinatal transmission of the human immunodeficiency virus in developing countries. N Engl J Med. 1997;337(12):853–6.

Macpherson CC. Climate change is a bioethics problem. Bioethics. 2013;27(6):305–8.

Macpherson CC. Research ethics guidelines and moral obligations to developing countries: capacity-building and benefits. Bioethics. 2019;33(3):399–405.

Mansour R, Naal H, Kishawi T, Achi NE, Hneiny L, Saleh S. Health research capacity building of health workers in fragile and conflict-affected settings: a scoping review of challenges, strengths, and recommendations. Health Res Policy Syst. 2021;19(1):84.

Matthews KR, Ho V. The grand impact of the Gates Foundation. Sixty billion dollars and one famous person can affect the spending and research focus of public agencies. EMBO Rep. 2008;9:409–12.

Mhalu FS. Burden of diseases in poor resource countries: meeting the challenges of combating HIV/AIDS, tuberculosis and malaria. Tanzan J Health Res [Internet]. 2006;7(3):179–84. Available from: https://www.ajol.info/index.php/thrb/article/view/14257

National Commission for the Protection of Human Subjects of Biomedical and Behavioral Research. *The Belmont report: ethical principles and guidelines for the protection of human subjects of research*. Washington, DC: The National Commission; 1978. p. 10.

Neufeld V, et al. The rich-poor gap in Global Health research: challenges for Canada. CMAJ. 2001;164:1158–9.

NIH Clinical Center. Ethics in clinical research: ethical guidelines [Internet]. Bethesda: MDL NIH Clinical Center; 2021 [updated 2021; cited 2021 Aug 4]. Available from:https://www.cc.nih.gov/recruit/ethics.html

Nuffield Council on Bioethics. Research in Global Health emergencies: ethical issues short report. London: Nuffield Council on Bioethics; 2020. p. 13.

OECD. Coronavirus (COVID-19) vaccines for developing countries: An equal shot at recovery [Internet]. OECD. [cited 2021 Sep 19]. Available from: https://www.oecd.org/coronavirus/policy-responses/coronavirus-covid-19-vaccines-for-developing-countries-an-equal-shot-at-recovery-6b0771e6/

Office for Human Research Protections U.S, Department of Health and Human Services. 2020 International Compilation of Human Research S.pdf [Internet]. [cited 2021 Sep 19]. Available from: https://www.hhs.gov/ohrp/sites/default/files/2020-international-compilation-of-human-research-standards.pdf

OHRP. DCO Activity Data. 2021. [cited 2021 Nov 10]. Available from: https://www.hhs.gov/ohrp/compliance-and-reporting/dco-activity-data/index.html

Ostlin P, Sen G, George A. Paying attention to gender and poverty in Health Research: content and process issues. Bull World Health Organ. 2004;82:740–5.

Pan American Health Organization. Guidance for ethics oversight of COVID-19 research in response to emerging evidence. 2020. [cited 2021 Nov 10]. Available from: https://iris.paho.org/handle/10665.2/53021

Pan American Health Organization/World Health Organization. Health in all policies. [cited 2021 Nov 10]. Available from: https://www3.paho.org/hq/index.php?option=com_content&view=article&id=9361:2014-welcome-health-all-policies&Itemid=40258&lang=en

Participants in the 2001 Conference on Ethical Aspects of Research in Developing Countries. Fair benefits for research in developing countries. Science. 2002;298(5601):2133–4.

Pillar C. Failure to protect? 2021. [cited 2021 Nov 10]. Available from: https://www.science.org/content/article/critics-say-childhood-asthma-study-unethically-withheld-care-and-see-troubling-trend

Pinto AD, Upshur REG. Global health ethics for students. Dev World Bioeth. 2009 Apr;9(1):1–10.

Pratt B. Exploring the ethics of global health research priority-setting. Br Med J [Internet]. 2018;19(1). Available from: https://bmcmedethics.biomedcentral.com/articles/10.1186/s12910-018-0333-y

Resnik DB. Glossary of commonly used terms in research ethics. 2015 [cited 2021 Nov 10]. Available from: https://www.niehs.nih.gov/research/resources/bioethics/glossary/index.cfm

Richardson HS, Belsky L. The ancillary-care responsibilities of medical researchers. An ethical framework for thinking about the clinical care that researchers owe their subjects. Hastings Cent Rep. 2004;34(1):25–33.

Rowson M, Willott C, Hughes R, Maini A, Martin S, Miranda JJ, Pollit V, Smith A, Wake R, Yudkin JS. Conceptualising global health: theoretical issues and their relevance for teaching. Glob Health. 2012;8:36. https://doi.org/10.1186/1744-8603-8-36.

Saenz C, Heitman E, Luna F, Litewka S, Goodman KW, Macklin R. Twelve years of Fogarty-funded bioethics training in Latin America and the Caribbean: achievements and challenges. J Empir Res Hum Res Ethics. 2014;9(2):80–91.

Schroeder D, Cook J, Hirsch F, Fenet S, Muthuswamy V, editors. Ethics dumping: case studies from north-south research collaborations. Basel: Springer International Publishing; 2018.

Scully JL. The responsibilities of the engaged bioethicist: scholar, advocate, activist. Bioethics. 2019;33(8):872–80.

Solomon M. Trust: the need for public understanding of how science works. Hastings Cent Rep. 2021;51(S1):S36–9.

The Council for International Organizations of Medical Sciences (CIOMS). International ethical guidelines for health-related research involving humans. Geneva: The Council for International Organizations of Medical Sciences; 2016. p. 119.

The Pan American Health Organization. Guidance for ethics oversight of COVID-19 research in response to emerging evidence [Internet]. PAHO; 2020 [cited 2021 Aug 6]. 7 p. Available from: https://iris.paho.org/bitstream/handle/10665.2/53021/PAHOIMSHSSCOVID-19200035_eng.pdf?sequence=1&isAllowed=y

The Tuskegee Timeline. U.S. Public Health Service Syphilis Study at Tuskegee. U.S. Centers for Disease Control and Prevention. Archived from the original on May 10, 2019. Retrieved December 18, 2020. It was called the "Tuskegee Study of Untreated Syphilis in the Negro Male".

The World Health Organization. Guidance for managing ethical issues in infectious disease outbreaks. Spain: World Health Organization; 2016.

TRUST Consortium. Global code of conduct for research in resource-poor settings [Internet]. European Union's Horizon 2020 Research and Innovation Programme; 2020 [cited 2021 Aug 6]. 4 p. Available from:

https://www.globalcodeofconduct.org/wp-content/uploads/2018/05/Global-Code-of-Conduct-Brochure.pdf

United Nations. World social report 2020: inequality in a rapidly changing world [Internet]. UN; 2020 [cited 2021 Sep 19]. Available from: https://www.un-ilibrary.org/economic-and-social-development/world-social-report-2020_7f5d0efc-en

Valles SA. Bioethics and the framing of climate change's health risks. Bioethics. 2015;29(5):334–41.

Wabnitz K-J, Gabrysch S, Guinto R, Haines A, Herrmann M, Howard C, et al. A pledge for planetary health to unite health professionals in the Anthropocene. Lancet. 2020;396(10261):1471–3.

White C. Global spending on health research still skewed towards wealthy nations. Br Med J [Internet]. 2004;329(7474) Available from: https://www.proquest.com/docview/1777625189

Winslow CE. The untilled fields of public health. Science. 1920;51(1306):23–33.

Wolff J, Atuire C, Bhan A, Emanuel E, Faden R, Ghimire P, et al. Ethical and policy considerations for COVID-19 vaccination modalities: delayed second dose, fractional dose, mixed vaccines. BMJ Glob Health. 2021;6(5):e005912.

World Health Organization. Immunization and vaccine-preventable communicable diseases. 2021a. Available from: https://www.who.int/data/gho/data/themes/immunization

World Health Organization. COVID-19 vaccination: supply and logistics guidance [Internet]. [cited 2021b Sep 19]. Available from: https://www.who.int/publications-detail-redirect/who-2019-ncov-vaccine-deployment-logistics-2021-1

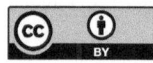

# Gender Equity in African Academia: An Implementation Science Evaluation of the Kenya Context

Christine Ngaruiya

*What we measure, we consider; what we consider, we address; what we address, brings change.*

## Abstract

Progress toward equity in the academic context in Africa continues to lag despite local, regional, and international calls for progress. Implementation science, "the scientific study of methods to promote the systematic uptake of research findings and other evidence-based practices into routine practice," provides a set of tools to dissect why this is the case. Implementation science is a discipline with theories, models, and frameworks that are applicable to generating sustainable interventions that can be applied to various problems and settings. Arguably, the "practice" of gender equity in global health and academic partnerships has not been routine in nature and, in large part, is still not evidence-based. Strategies on how to approach this plethora of problems and what to prioritize have not been well addressed, and there is a lack of recommendations based on the African sociocultural context. In this chapter, an analysis of the status quo of gender equity in academia and academic partnerships is addressed using the CFIR-ERIC tool—a well-established implementation science framework. The Consolidated Framework for Implementation Research (CFIR) domains are used to delineate the problem at different system levels. The associated Expert Recommendations for Implementing Change (ERIC) in the tool provide strategies ranked based on priority. The CFIR-ERIC tool was developed in Western contexts and so may have some limitations with generalizability to the Africa context. This initial analysis provides incipient guidance on action strategies. Also, it presents the need for implementation science and other methodologies to evaluate best practices for evidence-based strategies to close the gender gap.

## Keywords

Gender equity · Academia · Implementation science · Consolidated framework for implementation research · Africa

**Author Perspective**

I am a Kenyan-American female academic who has worked in the Africa and US continents for two decades. In this role, my observations on

C. Ngaruiya (✉)
Department of Emergency Medicine, Stanford School of Medicine, Stanford University, Stanford, CA, USA
e-mail: cngaruiy@stanford.edu

© The Author(s) 2024
A. Stewart Ibarra, A. D. LaBeaud (eds.), *Transforming Global Health Partnerships*, Sustainable Development Goals Series, https://doi.org/10.1007/978-3-031-53793-6_3

gender equity are one of the issues that give me the greatest pause. In turn, this has fueled a pursuit for effective means of narrowing pervasive equity gaps. In this chapter, I explore challenges to achieving gender equity in the African academic context using a well-established implementation science framework. This framework provides a transparent process for solution generation in a given context, and through it I aim to share strategies for implementation to help chip away at this Goliath problem.

---

**Key Tenets**

1. Gender equity in the African academic context and in global health partnerships is complex and requires intentional, evidence-based strategies to realize change
2. Implementation science provides a novel and appropriate approach for planning and evaluation of strategies to achieve gender equity in Africa and beyond
3. Foundational strategies such as implementing and equipping institutional champions for gender equity, conducting local assessments on readiness for implementation, and conducting consensus discussions are recommended for the Africa context as indicated by an analysis using the CFIR-ERIC tool
4. This chapter addresses the following SDGs: #3 Good health and well-being; #4 Quality Education; #5 Gender Equality; #8 Decent Work and Economic Growth; #10 Reduce Inequality; #16 Peace, Justice and Strong Institutions; #17 Partnership for the Goals.

---

# 1    Introduction

Equity in global health and development became an increasingly important focal point in the latter half of the twentieth century, as indicated by clear literature, policies, and associated movements around it. Margaret Whitehead's writings in the 1990s provide some of the earliest clarifying definitions of equity in global health as: "not only unnecessary and avoidable but, in addition… unfair and unjust." (Whitehead 1992) The United Nations general assembly's landmark adoption of the Universal Declaration of Human Rights in 1948 serves as another cornerstone for this change (Assembly 1948). This policy, highlighting equality in "dignity and rights," was the birthplace for multiple other equity efforts, including for gender equity, "without distinction of any kind, such as race, colour, sex, language, religion, birth or another status." The subsequent Beijing declaration of 1995 adopted at the fourth World Conference on Women, is highly acclaimed as the turning point for gender equity efforts in particular (UN 1955). This included priorities such as: "tak(ing) all necessary measures to eliminate all forms of discrimination against women and the girl child and remove all obstacles to gender equality and the advancement and empowerment of women…" as well as "promot(ing) women's economic independence, including employment."

Consequently, and most recently, the United Nations Sustainable Development Goals (SDGs)—a cluster of targets and indicators that guide global health and global development more broadly—demonstrate evidence of the continued pervasiveness and attentiveness towards gender equity in global health. In 2015, when the SDGs were released, an entire goal was dedicated to gender equity or more specifically: "achiev(ing) gender equality and empower(ing) all women and girls." This initiative too provides a foundation for transformative change, by aligning world leaders, policy-makers, practitioners and individuals alike to these consensus UN goals—the body to which all member states and its citizens voluntary subscribe to. In sum, targets and indicators guiding our resource allocation and development efforts should have focused on "end(ing) all forms of discrimination against all women and girls everywhere" (target 5.1) and "ensur(ing) women's full and effective participation and equal opportunities for leadership at all levels…"

(target 5.5). Yet, even though these and other efforts are laudable in their attainment, gaps persist in practicality, and the reach of their impact remains disparate.

This is also true in the African context, where the majority of my own personal and professional experiences have occurred. The advancement of "gender equity" in academia on the African continent remains widely under-prioritized and consistently unaddressed. According to a recent report by McKinsey and Company, as of 2019, progress towards gender parity in Africa had stagnated for the preceding four years, and the duration of time to parity stood at 140 years (McKinsey Global Institute 2019). While other regions had done marginally better, an urgent call for progress on the African continent was made. Without equity on the continent, it is a sequitur that equity and inclusion in partnerships will suffer.

Lack of gender parity in academics persists to date across the lifetime of girls and women, spanning entire careers. For example, in primary education, a lower proportion of girls enroll in school than boys despite government efforts to make elementary education free in some countries such as Kenya (Cherotish et al. 2014). These inequities are based on conventional cultural preferences for educating boys over girls, given their potential as economic contributors to the household, a disproportionate burden of domestic work being given to girls, lack of access to appropriate hygiene and sanitation during menstrual periods and early marriage.

This disparity in representation, however, pervades the education spectrum, including those pursuing advanced academic degrees. While limited evidence exists on the gender representation of women in academic positions, statistics on academic leadership that are available are a window into the problem. With only 40 female vice-chancellors across Africa and no record of current female chancellors that is available, the status quo is dismal (Naidu 2021). This under-representation of women at the highest tiers of leadership portends similarly poor representation of women at the junior and mid-career academic levels with implications for health, science and global health.

In addition to the leadership gap, women constitute less than a third of research scientists globally—including in sub-Saharan Africa (World Health Organization 2019). These issues, in turn, may be worse for those that are non-binary, transgendered, or who constitute other gender minorities in these spaces (Bilimoria and Stewart 2009).

In this chapter, the barriers and opportunities to succeeding as a woman academic in the Africa context are presented, through the Kenya lens, with the potential for shared lessons in similar settings. The status quo on gender equity is analyzed using well-established implementation science frameworks (the combined CFIR-ERIC tool) to provide recommendations rooted in generalizable paradigms. Solutions are framed based on the tool codified by perspectives from lived experiences of mid-career academic women active in global health with roles as academic clinician-scientists, in academic leadership, and in policymaking, with narratives of these experiences shared as case studies presented in the next chapter. For the sake of this chapter, the definition of "global health" used is "an area for study, research, and practice that places a priority on improving health and achieving health equity for all people worldwide," which was used initially by Koplan et al. (2009).

Global health practitioners and policy-makers alike would do well to recognize the leadership contributions of, advance training for, and ensure the advancement of women; effective global health partnerships will thrive off of it, and the closing of development goal gaps depends on it. These strategies are presented and discussed in detail later in the chapter.

## 2 Application of Implementation Science Frameworks to Gender Equity

In this chapter, I use an implementation science lens to evaluate the status quo on gender parity in the Africa context using input from existing literature on the topic and expert opinion. Implementation science pertains to an area of research that focuses, in part, on fine-tuning the who (such as who delivers it), what (what is its content), when (at what point in time: hour, day, week, month) and where (place or location) of "a thing" (typically an "intervention" such as an educational program) to ensure the most effective and sustainable impact of said "thing." While implementation science, the science of implementation of "things," doesn't necessarily purport that a given "thing" or intervention is wrong, it does critically analyze the components of said "thing" with the hypothesis that if any aspect of the strategy on how the "thing" is being implemented is not optimized for a given context, its impact will inevitably suffer.

I propose, then, that while substantial efforts aimed at affecting gender equity in African academia do exist, using an implementation science approach will enable us not only systematically to evaluate what gaps persist but also provide prioritized solutions or strategies for targeting them and add to the literature by guiding critical stakeholders in their actions. Gender equity and gender equity in academia agendas have received unprecedented attention in recent years. However, it is apparent that parity in access and outcomes continue to elude women; this is evidenced by relatively recent initiatives such as UN Women's ongoing efforts (UN Women 2022), the 2021 Executive Order by President Biden establishing the White House Gender Policy Council that was assumed by USAID (USAID 2022), and the re-upping of commitments at the Generation Equality Forum by WHO that also took place in 2021 (World Health Organization 2021); these initiatives foretell a persistently lingering gap in the 2030 agenda (Sustainable Development Goals 2022). It is apparent that either the choice of leading strategies or the approaches by which they are being implemented is ineffective; in addition, the types of strategies may be ineffective.

Two well-established implementation science frameworks have been used to guide this. The Consolidated Framework for Implementation Research (CFIR) Expert Recommendations for Implementing Change (ERIC) tool is used to identify and prioritize barriers and generate priority strategies for achieving gender equity in

academia and academic partnerships. CFIR is a well-established implementation science framework that consists of constructs arranged across five domains that can be used in pre-implementation planning, mid-implementation, or post-implementation evaluation (Consolidated Framework for Implementation Research 2022a). The five domains ("Intervention Characteristics," "Outer Setting," "Inner Setting," "Characteristics of Individuals," and "Process") provide a systematic approach to evaluating different components of the "thing" (or intervention), each with their barriers and facilitators for potential actionable change (see Box 1).

**Box 1: CFIR Domains and Descriptions**

| CFIR domain | Description |
|---|---|
| Intervention characteristics | The "thing" being implemented, e.g., a new clinical treatment, educational program, or city service. |
| Outer setting | The setting in which the inner setting exists, e.g., hospital system, school district, state. There may be multiple outer settings and/or multiple levels within the outer setting (e.g., community, system, state). |
| Inner setting | The setting in which the innovation is implemented, e.g., hospital, school, city. There may be multiple inner settings and/or multiple levels within the inner setting, e.g., unit, classroom, team. |
| Characteristics of individuals | The roles and characteristics of individuals. |
| Process | The activities and strategies used to implement the innovation. |

This evaluation, and associated outputs/recommendations that are provided as broken up by domain, can then: guide design (pre-implementation), guide modification depending on the effectiveness of status quo (mid-implementation), and guide sustainability or (later on) dissemination of the "thing" to other contexts (post-implementation). The domain "Inner Setting," by way of example, assesses "the setting in which the innovation is implemented, e.g., hospital, school, city," and in the evaluation for this paper, the academic institution (i.e., status quo of "things" or interventions targeting gender equity in partnerships at this level of institution). As part of the Inner Setting, constructs such as "climate" and "readiness for implementation" are evaluated. The "Outer Setting," is that in which the Inner Setting exists, e.g., hospital system, school district, state—this will be the country Kenya/ Kenya context in our case. This domain includes constructs such as "peer pressure" and "external policies and incentives" that might influence implementation. All domains and characteristics are defined in full on the CFIR website, an excellent resource with tips on applying the tool and generating a validated questionnaire to assess these constructs based on the CFIR principles. I propose the systematic evaluation, "mid-implementation," afforded by the CFIR will elucidate the next steps for effective implementation of strategies, or modifications to current strategies, to close the gender equity gap in global health and partnerships, particularly for the Kenya context, with potential for generalizability to similar settings.

The Expert Recommendations for Implementing Change (ERIC) consists of 73 implementation strategies identified through expert consensus encompassing previously poorly defined recommendations for key strategies to guide implementation approaches (Powell et al. 2015). These strategies are concise and discrete; examples include "Access new funding," "Capture and share local knowledge," and "Conduct ongoing training." Moreover, the combined CFIR-ERIC tool provides a "strategy-matching" mechanism using the CFIR to delineate and input key barriers for intervention implementation, then proposing optimal strategies from ERIC based on those barriers identified (Consolidated Framework for Implementation Research 2022b).

## 2.1   CFIR Barriers Identified

The newly developed CFIR-ERIC tool was used to identify barriers to gender equity in global health in the African context. This is based on existing literature on gender equity in the global health context and framed by personal experiences of women in African science like myself. The scoring tool uses a "1" to represent the presence of the characteristic and "0" to represent the absence of the characteristic. For intervention characteristics, domains identified as problematic were "intervention source", "evidence strength and quality", "relative advantage" and "adaptability" (see Table 1) regarding successful implementation of gender equity interventions and gender equitable partnerships. These are explained in the following paragraphs.

Many African cultures have long viewed gender equity as being outside or other, a concept of the West that leaders and even policy-makers are not necessarily willing to adapt (Kaganas and Murray 1994; Olatunji 2013; Msuya 2019). In the 1994 paper by Kaganas et al., they cited indigenous leaders refuting policy changes on gender equity, given traditional mores that women are not created equal to men. With a premise of skepticism and reticence on what may be perceived as imported principles, implementation will continue to suffer. These views on the intervention source confer a negative perception of the relative advantage of gender equity interventions over the status quo and, in turn, affect adaptability if these negative perceptions by stakeholders determine it not to be a good fit for local needs. In a more recent paper by Msuya, she highlights that "respect for cultural differences (can) exist simultaneously with the belief that cultural practices and beliefs can and do change over time," enforcing that responsive adaptation does not necessarily devalue cultural practices (Msuya 2019). As such, while there is the promise for change, including through increased representation of policy-makers who can directly contribute to change (Mutume 2005), global indicators, as discussed earlier, indicate that much is still needed. Perceptions of these

**Table 1** CFIR-ERIC tool "Intervention Characteristics" topics and related barriers for gender equity in global health in the Africa context

|   | Intervention characteristics | |
|---|---|---|
| 1 | Intervention source | Stakeholders have a negative perception of the innovation because of the entity that developed it and/or where it was developed. |
| 1 | Evidence Strength & Quality | Stakeholders have a negative perception of the quality and validity of evidence supporting the intervention. |
| 1 | Relative advantage | Stakeholders do not see the advantage of implementing the innovation compared to an alternative solution or keeping things the same. |
| 1 | Adaptability | Stakeholders do not believe that the innovation can be sufficiently adapted, tailored, or reinvented to meet local needs. |
| 0 | Trialability | Stakeholders believe they cannot test the innovation on a smaller scale within the organization or undo implementation if needed. |
| 0 | Complexity | Stakeholders believe that the innovation is complex based on their perception of duration, scope, radicalness, disruptiveness, centrality, and/or intricacy and number of steps needed to implement. |
| 0 | Design quality and packaging | Stakeholders believe the innovation is poor quality based on the way it is bundled, presented, and/or assembled. |
| 0 | Cost | Stakeholders believe the innovation costs and/or the costs to implement (including investment, supply, and opportunity costs) are too high. |

culture-shifting principles may need to be reconciled (see chapters "Role of Social Science in Infectious Disease Research: a Case Study of Partnering with Communities in Vector Control in a Kenyan Village" and "Gender Equity in Academia Thriving as a Clinician-Scientist, Establishing Partnerships, and Driving Policy for Change in the Kenya Context").

Additionally, it has been posited that the evidence base for best practices on gender equity interventions, such as "gender-responsive" policies that enforce equity without a quota or means of enforcing implementation, is still lacking (Gupta 2019). Without sufficient data, including economic data on proposed interventions (e.g., how much does it cost, or more importantly, how much money does it save in pursuing gender equity in an organization), proposals for implementation and adaptation of novel interventions to increase gender equity may be met with resistance.

Trialability (see Table 1) was not identified as a major barrier, as interventions are already occurring secondary to external pressures such as those from the SDGs, despite whether complexity, design quality, or cost have been considered. In sum, outside pressures have initiated or inspired some acceptance and trial implementa-

tions of changes related to gender equity, even if superficial and unsustainable (Kelan 2020). However, intervention implementation must be augmented by addressing identified barriers to intervention characteristics to realize greater success.

Barriers regarding the "outer setting" domain (see Box 1) that were identified as barriers to implementing actions to increase gender equity in an African context were: "cosmopolitanism"—organizations are not effectively sharing best practices or challenges in implementing these needed, yet novel, programs or interventions (see Table 2) (Lauer 2020). As such, ideas on successful interventions to increase gender equity, as well as best practices for implementing them, are not readily or regularly being exchanged. We also identified "peer pressure" as a limitation for similar reasons in that lack of exchange on what others (competing institutions) are doing is not routinely being publicized. Providing communities of practice that can share, exchange ideas, motivate, and challenge one another to do better will be beneficial in ensuring accountability in progress for gender equity in academia and partnerships. As has been mentioned previously, there is extensive literature on the need for gender equity in academia, including in Africa

**Table 2** CFIR-ERIC tool "Outer Setting" topics and related barriers for gender equity in global health in the Africa context

| | Outer setting | |
|---|---|---|
| 0 | Patient needs & resources | Patient needs, including barriers and facilitators to meet those needs, are not accurately known and/or this information is not a high priority for the organization. |
| 1 | Cosmopolitanism | The organization is not well networked with external organizations. |
| 1 | Peer pressure | There is little pressure to implement the innovation because other key peer or competing organizations have not already implemented the innovation nor is the organization doing this in a bid for a competitive edge. |
| 0 | External Policy & Incentives | External policies, regulations (governmental or other central entity), mandates, recommendations or guidelines, pay-for-performance, collaborative, or public or benchmark reporting do not exist or they undermine efforts to implement the innovation. |

(Mulwa 2021; Aina 2013; Okeke-Ihejirika 2012; Mama 2006; Tiedeu et al. 2019), as well as benchmarks set by multiple agencies, so we did not identify "patient" (end-user) needs or external policies as limitations.

Several barriers in the "inner setting" domain are proposed that affect the successful implementation of gender equity interventions in academia or academic partnerships (see Table 3). Culture and lack of accountability that were discussed previously encapsulate issues related to the factors: "culture," "implementation climate," "tension for change," "relative priority," "incentives," "feedback," and "leadership engagement." Later in this text, solutions to navigating some of these challenges are addressed. Additionally, issues of immature or poorly resourced organizations, such as may be the case for some in the global south, affects the capacity to identify, evaluate, address, or implement interventions even if the will is present to do so. This alludes to issues with "structural characteristics," "readiness for implementation," and "access to knowledge and information." As interventions are being proposed, resources on implementation should be made easily accessible and framed for the resource variable context; critiques against the SDGs in the past have supported this argument by highlighting targets for the global south set by external stakeholders that place lofty and unachievable goals without clear steps on how to achieve them (SDG Knowledge Hub 2017) or accounting for resource limitations in doing so (Gupta and Vegelin 2016). For example, a well-established recommendation for gender equity revolves around equity in pay across genders. However, if monitoring and evaluation infrastructure that tracks remuneration, such as annual financial reports from universities that summarize average pay by gender, is not implemented or updated regularly, the ability to effect change is a moot point (data2x 2022).

Building upon earlier discussion, within the "characteristics of individuals" domain, some barriers revolve around individual beliefs on gender equity (Msuya 2019) in academia and partnerships that are rooted in cultural mores within the Africa context. As a result, individuals with decision-making power (e.g., institutional leaders such as deans, senior professors, and lecturers) may hold on to conventions that impede a progressive gender equity agenda (Kaganas and Murray 1994; Olatunji 2013; Msuya 2019) (see Table 4). This lackluster buy-in from those with the influence and resources to effect institutional change translates into a lack of enthusiasm for sustained change. The persistent equity gaps evidence this. While motivation or willingness for change might be observed initially, this may be clouded by other priorities (e.g., curriculum development, purchasing of materials, and hiring and promotions process), particularly in the resource-variable setting. Additional institutional challenges, such as lack of appropriate staff, low wages, delays in payment, and labor strikes may also leave the gender equity agenda at the bottom of the priority list.

Self-efficacy (see Table 4) of implementation interventions is another barrier. This could be improved through education and access to

**Table 3** CFIR-ERIC tool "Inner Setting" topics and related barriers for gender equity in global health in the Africa context

| | Inner setting | |
|---|---|---|
| 1 | Structural characteristics | The social architecture, age, maturity, and size of an organization hinders implementation. |
| 0 | Networks & Communications | The organization has poor quality or non-productive social networks and/or ineffective formal and informal communications. |
| 1 | Culture | Cultural norms, values, and basic assumptions of the organization hinder implementation. |
| 1 | Implementation climate | There is little capacity for change, low receptivity, and no expectation that use of the innovation will be rewarded, supported, or expected. |
| 1 | Tension for change | Stakeholders do not see the current situation as intolerable or do not believe they need to implement the innovation. |
| 1 | Compatibility | The innovation does not fit well with existing workflows nor with the meaning and values attached to the innovation, nor does it align well with stakeholders' own needs and/or it heightens risk for stakeholders. |
| 1 | Relative priority | Stakeholders perceive that implementation of the innovation takes a backseat to other initiatives or activities. |
| 1 | Organizational Incentives & Rewards | There are no tangible (e.g., goal-sharing awards, performance reviews, promotions, salary raises) or less tangible (e.g., increased stature or respect) incentives in place for implementing the innovation. |
| 1 | Goals and feedback | Goals are not clearly communicated or acted upon, nor do stakeholders receive feedback that is aligned with goals. |
| 1 | Learning climate | The organization has a climate where: a) leaders do not express their own fallibility or need for stakeholders' assistance or input; b) stakeholders do not feel that they are essential, valued, and knowledgeable partners in the implementation process; c) stakeholders do not feel psychologically safe to try new methods; and d) there is not sufficient time and space for reflective thinking or evaluation. |
| 1 | Readiness for implementation | There are few tangible and immediate indicators of organizational readiness and commitment to implement the innovation. |
| 1 | Leadership engagement | Key organizational leaders or managers do not exhibit commitment and are not involved, nor are they held accountable for implementation of the innovation. |
| 0 | Available resources | Resources (e.g., money, physical space, dedicated time) are insufficient to support implementation of the innovation. |
| 1 | Access to knowledge and information | Stakeholders do not have adequate access to digestible information and knowledge about the innovation nor how to incorporate it into work tasks. |

**Table 4** CFIR-ERIC tool "Characteristics of Individuals" topics and related barriers for gender equity in global health in the Africa context

| | Characteristics of individuals | |
|---|---|---|
| 1 | Knowledge & Beliefs about the intervention | Stakeholders have negative attitudes toward the innovation, they place low value on implementing the innovation, and/or they are not familiar with facts, truths, and principles about the innovation. |
| 1 | Self-efficacy | Stakeholders do not have confidence in their capabilities to execute courses of action to achieve implementation goals. |
| 1 | Individual stage of change | Stakeholders are not skilled or enthusiastic about using the innovation in a sustained way. |
| 0 | Individual identification with organization | Stakeholders' are not satisfied with and have a low level of commitment to their organization. |

**Table 5** CFIR-ERIC tool "Process" topics and related barriers for gender equity in global health in the Africa context

| | Process | |
|---|---|---|
| 1 | Planning | A scheme or sequence of tasks necessary to implement the intervention has not been developed or the quality is poor. |
| 0 | Opinion leaders | Opinion leaders (individuals who have formal or informal influence on the attitudes and beliefs of their colleagues with respect to implementing the intervention) are not involved or supportive. |
| 1 | Formally appointed internal implementation leaders | A skilled implementation leader (coordinator, project manager or team leader), with responsibility to lead implementation of the innovation, has not been formally appointed or recognized within the organization. |
| 1 | Champions | Individuals acting as champions who support, market, or 'drive through' implementation in a way that helps to overcome indifference or resistance by key stakeholders are not involved or supportive. |
| 1 | External change agents | Individuals from an outside entity formally facilitating decisions to help move implementation forward are not involved or supportive. |
| 1 | Key stakeholders | Multi-faceted strategies to attract and involve key stakeholders in implementing or using the innovation (e.g., through social marketing, education, role modeling, training) are ineffective or non-existent. |
| 1 | Patients/customers | Multi-faceted strategies to attract and involve patients/customers in implementing or using the innovation (e.g., through social marketing, education, role modeling, training) are ineffective or non-existent. |
| 1 | Executing | Implementation activities are not being done according to plan. |
| 1 | Reflecting & evaluating | There is little or no quantitative and qualitative feedback about the progress and quality of implementation nor regular personal and team debriefing about progress and experience. |

resources on implementation strategies for gender equity programs and plans. This may look different for each institution but could include: building internal capacity by training faculty and staff on gender equity, mainstreaming implementation of gender equity related topics in curricula, or hiring expert consultants/ consultant organizations. However, training resources and tools are not widely accessible or widely deployed at this time.

Finally, regarding the "process" domain (see Box 1), we proposed that nearly all aspects could seek improvement (see Table 5). Planning is previously discussed in providing resources or guidelines for implementing novel interventions. Additionally, having formally appointed leaders or champions within each institution (a growing mainstay in Western institutions) is not commonplace in the African academic institution or organization (Bradley et al. 2022; Pihakis et al. 2019). The lack of accountability both internally and externally to institutions hampers effective and sustainable gender equity intervention implementation.

## 2.2 Eric Strategies Based on CFIR Inputs/Barriers

Based on the CFIR-ERIC inputs identified as barriers, as outlined by CFIR domains, the leading ERIC strategies that are proposed include: identifying and preparing champions, conducting assessments for the readiness of implementation of gender equity interventions, and identifying barriers and facilitators, as well as conducting local consensus discussions (see Table 6). Additional solutions include other foundational activities such as obtaining buy-in from local opinion leaders, building coalitions to support key stakeholders, and sharing local knowledge. We explore some of the top strategies in further detail with the understanding that context-specific approaches to implementing each of these strategies may differ. In contrast, at the bottom of the list are the tailoring of strategies, alluding to the fact that several foundational steps have not occurred as yet. The full list of ERIC strategies and their overall ranking as assessed by experts in implementation science (and that are

**Table 6** ERIC strategies based on CFIR-ERIC tool inputs (top 20 out of 73 shown)

|    | ERIC strategies |
|----|-----------------|
| 1  | Identify and prepare champions |
| 2  | Assess for readiness and identify barriers and facilitators |
| 3  | Conduct local consensus discussions |
| 4  | Inform local opinion leaders |
| 5  | Build a coalition |
| 6  | Conduct educational meetings |
| 7  | Alter incentive/allowance structures |
| 8  | Conduct local needs assessment |
| 9  | Create a learning collaborative |
| 10 | Facilitation |
| 11 | Capture and share local knowledge |
| 12 | Identify early adopters |
| 13 | Promote adaptability |
| 14 | Develop a formal implementation blueprint |
| 15 | Recruit, designate and train for leadership |
| 16 | Use advisory boards and workgroups |
| 17 | Audit and provide feedback |
| 18 | Conduct educational outreach visits |
| 19 | Involve executive boards |
| 20 | Tailor strategies |

not weighted based on context-specific needs as in our analysis) are available in the original publication by Powell et al. c These may provide a comparison for what the standard list of priorities might be, as opposed to those unique to this context. Limitations in the list of strategies include the expert panel that derived them as priorities (individuals came predominantly from the US and North America), as highlighted by the authors. Despite this, they provide an initial insightful approach to prioritizing action and devising a plan to address this systematically.

cate themselves to supporting, marketing, and driving through an implementation, overcoming indifference or resistance that the intervention may provoke in an organization." Of note, the creators of the CFIR-ERIC tool highlight that "champions are often distinguished from opinion leaders…" This may manifest such that individuals at the institution who are identified or employed as "champions" (ERIC strategy 1) may be, and maybe even should be, distinct from having existing offices or primary leadership positions.

Through the identification of local leaders within the organization that can help identify opportunities for, drive interventions to support and advocate for accountability on gender equity initiatives in the institution, there is an increased likelihood for implementation success and less likelihood of its priority being overshadowed by others, or completely forgotten (see Excerpt 1 *On leadership*). Such individuals have been named "diversity leaders," "diversity officers," "vice chairs for diversity," "deans for diversity and inclusion," and a plethora of other titles, and in turn, are also provided with the necessary resources and agency to conduct their jobs (VCU News Staff 2021; University of Reading 2022). In sum, they can be at any level of the academic hierarchy, from the departmental level to the university/campus-wide, with program implementers, administrative staff, and other personnel supporting their office. This infrastructure provides the necessary foundation to begin to implement the level of impactful programs needed to realize sustainable change.

## 3 Discussion/Strategies for Improving Gender Equity According to CFIR-ERIC Outputs and ERIC Strategies

### 3.1 Identify and Prepare Champions

According to the CFIR-ERIC tool, this first strategy (ERIC strategy 1, Table 6) encompasses "identifying and preparing individuals who dedi-

**Chapter 18, Excerpt 1: On Leadership**
I soon came to be known as "Dr Social Issues" as I consistently called out the fact that the only items represented on the agenda were matters on the economic pillar and seldom on the social pillar, which is where health lies. Consequently, it became my mission to push this important pillar to the forefront. I watched in dismay as time and again, our articulation of important

matters in the health sector were overlooked… Ultimately, it became apparent that in order to effectively communicate across this chasm, that they needed to hear the matters framed from a perspective of economic impact… I had to change how I framed health issues if ever they were to ever get to the policy table.

Training is important in onboarding and supporting these individuals for successful outputs. For example, it is shortsighted to place a woman in a role based on gender; it is critical to equip whoever is placed in such roles for success. Expertise in best practices and guidance will be needed. Training can be done through organizations or programs such as Women in Global Health or Women Leaders in Global Health; these organizations are also inclusive in supporting male allies for gender equity in global health and have various programming to support institutional or institutional leadership development. Activities that these champions and their respective offices might lead include: (i) conducting/leading assessments, (ii) advocacy for, and implementation of, increased professional development opportunities (48), and (iii) expanding mentorship opportunities for women in academia, among others.

Additionally, it is vital that institutions are intentional about ensuring more women have access to leadership positions. Availing more women in leadership, and mentoring them on how to lead effectively, begets increased opportunities to be mentors themselves. Furthermore, there needs to be increased awareness for men on the disparity in access to mentorship/ sponsorship among women. Training all staff/ faculty in leadership on how to mentor/ sponsor, specifically on the nuances of mentoring women (e.g., impostor syndrome, family balance, etc.) would be ideal. Mentorship should consider the unique challenges faced in different environments and develop strategies to help address these. These models should also be provided along the different career stages-early, mid- and late career. All

in all, the key to these champion roles includes appropriate incentivization and support/ supportive staff, as previously discussed, to help ensure success.

## 3.2 Assess for Readiness and Identify Barriers and Facilitators

ERIC defines readiness assessments as encompassing a wide variety of components. These may include the following factors to facilitate the implementation of gender equity intervention (adapted from the CFIR-ERIC guide):

- Agency finances
- Staffing level
- Material or logistical resources needed
- Availability of leadership support,
- Status quo of organizational priority for change, and
- Presence of successful experience with quality improvement techniques and change management in past

Ultimately, the conclusion from these readiness assessments should be to help guide whether or not to proceed with the implementation or to what extent, based on the readiness or feasibility of the organization at the time of assessment. Naturally, Powell et al. highlight that specific barriers may not be identified until implementation occurs (Powell et al. 2015). This is also why monitoring and evaluation, as highlighted previously, will be key.

Several tools for evaluating gender equity and diversity are widely accessible. They can be employed by academic institutions, global health organizations in Kenya or Africa, and global health organizations pursuing partnerships with Kenya or Africa. The accountability should be placed on stakeholders seeking out partnerships, in this case, such as a research team lead or organization director. Some of the tools available include the gender equality in academia and research (GEAR) assessment (European Institute for Gender Equality 2022), which provides a "step-by-step guide for all those seeking to implement measures in support of gender equality in research organizations, universities or other public bodies" and also provides next steps for gender equality programming in respective organizations. The UN Women's Gender Equality Capacity Assessment Tool provides individual-level assessments of employees and their capacity to respond to and effect change for gender equality in the organization (UN Women 2014). It also provides the next steps using outputs from the tool's assessment. The City of San Francisco in the USA proposes a set of guidelines to follow when conducting readiness or needs assessments that encourages beginning with aligning any assessment with the organization's specific vision/ mission, followed by identifying specific targets such as departments, services or programs that should be assessed, and then envisioning clear outcomes, in terms of the projected impacts on gender equality if programs or interventions are established (sfgov.org n.d.). Finally, they suggest ensuring a monitoring strategy is in place to assess the policies or interventions implemented, ensure appropriate reach of policy changes or interventions for both men and women in the organization, and ensure responsiveness to evaluations resulting from this monitoring. Additional tools proposed with the CFIR-ERIC tool are also available (Academic 2022; African 2022; Weggemans et al. 2019; Helfrich et al. 2009; Lehman et al. 2002; Weiner et al. 2008).

## 3.3    Conduct Local Consensus Discussions

Given the current apropos movement towards decolonizing global health (Abimbola and Pai 2020) (see chapter "Colonialism, Decolonization, and Global Health"), I cannot overemphasize the importance of consensus discussions that are inclusive and participatory in nature to drive effective and sustainable change for equity, including as it pertains to gender. I argue that these need to occur at the local, African institution level as well as in organizations that routinely engage in global health partnerships with

institutions in the Africa context that are outside of these institutions. Procedures for engagement, and relationship building, that are not only equitable but also transparent and subject to open critique are vital. As proposed by the CFIR-ERIC tool, agreeing on the problem—in this case, lack of gender equity in academia and partnerships—is the first step. Determining how this is addressed, though, will also require consensus. Finally, the tool also highlights that consensus discussions can have two different objectives: the first being whether the goal is to drive or build consensus around an issue in the given organization, and the second being to simply do an assessment of whether or not consensus exists on a given issue or strategy. In sum, depending on the nature of what is being pursued, consensus discussions may have different objectives. All the same, they should be occurring early and in a regular fashion.

Redefining, and gaining consensus on measures of academic success, for example, is critical (see Excerpt 2). Furthermore, means of ensuring equitable measurements of success for women faculty, who are impacted disproportionately by child care or prolonged leaves due to pregnancy or maternity leave (see Excerpt 3 on *The Pregnancy Penalty*), should also be accounted for.

For those seeking partnerships with African institutions that are outside of these organizations, we propose consensus discussions occur within these organizations and also potentially when engaging with African institutions to develop new partnerships. Opportunities might include ensuring equitable representation in research project initiatives, that ensure the appointment of women as lead Primary Investigators and/ or Co-investigators in projects, as well as equitable representation throughout the different levels of the research team. Community-Based Participatory Research provides an ideal approach to ensuring equitable presentation across multiple domains, including those of community members directly influenced by research programs or initiatives (Israel et al. 2001). Developing successful collaborations will require the appreciation of bidirectional learning and structures that help to

**Chapter 18, Excerpt 2: The African Academic Surgeon**

The role of the academic surgeon is an old one but perhaps not as well embraced in the Africa context. As an academic scientist there is the triple expectation of delivery in terms of clinical service to address the needs of patients, teaching and the inherent responsibility to train the next generation of surgeons with this new knowledge and in research meaning the opportunity to push the needle and generate new region specific, culturally appropriate data that will help to enhance patient care. The tensions invariably set in when these three factors come into direct competition. Sub-Saharan Africa has the greatest health workforce deficits and more than 2 million workers are needed to address the workforce deficits (6, 7). As such, many clinicians are faced with large patient volumes and often struggle to provide optimal care to patients… A lack of protected time to conduct research, lack of skills in basic research methodology and a failure of institutional and infrastructural support for many aspects of research such as grant applications and management, manuscript preparation, statistical support and data management frequently result in not as many faculty engaging in research.

**Chapter 18, Excerpt 3: The Pregnancy Penalty**

Clear actionable policies around maternity and paternity leave, ensure a balanced outlook and wellness for all staff. While policies around these exist in many large institutions, on an individual level there is still an amount of victimization. Anecdotally, cases have occurred where academic clinicians were forced to pay their institutions money, as a result of going on maternity leave, or being compelled to not sit their exams etc. as a result of falling pregnant even if they personally felt capable of doing so. Sadly, these cases are not unique (9, 10) and should all give us pause in the process of developing a more inclusive workforce.

support career progression for academics in both HICs and LMICS. These need to be linked to sustainable capacity-building efforts that will develop skillsets for women and other academicians in Africa. Implementation science research, in and of itself, also provides an opportunity to explore the best means for implementing these partnerships and assessing outcomes of collaborations as a result; the RE-AIM framework, for example, provides standardized tools to help ensure that equity is at the forefront of any intervention, project, and possibly even partnership and could be employed (Glasgow et al. 1999).

Strategies by organizations such as the African Union to provide guidelines for engagement and best practices for disseminating these guidelines are needed. This, and other organizations/ institutions or academic conferences, could also act as convening bodies for consensus-driving discussions so that opportunities are not missed. This could take place in the form of panel discussions on collaboration with the diaspora, perhaps providing lecture series on the topic, having sessions co-led/ supported by a diasporan to get them more engaged in an equitable fashion complementary to but not in place of Africa-based individuals.

Finally, measures of accountability to ensure consensus is tracked and evaluated should be put into place. For example, at the institutional level, reports on efforts made to increase diversity by the department during annual reviews could be mandated; these might include efforts to recruit and retain women faculty, efforts to support maternity leave or return to work, as well as highlight excellence in a uniform format that also gives women the opportunity to be spotlighted. Moreover, highlighting/ understanding why women leave, such as through institutional audits and exit interviews performed by unbiased parties, could be done. Finally, ensuring safe spaces for discussion are facilitated by the institution, such as at communal meetings where speakers or facilitators engage in discussions on gender equity, case examples from the institution might be tackled publicly, and solutions are generated in a participatory fashion.

# 4    Conclusions

There is a burgeoning role for women in the workplace, in global health, and in academic spaces, especially in Sub-Saharan Africa. To ultimately improve global public health outcomes, there is a need to build a diverse and inclusive workforce. Intentionality and deliberate efforts to develop institutional, national-level, regional, and international collaborations and strategies will be key to enabling the full participation of all genders in developing and implementing effective solutions for global health in the twenty-first century. These efforts must be supported through effective, context-sensitive strategies, including implementing institutional champions, conducting readiness assessments, and gaining organizational consensus through open discourse.

# Glossary

**Academic:** A member (such as a professor) of an institution of learning (such as a university) (Academic 2022).

**African:** A native or inhabitant of Africa; a person and especially a Black person of African ancestry; of, relating to, or characteristic of the continent of Africa or its people (African 2022).

**Clinician Scientist:** Clinician–scientists are commonly defined as health care professionals (e.g., physicians, nurses, physical and occupational therapists) who are expert in both research and clinical practice (Weggemans et al. 2019).

**Diaspora:** People settled far from their ancestral homelands (Diaspora 2022).

**Gender:** The behavioral, cultural, or psychological traits typically associated with one sex (Gender 2022).

**Gender equity:** Means fairness in addressing the different health needs of people according to their gender. Inequitable health outcomes based on gender are both avoidable and unacceptable. A concept of fairness recognizes that there are differences between the sexes and that resources must be allocated differentially to address unfair disparities (Global Health 5050 2022).

**Global health:** An area for study, research, and practice that places a priority on improving health and achieving health equity for all people worldwide (Koplan et al. 2009).

**"Global North" and "Global South":** The concept of a gap between the Global North and the Global South in terms of development and wealth; richer countries are almost all located in the Northern Hemisphere, with the exception of Australia and New Zealand. Poorer countries are mostly located in tropical regions and in the Southern Hemisphere. Despite very significant development gains globally which have raised many millions of people out of absolute poverty, there is substantial evidence that inequality between the world's richest and poorest countries is widening. There are many causes for these inequalities including the availability of natural resources; different levels of health and education; the nature of a country's economy and its industrial sectors; international trading policies and access to markets; how countries are governed and international relationships between countries; conflict within and between countries; and a country's vulnerability to natural hazards and climate change (Royal Geographical Society with IBG 2022).

**High-Income Countries (HICs) and "Low- and Middle-Income Countries" (LMICs):** Low-income economies are defined as those with a Gross National Income (GNI) per capita, calculated using the World Bank Atlas method, of $1085 or less in 2021; lower middle-income economies are those with a GNI per capita between $1086 and $4255; upper middle-income economies are those with a GNI per capita between $4256 and $13,205; high-income economies are those with a GNI per capita of $13,205 or more. The term country, used interchangeably with economy, does not imply political independence but refers to any territory for which authorities report separate social or economic statistics (The World Bank 2022).

# References

Abimbola S, Pai M. Will global health survive its decolonisation? Lancet. 2020;396(10263):1627–8.

"Academic." Merriam-Webster.com Dictionary, Merriam-Webster, https://www.merriam-webster.com/dictionary/academic. Accessed 9 Nov 2022.

"African." Merriam-Webster.com Dictionary, Merriam-Webster, https://www.merriam-webster.com/dictionary/African. Accessed 9 Nov 2022.

Aina O. Gender Equity and Higher Education in Africa. Lead Paper Presented at the 1st International Interdisciplinary Conference on Gender and Higher Education in Africa: Emerging Issues. In International Interdisciplinary Conference on Gender and Higher Education in Africa: Emerging Issues. 2013. Ibadan, Nigeria.

Assembly UNG. The universal declaration of human rights (UDHR). New York: United Nations General Assembly; 1948.

Bilimoria D, Stewart AJ. "Don't ask, Don't tell": the academic climate for lesbian, gay, bisexual, and transgender Faculty in Science and Engineering. NWSA J. 2009;21(2):85–103.

Bradley SW, et al. The impact of chief diversity officers on diverse faculty hiring. South Econ J. 2022;89(1):3–36.

Cherotish NV, Simatwa EMW, Ayodo TMO. Impact of free secondary education policy on genderequality in secondary school education in Kenya: a case study of Kericho County. Educ Res. 2014;5(3):83–97.

Consolidated Framework for Implementation Research. What is the CFIR? 2022a. [Nov 2022]; Available from: https://cfirguide.org

Consolidated Framework for Implementation Research. Strategy design. 2022b. [Nov 2022]. Available from: https://cfirguide.org/choosing-strategies/

data2x. Bridging the gap: mapping gender data availability in Africa. 2022.

"Diaspora." Merriam-Webster.com Dictionary, Merriam-Webster, https://www.merriam-webster.com/dictionary/diaspora. Accessed 9 Nov 2022.

European Institute for Gender Equality. Gender equality in academia and research. 2022. [Nov 2022]. Available from: https://eige.europa.eu/gender-mainstreaming/toolkits/gear/step-step-guide

"Gender." Merriam-Webster.com Dictionary, Merriam-Webster, https://www.merriam-webster.com/dictionary/gender. Accessed 9 Nov 2022.

Glasgow RE, Vogt TM, Boles SM. Evaluating the public health impact of health promotion interventions: the RE-AIM framework. Am J Public Health. 1999;89(9):1322–7.

Global Health 5050. Gender and global health (defining gender). 2022. [Nov 2022]; Available from: https://globalhealth5050.org/gender-and-global-health/

Gupta N. Research to support evidence-informed decisions on optimizing gender equity in health workforce policy and planning. Hum Resour Health. 2019;17(1):46.

Gupta J, Vegelin C. Sustainable development goals and inclusive development. Int Environ Agreem: Politics Law Econ. 2016;16(3):433–48.

Helfrich CD, et al. Organizational readiness to change assessment (ORCA): development of an instrument based on the promoting action on research in health services (PARIHS) framework. Implement Sci. 2009;4(1):38.

Israel BA, et al. Community-based participatory research: policy recommendations for promoting a partnership approach in health research. Educ Health (Abingdon). 2001;14(2):182–97.

Kaganas F, Murray C. The contest between culture and gender equality under South Africa's interim constitution. J Law Soc. 1994;21(4):409–33.

Kelan E. Why Aren't We Making More Progress Towards Gender Equity? 2020. [Nov 2022]. Available from: https://hbr.org/2020/12/why-arent-we-making-more-progress-towards-gender-equity. Accessed 9 Nov 2022

Koplan JP, et al. Towards a common definition of global health. Lancet. 2009;373(9679):1993–5.

Lauer M. NIH Challenges Academia to Share Strategies to Strengthen Gender Diversity. 2020. [Nov 2022]. Available from: https://nexus.od.nih.gov/all/2020/11/16/nih-challenges-academia-to-share-strategies-to-strengthengender-diversity/.

Lehman WE, Greener JM, Simpson DD. Assessing organizational readiness for change. J Subst Abus Treat. 2002;22(4):197–209.

Mama A. Pursuing gender equality in the African university. Int J African Renaiss Stud Multi Inter Transdiscip. 2006;1(1):53–79.

McKinsey Global Institute. The power of parity: advancing women's equality in Africa. 2019.

Msuya NH. Concept of culture relativism and women's rights in sub-Saharan Africa. J Asian Afr Stud. 2019;54(8):1145–58.

Mulwa M. The Gender Gap in Universities and Colleges in sub-Saharan Africa. E.S.S. Africa., Editor. 2021.

Mutume G. African women battle for equality. Africa Renewal, 2005.

Naidu E. Long walk to gender equality in African university leadership. 2021. [Nov 2022]. Available from: https://www.iol.co.za/sundayindependent/news/long-walk-to-gender-equality-in-african-university-leadership-b420e0b8-8033-4b0d-b869-fd827c8f9d87

Okeke-Ihejirika P. Gender Equity in Africa's Institutions of Tertiary Education. In Decolonizing philosophies of education. 2012. SensePublishers. p. 147–61.

Olatunji C-MP. An argument for gender equality in Africa. CLCWeb Comparat Literat Cult. 2013;15(1) https://doi.org/10.7771/1481-4374.2176.

Pihakis J, Paikeday TS, Armstrong K. The emergence of the chief diversity officer role in higher education. In Insights R, Editor. 2019.

Powell BJ, et al. A refined compilation of implementation strategies: results from the expert recommendations for implementing change (ERIC) project. Implement Sci. 2015;10(1):21.

Royal Geographical Society with IBG. A 60 second guide to… The Global North/South Divide. 2022.;

Available from: https://www.rgs.org/CMSPages/GetFile.aspx?nodeguid=9c1ce781-9117-4741-af0a-a6a8b75f32b4&lang=en-GB

SDG Knowledge Hub. Making SDG implementation easier: thinking about goals as means. 2017. [No 2022]. Available from: http://sdg.iisd.org/commentary/guest-articles/making-sdg-implementation-easier-thinking-about-goals-as-means/

sfgov.org. Gender analysis guidelines. City and County of San Francisco: Department on the Status of Women. Available from: https://sfgov.org/dosw/gender-analysis-guidelines

Sustainable Development Goals. Goal 5: Achieve gender equality and empower all women and girls. 2022. [Nov 2022]. Available from: https://www.un.org/sustainabledevelopment/gender-equality/

The World Bank. World Bank Country and Lending Groups 2022 Nov 2022.; Available from: https://datahelpdesk.worldbank.org/knowledgebase/articles/906519-world-bank-country-and-lending-groups

Tiedeu BA, Para-Mallam OJ, Nyambi D. Driving gender equity in African scientific institutions. Lancet. 2019;293:504–6.

UN. United Nations Beijing Declaration and Platform of Action, adopted at the Fourth World Conference on Women. 1955.

UN Women. Gender equality capacity assessment tool. 2014. [Nov 2022]. Available from: https://www.unwomen.org/en/digital-library/publications/2014/6/gender-equality-capacity-assessment-tool

UN Women. Commission on the status of women. 2022. [Nov 2022].

University of Reading. Diversity champions. Diversity. 2022. [Nov 2022]. Available from: https://www.reading.ac.uk/diversity/diversity-and-inclusion-team/diversity-champions

USAID. Gender Equality and Women's Empowerment. 2022. [Nov 2022]; Available from: https://www.usaid.gov/what-we-do/gender-equality-and-womens-empowerment

VCU News Staff. VCU receives 2021 Higher education excellence in diversity award. VCU News, 2021.

Weggemans MM, et al. Critical gaps in understanding the clinician-scientist workforce: results of an international expert meeting. Acad Med. 2019;94(10):1448–54.

Weiner BJ, Amick H, Lee SY. Conceptualization and measurement of organizational readiness for change: a review of the literature in health services research and other fields. Med Care Res Rev. 2008;65(4):379–436.

Whitehead M. The concepts and principles of equity in health. Int J Health Serv. 1992;22:429–45.

World Health Organization. Celebrating women leaders in science and health. 2019. [Nov 2022]. Available from: https://www.who.int/news-room/feature-stories/detail/celebrating-women-leaders-in-science-and-health

World Health Organization. WHO pledges extensive commitments towards women's empowerment and health. 2021. [Nov 2022]. Available from: https://www.who.int/news/item/05-07-2021-who-pledges-extensive-commitments-towards-women-s-empowerment-and-health

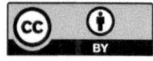

# A Holistic Systems Approach to Global Health Research, Practice, and Partnerships

Mercy Borbor-Cordova, Sadie Ryan, Rachel Lowe, Rosa von Borries, and Anna Stewart Ibarra ⓘ

*There are four revolutions currently transforming health and health systems: (a) life sciences; (b) information and communications technology; (c) social justice and equity; and (d) systems thinking to transcend complexity.*

Frenk J. "Acknowledging the Past, Committing to the Future".
Delivered September 5, 2008.

## Abstract

Emerging and persistent infectious diseases are global threats that have evidenced the interconnectedness and interdependence of the environment, animal, and human systems. To identify solutions to these complex real-world challenges, a systemic approach is needed to understand the interactions among natural and human systems. Collaborative partnerships among researchers from diverse disciplines with policy practitioners and societal actors are also key. Research and public health practice frameworks based on systems thinking approaches have been developed to address the complexity of infectious diseases

M. Borbor-Cordova (✉)
Faculty of Maritime Engineering and Sea Sciences, Escuela Superior Politécnica del Litoral (ESPOL), Guayaquil, Ecuador

Pacific International Center for Disaster Risk Reduction (PIC-DRR, ESPOL), Guayaquil, Ecuador
e-mail: meborbor@espol.edu.ec

S. Ryan
Department of Geography and the Emerging Pathogens Institute, University of Florida, Gainesville, FL, USA

College of Life Sciences, University of KwaZulu Natal, Pietermaritzburg, South Africa
e-mail: sjryan@ufl.edu

R. Lowe
Barcelona Supercomputing Center (BSC), Barcelona, Spain

Catalan Institution for Research and Advanced Studies (ICREA), Barcelona, Spain

Centre for Climate Change and Planetary Health and Centre for Mathematical Modelling of Infectious Diseases, London School of Hygiene & Tropical Medicine, London, UK
e-mail: rachel.lowe@bsc.es

R. von Borries
World Meteorological Organization, Geneva, Switzerland

Charité Universitätsmedizin Berlin, Berlin, Germany
e-mail: rosa.von-borries@charite.de

A. Stewart Ibarra
Inter-American Institute For Global Change Research (IAI), Panama City, Panama
e-mail: anna.stewart@dir.iai.int

© The Author(s) 2024
A. Stewart Ibarra, A. D. LaBeaud (eds.), *Transforming Global Health Partnerships*, Sustainable Development Goals Series, https://doi.org/10.1007/978-3-031-53793-6_4

51

and other global health threats from local to global scales. For example, the Planetary Health framework focuses on human health and the interactions with the natural systems upon which it depends, stating that the health of human civilization depends on a healthy planet. The One Health approach aims to achieve optimal health and well-being outcomes by recognizing the interconnections between people, animals, plants, and their shared environment. Indigenous Peoples recognize that humans are inextricably interconnected with all life on the planet. Accordingly, the climate crisis and disease threats constitute a "relationship problem." These holistic knowledge paradigms support a better understanding of infectious disease risks and the development of context-specific interventions to reduce disease transmission through transdisciplinary research and strong multinational partnerships. The theoretical concepts of these perspectives are described in this chapter and illustrated by the authors' experiences co-developing research approaches for zoonotic and vector-borne diseases, including early warning systems for dengue fever.

### Keywords

Systems thinking · Systems framework · Planetary health · One Health · Traditional knowledge · Transdisciplinary research · Global health · Infectious disease · Health disparities

### Author Perspective

We are women scientists and policy practitioners working at the climate, environment, and global health nexus. We are originally from Ecuador, the UK, the USA, and Germany, and we currently live across three continents in the North and South. Our backgrounds include ecology, medicine, public health, public administration, geography, meteorology, oceanography, epidemiology, and mathematics. We have all worked at the science-policy interface, directly in national or intergovernmental bodies or as scientists co-creating transformable knowledge and evidence

to inform decision-making. Four of us have worked together closely for over a decade, navigating many co-developed projects and transdisciplinary team dynamics. Our joint work approach has allowed us to develop integrated science but most importantly, embark on a joyful journey from recognizing our diversity to creating a common vision of interconnectedness. We value transdisciplinary collaboration and applied research grounded on equity considerations aimed at contributing to societal benefits.

**Key Tenets for Systems Thinking in Global Health Research and Practice**

1. Infectious diseases are influenced by multiple social and biophysical drivers interacting as elements of an interconnected system. Systems thinking and general systems theory provide a framework for understanding these complex dynamics.

2. Global environmental changes and infectious disease threats are interconnected and interdependent; these complex real-world issues require a systemic approach integrating natural and human systems.

3. One Health and Planetary Health are research frameworks and movements that address global health issues from an integrated systems approach.

4. Human health is intrinsically linked to the planet's health and ecosystems, highlighting the need to integrate Western and non-Western scientific knowledge to better understand these complex interactions.

5. Transdisciplinary and international research partnerships with multisectoral stakeholders can support the successful co-creation and implementation of context-specific global health interventions.

6. This chapter addresses the following SDGs: #3: Ensure healthy lives and promote well-being for all at all ages; #10:

Reduce inequality within and among countries; #13: Take urgent action to combat climate change and its impacts; #17: Strengthen the means of implementation and revitalize the Global Partnership for Sustainable Development.

# 1 Introduction

Global health focuses on "improving human health while achieving equity in health for all people worldwide" (Koplan et al. 2009), or "achieving better health outcomes for vulnerable populations and communities around the world" (Chen et al. 2020). Those working in the field of global health are faced with responding to mounting challenges: emerging infectious disease threats in the context of climate change, growing social inequalities, biodiversity loss, and the degradation and pollution of air, soils, and waters, to name a few. These crises are interwoven, resulting from interactions among complex social and biophysical systems and the poor relationships between humanity and life on this planet, as clearly articulated by Indigenous scholars (see Chapter "Transforming the Planetary Health Crisis Through an Indigenous Land-Based Meta-Narrative").

Identifying solutions to these urgent issues require collaborative and often international partnerships among researchers from diverse disciplines, policy practitioners, health workers, and actors from civil society. Those most affected by the health issues, with deep local knowledge, are central to the research partnership, such as frontline health workers and Indigenous and local communities. By valuing and bringing together different ways of knowing, systems approaches provide a framework to guide global health partnerships.

The first part of this chapter introduces systems thinking in global health and presents the Planetary Health and One Health frameworks.

Brief examples of mosquito-borne and zoonotic diseases are shared to elucidate these frameworks. In the second part of the chapter, systems approaches are explained through transdisciplinary research approaches, with real-world examples related to the co-creation of early warning systems for dengue fever.

# 2 Systems Approaches in Global Health

Systems approaches can broadly be defined as "A paradigm or perspective that considers connections among different components [of a system], plans for the implications of their interactions, and requires transdisciplinary thinking as well as active engagement of those who have a stake in the outcome to govern the course of change (Leischow and Milstein 2006) p. 403." Holistic and systems approaches have been proposed to address the complexities of global health threats spanning global, regional, and local levels (Leischow and Milstein 2006; Peters 2014). Systems approaches have been used to study tobacco control (Best et al. 2007), tuberculosis (Sternberg 2015), infectious diseases (Xia et al. 2017), mosquito-borne diseases, and other health issues. Key concepts for systems approaches are shared in the glossary.

Infectious diseases are influenced by multiple social and biophysical factors interacting as system elements. The dynamic behavior of mosquito-borne disease transmission, for example, may include interactions among co-evolving pathogens and vector species, changing socio-ecological environments, and human behaviors. In addition, global interconnectedness and massive human migration can lead to the expansion of infectious diseases to new geographical regions. However, globally it is evident that certain regions, countries, and communities are more vulnerable to infectious diseases than others. Determinants of those health disparities are related to social injustice, poverty, environmental degradation, climate change, among other factors (Box 1).

**Box 1: Systems Thinking Origins**

Since the inception of Western scientific systems approaches, interdisciplinary partnerships have been key enabling factors for enhancing integrated and holistic approaches. A group of thinkers including Norbert Wiener (mathematician), von Ludwig Bertalanffy (biologist), Ross Ashby (psychiatrist), Gregory Bateson (anthropologist), Heinz van Foerster (polymath), Donella H. Meadows (systems scientist), and others, established the foundations for systems science thinking through a series of interdisciplinary meetings (Heylighen F.) going beyond their scientific disciplinary boundaries to seek a broader perspective and identify convergences and differences between disciplines, aiming to identify common principles to understand the complexity of the real world.

The fascinating and inspiring history of these thinkers is the story of their exchange of ideas, with philosophical, epistemological, ontological, and ethical inquiries, each coming from very different disciplines to reach a meta-scientific framework using a general systematology, which would "lead to a much-needed integration in scientific education" (Von Bertalanffy 1972). In this context, many scientists recognized the importance and functions of their work in the "border fields" of scientific disciplines, leading to the birth of interdisciplinary and even transdisciplinary sciences (Klein 2008).

It is important to note that systems thinking approaches and the fundamental and complex interconnectedness of life systems were deeply understood and practiced through Traditional Indigenous knowledge systems long before Western science (see Chapter "Transforming the Planetary Health Crisis Through an Indigenous Land-Based Meta-Narrative"). The Traditional Indigenous knowledge systems are based on sacred Natural laws (Redvers et al. 2022), providing a framework for both Western and non-Western ways of knowing and healing. Although Indigenous knowledge systems are beyond the scope of this chapter, people from Indigenous and local communities must be centered in global health research partnerships. Non-Western systems approaches should be elevated and valued in global health discourses such as One Health and Planetary Health (Redvers et al. 2022), particularly considering colonial legacies that perpetuate the hegemony of Western scientific discourses (see Chapter "Colonialism, Decolonization, and Global Health").

Interdisciplinary and transdisciplinary approaches allow research teams to apply systems thinking to address specific health issues (Fig. 1). Interdisciplinarity creates knowledge by transferring methods from one discipline to another or working across and between disciplinary boundaries (Fiore et al. 2008). Transdisciplinarity goes further by creating knowledge by constructing a common base of methods and concepts through the participation of a wide variety of actors, including researchers, practitioners, civil society, and others affected by the research, during a dynamic co-creation process that builds relationships and trust (Peters 2014; Max-Neef 2005; Lawrence et al. 2022). Transdisciplinarity is an applied science focused on solving urgent problems by spanning disciplines and different kinds of knowledge to identify solutions. General System Theory (GST) and systems science are well aligned with transdisciplinary science when they move beyond academic expertise to co-develop solutions with diverse actors (Peters 2014; Xia et al. 2017; Rüegg et al. 2018; de Savigny and Adam 2009). Transdisciplinarity is described in detail later in this chapter.

In the field of global health, One Health and Planetary Health have emerged as inter- and trans-disciplinary systems-based research and

## Systems Thinking in practice

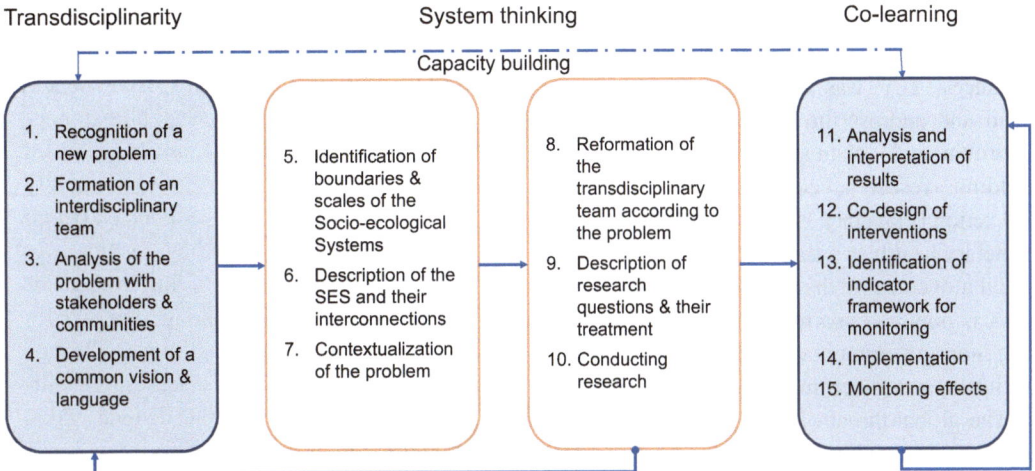

**Fig. 1** Diagram of some activities during a transdisciplinary process guided by systems thinking to address complex socio-ecological systems (SES). From the authors' experiences, this process is not linear, with outcomes from each stage feeding back to inform and modify earlier stages. Some stages may be reordered, skipped, or modified depending on the issue and local context. (Source: Wilcox et al. 2019)

practice paradigms, frameworks, or movements within Western science. These frameworks share the need for transdisciplinary approaches to address human health interactions with social, environmental, and political systems across regions, countries, and communities. These frameworks focus on specific principles and concepts to be implemented in the real world. In the following sections, those frameworks are illustrated using examples from the authors' research on infectious diseases in different contexts.

### 2.1 Planetary Health: Recognizing that Human Health Depends on the Health of the Planet

Planetary Health goes beyond seeking equal access to health care worldwide, highlighting the interdependence of human health and the health of the total environment. Planetary Health focuses on analyzing and addressing the impacts of human disruptions to Earth's natural systems on human health and all life on Earth (Planetary Health 2023). The Rockefeller Foundation-Lancet Commission on Planetary Health launched the concept in 2015, defining Planetary Health as "the health of human civilization and the state of the natural systems on which it depends" (Whitmee et al. 2015). Planetary boundaries represent a key Planetary Health concept representing safe environmental limits of Earth's natural systems within which humanity can flourish (Steffen et al. 2015).

The Planetary Health approach provides new ways to address complex issues that ultimately impact human health (Pongsiri et al. 2017). Climate change, biodiversity loss, and globalization generate intertwined risks such as the re-emergence and emergence of infectious diseases. Some examples of these interconnections are evidenced by emerging outbreaks of infectious diseases associated with land use change, such as malaria (Santos and Almeida 2018), dengue (Charlesworth et al. 2022; Lowe et al. 2011), and waterborne diseases (Herrera et al. 2017). In places where land use change is associated with agriculture, there are implications for food security and nutrition (Hickey et al. 2016). The Planetary Health approach recognizes multilevel determinants of human health, considering biological, social, and environmental causes, and seeks to identify non-linear and irreversible changes in natural systems with implications for human health (Pongsiri and Bassi 2021).

To support these efforts, the Planetary Health Alliance (PHA) was founded in 2015 to understand and address the health impacts of global environmental change through community-building, research, education, mainstreaming, and action (Planetary Health 2023). PHA defines planetary health as a transdisciplinary field and a social movement to drive societal transformation. PHA is now a consortium of over 300 universities, non-governmental organizations, research institutes, and governmental entities worldwide.

The global threat of climate change is a case for planetary health. It is a global-scale problem whose local impacts are unequally distributed, with the most vulnerable populations suffering the greatest harm. In the sixth Climate Change Assessment Report, the Intergovernmental Panel on Climate Change (IPCC) concluded that climate change has adversely affected the physical and mental health of people globally, mediated through natural and human systems, including social and health inequalities (Pörtner et al. 2022). In terms of infectious diseases, in regions like Latin America and the Caribbean, the incidence of vector-borne diseases has increased in part due to the expansion of the range of mosquito vectors and/or increased reproduction of disease vectors associated with more suitable climate conditions (Pörtner et al. 2022; Castellanos et al. 2022) (Box 2).

whole country, at sub-national levels, under different climate change scenarios. The data integration of larval mosquito (*Aedes aegypti*) surveillance records, land use and land cover, climate, elevation, human population data, and other social data allowed for a more holistic approach to suitability modeling than previously conducted (Lippi et al. 2019). The modeling results suggested that communities living in areas of transitional elevation along the Andes mountains and subtropical areas will face an increased risk of viral diseases transmitted by *Aedes aegypti*, like dengue, Zika, and chikungunya, in the coming decades.

From a planetary health perspective, multiscalar climate scenarios developed across global to local scales can provide important information about future health risks for climate and health adaptation planning. These models can be converted into interactive tools to support the health sector in planning for the effects of climate change. For example, the tool could highlight the need to increase public health surveillance efforts in zones with a high risk of disease emergence during certain seasons. Integrated systems-based modeling approaches can connect global scale phenomena and impacts to the regional and subnational scales where decision-making occurs.

**Box 2: Planetary Health to Address the Impacts of Climate Change on the Increasing Distribution of Mosquito-Borne Diseases**

As an example of global to local interconnections, the authors of this chapter are investigating how future climate scenarios can affect the range of vector-borne diseases in Ecuador. Applying a multi-faceted ecological niche model, and space-time analysis, predicted mosquito distributions by the year 2050 were visualized for the

## 2.2 One Health: The Interdependence of Human Health, Animal Health and the Health of the Environment

One Health is a "collaborative, multisectoral and transdisciplinary approach—working at local, regional, national and global level—to achieve optimal health and well-being outcomes recognizing the interconnections between people, animals, plants, and their shared environment (One Health Basics 2022)." The term One Health gained prominence in the twenty-first century; however, the concept's origins can be traced back to the 1800s when the German physician Rudolf Virchow stated: "Between animal and human medicine there is no dividing line – nor should there be. The object is different, but the experience obtained constitutes the basis of all medicine" (Eyre 2015).

Human and animal (veterinary) medicine were practiced separately until the twentieth century, despite observations by Western scientists in the 1800s of similarities between animal and human disease processes. In 2008, international agencies, including the United Nations Food and Agricultural Organization (FAO), the World Organization for Animal Health (WOAH), previously called the International Office of Epizootics (OIE), the World Health Organization (WHO), World Bank, UNICEF, and the United Nations System Influenza Coordination (UNSIC) developed a joint Strategic Framework in response to the evolving risk of emerging and re-emerging infectious diseases which led to substantial progress in implementing One Health principles at a global scale. In 2022, FAO, WHO, WOAH, and UNEP launched the first One Health Joint Plan of Action (2022–2026), which seeks to create "a world better able to prevent, predict, detect and respond to health threats and improve the health of humans, animals, plants and the environment while contributing to sustainable development." (WHO 2022) The One Health concept focuses on interactions of humans and animals, bringing together professions such as public health practitioners, doctors, epidemiologists, veterinarians, ecologists, and wildlife experts to address key challenges such as zoonotic diseases, antimicrobial resistance, and vector-borne diseases (Fagre et al. 2022) (Box 3).

---

**Box 3: One Health in the South African Landscape: Learning in a Multi-actor Complex System**

A story of learning through the One Health approach is the case of bovine tuberculosis (bTB) in the Kruger National Park landscape in South Africa. Sadie Ryan, as an early career conservation biologist and ecologist, started her doctoral research in the ecology of African buffalo (*Syncerus caffer*) and the spread of bovine tuberculosis. bTB is an infectious disease caused by the bacteria *Mycobacterium bovis*, which impacts cattle production but also affects wildlife where spillover and spread occur. The disease spread among the buffalo herds in the park, likely introduced by cows on the southern park border (animal system). Lions and other carnivores are susceptible to systemic bTB, of which one major manifestation is swelling of the joints, making them unable to hunt, leading to starvation. Other wild bovids, elephants, and rhinos were also at risk. This was a major problem for the managers of protected fauna. The disease also jeopardized tourism revenue for the park and the economy of the local people. People were also at risk of contracting bovine tuberculosis through consuming infected raw milk, encountering bTB at slaughter, and, when immune response permits, via aerosol transmission from a cow coughing. The rates of bTB as the causative agent for human TB cases remains a massive question in managing human tuberculosis (human system). Public health surveillance for bTB among human cases is rare, and TB treatment, while vastly improved in its global quality and distribution, is often unavailable (health system).

The case of bTB in the larger Kruger Park landscape exemplifies a One Health framing of an interconnected systems problem. The multiple actors, decision-makers, those directly impacted, those affected, and those able to approach this from various perspectives, included e.g. cattle interests, their ability to sell, export, or even use their animal products; subsistence-level populations around the park at risk of both potential health impacts, and livelihood impact via cattle holdings; the park's economic well-being and ability to maintain a healthy

(continued)

tourism-driven business model; rangers, monitoring the wildlife, the landscape, and vigilant for poacher activity; researchers, from multiple countries, providing evidence to support or contradict assumptions and knowledge about the interacting system. These diverse actors interacted within complex human-animal and institutional systems.

Sadie's work began by gathering ecological data on how buffalo move around and use managed savanna landscapes. This groundwork supported the creation of dynamic models of those landscapes and informed the more significant questions of bTB prevention and control facing managers and actors. This story acknowledges the relevance of generating local evidence with diverse actors to understand disease ecology on local landscapes, which can inform processes across larger landscapes. Understanding One Health systems locally and globally is key to reducing the risk of future diseases. Over the subsequent 20 years, Sadie brought this approach to tackle diverse infectious diseases such as dengue, malaria, anthrax, foot-and-mouth disease, blue tongue virus, and citrus greening.

## 2.3    Common Challenges

Challenges are often encountered when researchers begin to apply systems frameworks in the real world, many of which are shared in the case studies of this book. Some of these challenges are described below, including institutional/political factors, resource limitations, and building solid partnerships.

Public health agencies often lack a specific mandate at the national level to address One Health and Planetary Health issues through intersectoral coordination. The traditional mandate of public health institutions focuses on competencies and challenges within their health systems.

As a result, health sector responses remain siloed and coordinated action is limited with agencies such as disaster risk reduction authorities, local governments, national institutes of meteorology, and ministries of the environment. This also results in limited sharing of data and health impact analysis (e.g., epidemiological data, urban vulnerability, and biological hazards) between different sectors due to a lack of formal data-sharing agreements between institutions. The data sources gathered by different sectors are often available at different spatiotemporal resolutions, which need to be harmonized to understand infectious disease dynamics better. Without collaboration mechanisms, there is often a lack of sustained funding and dedicated personnel to implement solutions. In some countries, the high turnover rate of government officials and staff present additional challenges.

Another common challenge is the significant time commitment needed to build solid, trusting relationships that enable co-learning and co-creation processes among scientists, public health practitioners, decision-makers, and other stakeholders. At the beginning of the partnership, there may be a mismatch between the timing and priorities of researchers and practitioners (see Chapter "Team Science and Infectious Disease Work: Exploring Challenges and Opportunities"). Public health practitioners have busy jobs, decision-makers have little time to interact with researchers, and researchers are often assessed by rapid scientific outputs and survive on short-term and fragile funding streams. It may also be challenging for public health practitioners and decision-makers to use research results due to established protocols and decision-making processes in health systems that are hard to change. Developing shared expectations of realistic timelines and outcomes is a critical part of the partnership process (see Chapter "Team Science and Infectious Disease Work: Exploring Challenges and Opportunities").

The following section describes transdisciplinary approaches to address these common challenges, with examples from the authors' work to develop early warning systems for dengue fever.

## 3 Transdisciplinary Approaches to Put Systems Frameworks into Practice

### 3.1 Introduction to Transdisciplinary Approaches

Transdisciplinary science approaches can support the application of One Health, Planetary Health, and other systems frameworks to address urgent real-world global health challenges. Transdisciplinary research brings together diverse non-academic actors with researchers from natural and social sciences to form a collaborative research partnership. Those who will use or apply the final outputs/tools/information from the research are engaged in co-creating scientific knowledge across the stages of the research process, increasing the likelihood that the outcomes of the research process are relevant and useful. Research questions and methodologies are more likely to be ethical and appropriate for specific cultural, social, and political contexts (Sibbald et al. 2019) (see Chapter "Ethical Challenges in Global Health Research" on ethics). Members of a scientific transdisciplinary team are involved in a co-learning process across disciplines and often sectors, creating a common language, timeframe, expectations, and collaborative model to address a health issue in a specific system (Leischow and Milstein 2006; Pongsiri and Bassi 2021; Sibbald et al. 2019; Iyer et al. 2021).

### 3.2 Introduction to Early Warning Systems for Health Sectors

Research to support developing and implementing an early warning system for a health issue is an excellent example of a transdisciplinary process. Early Warning Systems (EWS) are being developed for climate-sensitive health issues (e.g., heat/cold waves, water- and vector-borne infectious diseases). The research questions are problem-driven and solution-oriented. An EWS can assist the public health sector in preventing outbreaks and saving lives.

Health sectors worldwide are developing EWSs to adapt to changing climate conditions. The 6th report of the Intergovernmental Panel on Climate Change (IPCC AR6) states that anthropogenic climate change is unequivocal, impacting the well-being and the health of the planet (Pörtner et al. 2022). Moreover, extreme climatic events will increase in intensity and frequency, impacting climate-sensitive infectious diseases particularly amongst the most vulnerable populations (Pörtner et al. 2022).

Systems-based research approaches can integrate climate, environment, animal, and human systems data with forecasting and communication technologies. A climate-driven EWS uses climate information, such as seasonal forecasts, with epidemiological information and other variables to predict the likelihood of a dengue outbreak in the future. With enough lead time, public health practitioners can deploy early intervention measures to reduce disease transmissions, such as vector control, education for frontline health workers and communities, and ordering/stocking of critical diagnostic and therapeutic supplies (Lowe et al. 2011; Degallier et al. 2010; Stewart-Ibarra et al. 2022).

Partners in the collaborative research process may include public health staff (prevention offices, epidemiological surveillance, vector control), weather/climate staff of the national meteorological services, researchers, other actors in local government, communities, and the private sector. To create an enabling environment for these partnerships, it is important to identify the shared priorities and expectations, research needs, current capabilities, and capacity gaps (Borbor et al. 2016). This co-creation process requires careful coordination and clear communication to build trust, the foundation for sustained engagement (Stewart-Ibarra et al. 2022).

### 3.3 Example of Transdisciplinary Collaborations for Dengue Early Warning

In the following section, the authors will briefly share their experience with transdisciplinary collaboration to study dengue fever and develop early warning tools for the public health sector.

In 2007, Ecuadorian scientists Anna Stewart Ibarra (environmental scientist) and Mercy Borbor-Cordova (oceanographer) met for the first time in Ecuador when Anna began her doctoral research. dengue fever, a mosquito-borne viral disease, which had emerged over the last two decades and become hyper-endemic in coastal urban areas. They discussed the importance of initiating dengue research in Ecuador, as little was known about the local disease transmission dynamics; however, it was clear that climate conditions and social inequities were significant drivers, and a systems approach was needed to provide evidence supporting disease control strategies. They discussed the feasibility of data collection, identified local partners, and devel-

oped a strategy to work with multiple sectors and high-risk communities in the coastal region. Research questions aimed to understand the dynamics of dengue transmission, the ecology of the vector *Aedes aegypti*, and the interactions with the climate and human systems to inform public health interventions.

In 2011, the team grew to include the expertise of Sadie Ryan, a conservation biologist and quantitative ecologist, who applied a One Health approach to understanding dengue transmission across landscapes. The same year, Rachel Lowe, a meteorologist and public health expert, also joined the team, providing her expertise in climate and statistical modeling to forecast dengue outbreaks. Over the next decade, their collaboration blossomed into a long-lasting partnership and friendship, which has expanded into diverse systems approaches across disciplines and geographic areas.

Together they applied socio-ecological systems (SES) and modeling frameworks to understand the drivers of dengue transmission (Fig. 2). They integrated information from epidemio-

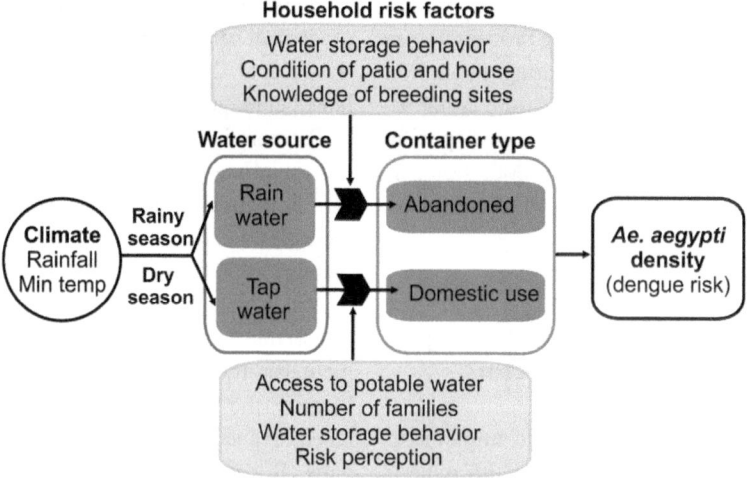

**Fig. 2** This figure illustrates how climate and environmental factors interact with socio-ecological systems at the city and household level to influence the risk of dengue transmission in peri-urban neighborhoods in southern coastal Ecuador. Factors were identified through an entomological field surveillance study and modeling. Containers with standing water were surveyed around homes. Water source refers to the water in the container, and container type refers to whether the container was rubbish/abandoned or whether it was currently in use by the household. Household risk factors were identified via surveys with the heads of household. (Source: Stewart-Ibarra et al. 2014)

logical and entomological field surveillance studies, weather stations, and demographic census data to understand drivers and hotspots of dengue on the landscape in Ecuador and later in the Caribbean (Lippi et al. 2019; Lippi et al. 2020). They provided the first evidence for the impacts of El Niño events on dengue outbreaks in Ecuador (Stewart-Ibarra and Lowe 2013) and developed methods for (sub)seasonal dengue forecasting, using weather data and El Niño indices as potential triggers of dengue outbreaks (Lowe et al. 2017). Different timeframes and forecasting horizons were explored to assess the impact of extreme climatic events (El Niño, droughts, etc.) and long-term climate change (Tompkins et al. 2019) and to support public health interventions in the short, medium, and long run (Stewart-Ibarra et al. 2014).

Engaging with government and community partners in Ecuador was a critical part of the collaborative research process. Mercy, in her role as an officer and ministerial-level decision-maker in the government of Ecuador, guided the team in effective engagement with decision-makers from the health and climate sectors. Individuals from climate and health institutions were central team members, contributing expertise, innovations, field and laboratory resources, local credibility, and connection to communities and authorities to ensure that the research supported public health priorities (WMO 2014; Stewart-Ibarra et al. 2019a). Dozens of scientific articles were jointly authored with climate and health sector partners; however, they had difficulty making headway in implementing an operational EWS for dengue in Ecuador due in part to an ever changing political landscape and institutional challenges.

In 2017, they began a fruitful collaboration with public health and climate sector partners in Barbados (Stewart-Ibarra et al. 2022) in the Eastern Caribbean region to co-develop a dengue EWS. As in Ecuador, strong intersectoral partnerships, particularly between the national climate and health sectors, have been a critical component of the research and development process, which is ongoing (Lowe et al. 2020). Equitable and effective collaboration, emphasizing co-learning, has created an environment that

enables the translation of scientific knowledge into public health action.

In Ecuador and Barbados, the transdisciplinary process strengthened the co-production of knowledge on adaptation measures for vector-borne disease control (Stewart-Ibarra et al. 2019b). An important lesson was that developing trust and strong partnerships required time and a common vision during the co-production process. Over several years, the team validated and improved the early warning model and visualization according to the needs of sectoral partners, increasing a sense of ownership, legitimacy, and utility. Policy outcomes include contributions to the Third National Communication of Climate Change in Ecuador and inclusion in the Caribbean Health-Climatic Bulletin in 2020. The team has also supported capacity-building activities for students, scientists, and practitioners.

This long-term partnership of 'systems thinkers' was built through sustained dialogue, co-design of transdisciplinary research tools, fieldwork campaigns, scientific publications, and joint trainings with health and climate practitioners. Beyond scientific work, a joyful camaraderie has strengthened the bonds of the team during many years of working together on projects.

## 4    Conclusions

Moving beyond the boundaries of Planetary Health and One Health, people identifying with one or several of these concepts are encouraged to engage with each other to consider the diverse perspectives, expertise, and experiences within and across these concepts. Researchers and practitioners should regularly interrogate underlying assumptions and beliefs and question power structures and dominant scientific and global health narratives (Buse et al. 2018), such as the colonial legacies of global health (see Chapter "Colonialism, Decolonization, and Global Health"). There are significant contributions from the social sciences, such as team science (see Chapter "Team Science and Infectious Disease Work: Exploring Challenges and Opportunities"), to guide critical reflections and good practices in applying systems thinking to stakeholder engagement and equitable partnerships (Lawrence et al. 2022; Smith et al. 2019).

## Glossary

**Autoregulation:** Through feed-back, the system is maintained at a certain level of functioning. One example is. the autoregulation of parasite-host systems (Tompkins and Begon 1999) and the mechanisms of development of an epidemic process.

**Dynamic complexity:** Systems are constantly changing, adjusting and readjusting over time scales. For example, the effect of climate on disease transmission may be non-linear and vary in space and time.

**Functionality:** Ensuring a correlation between inputs and outputs to generate an expected result. Infectious diseases are complex systems (and subsystems) which are functionally organized and can be resolved in each level of organization and within temporal and spatial scales.

**General Systems Theory (GST):** GST is a holistic approach, in this case that allows infectious disease research to be addressed from global to local levels identifying interactions of environmental and human systems

**Hierarchy:** A system formed by several subsystems organized according to a level structure, for example on the risk of infectious disease, the reservoir of infection, the route of transmission and related factors, and the prevention and control measures.

**Integrality:** The modification of one part of the system leads to the change of the other components and of the whole; for example, modifying or controlling the route of transmission can reduce risk of infectious disease.

**Interdependency:** The components of a system are interrelated by enabling the emergence of some overall combined properties.

**Interdisciplinary Research:** Research efforts conducted by investigators from different disciplines based upon a conceptual model that links or integrates theoretical frameworks, study designs and methodologies from these disciplines, and requires the use of perspectives and skills of the involved disciplines throughout multiple phases of the research process (Aboelela et al. 2007).

**One Health:** Transdisciplinary approach to achieve optimal health and well-being recognizing the interconnections between people, animals, plants, and their shared environment (WHO 2017).

**Planetary Health:** Solutions-oriented, transdisciplinary field and social movement focused on analyzing and addressing the impacts of human disruptions to Earth's natural systems on human health and all life on Earth (Lerner and Berg 2017).

**Processes:** The components or activities within the system that work together to make it function. The control and prevention of infectious diseases relies on a thorough understanding of the factors determining transmission and their processes.

**Self-organization:** The system has the capacity to create new stable states through self-reinforcing mechanisms. For example, infectious disease systems persist and spread due to formation of cycles/loop between the host subsystem, the pathogen subsystem, and the environmental subsystem (Garira 2020; Angelstam et al. 2013).

**Systems Thinking:** Conceptual framework that organizes the understanding of complex systems using four rules: organizing ideas by distinctions, systems, relationships, and perspectives. In this framework, distinctions refer to how elements in a system have identified and can be grouped by what they are not, systems refer to elements that may be parts or a whole, relationships refer to associations between elements and their causal ordering, and perspectives refers to the viewpoint from which elements are analyzed (Cabrera and Cabrera 2018).A paradigm or perspective that considers connections among different components [of a system], plans for the implications of their interactions, and requires transdisciplinary thinking as well as active engagement of those who have a stake in the outcome to govern the course of change (Leischow and Milstein 2006) p. 403.

**Traditional Knowledges:** Systems of knowledge, know-how, skills and practices that are developed, sustained and passed on from generation to generation within a community, often forming part of its cultural or spiritual identity (Keats and Evans 2020).

**Transdisciplinary Research:** Research efforts conducted by investigators from different disciplines working jointly to create new conceptual, theoretical, methodological, and translational innovations that integrate and move beyond discipline-specific approaches to address a common problem (Lawrence et al. 2022; Angelstam et al. 2013; Brandt et al. 2013; Pohl and Hadorn 2008).

# References

Aboelela SW, Larson E, Bakken S, Carrasquillo O, Formicola A, Glied SA, et al. Defining interdisciplinary research: conclusions from a critical review of the literature. Health Serv Res. 2007;42(1 Pt 1):329–46. https://doi.org/10.1111/j.1475-6773.2006.00621.x.

Angelstam P, Andersson K, Annerstedt M, Axelsson R, Elbakidze M, Garrido P, et al. Solving problems in social–ecological systems: definition, practice and barriers of transdisciplinary research. Ambio. 2013;42(2):254–65. https://doi.org/10.1007/s13280-012-0372-4.

Best A, Clark PI, Leischow SJ, Trochim WM. Greater than the sum systems thinking in tobacco control, NCI tobacco control monograph series. U.S. Department of Health & Human Services, National Institutes of Health, National Cancer Institute; 2007.

Borbor MJ, Ayala EB, Cárdenas WB, Endy TP, Finkelstein JL, León R, et al. Chapter 5: Developing and delivering health-tailored climate products and services, case study 5.C vector-virus microclimate surveillance system for dengue control in Machala, Ecuador. In: Climate Services for Health: global case studies of enhancing decision support for climate risk management and adaptation. Geneva: World Health Organization/World Meteorological Organization; 2016. p. 106–9.

Brandt P, Ernst A, Gralla F, Luederitz C, Lang DJ, Newig J, et al. A review of transdisciplinary research in sustainability science. Ecol Econ. 2013;92:1–15. Available from: https://www.sciencedirect.com/science/article/pii/S0921800913001377

Buse CG, Oestreicher JS, Ellis NR, Patrick R, Brisbois B, Jenkins AP, et al. Public health guide to field developments linking ecosystems, environments and health in the Anthropocene. J Epidemiol Community Health. 2018;72(5):420–5. https://doi.org/10.1136/jech-2017-210082.

Cabrera D, Cabrera L. Systems thinking made simple: new Hope for solving wicked problems. 2nd ed. Plectica LLC; 2018. 222 p. Available from: https://play.google.com/store/books/details?id=lfEwugEACAAJ

Castellanos EJ, Lemos MF, Astigarraga L, Chacón N, Cuvi N, Huggel C, et al. Central and South America. In: Pörtner H, Roberts D, Tignor M, Poloczanska E, Mintenbeck K, Alegria A, et al., editors. Climate change 2022: impacts, adaptation and vulnerability contribution of working group II to the sixth assessment report of the intergovernmental panel on climate change. Cambridge University Press; 2022. p. 1689–816. Available from: https://repositorio.inta.gob.ar/handle/20.500.12123/12589

Charlesworth SM, Kligerman DC, Blackett M, Warwick F. The potential to address disease vectors in favelas in Brazil using sustainable drainage systems: Zika, drainage and greywater management. Int J Environ Res Public Health. 2022;19(5):2860. https://doi.org/10.3390/ijerph19052860.

Chen X, Li H, Lucero-Prisno DE 3rd, Abdullah AS, Huang J, Laurence C, et al. What is global health? Key concepts and clarification of misperceptions: report of the 2019 GHRP editorial meeting. Glob Health Res Policy. 2020;5:14. https://doi.org/10.1186/s41256-020-00142-7.

de Savigny D, Adam T, editors. Systems thinking for health systems strengthening, vol. 26. Alliance for Health Policy and Systems Research & World Health Organization; 2009. p. 107–8.

Degallier N, Favier C, Menkes C, Lengaigne M, Ramalho WM, Souza R, et al. Toward an early warning system for dengue prevention: modeling climate impact on dengue transmission. Clim Chang. 2010;98(3):581–92. https://doi.org/10.1007/s10584-009-9747-3.

Eyre P. Combined veterinary-human medical education: a complete one health degree? J Vet Med Educ. 2015;42(4):283. https://doi.org/10.3138/jvme.0615-093.

Fagre AC, Cohen LE, Eskew EA, Farrell M, Glennon E, Joseph MB, et al. Assessing the risk of human-to-wildlife pathogen transmission for conservation and public health. Ecol Lett. 2022;25(6):1534–49. https://doi.org/10.1111/ele.14003.

Fiore SM, Rosen M, Salas E, Burke S, Jentsch F. Processes in complex team problem-solving: parsing and defining the theoretical problem space. In: Letsky M, Warner N, Fiore SM, Smith C, editors. Macrocognition in teams. CRC Press; 2008. p. 21.

Garira W. The research and development process for multiscale models of infectious disease systems. PLoS Comput Biol. 2020;16(4):e1007734. https://doi.org/10.1371/journal.pcbi.1007734.

Health Organization W. One health joint plan of action, 2022–2026. World Organisation for Animal Health (WOAH) (founded as OIE): FAO; UNEP; WHO; 2022. Available from: https://apps.who.int/iris/bitstream/handle/10665/363518/9789240059139-eng.pdf?sequence=1

Herrera D, Ellis A, Fisher B, Golden CD, Johnson K, Mulligan M, et al. Upstream watershed condition predicts rural children's health across 35 developing countries. Nat Commun. 2017;8(1):811. https://doi.org/10.1038/s41467-017-00775-2.

Hickey GM, Pouliot M, Smith-Hall C, Wunder S, Nielsen MR. Quantifying the economic contribution of wild food harvests to rural livelihoods: a global-comparative analysis. Food Policy. 2016;62:122–32. https://doi.org/10.1016/j.foodpol.2016.06.001.

Iyer HS, DeVille NV, Stoddard O, Cole J, Myers SS, Li H, et al. Sustaining planetary health through systems thinking: public health's critical role. SSM Popul Health. 2021;15:100844. https://doi.org/10.1016/j.ssmph.2021.100844.

Keats B, Evans P. Traditional knowledge and resource management in the northwest territories, Canada: definitions, disciplinary divides, and reasons for decisions. Extr Ind Soc. 2020;7(4):1309–18. Available from: https://www.sciencedirect.com/science/article/pii/S2214790X20302495

Klein JT. Evaluation of interdisciplinary and transdisciplinary research: a literature review. Am J Prev Med. 2008;35(2 Suppl):S116–23. https://doi.org/10.1016/j.amepre.2008.05.010.

Koplan JP, Bond TC, Merson MH, Reddy KS, Rodriguez MH, Sewankambo NK, et al. Towards a common definition of global health. Lancet. 2009;373(9679):1993–5. https://doi.org/10.1016/S0140-6736(09)60332-9.

Lawrence MG, Williams S, Nanz P, Renn O. Characteristics, potentials, and challenges of transdisciplinary research. One Earth. 2022;5(1):44–61. Available from: https://www.sciencedirect.com/science/article/pii/S2590332221007284

Leischow SJ, Milstein B. Systems thinking and modeling for public health practice. Am J Public Health. 2006;96(3):403–5. https://doi.org/10.2105/AJPH.2005.082842.

Lerner H, Berg C. A comparison of three holistic approaches to health: one health, EcoHealth, and planetary health. Front Vet Sci. 2017;4:163. https://doi.org/10.3389/fvets.2017.00163.

Lippi CA, Stewart-Ibarra AM, Loor MEFB, Zambrano JED, Lopez NAE, Blackburn JK, et al. Geographic shifts in Aedes aegypti habitat suitability in Ecuador using larval surveillance data and ecological niche modeling: implications of climate change for public health vector control. PLoS Negl Trop Dis. 2019;13(4):e0007322. https://doi.org/10.1371/journal.pntd.0007322.

Lippi CA, Stewart-Ibarra AM, Romero M, Lowe R, Mahon R, Van Meerbeeck CJ, et al. Spatiotemporal tools for emerging and endemic disease hotspots in small areas: an analysis of dengue and chikungunya in Barbados, 2013–2016. Am J Trop Med Hyg. 2020;103(1):149–56. https://doi.org/10.4269/ajtmh.19-0919.

Lowe R, Bailey TC, Stephenson DB, Graham RJ, Coelho CAS, Sá Carvalho M, et al. Spatio-temporal modelling of climate-sensitive disease risk: towards an early warning system for dengue in Brazil. Comput Geosci. 2011;37(3):371–81. [cited 2015 Jul 8]. Available from: https://www.sciencedirect.com/science/article/pii/S0098300410001445

Lowe R, Stewart-Ibarra AM, Petrova D, García-Díez M, Borbor-Cordova MJ, Mejía R, et al. Climate services for health: predicting the evolution of the 2016 dengue season in Machala, Ecuador. Lancet Planet Health. 2017;1(4):e142–51. https://doi.org/10.1016/S2542-5196(17)30064-5.

Lowe R, Ryan SJ, Mahon R, Van Meerbeeck CJ, Trotman AR, Boodram L-LG, et al. Building resilience to mosquito-borne diseases in the Caribbean. PLoS Biol. 2020;18(11):e3000791. https://doi.org/10.1371/journal.pbio.3000791.

Max-Neef MA. Foundations of transdisciplinarity. Ecol Econ. 2005;53(1):5–16. https://doi.org/10.1016/j.ecolecon.2005.01.014.

One Health Basics. [cited 2023 Feb 18]. 2022. Available from: https://www.cdc.gov/onehealth/basics/index.html

Peters DH. The application of systems thinking in health: why use systems thinking? Health Res Policy Syst. 2014;12(1):51. https://doi.org/10.1186/1478-4505-12-51.

Planetary Health. Planetary Health Alliance. [cited 2023 Feb 18]. Available from: https://www.planetaryhealthalliance.org/planetary-health

Pohl C, Hadorn GH. Core terms in transdisciplinary research. In: Hadorn GH, Hoffmann-Riem H, Biber-Klemm S, Grossenbacher-Mansuy W, Joye D, Pohl C, et al., editors. Handbook of transdisciplinary research. Dordrecht: Springer Netherlands; 2008. p. 427–32. https://doi.org/10.1007/978-1-4020-6699-3_28.

Pongsiri MJ, Bassi AM. A systems understanding underpins actions at the climate and health nexus. Int J Environ Res Public Health. 2021;18(5):2398. https://doi.org/10.3390/ijerph18052398.

Pongsiri MJ, Gatzweiler FW, Bassi AM, Haines A, Demassieux F. The need for a systems approach to planetary health. Lancet Planet Health. 2017;1(7):e257–9. https://doi.org/10.1016/S2542-5196(17)30116-X.

Pörtner H-O, Roberts DC, Poloczanska ES, Mintenbeck K, Tignor M, Alegría A, Craig M, Langsdorf S, Löschke S, Möller V, Okem A. IPCC, 2022: Summary for policymakers. In: Pörtner HO, Roberts DC, Tignor M, Poloczanska ES, Mintenbeck K, Alegría A, Craig M, Langsdorf S, Löschke S, Möller V, Okem A, Rama B, editors. Climate change 2022: impacts, adaptation, and vulnerability contribution of working group II to the sixth assessment report of the intergovernmental panel on climate change. Cambridge/New York: Cambridge University Press; 2022. p. 3–33. https://doi.org/10.1017/9781009325844.001.

Redvers N, Celidwen Y, Schultz C, Horn O, Githaiga C, Vera M, et al. The determinants of planetary health: an indigenous consensus perspective. Lancet Planet Health. 2022;6(2):e156–63. https://doi.org/10.1016/S2542-5196(21)00354-5.

Rüegg SR, Nielsen LR, Buttigieg SC, Santa M, Aragrande M, Canali M, et al. A systems approach to evaluate one health initiatives. Front Vet Sci. 2018;5:23. https://doi.org/10.3389/fvets.2018.00023.

Santos AS, Almeida AN. The impact of deforestation on malaria infections in the Brazilian Amazon. Ecol Econ. 2018;154:247–56. https://doi.org/10.1016/j.ecolecon.2018.08.005.

Sibbald SL, Kang H, Graham ID. Collaborative health research partnerships: a survey of researcher and knowledge-user attitudes and perceptions. Health Res Policy Syst. 2019;17(1):92. https://doi.org/10.1186/s12961-019-0485-3.

Smith L, Pihama L, Cameron N, Mataki T, Morgan H, Te Nana R. Thought space Wānanga—A Kaupapa Māori decolonizing approach to research translation. Genealogy. 2019;3(4):74. [cited 2023 Feb 20]. Available from: https://www.mdpi.com/2313-5778/3/4/74

Steffen W, Richardson K, Rockström J, Cornell SE, Fetzer I, Bennett EM, et al. Sustainability. Planetary boundaries: guiding human development on a changing planet. Science. 2015;347(6223):1259855. https://doi.org/10.1126/science.1259855.

Sternberg LS. Tuberculosis and one health – what is in a name? Front Vet Sci. 2015;2:54. https://doi.org/10.3389/fvets.2015.00054.

Stewart-Ibarra AM, Lowe R. Climate and non-climate drivers of dengue epidemics in southern coastal Ecuador. Am J Trop Med Hyg. 2013;88(5):971–81. https://doi.org/10.4269/ajtmh.12-0478.

Stewart-Ibarra AM, Muñoz ÁG, Ryan SJ, Ayala EB, Borbor-Cordova MJ, Finkelstein JL, et al. Spatiotemporal clustering, climate periodicity, and social-ecological risk factors for dengue during an outbreak in Machala, Ecuador, in 2010. BMC Infect Dis. 2014;14(1):610. https://doi.org/10.1186/s12879-014-0610-4.

Stewart-Ibarra AM, Henderson RR, Heydari N, Borbor-Cordova MJ, Fujii Y, Bardosh K. Tracking Aedes aegypti in a hotter, wetter, more urban world. In: Locating Zika. London: Routledge; 2019a. p. 128–49. https://doi.org/10.4324/9780429456558-6.

Stewart-Ibarra AM, Romero M, Hinds AQJ, Lowe R, Mahon R, Van Meerbeeck CJ, et al. Co-developing climate services for public health: stakeholder needs and perceptions for the prevention and control of Aedes-transmitted diseases in the Caribbean. PLoS Negl Trop Dis. 2019b;13(10):e0007772. https://doi.org/10.1371/journal.pntd.0007772.

Stewart-Ibarra AM, Rollock L, Best S, Brown T, Diaz AR, Dunbar W, et al. Co-learning during the co-creation of a dengue early warning system for the health sector in Barbados. BMJ Glob Health. 2022;7(1):e007842. https://doi.org/10.1136/bmjgh-2021-007842.

Tompkins DM, Begon M. Parasites can regulate wildlife populations. Parasitol Today. 1999;15(8):311–3. https://doi.org/10.1016/s0169-4758(99)01484-2.

Tompkins AM, Lowe R, Nissan H, Martiny N, Roucou P, Thomson MC, et al. Chapter 22: Predicting climate impacts on health at sub-seasonal to seasonal timescales. In: Robertson AW, Vitart F, editors. Sub-seasonal to seasonal prediction. Elsevier; 2019. p. 455–77. Available from: https://www.sciencedirect.com/science/article/pii/B978012811714900022X.

Von Bertalanffy L. The history and status of general systems theory. Acad Manag J. 1972;15(4):407–26. https://doi.org/10.2307/255139.

Whitmee S, Haines A, Beyrer C, Boltz F, Capon AG, de Souza Dias BF, et al. Safeguarding human health in the Anthropocene epoch: report of the Rockefeller Foundation-lancet commission on planetary health. Lancet. 2015;386(10007):1973–2028. https://doi.org/10.1016/S0140-6736(15)60901-1.

WHO. One health. WHO AIDS Tech Bulletin; 2017. Available from: https://www.otago.ac.nz/wellington/otago635537.pdf

Wilcox BA, Aguirre AA, De Paula N, Siriaroonrat B, Echaubard P. Operationalizing one health employing social-ecological systems theory: lessons from the greater Mekong sub-region. Front. Public Health. 2019;7:85. https://doi.org/10.3389/fpubh.2019.00085.

WMO. Implementation plan of the global framework for climate services. World Meteorological Organization; 2014. [cited 2022 Aug 3]. Available from: http://www.wmo.int/gfcs/sites/default/files/implementation-plan//GFCS-IMPLEMENTATION-PLAN-FINAL-14211_en.pdf

Xia S, Zhou X-N, Liu J. Systems thinking in combating infectious diseases. Infect Dis Poverty. 2017;6(1):144. https://doi.org/10.1186/s40249-017-0339-6.

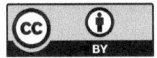

# Team Science and Infectious Disease Work: Exploring Challenges and Opportunities

Sonia Alvarez, Maritza Salazar,
and A. Desiree LaBeaud ⓘ

*Compassionate people are geniuses in the art of living, more necessary to the dignity, security, and joy of humanity than the discoverers of knowledge.*

Albert Einstein

## Abstract

Collaborative global health research has been growing rapidly for approximately three decades now. This type of collaborative research, in contrast with a sole researcher approach, predominant in the past, has called for the integration of investigators, clinicians, practitioners, and others from outside of academia, often from different nations, in search of answers to a multitude of complex health problems. Team science is a novel way to conduct scientific research on individual and public health problems. Most areas of scientific inquiry today are multi-dimensional, and so are the teams studying them. Cross-disciplinary teams search for global applications of scientific advances to allevi-ate or eradicate human illness and suffering. These applications require consideration of social, political, and economic contexts across geographical boundaries. Integration of various bodies of knowledge, methods, approaches, and participating institutions' protocols demand a new set of practices and considerations to improve the integrity of researchers as they operate within teams and the quality of scientific production. This chapter includes an overview of relevant team science topics and the study of team science research. It presents evidence of practices and elements that contribute to the integration and success of research teams. Concurrently, it narrates the experience of one laboratory team in their quest to anticipate and eventually integrate team science elements into their daily scientific and social practice. The authors believe that embracing team science practices is equally time-consuming and worthwhile, as both scientific production, research impact, and team members' professional quality of life are maintained and improved. In addition, team members experience personal satisfaction and joy in establishing and maintaining trusting relationships.

S. Alvarez (✉)
Stanford School of Medicine, Stanford University, Stanford, CA, USA

M. Salazar
UCI Paul Merage School of Business, University of California Irvine, Irvine, CA, USA
e-mail: Campomaritza.salazar@uci.edu

A. D. LaBeaud
Department of Pediatrics, Division of Infectious Diseases, Stanford University, Stanford, CA, USA
e-mail: dlabeaud@stanford.edu

© The Author(s) 2024
A. Stewart Ibarra, A. D. LaBeaud (eds.), *Transforming Global Health Partnerships*, Sustainable Development Goals Series, https://doi.org/10.1007/978-3-031-53793-6_5

**Keywords**

Team science · Science of team science · Collaborative science · Global health research · International collaboration · Cross-disciplinary · Interdisciplinary · Transdisciplinary research

**Author Perspective**

We are women scientists with diverse backgrounds that converge exceptionally in the writing of this chapter. Originally from Cuba, Mexico, and the USA, we currently live and work in California, USA. We are co-authors for the first time. Our professional backgrounds include psychology, social-community psychology, community development, public health, social work, business administration and management, biology, pediatric medicine, global health, infectious disease, clinical research, and arbovirus epidemiology. The diversity of our backgrounds is integrated by a set of core values, interests, and global goals: namely, the betterment of human experiences through scientific discoveries, excellence and effectiveness, curiosity about individual and group processes, human diversity, collaboration, equity, and justice. In addition, we share concerns for the environment and the protection of our planet.

**Key Tenets**

1. Team success ought to be measured not only by scientific results but by the quality and satisfaction of the interactions/partnerships of members of scientific teams.
2. The team leader must guide the team in establishing a trusting environment.
3. Self-awareness and the cultivation of a 'diversity mentality' are key to success in team science.
4. The definition of a shared vision and mission contributes to group cohesion and commitment to excellence.

5. Effective communication skills are critical for the internal routine exchange of information and the external communication of scientific results.
6. The chapter addresses the following SDGs: #3 Good Health and Well-Being, #5 Gender Equality, #10 Reduced Inequalities, #16 Peace, Justice and Strong Institutions, # 17 Partnerships for the Goals

# 1　Introduction

## 1.1　Team Science

The predominance of collaborative teamwork in public health research and practice requires a closer look at the factors that make teams effective. As "collectives who exist to perform organizationally relevant tasks" (Kozlowski and Bell 2003, p. 334), public health teams are often required to tackle seemingly intractable biomedical and societal problems, like the COVID-19 pandemic or endemic malaria transmission. Public health teams, as a result, tend to be composed of individuals who have the breadth and depth of expertise, experience, training, and education necessary to accomplish diverse aims. Global health involves many disciplines that function within public health teams but takes a wider geographical approach that includes working on transnational health problems and solutions.

The reliance on teamwork in the field of global health is necessary in a complex global work environment (e.g., Fiore et al. 2001; Hackman and Morris 1975), which includes health problems driven by interconnected micro- and macro- biophysical and social factors. Addressing these challenges requires research collaborations that span across disciplinary, organizational, geopolitical, and cultural boundaries. These features of global health teams present undeniable obstacles to effective teamwork due to the heightened burden imposed by the challenges of coordination, communication, and project execution (Emmanuelides 1993; Olson et al. 1995). Simultaneously, rapid changes in science and technology, including an increase in the speed of global scientific output, data capture, and computing capabilities, create both opportunities and challenges as teams have more tools at their disposal, but also greater demands to coordinate a large body of specialized knowledge. In addition, the current system of academic science in the Global North overvalues individual effort and undervalues collaborative team science during the formal academic promotions and tenure process. An overhaul of this process and more equitable collaborations and authorship models are recommended to foster the rebalancing of power among team members to promote equity amongst global health teams (Hedt-Gauthier et al. 2018). These factors are important to consider when exploring facilitators and inhibitors to effective teamwork in the field of global health.

## 1.2 The Science of Team Science

The Science of Team Science (SciTS) is one body of knowledge that seeks to provide guidance for complex collaborations that are increasingly common in global health (Wuchty et al. 2007). Team science or convergence science refers to a growing field of expertise that examines the processes by which small and large teams, research centers, and institutes communicate and conduct research together across disciplines, institutions, and geographies. A fundamental assumption of team science is that scholarly progress on complex problems requires drawing together and integrating diverse expertise, tools, and technologies. Being able to leverage vastly different sources of expertise is rapidly becoming a prerequisite to solving complex problems (Ancona and Caldwell 1992; Cronin and Weingart 2007), and the examination of what factors and conditions foster the integration of knowledge across boundaries is essential for scientific advancement in global health.

Recent reviews of the SciTS literature reveal significant advances in understanding the facilitators and impediments to team functioning (Hall et al. 2020). Greater insight into the value of diversity, the role of team size, and the effects of critical team processes (e.g., communication and coordination) on outcomes of scientific teams have important implications for teams engaged in global health research. In examining the applicability of team science research findings to global health teams, we also identify several areas of inquiry that remain underexplored. The focus of this chapter is to highlight where team science provides key guidance for global health teams, while also highlighting gaps for future research.

Throughout this chapter, we will refer to the LaBeaud Lab (see Box 1), an infectious disease research laboratory at Stanford University School of Medicine, to illustrate the application of team science concepts and strategies.

### Box 1: The LaBeaud Lab Experience

The primary aim of our academic research lab, based at Stanford University (USA), is to understand arboviral infections and their long-term implications. As such, the lab investigates dengue, chikungunya, Zika, yellow fever, and Rift Valley fever viruses in Kenya, Grenada, and Brazil.

Working with researchers, students, trainees, and global community partners, we hope to optimize control strategies to prevent emerging infections and improve the health of communities all over the world. For each section below, we will connect foundational concepts in team science to the experience of applying such concepts in the LaBeaud laboratory.

As we start narrating our team experience, we realize and acknowledge our privileged position by virtue of operating within an elite university in the Global North which encourages work/life balance and provides internal resources for exploration and contemplation of alternate practices. Groups lacking these resources might struggle to embark in humanistic exploration as mentioned in this chapter. At the same time, however, we wonder what other types of social capital prevalent in other cultures are effective in creating trust, cohesiveness, and satisfaction in teamwork.

## 2    Performance Outcomes of Global Health Teams

Team performance results from how the team members "think, do, and feel" (Day et al. 2004, p. 863). Traditional models of teamwork often reflect work units engaged in more routine and simpler tasks than those required by global health research. As such, these models do not adequately reflect a large portion of teamwork conducted today by knowledge workers (Davenport et al. 2002; Drucker 1999), such as global health teams, where the work is complex, ambiguous, and ever evolving. In scientific collaborations or teams, the nature of team performance *itself* diverges from efficacy and efficiency, as teams are not only producing concrete scientific results as quickly as they can in the form of publication and reports, but scientific results and new insights regarding the public and global health issues under investigation are also frequently changing and very dynamic.

Several conceptual frameworks and scales exist to measure the impact of research and clinical practices under the discipline of Translational Research; the type of research whose aim is to investigate and apply results to solve real problems. A considerable amount of literature exists about its benefits both for science and communities (Luke et al. 2018; Dembe et al. 2014). Although traditional assessments of scientific productivity, including the creation of knowledge products such as grant funding, manuscripts, or patents, are relevant to scientific collaborations, other performance outcomes are also important (Box 2). In global health work, performance outcomes might include shifts in behaviors and attitudes among the populations engaged in a community-based health program. Other outcomes could include contributing to national or global policies related to evidence-based management of infectious diseases. Longer-term outcomes of global health teams can include implementation programs that effectively increase the acceptance and uptake of health-related behaviors and protocols that positively impact population health.

---

**Box 2: A Multi-dimensional Team Approach**

Members of the LaBeaud lab adhere to the notion that the value of scientific outcomes must be measured by their usefulness in real-life community settings and the improved health status of populations served by the work.

Engagement through collaborative work is intrinsically tied to success by leveraging expert knowledge from different disciplines and cultural settings. **Success**, in turn, is defined in terms of the impact that scientific discoveries could have on individuals in the communities where research takes place, the scientific quality of such research, and the team members' personal and professional growth. Team members recognize and value the connection between the human side of the scientific endeavor and the ultimate quality of its outcomes (Berger and Luckmann 1966; Kuhn 1962).

---

## 2.1    Characteristics of Global Health Teams

The quest to address the health challenges affecting communities around the world can elicit very different patterns of team formation. Although all collaborations require drawing together specialists from different disciplines, specialties, and localities, as well as stakeholders and policy makers, the urgency of the situation may sometimes demand the rapid formation of temporary collaborations. Individual specialists may be drawn together quickly to address an infectious disease outbreak, as seen in several case studies presented in this book. In this context, learning to work together, adapting to one another, and gaining confidence as a group requires a more rapid, dynamic approach (Wageman et al. 2012). In less urgent situations, global health teams can form slowly, and team members have the time to establish common ground and build trust, including developing a shared language and understanding of their joint processes through ongoing interaction. In these long-term and stable teams, such as the LaBeaud lab example shared in this chapter, team functioning will require different insights from the field of team science than in situations where individual experts come together rapidly around a common public health challenge or question.

## 2.2 Inputs to Team Performance

### 2.2.1 Disciplinary Diversity

The value of diversity among members of scientific teams has been well-documented (Guan et al. 2015; Lee et al. 2015). Although research on innovation suggests that spanning disciplines is beneficial because it allows scientists to see connections across fields (Fleming 2001; Schiling 2005), other scholarly work highlights that doing work across disciplinary domains can also be cumbersome and that scholars that choose to do so are often less productive due to the cognitive, communication, and coordination costs incurred (Leahey et al. 2017). If done successfully, however, working across disciplines can be a high-risk and high-reward endeavor as the impact of such work can be greater in the long term (Leahey et al. 2017) (Box 3).

### 2.2.2 Ethnic and Cultural Diversity

Global health collaborations usually include individuals from different countries and cultures. Team science research provides limited guidance about the role of cultural and ethnic diversity in science teams. The lack of work on the role of ethnic and cultural diversity limits our understanding of how to maximize the benefits of differences in cultural backgrounds, languages, or customs. Other research on multicultural experience suggests that collaborators who have lived or worked in another nation, including in the field of international public health work, show increased levels of trust, communication competence, and leadership effectiveness (Maddux et al. 2021). Similarly, shared team identity can

> **Box 3: Disciplinary and Knowledge Diversity**
> Over the last decade, the LaBeaud lab has established collaborations with individuals from diverse professions, including virologists, epidemiologists, pediatric and adult clinicians, anthropologists, entomologists, veterinarians, biostatisticians, biologists, microbiologists, environmentalists, diagnosticians, ecologists, artists, bioengineers, climate scientists, electrical and computer engineers, communications experts, geographers, policy experts, health educators, behavioral and organizational scientists, sociologists, ministers of health and community residents and leaders.
>
> Disciplinary diversity has helped our lab amplify the perspective of research projects. Discussions that start from a specific aspect of the study or lab procedure, often progress to rich discussions about different elements such as clinical, cultural, institutional, environmental, social, and other real-life dimensions. What may start as a concrete scientific finding, often results in a meaningful community intervention or a new strategy for system change. This is possible when various disciplines including community members' perspectives are included and valued.

support team creativity when ethnic differences are salient within teams (Salazar et al. 2017). Unifying culturally diverse teammates around shared work aims and a team mission can help to bring teammates together and foster joint, collective effort, toward goal accomplishment. Moreover, as team members from different countries and cultures interact, they grow in their understanding of one another and their diverse backgrounds. Such personal development of individual team members is an important benefit of teamwork in global collaborations, and as such, it deserves more attention and deliberate incorporation into the process of team science (Box 4).

**Box 4: Ethnic and Cultural Diversity**

Despite the frequent changes in team size and composition of the LaBeaud lab, at any time most team members claim their heritage from different parts of the world. The majority speak their native language. We have representatives from South America, the Caribbean, North America, Asia, the Middle East, Africa, and Europe who have lived in their places of origin or are integrated within their culture of origin. This allows our team to bring to the forefront of our practice elements of justice, diversity, equity, and inclusion, what has recently been called a JEDI framework for scientific collaborations.

Likewise, these individuals range from curious high school students to internationally renowned expert professionals. The team also includes a wide spectrum of ages, gender identities, sexual orientations, nationalities, ethnic backgrounds, religions, political persuasions, and socioeconomic backgrounds.

ity, and ability, resulting in structural marginalization and disadvantage, known as *intersectionality* (Crenshaw 1989). Female scientists encounter greater barriers to career advancement than men, although women have increased their participation in higher education (Castillo et al. 2014; Huan et al. 2020; Bloodhart et al. 2020; McKinnon and O'Connell 2020; O'Connell and McKinnon 2021). In some regions, the barriers to training and professional advancement in global health research and practice are even greater (see chapters "Gender Equity in African Academia: An Implementation Science Evaluation of the Kenya Context" and "Gender Equity in Academia Thriving as a Clinician-Scientist, Establishing Partnerships, and Driving Policy for Change in the Kenya Context"). The role of women in science warrants further attention, considering that no country in the world has achieved one hundred percent gender equality and closed the gender gaps on economic, political, education, and health-based criteria. Iceland, the country with the highest gender equality index of 0.91 (World Economic Forum, 2022), is close but has not yet achieved full equality. In contexts where deep gender biases persist, teams may struggle to achieve and benefit from gender diversity.

### 2.2.3 Gender Diversity

The SciTS literature provides insight into the value of gender diversity in scientific collaboration. This body of research highlights that having teams that include women is advantageous. Gender diversity can improve intra-team dynamics that support cognitive and social integration (Woolley et al. 2015) and more effective collaboration among team members. Most studies have focused on binary gender (men and women) perspectives in Western contexts. This suggests the need for team science studies to address the experience of non-binary and transsexual individuals, and gender dynamics in non-Western team settings. Gender identity qualifies our life and professional experiences and, as such, could bring a valuable perspective to transdisciplinary scientific work. Gender intersects with other social identities and stratifiers such as age, socioeconomic status, race, ethnicity, nationality, religion, disabil-

### 2.2.4 Temporal Diversity

Another important source of diversity in global health teams is temporal diversity. Temporal differences include pacing style, e.g., pattern of effort distribution over time in working toward deadlines (Gevers et al. 2009, 2016) and time urgency e.g., chronic hurriedness (Mohammed and Angell 2004; Mohammed and Nadkarni 2011; Mohammed et al. 2017). In research today, where effective time management is critical for team performance, an emerging literature is demonstrating that time is an ever-present performance factor for teams (Ancona and Chong 1999; Bluedorn and Denhardt 1988) and that temporal differences have important implications for conflict (Bakker et al. 2013; Mohammed et al. 2017; Mohammed and Angell 2004), collaboration (Gevers et al. 2016), performance (Mohammed and Nadkarni 2011, 2014), and timeliness (Gevers et al. 2009). In global health teams, mismatches in pacing and time urgency can create chasms between members in terms of how to complete work, leading to coordination challenges and conflict. If the work is not completed at the same pace and urgency as a collaborator might want, conflict, frustration, and a breakdown in collaborations may result, despite the motivation to work together to solve an important health issue. (Box 5).

---

**Box 5: Diversity across dimensions in the LaBeaud Lab**

Geographical, institutional, and political diversity has been prominent in the LaBeaud Lab. We conduct research in three continents on many different viruses and the various diseases they cause to serve different communities and populations. This has added more complexity to coordination of research activities, administration, and financial transactions.

Social activities and sharing of personal experiences have helped us understand and respect different cultural backgrounds. At the time of writing this chapter, with a team of 15 members, ten different home countries are represented.

Given this complex composition, it became clear that our lab team members at Stanford would need to have greater self-awareness to improve our agility to respond to changing circumstances, foster a high toleration to frustration, and support greater humility and respect to accommodate cultural differences in temporal perceptions. We have learned to recognize and validate differences in perception and expression of a sense of urgency across countries and continents. Time management and planning practices also differ across cultures. We learned quickly that when these differences are not understood, validated, anticipated, and negotiated, unnecessary conflict and resentment can easily arise.

---

### 2.2.5 Diversity Mindset

Research suggests that people's thoughts and attitudes about diversity can shape the integration of diverse information, viewpoints, and perspectives (van Knippenberg and Haslam 2003) (Box 6). Team members' attitudes about the value of diversity in collective settings has been examined at the group level (Ely and Thomas 2001). The development of diversity mindsets is important and pro-diversity beliefs were previously found to stimulate the use of differences in teams, such as varied perspectives and suggestions, while also limiting intergroup bias—favoritism toward fellow group members and bias towards outgroup members or those with whom they do not perceive as sharing a common affiliation (e.g., van Knippenberg and Schippers 2007; van Knippenberg et al. 2013). (Box 6)

---

**Box 6: Diversity Mindset**

In addition to having individuals who value diversity, the LaBeaud lab considered it was important to maintain a group's diversity mindset by incorporating conscious and deliberate appreciation of diversity in the team. It is easier to appreciate others' differences and idiosyncrasies when your own are being respected and celebrated. During weekly meetings team members not only make presentations about ongoing research but also allow time on the meeting agenda for voluntary sharing of an inspirational quote and a question of the week. These seemingly simple practices allow for personal expression and storytelling resulting in stronger social bonds. These recurrent combinations of professional presentations and personal sharing facilitate the exchange of knowledge, appreciation of the scientific work of others, scientific analyses of lab tests and data as well as personal disclosure of personal stories and idiosyncrasies within a psychologically safe space.

---

(continued)

**Box 6** (continued)

Most members of the LaBeaud lab team interact with members of local research teams in Kenya, Grenada, and Brazil. Each group operates within different academic, governmental, and philanthropic institutions; each with their own set of operational standards. These groups have their distinct set of characteristics and ways to approach research tasks that may conflict with the Stanford team's working style and preferences. Some examples are differences in work standards, communication styles, perception of time, sense of urgency, and conflict resolution style. To avoid unnecessary and unproductive conflict within and between the Stanford team and our offsite teams, we have done work to acknowledge our own default conflict styles and those of our partners so that we are able to approach conflict thoughtfully when it arises.

### 2.2.6   Dynamic Diversity

The problems that global health teams seek to address are ever evolving. As new research findings emerge, the expertise required to solve the seemingly intractable problem can shift, requiring the addition of new specialists or the use of new tools and techniques. The permeability of team membership, dependent on the ever-changing nature of the problem itself, means that the team, its goals, and the roles and responsibilities of its members are often in flux (Box 7). Few studies in the field of team science have examined the effects of bringing new members, with different expertise, into existing collaborations. Although research on groups and teams highlights how a shared identity and sense of belonging facilitate knowledge transfer and exploratory learning processes among existing team members and new members joining the group (Kane 2010), future research should explore the factors that support the onboarding of new team members in global health collaborations across different phases of the project work.

**Box 7: Dynamic Diversity**

One of the main characteristics of the LaBeaud team is its dynamic diversity. Recruitment of personnel has sometimes been planned and many times unplanned; often in response to students and professionals interested in learning or collaborating on the research and, also due to the evolution of the research itself. Every year we welcome new members and see others move forward onto their next professional endeavors.

As the LaBeaud lab team size increased, so did its operational and administrative structure. This growth called for practical tools to onboard new members and orient prospective members. A 26-page Onboarding Booklet has been very useful for us to integrate new members and most recently, a Lab Portal, allows new and current members find important documents and useful links to facilitate efficient uptake of study knowledge, communication, and administrative procedures. These practical tools help minimize anxiety and confusion that comes from lack of information and clarity.

Cross training and mechanisms for knowledge sharing has helped our lab to leverage expertise and avoid gaps in know-how when staff or mentees departed the lab upon completion of their degree or to pursue their own career aims. Such internal collaboration and cross training have helped maintain productivity amidst recurrent personnel transition during projects.

Key to this process has been keeping documentation and written protocols ranging from administrative to lab assay protocols and effective presentation formats. In addition, our lab allocates time for group sessions on effective communication, cultivation of a learning mindset, and agility in utilizing available human, educational and technical support resources.

# 3     Intervening Processes

Scientific teams can be strengthened by increasing the decision making and communication competencies of team members to enhance mutual understanding and the inclusion of diverse ideas and values (McGreavy et al. 2015) (see chapter "Foundations and Future Directions of Global Health Communication"). Among established teams, frequent face-to-face meetings (in person or online), whether for team coordination or substantive discussions, supports effective communication and contributes to increased productivity (Vasileiadou and Vliegenthart 2009) and greater research impact (Jeong and Choi 2015; Verbree et al. 2015). Coordination behaviors, including division of responsibility for tasks and knowledge transfer among researchers predict a range of project outcomes, such as producing new knowledge, creating new tools, and training students (Cummings and Kiesler 2007) (Box 8). Establishing clear decision-making processes and coordination of tasks can be particularly valuable when tackling global health challenges that involve collaborators spanning different institutions and continents, especially during an urgent public health crisis.

The use of technology to communicate (e.g., e-mail, phone, and video conferences) may be very useful for some project outcomes (e.g., development of new ideas and knowledge) yet may not give scientists an added advantage for other coordination outcomes e.g., track project progress over time, simultaneous group decision making, direct supervision of students) (Cummings and Kiesler 2005). Perhaps surprisingly, the use of emails, specifically, has not been found advantageous in terms of research productivity, and in some cases, it has been found detrimental due to information overload (Vasileiadou and Vliegenthart 2009). Studies on the use of social media and its effectiveness for various types of collaborations, including scientific collaborations, point to various considerations. Some studies indicate that the use of social media, although very effective and widely used for information exchange and coordination, lacks face-to-face interactions, and can be perceived as

**Box 8: Operational Structure**

The growth in size and diversity in the LaBeaud lab between 2014 and 2016 demanded coordinating structures and a shared identity to facilitate the collaboration with other research teams and to strengthen the Stanford team's operations.

Adding a project manager to the LaBeaud lab team allowed the creation of basic, yet critical pieces of an organizational and operational office structure. In addition to streamlining tasks and monitoring task completion, some elements had a less obvious objective: to make the environment for scientific pursuit one that would nurture the scientists themselves.

One of the earliest team building tasks was the articulation of the lab's identity through individual and group activities around values clarification, definition of the lab's work ethics, and conceptualizing our mission and vision, along with a directory of collaborators and a biyearly newsletter.

Such process culminated with collective definitions of "who we are", "what we intend to do", "why we do it", "which values guide us", and "how we do it". Each year we review these definitions to ensure our "who", "what", "why", and "how" are aligned with our collective actions and intended plans.

less effective in fostering community collaborations (Murthy and Lewis 2015).

## 3.1     Conflict

Research on conflict suggests that it can have both a positive and negative influence on the relationship between team collaboration and performance. For instance, task conflict (i.e., disagreements about the best way to accomplish work tasks) and relationship conflict (i.e., perceptions of interpersonal differences between people) can influence team performance and satisfaction in a negative manner (De Dreu and Weingart 2003). Process conflict, which is the disagreement over the procedures or methods the group should use for completing its joint work, can foster lower levels of team performance, satisfaction, and team coordination (Behfar et al. 2011). Examples of process conflict include disagreement concerning who is responsible for what work, how work should be completed, or when work should be accomplished (Jehn 1997). In teams composed of individuals who represent different national cultures, such as global health teams, process conflict may occur during discussion of when to show up for meetings or whether it is better to deal with conflict directly or indirectly (Behfar et al. 2006). Additionally, teams composed of individuals from diverse professional communities may also encounter process conflict because the approach to address problems may vary based on the heterogeneity of their training, tools, and methodologies (Stokols et al. 2008).

On the other hand, scholars suggest that moderate levels of task conflict can improve team creativity (Farh et al. 2010) and foster innovation (De Dreu 2006). Team creativity research suggests that knowledge creation endeavors often consist of and require combining existing knowledge that initially appeared unrelated or irrelevant to one another (Guilford 1959; Rietzschel et al. 2007). When focusing on the verbal exchange among individuals, the combination of perspectives and ideas can result from a process by which parties' conflict about their differences and affirm their areas of agreement. A consequence can be the creation of an outcome that is different from that which either party conceived of previously (Bartunek and Moch 1987; Van de Ven and Poole 1995). Research by Salazar and Lant (2018) suggests that scientific leaders can foster the combination of ideas, suggestions, and creativity by presenting shared problems that contain overlapping elements that intersect with the interests and expertise of the individual members and by communicating that the contributions of all diverse experts in the team are valued (Box 9).

### Box 9: Group Dynamics: Roles of the Leader and Team Members

The role of the leader for the Stanford team, overseas teams, and individual partners has been essential for coordinating, mediating, solving, and restoring team productivity and balance. Team science requires time, emotional and mental energy, transparency, and consistency. Mechanisms to lead groups processes that require their time and effort, take time to incorporate into routine operations. The leader's commitment to advance an agenda of team development becomes the positive force to counter dividing forces such as large workloads, non-productive conflict, and stress.

An example of such an initiative in the LaBeaud lab is the delivery of a series of team building sessions to foster self-awareness among members of the group. This step was considered the basis of any significant and lasting change for working relationships. Team members have discussed what group dynamics entail, the role of leadership in fostering a trustful and fair environment, individual personality traits and work styles (Myers-Briggs Type Assessment, Thomas-Kilmann Conflict Mode Instrument, and the Gallup Strengths Assessment), conflict resolution, and communication styles.

As a result of these sessions, the group arrived at a set of principles for effective communication to foster clarity and to avoid unnecessary and non-productive conflict in future interactions. This set of principles became our Communication Agreement document and now serves to guide effective communication among team members.

## 3.2 Coordination

Coordination has been defined as orchestrating interdependent actions (Marks et al. 2001). Transdisciplinary teams working on generating new scientific knowledge across disciplinary boundaries pose a particular challenge for coordination because knowledge and expertise are distributed across team members (Cannon-Bowers et al. 1993; Faraj and Sproull 2000) and geographic locations. Such complex collaborations may require more robust resources and greater attention to coordination strategies. Without sufficient resources to support teams, productivity can decline, yet projects with greater numbers of partner institutions tend to use fewer coordination mechanisms (Cummings and Kiesler 2007). Furthermore, multi-university projects that use fewer coordination mechanisms yield poorer outcomes (Cummings and Kiesler 2007). The observed coordination costs of large teams, especially those that are cross-disciplinary or span multiple sites, countries and time zones, may be due to the extended time and effort needed to develop shared knowledge of one another's disciplinary contributions to the project, shared terminology for the collaborative science, and a mutually agreed-upon conceptual model.

These above-mentioned coordination costs warrant the need for leadership, management, and communication practices to bridge institutional cultures, policies, and procedures across boundaries (Fiore 2008; Hall et al. 2012; Vogel et al. 2014) (Box 9). The behaviors of leaders that support coordination when engaged in creative ventures are important to consider (Mumford et al. 2012). The leader's social skills (i.e., persuasion, perspective taking, group facilitation) and the ability to create shared understanding (i.e., concrete production missions: planning the structure and timing of a task, but not the conduct of the work) are at the center of influence within the team's workflow. A leader can facilitate the awareness of who knows what by forming and fostering connections between members who may be unfamiliar with one another. This assists the team in open communication across boundar-

> **Box 10: The Stanford Team Structure and Coordination**
>
> Although the LaBeaud Lab team has established open communication and shared decision-making practices, there is a formal basic operational structure composed of a Principal Investigator, a Lab Manager, a Data Manager, and a Projects Manager.
>
> Coordination among these four lead roles has proven essential for the effective advancement of the various research projects that take place at any given time. Clear, timely, and effective communication has been key for success. Historically, instances of flaws in coordination and communication led to conflicts in our lab. We learned that those conflicts negatively impact the group dynamics even if in subtle ways.
>
> Direct and frequent communications, consultations, feedback, and sharing of ideas and resources with peers, staff, leaders, mentors, and community members have become standard processes in our transdisciplinary research projects.
>
> Hierarchies do exist due to levels of knowledge and expertise as well as established by institutional structures and economic/political realities but a conscious effort for horizontal interactions and inclusive decision making prevails for us as a principle and as the norm.

ies while buffering them from competing time demands (Ancona and Caldwell 1992) (Box 10).

## 3.3 Macro Factors

External features can include general dimensions such as the type of task and its complexity (e.g., high technology product development), the organization that employs the team (Cohen and Bailey 1997; Kozlowski et al. 1999; Salazar et al. 2012) and the national context. The impact of these external influences on teamwork and team performance cannot be understated (Hackman 1987). The science of team science literature suggests that researchers tend to collaborate with members from their research institutions (Dhand et al. 2016; Mayrose and Freilich 2015). When difficulties arise, it is often because of the geographic distance between collaborators involved in scientific collaborations (Harris et al. 2012). Yet, despite such challenges, scientific collaborations spanning organizational and regional boundaries are beneficial and often necessary when phenomena, such as infectious diseases, transcend geographic territories.

Global health collaborations, by their very nature, operate across distinct localities around the globe. The consequence is that scientific collaboration is influenced by the cultures of the country and the distinct norms, rules, laws, and practices that define the various regions from which collaborators hail. The various infrastructural differences between nations can, at times, create bottlenecks in the workflow of taskwork due to transferring funds, establishing non-disclosure agreements, or gaining access to local resources and intended populations. Sometimes a global health initiative or project can be hindered by the dynamics between nations as macro-level policies shape how science and public health interventions can proceed. Interacting and partnering with regional centers that support cross-boundary work, such as the African Union, are critical as these unifying bodies can support effective articulation with national or local partners, who may be fragmented.

When working together in a global health team, each member is influenced by socio-economic-political environments in which they grew up, the academic institutions where they acquired their formal education, the requirements imposed by the sources of funding they use to conduct the research, and other influences (Box 11). These macro factors influence how we relate to the persons with whom we participate in our research projects. Most, if not all our decisions, are influenced by social, economic, and political contexts that shape our beliefs, choices and decisions in addition to our personal needs and preferences.

> **Box 11: Macro Factors**
>
> The LaBeaud lab team has recognized macro factors as real and impactful, while at the same time remaining committed to rigorous and systematic checks and balances, to stick to data-driven and rational conclusions.
>
> Our team contends with personal, social class and geopolitical privilege by virtue of operating within an economically and technologically advanced country. Individually and as a group our team is committed to assess recurrently if and how our privileges influence our thoughts, assumptions, and behavior when interacting with collaborators outside the United States.
>
> We understand that we must be vigilant to counter colonizing tendencies in our research. We deeply believe in our community partners' self-determination and empowerment. Moreover, we believe that non-Western and non-academic ways of knowing are to be valued and incorporated into our research and considered as part of valid scientific outcomes.
>
> This vigilance takes place both at the personal level and at the institutional level when our beliefs and values clash with established bureaucratic and financial systems of both grantors and recipient institutions that do not mirror the realities of global health research and support equitable solutions.

## 4    Conclusion & Discussion

The science of team science (SciTS) is an emerging field of research that has recognized the need for research teams to develop a capacity for equitable and impactful transdisciplinary collaboration. Although attempts have been made to draw upon and apply theoretical frameworks to interdisciplinary teamwork (Fiore 2008), many questions remain about its implications for global health scientific collaborations. The focus of this chapter is to bring together the insights gathered from the SciTS and highlight how they can guide scholars engaged in global health research. This chapter also sheds light on new areas of investigation that are needed, such as best practices to support diversity and team productivity and effective practices to onboard new team members into new and established groups of scientific collaborators.

Ultimately, global health practitioners are working to generate knowledge that can alleviate human suffering. The technical, scientific tools to pursue that goal are often the focus of scientists' conversations; however, the tools to foster effective social interactions, although equally important, are seldom discussed, investigated, or purposefully implemented. SciTS helps to address this gap by shedding light on best practices to foster productive and satisfying teams in global health that integrate the scientist into the science.

## Glossary

**Collective intelligence:** Knowledge that arises from a group collaboration that would not normally have come about if the individuals had not exchanged information and expertise with one another on a topic (Woolley et al. 2010).

**Convergence:** "Convergence comes as a result of the sharing of methods and ideas by chemists, physicists, computer scientists, engineers, mathematicians, and life scientists across multiple fields and industries. It is the integration of insights and approaches from historically distinct scientific and technological disciplines" (Committee on Key Challenge Areas for Convergence and Health 2014; p. 8.).

**Cross-disciplinary:** Any collaboration between groups from more than one discipline. An overarching term that encompasses multi-, inter- and trans-disciplinary collaborations (Stokols et al. 2008). See individual definitions of these terms.

**Interdisciplinary:** Research collaboration between two or more disciplines undertaken jointly between two or more individuals from each discipline, in a way that integrates information, data, and concepts (Stokols et al. 2008).

**Multidisciplinary:** Research collaboration between groups belonging to two or more disciplines that is performed in a sequential, additive manner where each group contributes independently to achieve the result (Stokols et al. 2008).

**Team science:** Collaborative scientific research conducted in an interdependent manner by individuals working in small teams or larger groups (Cooke and Hilton 2015).

**Transdisciplinary:** A collaboration between two or more disciplines that integrates concepts and methods to an extent that transcends each, leading to the creation of a new discipline (Stokols et al. 2008; Falk-Krzesinski et al. 2010; National Research Council 2014) Transdisciplinary research is marked by the inclusion of non-academic participants, particularly those most affected by the issue addressed in the research (Stock and Burton 2011).

## References

Ancona DG, Caldwell DF. Demography and design: Predictors of new product team performance. Organ Sci. 1992;3:321–241.

Ancona DG, Chong C. Cycles and synchrony: The temporal role of context in team behavior. Res Manag Groups Teams. 1999;2:33–48.

Bakker RM, Boros S, Kenis P, Oerlemans LAG. It's only temporary: Time frame and the dynamics of creative project teams. Br J Manag. 2013;24(3):383–97.

Bartunek JM, Moch MK. First-order, second-order, and third-order change and organization development interventions: a cognitive approach. J Appl Behav Sci. 1987;23(4):483–500.

Behfar KJ, Kern M, Brett J. Managing challenges in multicultural teams. In: Chen Y-R, editor. National culture and groups, Research on Managing Groups and Teams, vol. 9. Bingley: Emerald Group Publishing Limited; 2006. p. 233–62.

Behfar KJ, Mannix EA, Peterson RS, Trochim WM. Conflict in small groups: The meaning and consequences of process conflict. Small Group Res. 2011;42(2):127–76.

Berger PL, Luckmann T. The social construction of reality: A treatise in the sociology of knowledge. Garden City: Anchor Books; 1966.

Bloodhart B, Balgopal MM, Casper AMA, McMeekin LBS, Fischer EV. Outperforming yet undervalued: Undergraduate women in STEM. PLoS One. 2020;15:e0234685.

Bluedorn AC, Denhardt RB. Time and organizations. J Manag. 1988;14(2):299–320.

Cannon-Bowers, J. A., Salas, E., & Converse, S. (1993). Shared mental models in expert team decision making. In N. J. Castellan, Jr. (Ed.), Individual and group decision making: Current issues (pp. 221–246). Lawrence Erlbaum Associates, Inc.

Castillo R, Grazzi M, Tacsir E. Women in science and technology: What does the literature say? Inter-American development bank, Technical note no. IDB-TN-637; 2014.

Cohen SG, Bailey DE. What makes teams work: Group effectiveness research from the shop floor to the executive suite. J Manag. 1997;23:239–90.

Committee on Key Challenge Areas for Convergence and Health. 2014; p. 8.

Cooke NJ, Hilton ML, National Research Council. Overview of the research on team effectiveness. In: Enhancing the effectiveness of team science. National Academies Press (US); 2015. https://doi.org/10.17226/19007.

Crenshaw K. Demarginalizing the intersection of race and sex: a Black feminist critique of antidiscrimination Doctrine, feminist theory, and antiracist politics. University of Chicago Legal Forum; Issue 1, Article 8; 1989.

Cronin MA, Weingart LR. Representational gaps, information processing, and conflict in functionally diverse teams. Acad Manag Rev. 2007;32:761–73.

Cummings JN, Kiesler S. Collaborative research across disciplinary and organizational boundaries. Soc Stud Sci. 2005;35(5):703–22.

Cummings JN, Kiesler S. Coordination costs and project outcomes in multi-university collaborations. Res Policy. 2007;36(10):1620–34.

Davenport TH, Thomas RJ, Cantrell S. The mysterious art and science of knowledge worker performance. Sloan Manag Rev. 2002;44:23–30.

Day DV, Gronn P, Salas E. Leadership capacity in teams. Leadersh Q. 2004;15:857–80.

De Dreu CKW. When too little or too much hurts: evidence for a curvilinear relationship between task conflict and innovation in teams. J Manag. 2006;32(1):83–107.

De Dreu CKW, Weingart LR. Task versus relationship conflict, team performance, and team member satisfaction: A meta-analysis. J Appl Psychol. 2003;88:741–9.

Dembe AE, Lynch MS, Gugiu PC, Jackson RD. The translational research impact scale: development, construct validity, and reliability testing. Eval Health Prof. 2014;37(1):50–70.

Dhand A, Luke DA, Carothers BJ, Evanoff BA. Academic cross-pollination: the role of disciplinary affiliation in research collaboration. PLoS One. 2016;11(1):e0145916.

Drucker PF. Knowledge-worker productivity: the biggest challenge. Calif Manag Rev. 1999;41:78–94.

Ely RJ, Thomas DA. Cultural diversity at work: the effects of diversity perspectives on work group processes and outcomes. Adm Sci Q. 2001;46(2):229–73.

Emmanuelides PA. Towards an integrative framework of performance in product development projects. J Eng Technol Manag. 1993;10:363–92.

Falk-Krzesinski HJ, Börner K, Contractor N, Fiore SM, Hall KL, Keyton J, Uzzi B. Advancing the science of team science. Clin Transl Sci. 2010;3(5):263–6.

Faraj S, Sproull L. Coordinating expertise in software development teams. Manag Sci. 2000;46:1554–68.

Farh JL, Lee C, Farh CIC. Task conflict and team creativity: aquestion of how much and when. J Appl Psychol. 2010;95(6):1173–80.

Fiore S. Interdisciplinarity as teamwork: How the science teams can inform team science. Small Group Res. 2008;39:251–77.

Fiore S, Salas E, Cannon-Bowers JA. Group dynamics and shared mental model development. In: London M, editor. How people evaluate others in organizations. Laurence Erlbaum Associates, Inc; 2001. p. 309–36.

Fleming ND. Teaching and learning styles: VARK strategies. Christchurch: Neil Fleming; 2001.

Gevers JMP, van Eerde W, Rutte CG. Team self-regulation and meeting deadlines in project teams: Antecedents and effects of temporal consensus. Eur J Work Organ Psy. 2009;18(3):295–321.

Gevers JMP, Rispens S, Li J. Pacing style diversity and team collaboration: the moderating effects of temporal familiarity and action planning. Group Dyn Theory Res Pract. 2016;20(2):78–92.

Guan J, Yan Y, Zhang J. How do collaborative features affect scientific output? Evidences from wind power field. Scientometrics. 2015;102:333–55.

Guilford JP. Traits of creativity. In: Anderson HH, editor. Creativity and its cultivation. New York: Harper & Row; 1959. p. 142–61.

Hackman JR. The design of work teams. In: Lorsch JW, editor. Handbook of organizational behavior. Prentice-Hall; 1987. p. 315–42.

Hackman JR, Morris CG. Designing work for individuals and groups. In: Hackman JR, Suttle JL, editors. Improving life at work: Behavioral science approaches to organizational change. Goodyear; 1975. p. 242–58.

Hall KL, Vogel AL, Stipelman B, Stokols D, Morgan G, Gehlert S. A four-phase model of transdisciplinary team-based research: Goals, team processes, and strategies. Transl Behav Med. 2012;2:415–30.

Hall KL, Vogel AL, Croyle RT, editors. Strategies for Team Science Success. Handbook of evidence-based principles for cross-disciplinary science and practical lessons learned from health researchers. Cham: Springer Nature; 2020.

Harris JK, Provan KG, Johnson KJ, Leischow SJ. Drawbacks and benefits associated with inter-organizational collaboration along the discovery-development-delivery continuum: a cancer research network case study. Implement Sci. 2012;7(1):1–13.

Hedt-Gauthier B, Airhihenbuwa CO, Bawah A, Burke KS, Cherian T, Connelly MT, Hibberd PL, Ivers LC, Jerome JG, Kateera F, Manabe YC, Maru D, Murray M, Shankar AJ, Shuchman M, Volmink J. Academic promotion policies and equity in global health collaborations. Lancet. 2018;392(10158):1607–9.

Huan J, Gates AJ, Sinatra R, Barabasi A-L. Historical comparison of gender inequality in scientific careers across countries and disciplines. Proc Natl Acad Sci USA. 2020;117(9):4609–16.

Jehn KA. A qualitative analysis of conflict types and dimensions in organizational groups. Adm Sci Q. 1997;42:530–57.

Jeong S, Choi JY. Collaborative research for academic knowledge creation: How team characteristics, motivation, and processes influence research impact. Sci Public Policy. 2015;42(4):460–73.

Kane AA. Unlocking knowledge transfer potential: Knowledge demonstrability and superordinate social identity. Organ Sci. 2010;21:643–60.

Kozlowski SWJ, Bell BS. Work groups and teams in organizations. In: Borman WC, Ilgen DR, Klimoski RJ, editors. Handbook of psychology: Industrial and organizational psychology. London: Wiley; 2003. p. 333–75.

Kozlowski SWJ, Gully SM, Nason ER, Smith EM. Developing adaptive teams: a theory of compilation and performance across levels and time. In: Ilgen DR, Pulakos ED, editors. The changing nature of performance: implications for staffing, motivation, and development. Jossey-Bass; 1999. p. 240–92.

Kuhn T. The structure of scientific revolutions. Chicago: University of Chicago Press; 1962.

Leahey E, Beckman CM, Stanko TL. Prominent but less productive: The impact of interdisciplinarity on scientists' research. Adm Sci Q. 2017;62(1):105–39.

Lee Y, Walsh JP, Wang J. Creativity in scientific teams: Unpacking novelty and impact. Res Policy. 2015;44(3):684–97.

Luke DA, Sarli CC, Suiter AM, Carother BJ, Combs TB, Allen JL, Beers CE, Evanoff BA. The translational science benefits model: a new framework for assessing the health and societal benefits of clinical and translational sciences. Clin Transl Sci. 2018;11(1):77–84.

Maddux WW, Lu JG, Affinito SJ, Galinsky AD. Multicultural experiences: a systematic review and new theoretical framework. Acad Manag Ann. 2021;15(2):345–76.

Marks MA, Mathieu JE, Zaccaro SJ. A temporally based framework and taxonomy of team processes. Acad Manag Rev. 2001;26:356–76.

Mayrose I, Freilich S. The interplay between scientific overlap and cooperation and the resulting gain in co-authorship interactions. PLoS One. 2015;10(9):e0137856.

McGreavy B, Lindenfeld L, Bieluch KH, Silka L, Leahy J, Zoellick B. Communication and sustainability science teams as complex systems. Ecol Soc. 2015;20(1)

McKinnon M, O'Connell C. Perceptions of stereotypes applied to women who publicly communicate their STEM work. Human Soc Sci Commun. 2020;7(160)

Mohammed S, Angell LC. Surface- and deep-level diversity in workgroups: examining the moderating effects of team orientation and team process on relationship conflict. J Organ Behav. 2004;25:1015–39.

Mohammed S, Nadkarni S. Temporal diversity and team performance: the moderating role of team temporal leadership. Acad Manag J. 2011;54(3):489–508.

Mohammed S, Nadkarni S. Are we all on the same temporal page? The moderating effects of temporal team cognition on the polychronicity diversity–team performance relationship. J Appl Psychol. 2014;99(3):404–22.

Mohammed S, Alipour KK, Martinez P, Livert D, Fitzgerald D. Conflict in the kitchen: temporal diversity and temporal disagreements in chef teams. Group Dyn. 2017;21:1–19.

Mumford MD, Friedrich TL, Vessey WB, Ruark GA. Collective leadership: Thinking about issues vis-a`-vis others. Indus Org Psychol. 2012;5:408–11.

Murthy D, Lewis JP. Social media, collaboration, and scientific organizations. Am Behav Sci. 2015;59(1):149–71.

National Research Council. Convergence: facilitating transdisciplinary integration of life sciences, physical sciences, engineering, and beyond. Washington, DC: The National Academies Press; 2014.

O'Connell C, McKinnon M. Perceptions of barriers to career progression for academic women in STEM. Societies. 2021;11(2):27. https://doi.org/10.3390/soc11020027.

Olson EM, Walker OC, Reukert RW. Organizing for effective new product development: the moderating role of product innovativeness. J Mark. 1995;59:48–62.

Rietzschel EF, Nijstad BA, Stroebe W. Relative accessibility of domain knowledge and creativity: the effects of knowledge activation on the quantity and originality of generated ideas. J Exp Soc Psychol. 2007;43(6):993–46.

Salazar MR, Lant T. Facilitating Innovation in Interdisciplinary Teams: The role of leaders and integrative communication. InformSci. 2018;21:157–78.

Salazar MR, Lant TK, Fiore SM, Salas E. Facilitating innovating in diverse science teams through integrative capacity. Small Group Res. 2012;43:527–58.

Salazar MR, Feitosa J, Salas E. Diversity and team creativity: Exploring underlying mechanisms. Group Dynamics. Theory Res Pract. 2017;21(4):187–206.

Schiling MA. Strategic management of technological innovation. New York: McGraw-Hill; 2005.

Stock P, Burton RJF. Defining terms for integrated (multi-inter-trans-disciplinary) sustainability research. Sustainability. 2011;3(8):1090–113. https://doi.org/10.3390/su3081090

Stokols D, Misra S, Moser RP, Hall KL, Taylor BK. Ecology of team science: understanding contextual influence on transdisciplinary collaboration. Am J Prev Med. 2008;35:S96–S115.

Van de Ven AH, Poole MS. Explaining development and change in organizations. Acad Manag Rev. 1995;20(3):510–40.

van Knippenberg D, Haslam SA. Realizing the diversity dividend: Exploring the subtle interplay between identity, ideology, and reality. In: Haslam SA, van Knippenberg D, Platow MJ, Ellemers N, editors. Social identity at work: Developing theory for organizational practice. Psychology Press; 2003. p. 61–77.

van Knippenberg D, Schippers MC. Work group diversity. Annu Rev Psychol. 2007;58:515–41.

van Knippenberg D, van Ginkel WP, Homan AC. Diversity mindsets and the performance of diverse teams. Organ Behav Hum Decis Process. 2013;121:183–93.

Vasileiadou E, Vliegenthart R. Research productivity in the era of the internet revisited. Res Policy. 2009;38(8):2009.

Verbree M, Horlings E, Groenewegen P, der Weijden IV, van den Besselaar P. Organizational factors influencing scholarly performance: a multivariate study of biomedical research groups. Scientometrics. 2015;102:25–49.

Vogel AL, Stipelman BA, Hall KL, Nebeling L, Stokols D, Spruijt-Metz D. Pioneering the transdisciplinary Team Science approach: Lessons learned from National Cancer Institute grantees. J Transl Med Epidemiol. 2014;2:1027.

Wageman R, Gardner H, Mortensen M. The changing ecology of teams: new directions for teams research. J Organ Behav. 2012;33:301–15.

Woolley AW, Chabris CF, Pentland A, Hashmi N, Malone TW. Evidence for a collective intelligence factor in the performance of human groups. Science. 2010;330(6004):686–8.

Woolley AW, Aggarwal I, Malone TW. Collective intelligence and group performance. Curr Dir Psychol Sci. 2015;24(6):420–4.

World Economic Forum. Global gender gap report. 2022. Retrieved from http://reports.weforum.org/globalgender-gap-report-2022

Wuchty S, Jones BF, Uzzi B. The increasing dominance of teams in the production of knowledge. Science. 2007;316:1036–9.

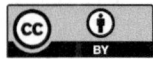

# Foundations and Future Directions of Global Health Communication

Maya Adam, Jennifer Gates, Nokwanele Mbewu, and Till Bärnighausen

*Communicating health messages to global audiences involves meeting people where they are and engaging them with equal parts science, compassion, and inspiration.*

## Abstract

Globally, lack of equitable access to easy-to-understand health information leaves many people poorly equipped to understand their health—and vulnerable to misinformation. In response to this need, health communication specialists must develop innovative, theory-driven approaches to engaging diverse populations with compelling messages. As we develop our approaches to health communication, we must address the needs of our audience, taking into account their education, language, literacy level, or cultural affiliations. If our goal is to reach the broadest spectrum of people worldwide, the guiding question for anyone designing global health messages should be: How do we make science-based health messages accessible to diverse, global audiences, some of whom rarely seek out health information through traditional public health platforms? In this chapter, we will explore the need for global health communication, some basic theoretical foundations of health communication, and recent innovations in this arena. We hope you will feel our passion for this exciting field and consider building it into your career. Helping our fellow global citizens to be engaged and informed participants in the care of their health is a critical step towards improving health outcomes. This is the primary goal of effective global health communication.

M. Adam (✉)
Department of Pediatrics, Stanford School of Medicine, Stanford University, Stanford, CA, USA

Heidelberg University, Heidelberg Institute of Global Health (HIGH), Heidelberg, Germany
e-mail: madam@stanford.edu

J. Gates
Icahn School of Medicine at Mt. Sinai, New York, NY, USA
e-mail: jennifer.gates@icahn.mssm.edu

N. Mbewu
The DG Murray Trust, Cape Town, South Africa

T. Bärnighausen
Heidelberg University, Heidelberg Institute of Global Health (HIGH), Heidelberg, Germany

Department of Global Health and Population, Harvard T. H Chan School of Public Health, Cambridge, MA, USA

Africa Health Research Institute, AHRI, Somkhele, KwaZulu-Natal, South Africa
e-mail: till.baernighausen@uni-heidelberg.de

## Keywords

Health communication · Global health · Health equity · Health literacy

## Author Perspective

We are scientists, caregivers, teachers and life-long learners who share a deep fascination with global health communication. Our diverse professional pathways allow us to bring different perspectives to this chapter. In Germany, Till Bärnighausen leads a large global health institute and studies the impact of global health interventions on human health outcomes. In South Africa, Nokwanele Mbewu helps community health workers to communicate health messages to their clients effectively. In the US, Jennifer Gates evaluates innovations in global health communications while completing her residency in Pediatrics. Designing interventions for global audiences, Maya Adam experiments with new health communication approaches at the intersection of education and entertainment. We came together through health communications collaborations spanning 7 years and three continents. These collaborations emerged from a shared passion for developing, testing and delivering

**Key Tenets**

1. Effective global health communication interventions engage diverse groups by being accessible, culturally inclusive and tailored to the health literacy level of the audience.
2. In order to reach our target audiences, we need to meet them where they are, via the channels through which they regularly consume information.
3. Storytelling and incorporating best practices from the arts and entertainment can help us to make global health messages more engaging and more effective, especially for hard-to-reach audiences.
4. Effective global health communication relies on effective communication within and across the teams creating and distributing global health messages.
5. This chapter addresses SDG #3, Good Health and Wellbeing.

impactful global health communication interventions—a passion we hope to share with you.

# 1 Introduction to Health Communication

## 1.1 Why Do We Need Effective Global Health Communication?

The science underlying health is a bit like the ocean: It's deep and wide and dark in many places. Unless you're a trained deep-sea diver, it can be scary and seem almost impossible to find your way around underneath the surface. Health research and the health systems that rely on it can feel similarly overwhelming—especially for people who face language or literacy barriers. Even experts in other fields of study can find it hard to understand and navigate the field of health sciences. This presents a real problem because, when it comes to our health, misinformation or even ineffective communication of key health messages can have serious consequences for people living all over the world. Finally, as discoveries—or new health challenges—emerge, we rely on effective global health communication to rapidly share that information with the public. This can be critical for managing acute health threats and supporting our fellow global citizens in understanding how they can live longer, healthier lives. In this chapter, we'll explore some of the theoretical frameworks for health communication and how different approaches to health communication have helped facilitate behavior change. We will also share how our modern digital environment is catalyzing innovations in health communication that are likely emerging as you read this. If you enjoy learning, teaching, counseling, or simply touching the lives of others in ways that could meaningfully improve their health, the field of health communication might be a professional area of interest for you. Join us as we explore the foundations and future directions for global health communication.

## 1.2 What Is Health Communication and What Are the Major Challenges to Effective Health Communication?

Health communication has been defined as: "the study and use of communication strategies to inform and influence decisions and actions to improve health" (Prevention CfDCa 2020). The content itself varies greatly, and any form of science-driven (evidence-based) health message—from a public service announcement aired around the world to a pamphlet handed to a new mother by her community health worker—qualifies as health communication. The main goal is to take a complex idea or recommendation that has been vetted by research within the scientific community and present it in a way that is accessible to everyone, especially the intended or "target" audience.

Sounds simple, right? Prepare to be surprised! While simplifying and conveying accurate health messages to the public *sounds* straightforward, there are significant practical challenges to effective health communication. Let's explore a few of them.

(a) **Low health literacy**: Differential access to health information, language and literacy barriers can contribute to low health literacy. In the health communication field, health literacy is defined as "the ability of an individual to obtain and translate knowledge and information in order to maintain and improve health in a way that is appropriate to the individual and system contexts." (Liu et al. 2020) Low health literacy is one of the biggest, real-world challenges to health communication. People who struggle to read, understand or apply health recommendations are far less likely to make informed health-related decisions (Schiavo 2013). The best, science-driven information, presented accurately to the public, can have little benefit for people who struggle to understand or apply it to their lives.

(b) **Audience diversity**: As health communicators, we sometimes need to create health messages that can scale quickly across audiences. In these situations, we generally reach more people when we create content that can benefit audiences from various cultures, geographic regions, languages, education, and literacy levels. For interventions to be effective globally, they need to thoughtfully integrate these audience characteristics and, ideally, be "glocalizable". Glocalization is the adaptation of globally accessible content for local resonance. By designing the health messages, stories, and visual elements of our content with the broadest possible audience in mind, we make it more likely that our health communication interventions will be easily adaptable for different settings—and more likely to resonate with diverse audiences. If our goal is to distribute important health messages globally, including reaching marginalized audiences, we are more likely to succeed if we design health communication content—from the outset—with an appreciation for audience diversity (Adam et al. 2021a). At the other end of the spectrum, health messages that are intended to reach narrower target audiences—especially those who share specific cultural norms or practices—are likely to be more successful if they feature characters who look and speak in ways that are familiar to those audiences. The take-home message here is that it's essential to define your intended target audience before designing the communication tools to reach them optimally.

(c) **Distribution**: The most rigorously researched, science-driven health messages can't do much to promote healthy behaviors if they never reach their target audiences. Distribution is one of the greatest challenges facing health communicators, yet it's often a problem we fail to consider until it's too late.

The temptation, all too often, is to think that if we create sound, sensible health messages, people will somehow find their way to the content. Ironically, audiences with the most to gain from preventive health messages are often the least likely to seek them out or bring them to attention. This results from the fact that marginalized and underserved populations are less likely to have access to health services where medical professionals routinely distribute health communication. Furthermore, public health programs delivered through schools and other community organizations are less likely to be adequately funded in communities that don't have the luxury of prioritizing preventive health measures. A lack of reliable internet access can translate into a lower likelihood of health messages reaching the people that need them the most. Distribution of health communication content remains a significant challenge and needs to be considered early on in the intervention development process (Aronson 2004; Pakenham-Walsh et al. 1997).

(d) **Reactance**: Have you ever been told you're not supposed to do something, only to find yourself wanting to engage in precisely that behavior? If someone tells you to reduce the amount of sugar in your diet, do you find yourself craving chocolate cake? Well, you're not alone. One of the reasons why persuasive health messages fail is that they can arouse motivations to reject them. This phenomenon is called *reactance,* and research exploring psychological reactance suggests that overly directive/restrictive health messages can leave the recipient of the message feeling like their freedom is being threatened (Brehm and Brehm 2013). To restore that freedom, people will sometimes actively engage in "bad behavior." Luckily, research also suggests that reactance can be partially overcome by using specific message design strategies. For example, when the person delivering the health recommendation is perceived as familiar or likable, the message's recipient is less likely to experience reactance (Silvia 2005). Similarly, when the health message is embedded in a story, reactance to the recommendation can be reduced.

(e) **Engagement**: Time use surveys and patterns of leisure time consumption suggest that people are increasingly feeling pressured for time, even during their limited periods of so-called "leisure time." An increasing number of people around the world now *identify* time as their most precious resource. In many countries, people spend more and more of their time on screen-based activities. The rapid expansion of content choices makes it increasingly challenging to engage target audiences with content related to their health (Glorieux et al. 2010; Schwartz 2004). So, not only do health communicators need to create content that is science-driven and accessible to their audiences, they need to make content that is engaging enough to compete with a multitude of other media options for a limited attention span (Fig. 1).

These challenges can all be overcome—and we'll explore approaches for doing so later in this chapter. But whenever we work to overcome challenges, we need a driver—a guiding goal or reason for getting better at what we do. In the case of designing more effective health communication interventions, the reason is health equity—giving each person a fair chance to reach their full health potential. All too often, the challenges described above contribute to health disparities. 'Health disparities' is a term used to describe the tendency for specific diseases or health conditions to be more common and more severe in vulnerable or underserved populations (Schiavo 2013). Health disparities result in major differences in health outcomes across populations. In some groups of people, diseases that are relatively easy to treat or prevent end up causing serious health problems—partly because health messages don't reach everyone in ways that are accessible to them.

This imbalance, or inequity, can be partially addressed by designing health communication

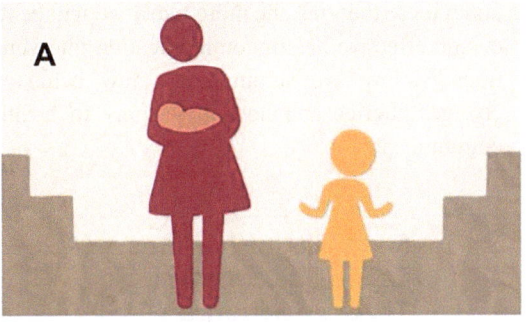

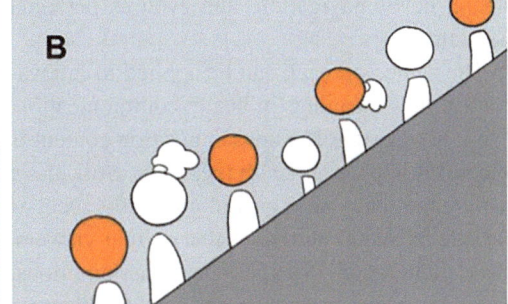

Fig. 1 Examples of culturally accessible character designs

A.  This animation prototype was used in a breastfeeding campaign for mothers from diverse cultural backgrounds living in South Africa
B.  This animation prototype was used for a global COVID-19 awareness video
C.  This animation prototype was used for a global nutrition education program

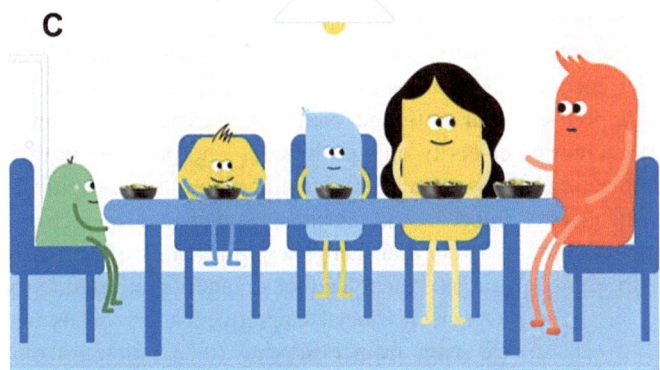

**Fig. 1** Examples of culturally accessible character designs (**a**) This animation prototype was used in a breastfeeding campaign for mothers from diverse cultural backgrounds living in South Africa (**b**) This animation prototype was used for a global COVID-19 awareness video (**c**) This animation prototype was used for a global nutrition education program

content to reach underserved or vulnerable groups. In some cases, this can be more easily achieved by involving members of an underserved group in designing their health messages. Human-centered design (HCD) is an approach that involves target audiences and local stakeholders in the design and production of their health content (Adam et al. 2018; Holeman and Kane 2020). When this approach is used authentically, it can increase the likelihood that the intended health messages will resonate with their target audience. HCD can also foster a sense of ownership that facilitates broader distribution within the target audience.

Human-centered design may be an especially useful approach for tailoring health communication interventions to specific communities. Other approaches may be equally powerful when the goal is to rapidly reach diverse audiences—sometimes even on a global scale. The concept of design-driven innovation—also called *innovation of meaning*—was first described by Roberto Verganti (Verganti 2018; Verganti and Öberg 2013). What is innovation of meaning? Consider this: every product or service we engage with has both an obvious function and a deeper meaning or significance in our lives. Verganti uses the example of candles. Their overt function (their original purpose) was to provide light, but for many people, candles have come to signify much more—relaxation, romance, or celebration, for example. The first mobile phones were invented to allow us to make calls from outside the home. Apple introduced an innovation of meaning with the iPhone by assigning the cellphone a new meaning—a new significance—in our lives. We now increasingly use our phones for entertainment, social media, news, navigation, and even as personal assistants.

The same approach can be applied to innovation for new meanings in health communication. The function of health communication content is to convey important health messages. Still, if we can embed these messages in culturally accessible (glocalizable) narratives that delight viewers, make them laugh, or experience other emotions, we assign new meaning to traditional health communication. The result of such innovation can maximize audience engagement, minimize reactance and support spontaneous sharing (ie: audience-led distribution) across social media and other platforms (Adam et al. 2020). Applying these frameworks can help us get closer to achieving the greater goals of health communication: improved health literacy, positive behavior change, better health outcomes for more people around the world and ultimately, health equity (Schiavo 2013).

## 2 An Overview of Behavior Change Theories

Successful health communication interventions raise awareness about health behaviors and shift social norms towards healthier outcomes. As designers of health communication interventions, we can more successfully support behavior change when we have a basic understanding of some key behavior change theories. These theories can provide a framework for identifying and understanding the factors that influence people's decisions about their health behaviors. For example, a person's beliefs about a given health behavior are one of the most critical determinants of whether or not they will perform it. A person who doesn't believe that flossing their teeth will prevent cavities and gum disease is unlikely to get out the floss each night before bed. Understanding and applying behavioral theories can help to identify the beliefs that need to be changed to promote healthier behaviors. The more we know

about these theories, the more likely we will be to design effective health communication interventions. Below, we summarize a few behavior change theories and how they apply to health communication.

## 3 Social Cognitive Theory (Also Called Social Learning Theory) (Bandura 1985; Bandura and Walters 1977)

Have you ever watched a healthy cooking show and felt inspired to go to the kitchen and get out your pots and pans? Or maybe you follow a celebrity on social media who posts about their new exercise regimen and how it has positively impacted their health. You do some research and find out that there's a similar class offered near you, and then you feel strangely motivated to try it yourself. Social Cognitive Theory posits that we learn from observing (then imitating) others—through social interactions, exposure to media, or other experiences.

The key components of social cognitive theory are:

(a) Attention: The behavior captures our attention; we notice it for some reason.
(b) Retention: At a later point in time, we remember the behavior that was modeled.
(c) Reproduction: We look for ways to copy the behavior—by seeking the resources we need in our environment to make it happen.
(d) Motivation and performance: We feel an internal impulse to continue performing the behavior regularly.
(e) Self-efficacy: We feel confident that we can continue to perform the behavior, even without the initial stimulus that triggered its adoption.

People learn by watching others—especially those they like, respect or admire—in conducive environments. For designers of health communication interventions, it's often more powerful to show a desirable behavior being enacted (ideally after establishing an affinity for the person performing the behavior) instead of simply telling your audience why that behavior will be good for them.

## 4    Transtheoretical Model of Behavior Change (Prochaska et al. 2009)

Also called the Stages of Behavior Change Model, the Transtheoretical Model of Behavior Change helps us to understand and view behavior change as a process with defined stages. Each stage is characterized by a different level of motivation or readiness. The five stages are:

(a) Pre-contemplation: In this stage, a person may be exposed to information about a given health behavior, but they have no intention of adopting it.
(b) Contemplation: A person enters this stage when they begin to consider adopting a given health behavior.
(c) Decision: In this stage, the person decides to adopt the health behavior.
(d) Action: During this stage, a person tries to adopt the health behavior in the short term.
(e) Maintenance: This stage is achieved when a person has managed to sustain the performance of the health behavior—usually for 6 months or longer.

Health communication specialists can use this model to segment target audiences into groups based on their stage of behavior change. Targeted messages can then be designed to support specific stages. For example, at the beginning of the COVID-19 pandemic, social distancing was an unfamiliar practice for many worldwide populations. Many people were in the early stages of change, learning about the benefits and/or con-

sidering the rationale and feasibility of staying apart from others. Health messages during this phase needed to emphasize why they made sense, as well as modeling it in action by likable, trusted, or respected role models. As the pandemic dragged on and pandemic fatigue set in, maintaining this health behavior emerged as a related but separate priority. By understanding where our audience is on their behavior change journey, we can design communication tools that will optimally support them.

## 5    Theory of Reasoned Action (Fishbein 1979; Madden et al. 1992)

Simply stated, this theory posits that a person's likelihood of performing a given health behavior is proportional to the strength of their intention to perform that behavior. The strength of their intention depends on their *attitude* towards the behavior and *subjective norms* (i.e., the attitudes of influential individuals around them towards the behavior). For example, suppose I have a negative attitude toward eating vegetables. Let's say I generally don't like them. Then let's say I spend much time with friends who wouldn't dream of missing out on their peas, carrots, and kale. They find my aversion to vegetables a major character flaw, and I can feel them judging me every time we eat together. According to the Theory of Reasoned Action, these two forces will factor significantly in my ultimate decision of whether or not I will order (and eat) that salad.

For designers of health communication interventions, the Theory of Reasoned Action can be useful for identifying factors that influence people's core attitudes, for profiling target audiences (those who would most benefit from the intervention), and for conducting program evaluations. Having said that, it's important to remember that while behavioral intent is a predictor of a given health behavior, we need to be careful about assuming that intention to adopt a behavior will translate into the *actual* adoption of that behavior. Behavioral intent is a good marker but not a direct measure of behavior change. Having said that, behavior change theorists highlight a subset of variables that are believed to have a direct and significant influence on the strength of behavioral intentions within any given target audience:

(a) Attitude: How positive am I towards the behavior and the idea of me, as an individual, enacting the behavior? An example: my doctor recommends that I get a mammogram to screen for early signs of breast cancer. I feel positive about the technology, and I understand the scientific basis for this health screening. On the other hand, I don't love

going *in* for a mammogram, but overall, I feel that the benefits of getting it done outweigh the discomfort, so I decide to do it.

(b) Perceived norms: How does my support structure feel about the behavior? My friends are all pretty health-conscious, so they have all gone to get mammograms. If I don't get mine (and admit it to them), they might judge me or think of me as someone who doesn't believe in science. Social norms can be a powerful motivator for behavior change.

(c) Personal agency: Continuing with this example, how confident do I feel that I will be able to make the appointment, make time in my work schedule to attend the appointment, and find my way to the clinic where I'll get my mammogram done? Many populations,

**Fig. 2** Overview of factors affecting behavior change

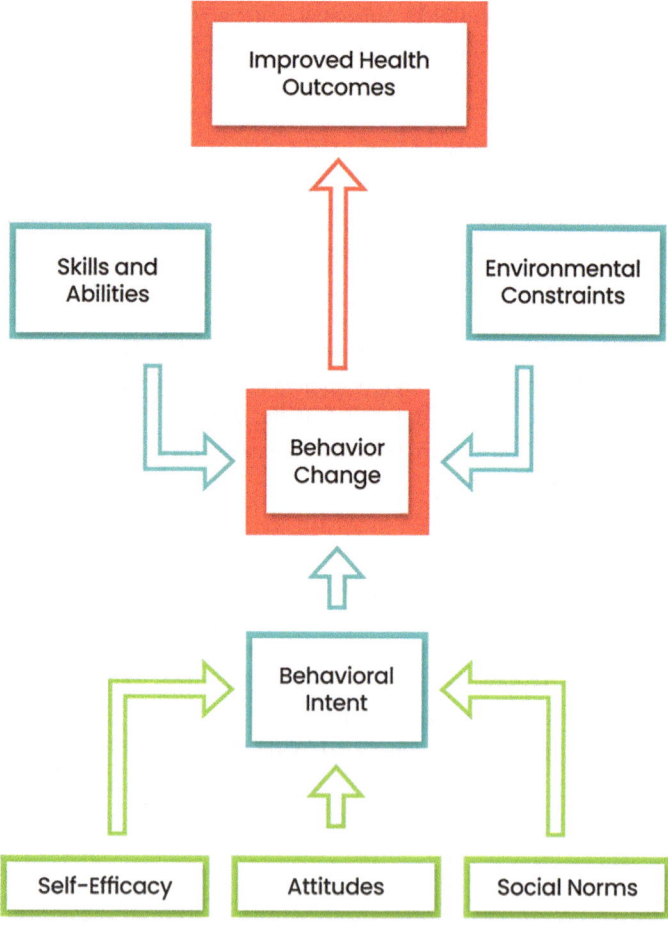

especially those struggling with low health literacy or language barriers, struggle to access services or adopt health behaviors even if these seem readily available to them. For this reason, health communication content that enhances personal agency can have a meaningful positive impact on health behaviors (Fig. 2).

## 6    Theoretical Foundations for Entertainment-Education

Entertainment-Education (E-E) is an approach to health communication in which narratives are built around key health messages. The goal of the resulting content (traditionally soap operas and radio dramas) is to entertain and educate target audiences. Academics like Dr. Arvind Singhal, widely considered one of the gurus of E-E, have documented the impact of the approach, suggesting that this mode of health communication can be a powerful way of engaging audiences in health messages and shifting their attitudes and behaviors (Singhal and Rogers 2012, 2002). By building compelling narratives around essential health messages, they can be delivered in ways that engage hard-to-reach audiences, increasing their knowledge, improving their attitudes and changing their health behaviors. Capitalizing on the broad appeal of entertainment, E-E interventions are grounded in *Social Cognitive Theory*. By showing people how they can live safer, healthier, and happier lives, social norms and attitudes shift. Other theoretical foundations of E-E include:

(a) *Elaboration Likelihood Model*: This model defines two contributing pathways toward attitude shifts that predict behavior change. The first "central route" is influenced by an individual's motivation and ability to understand the information presented. For designers of health communication content, this translates into essential decisions about the length of the content and the kind of language used. Getting these things right makes it much more likely that viewer attitudes will

be impacted via the central route. The second "peripheral route" involves cues that are embedded in the content and contribute to its acceptability to the viewer. Positive, peripheral cues, like compelling characters and an emotion-driven storyline, can enhance peripheral attitude changes. While these changes may be less enduring than central attitude changes, they can increase a person's motivation to process health messaging via the central route (Petty and Cacioppo 1986).

(b) *Drama Theory*: This theory suggests that, as a plot unfolds, the viewers' emotional involvement with the main characters facilitates identification with them. When we start to see ourselves or the people we care about in the characters of a narrative, it becomes much more likely that we will consider adopting the behaviors demonstrated by those characters (Sood et al. 2003) (Fig. 3).

## 7    Future Directions in Health Communication

To reach our target audiences, we need to understand where they are—and then meet them there. This means communicating in ways that are both accessible and compelling (i.e., meeting people where they are cognitively) and meeting our audiences on the platforms they regularly use—more and more via online interactions and social media. Research suggests that screen time and social media use are increasing around the world (Bucksch et al. 2016; Ernest et al. 2014). While this trend may have some negative health implications for society, these platforms also provide a powerful forum for health communicators to engage hard-to-reach audiences. They can help us to facilitate rapid, spontaneous (sometimes viral) dissemination of important, science-driven messages (Guadagno et al. 2013; Lutkenhaus et al. 2020). For preventive health messages, we must remember that many people don't search for health information until they get sick. This means that we need to find ways of making our content so compelling that it can compete with an enormous body of non-health-related content

**Fig. 3** Elaboration
likelihood model

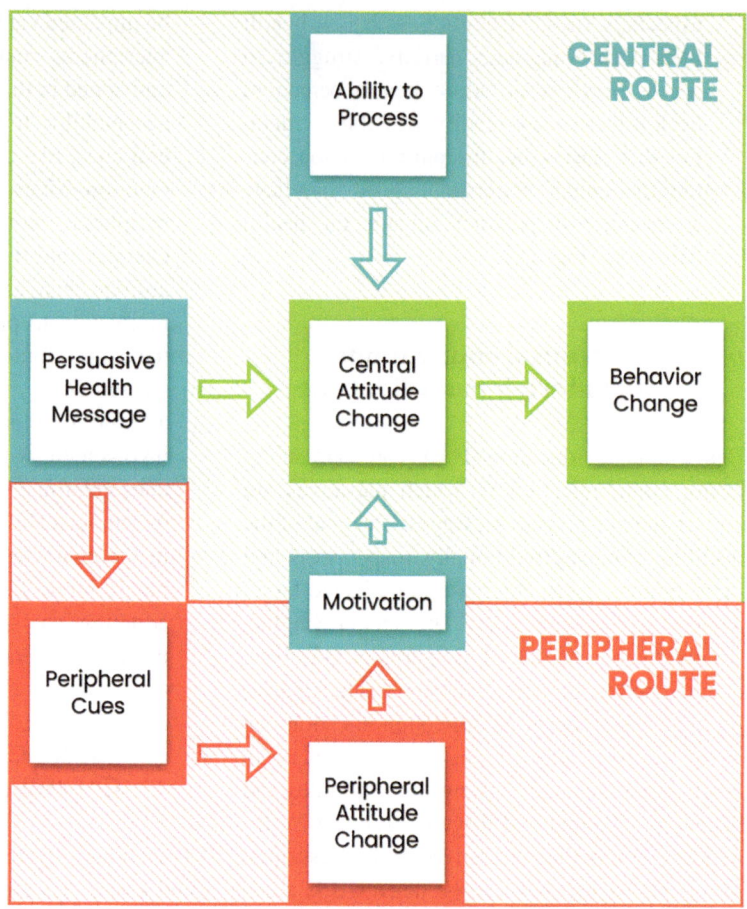

continuously vying for the attention of audiences whose discretionary time is limited.

The global experience of the COVID-19 pandemic underscored the urgent need for more innovative approaches to health communication. Public health agencies at all levels felt immense pressure to develop and deploy health messages without the delays often associated with sluggish public health campaigns. Early in the pandemic, these delays left a vacuum on social media that was filled by a sea of misinformation. We watched as the social media stratosphere exploded with anecdotal health recommendations—many of which played upon a sense of widespread fear and insecurity. This misinformation was ineffective at best and life-threatening at worst (Brennen et al. 2020; Kouzy et al. 2020).

For effective, science-driven health communication interventions to rise above this anecdotal noise, they need to be equally (or ideally, more) engaging than the competing content offerings. While our health messages often need to be developed on lower budgets, research into the characteristics of "viral" content can provide valuable insights for those wishing to create compelling health content. The main strategy, often overlooked by health communicators and educators in all fields, is the compelling nature of content that arouses emotions (Guadagno et al. 2013). When we see something that moves us— or even makes us laugh—we are more likely to pay attention to that content and decide to share it with others. This desire—to share our emotional state with others—falls under the umbrella of a phenomenon called emotional contagion, which can also involve sharing emotional experiences indirectly (for example, by forwarding a short health-related video). By creating content that

**Case Study: Innovation in Global Health Communication during COVID-19**

During the COVID-19 pandemic, a team of health communication specialists developed a collection of short, engaging videos created for a global audience so they could spread rapidly and organically via social media. To facilitate sharing, all of the content was open access and freely available for organizations of all types to re-post. They urgently needed to a) combat the misinformation that was going viral on social media and b) engage hard-to-reach audiences, including those who shy away from health communications—often because they perceive these to be too didactic or prescriptive. In the United States, the COVID-19 pandemic also fueled a polarization of public opinion, including beliefs about important health interventions like vaccination. Globally, lack of equitable access to easy-to-understand health information left many people in the dark about the pandemic—and more vulnerable to misinformation. In developing this approach to health communication, we were trying to address the needs of all people, regardless of their education, language, literacy level, or cultural affiliations.

An early challenge the team faced was how to design characters, settings, and narratives that would translate globally. They had done some research exploring the acceptability of culturally neutral animated characters with global audiences (Adam et al. 2021a). In response to this data, they decided to design characters that were so simple, they could resonate universally. Some videos, created especially for children, needed characters with facial features and other details. The content creators featured collections of diverse characters, including children from different countries and ethnicities. Using a wordless approach was one of the most exciting innovations. The team's first wordless pilot film went viral—reposted by public health agencies and media outlets in more than 12 countries—indicating that this was a compelling direction for global messaging. The Journal of Global Health published a commentary where the approach was called "designing for extreme scalability (Adam et al. 2020)." This experiment, motivated by an urgent real-world need, suggested that it was possible to create and organically spread content that showed more than telling.

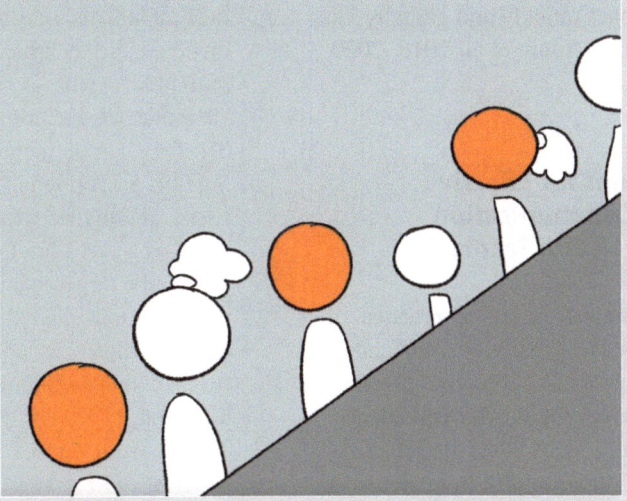

moves people and capitalizing on the human desire to share our emotional experiences with others, we can boost the dissemination of science-driven, reliable health messages while reducing reactance to those messages (Dillard and Pfau 2002; Gardner and Leshner 2016).

Short, animated story-based videos (SAS videos) designed for broad distribution via social media have shown promise for increasing behavioral intent to practice healthy behaviors and enhancing audience engagement. One of the exciting "future directions" for global health communication, these short, culturally accessible health communication interventions are readily glocalizable—they can quickly and easily be adapted for many global settings. Incorporating best practices from entertainment-education, communication theory, and the animation industry, such innovations can help to overcome the major challenges we explored at the beginning of this chapter (including low health literacy, audience diversity, distribution, reactance, and engagement) (Kincaid 2002; Slater 2002; Yoon and Malecki 2010). Research from Stanford University and the Heidelberg Institute of Global Health suggests that further experimentation with rapidly designed, broad-reaching health communication interventions is urgently needed and demonstrates the exciting potential for spreading critical health messages quickly and globally via social media networks (Adam et al. 2019, 2020, 2021a, b).

## 7.1 Foundations for Effective Internal Communication in Global Health Teams

At its core, communication is the practice of exchanging thoughts, ideas, emotions, and understanding between people. Like any practice, effective communication needs to have a cadence, be assessed frequently to evaluate its effectiveness, and be revised thoughtfully in response to the changing needs of the people involved. In this chapter, we have explored the most effective ways of communicating our global health messages to the world. We also need to remember the

---

**Best Practices for Internal Communication within and across Teams (Quintanilla and Wahl 2018; Perkins 2008)**

Several practices have been shown to support effective internal communication when practiced consistently in various professional sectors, including global health research. These are summarized below:

1. **Regular meetings**

   Finding the right cadence for regular team strategy meetings is as important as ensuring they occur. This is usually an iterative process involving feedback from all participants, especially as the cadence is being established. Team meetings allow everyone to stay informed of (and involved with) the activities, challenges, and achievements of the team. Running meetings efficiently by designating a timekeeper and setting an agenda supports their ongoing value to the team. Avoiding long meetings (over 50 min) communicates to all participants that their time is valued.

2. **Inclusive Environments**

   Invitations to attend regular meetings should include all team members involved in the project. In the case of individuals who serve as peripheral advisors but are not directly responsible, they can be invited to attend meetings on an "optional" or "if available" basis. If smaller groups in a project meet separately, brief updates should be sent to the larger team or meeting notes uploaded to a shared project hub, especially when critical decisions are reached that will impact the project's direction.

3. **Transparency and Clarity**

   Clear and concise communication within and between teams fuels the progress of any project. Consider the type, audience, and purpose of your communications.

(continued)

(a) *Type*: When might it be better to schedule a call with a collaborator instead of sending a lengthy email? When is a face-to-face meeting the best option? Choose the best type of communication using a cost-benefit analysis. Select the format that yields the most beneficial exchange of information (for all parties involved) using the available resources—including time.

(b) *Audience*: How well does the sender know the recipients of the information, and how would the audience prefer to receive it? What are the competing time pressures on your audience, and how can your communications integrate as seamlessly as possible into their daily informational inputs?

(c) *Purpose*: Is the main goal of the communication to share key information with many people or to brainstorm a solution for an acute challenge with just one person? These differing purposes will require different communication approaches.

4. **Respect**

Across different roles, and regardless of hierarchy, all team members should commit to communicating with respect for each other and for collaborators outside of the team. Leaders who model this behavior end up with teams that function more cohesively and productively.

5. **Online Collaboration Tools**

Across many different sectors, including academic research, teams are increasingly relying on methods of internal communication that are social, collaborative, and virtual. This trend has catalyzed the growing use of enterprise social media (ESM) platforms for many organizations. Used sensibly, these platforms can help connect people, their ideas and the information needed to implement them collaboratively within various types of teams (Anders 2016).

importance of establishing strong communication channels within and between the research teams who will be discovering, defining, and communicating critical global health messages (also see Chapter "Team Science and Infectious Disease Work: Exploring Challenges and Opportunities").

## 7.2    In Conclusion

As teachers, researchers, healthcare providers, and global citizens, we have a responsibility to create windows into an enormous vault of health science research so that people around the world can understand it and apply it to their lives. Gone are the days when health science and the research underlying it were intended only for experts in this field. Around the globe, people enjoy better health outcomes when they take an active role in understanding, managing, and promoting their health. Creating compelling, accessible, and engaging health communication content can support the citizens of our world as we strive to live happier healthier lives.

We include the following reflection questions for readers who are considering a role or actively engaged in health communication, but the exercise can be beneficial to anyone. These questions highlight how we engage with health communication in daily life and how we can increase our awareness and apply these concepts to benefit our health and the health of others.

1. Think back to a health message that impacted your behavior. It can be anything from a school-based health message to a social media post. What was your experience of consuming that health communication content? What were the characteristics of the content that likely changed your attitude and affected your behavior? Was the change enduring, and why do you think it was or wasn't effective in the longer term?

2. Think about how you receive information daily, from social media news alerts to discussions with your neighbor. Make a list of these different sources of information and then think about ways they would (or would not)

be suited to distribute health messages to the public. Think about how you might best extend messages to vulnerable or hard-to-reach communities. Now you're thinking like a health communicator!

3. Think back to a story you heard that was not intended to be a health message, but it nevertheless impacted your health decision-making. Why do you think that story affected your health behaviors? If you worked in the health communication field, would you consider incorporating stories into the design of your interventions? Why or why not?

## Glossary

**Health communication:** The study and use of communication strategies to inform and influence decisions and actions to improve health (CDC 2020).

**Health literacy:** The ability of an individual to obtain and translate knowledge and information in order to maintain and improve health in a way that is appropriate to the individual and system contexts (Liu et al. 2020).

**Reactance:** A phenomenon wherein overly directive/restrictive health messages leave the recipient of the message feeling like their freedom is being threatened. In response, they will be more likely to practice the forbidden behavior to re-establish their perceived freedom (Brehm and Brehm 2013).

**Health disparities:** A term used to describe the tendency for certain diseases or health conditions to be more common and more severe in vulnerable or underserved populations (Schiavo 2013).

**Human-centered design:** An approach to intervention/product development that involves target audiences and local stakeholders in the design and production of their own health content/products (Adam et al. 2018).

**Design-driven innovation (innovation of meaning):** An approach to innovation wherein the central goal is not just to make an intervention or product more effective, but also to confer one or more new functions/purposes upon it (Verganti et al. 2018).

## References

Adam M, McMahon S, Prober C, Bärnighausen T. Human-centered design of video-based health education: an iterative, collaborative, community-based approach. J Med Internet Res. 2018;21(1):e12128.

Adam M, Tomlinson M, Le Roux I, LeFevre AE, McMahon SA, Johnston J, et al. The Philani MOVIE study: a cluster-randomized controlled trial of a mobile video entertainment-education intervention to promote exclusive breastfeeding in South Africa. BMC Health Serv Res. 2019;19(1):211.

Adam M, Barnighausen T, McMahon SA. Design for extreme scalability: a wordless, globally scalable COVID-19 prevention animation for rapid public health communication. J Glob Health. 2020;10(1):010343.

Adam M, Chase RP, McMahon SA, Kuhnert KL, Johnston J, Ward V, et al. Design preferences for global scale: a mixed-methods study of "glocalization" of an animated, video-based health communication intervention. BMC Public Health. 2021a;21(1):1223.

Adam M, Johnston J, Job N, Dronavalli M, Le Roux IM, N Mkunqwana, N Tomlinson, M McMahon, SA LeFevre, A Vandomael, KL Kuhnert, P Suri, et al. The Philani MOVIE study of a community-based mobile video breastfeeding intervention in Khayelitsha, South Africa: A cluster-randomized controlled trial. [Original research manuscript]. In press 2021b

Anders A. Team communication platforms and emergent social collaboration practices. Int J Bus Commun. 2016;53(2):224–61.

Aronson B. Improving online access to medical information for low-income countries. N Engl J Med. 2004;350(10):966–8.

Bandura A. Model of causality in social learning theory. In: Cognition and psychotherapy. Springer; 1985. p. 81–99.

Bandura A, Walters RH. Social learning theory. Englewood Cliffs: Prentice Hall; 1977.

Brehm SS, Brehm JW. Psychological reactance: a theory of freedom and control. Academic; 2013.

Brennen JS, Simon F, Howard PN, Nielsen RK. Types, sources, and claims of COVID-19 misinformation. Reuters Institute. 2020;7(3):1.

Bucksch J, Sigmundova D, Hamrik Z, Troped PJ, Melkevik O, Ahluwalia N, et al. International trends in adolescent screen-time behaviors from 2002 to 2010. J Adolesc Health. 2016;58(4):417–25.

CDC. Gateway to Health Communication: USA.gov; 2020 [Available from: https://www.cdc.gov/health-communication/. Accessed Jan 13th 2023.

Dillard JP, Pfau M. The persuasion handbook: developments in theory and practice. Sage; 2002.

Ernest JM, Causey C, Newton AB, Sharkins K, Summerlin J, Albaiz N. Extending the global dialogue about media, technology, screen time, and young children. Child Educ. 2014;90(3):182–91.

Fishbein M. A theory of reasoned action: some applications and implications. 1979

Gardner L, Leshner G. The role of narrative and other-referencing in attenuating psychological reactance to diabetes self-care messages. Health Commun. 2016;31(6):738–51.

Glorieux I, Laurijssen I, Minnen J, van Tienoven TP. In search of the harried leisure class in contemporary society: time-use surveys and patterns of leisure time consumption. J Consum Policy. 2010;33(2):163–81.

Guadagno RE, Rempala DM, Murphy S, Okdie BM. What makes a video go viral? An analysis of emotional contagion and internet memes. Comput Hum Behav. 2013;29(6):2312–9.

Holeman I, Kane D. Human-centered design for global health equity. Inf Technol Dev. 2020;26(3):477–505.

Kincaid DL. Drama, emotion, and cultural convergence. Commun Theory. 2002;12(2):136–52.

Kouzy R, Abi Jaoude J, Kraitem A, El Alam MB, Karam B, Adib E, et al. Coronavirus goes viral: quantifying the COVID-19 misinformation epidemic on Twitter. Cureus. 2020;12(3):e7255.

Liu C, Wang D, Liu C, Jiang J, Wang X, Chen H, et al. What is the meaning of health literacy? A systematic review and qualitative synthesis. Fam Med Community Health. 2020;8(2):e000351.

Lutkenhaus RO, Jansz J, Bouman MPA. Toward spreadable entertainment-education: leveraging social influence in online networks. Health Promot Int. 2020;35(5):1241–50.

Madden TJ, Ellen PS, Ajzen I. A comparison of the theory of planned behavior and the theory of reasoned action. Personal Soc Psychol Bull. 1992;18(1):3–9.

Pakenham-Walsh N, Priestley C, Smith R. Meeting the information needs of health workers in developing countries: a new programme to coordinate and advise. British Medical Journal Publishing Group; 1997.

Perkins PS. The art and science of communication: tools for effective communication in the workplace. Wiley; 2008.

Petty RE, Cacioppo JT. The elaboration likelihood model of persuasion. In: Communication and persuasion. Springer; 1986. p. 1–24.

Prevention CfDCa. Gateway to Health Communication: USA.gov; 2020. Available from: https://www.cdc.gov/healthcommunication/

Prochaska JO, Johnson S, Lee P. The transtheoretical model of behavior change. 2009

Quintanilla KM, Wahl ST. Business and professional communication: keys for workplace excellence. Sage Publications; 2018.

Schiavo R. Health communication: from theory to practice. Wiley; 2013.

Schwartz B. The paradox of choice: why more is less. Ecco, New York; 2004.

Silvia PJ. Deflecting reactance: the role of similarity in increasing compliance and reducing resistance. Basic Appl Soc Psychol. 2005;27(3):277–84.

Singhal A, Rogers EM. A theoretical agenda for entertainment—education. Commun Theory. 2002;12(2):117–35.

Singhal A, Rogers E. Entertainment-education: a communication strategy for social change. Routledge; 2012.

Slater MD. Entertainment education and the persuasive impact of narratives. 2002

Sood S, Menard T, Witte K. The theory behind entertainment-education. Entertainment-Education and social change: Routledge; 2003. p. 139–72.

Verganti R. Overcrowded: designing meaningful products in a world awash with ideas. MIT Press; 2018. p. 48.

Verganti R, Öberg Å. Interpreting and envisioning—a hermeneutic framework to look at radical innovation of meanings. Ind Mark Manag. 2013;42(1):86–95.

Yoon H, Malecki EJ. Cartoon planet: worlds of production and global production networks in the animation industry. Ind Corp Chang. 2010;19(1):239–71.

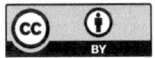

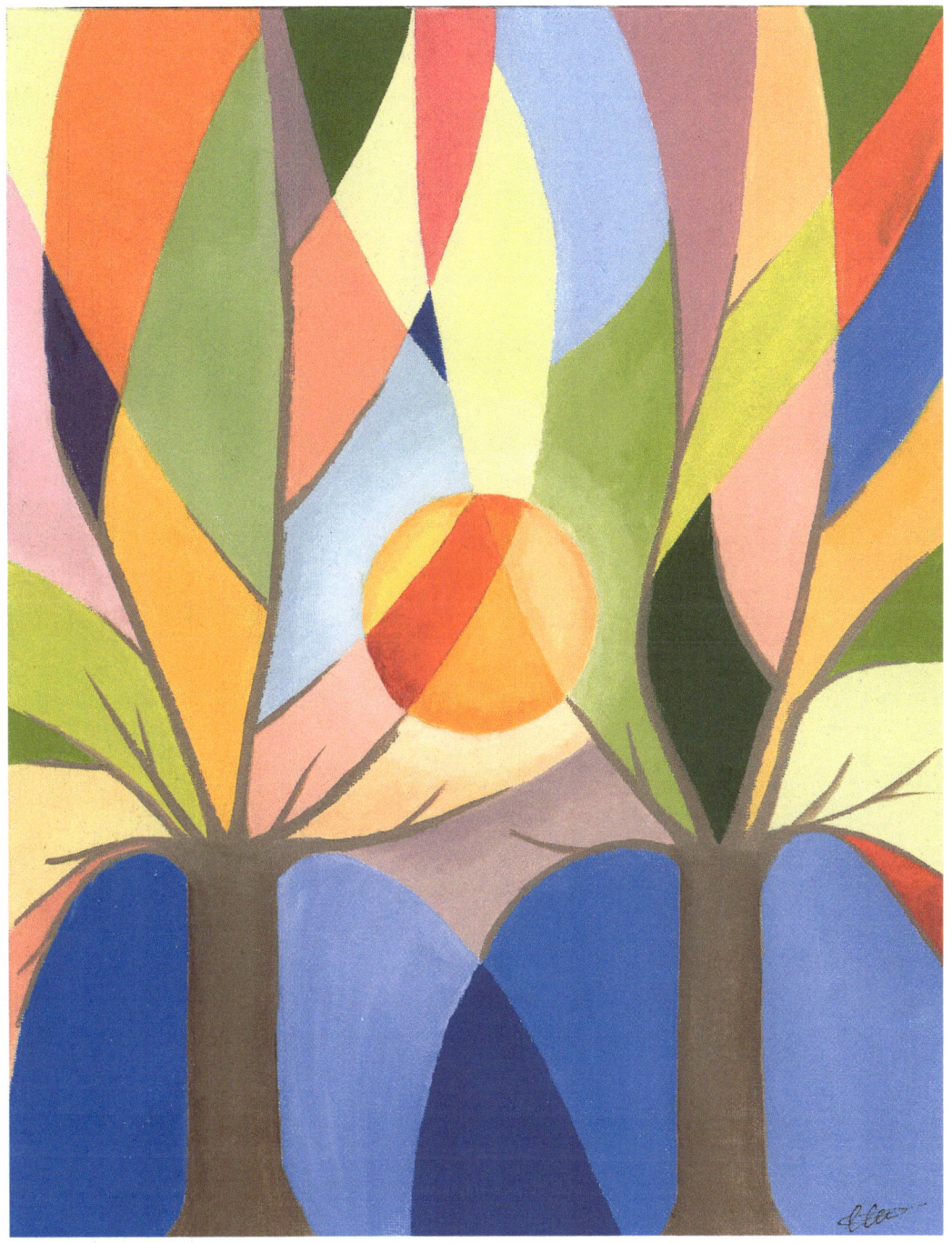

"Seeking Sun" by Mira Cheng

# Collective Learning: Power and Trust in Partnerships in the 3D Program for Girls and Women in Rural Pune District, India

Sia Nowrojee and Manisha Gupte

*There is no thing as a single-issue struggle because we do not live single-issue lives.*

Audre Lorde, Black, lesbian, mother, warrior, poet (1934–1992)

## Abstract

This chapter describes lessons learned through the partnerships jointly facilitated by the 3D Program for Girls and Women and Mahila Sarvangeen Utkarsh Mandal (MASUM) in rural Pune District, India, from 2017 to 2021. The analysis is done from our different perspectives, as one partner based in India and the other in the United States. We describe our process of joint learning as we navigated our own North-South partnership and other multisectoral partnerships; advanced gender equality by putting girls and women at the center of partnerships and decision-making; held those in power accountable to protect the rights of girls and women; adapted through COVID-19; and worked together intentionally on different 'sides' of our partnership. We explore power and trust within our own partnership and in the other partnerships we facilitated to address social determinants of health and advance gender equality. We highlight how different priorities and needs among stakeholders enriched the process when power differentials were managed in a spirit of trust and camaraderie, within a process of identifying and working towards shared commitments. Based on this analysis, we share lessons we learned and key tenets for global health and international development partnerships.

## Keywords

Partnerships · Power · Trust · Feminism · Gender equality

## Author Perspective

We are two feminists, one based in India, the other in the United States, who share a strong commitment to gender equality and social justice. We believe that girls and women should be at the center of the policies and programs that impact them; that they are best served when typical development and global health siloes are challenged, so that stakeholders can work together within a wholistic human rights framework to address structural inequalities and injustices; and that within that framework, diverse stakeholders can bring different perspectives and resources that add value to partnerships and programs.

S. Nowrojee (✉)
United Nations Foundation, Washington, DC, USA
e-mail: snowrojee@unfoundation.org

M. Gupte
Mahila Sarvangeen Utkarsh Mandal (MASUM),
Pune, Maharashtra, India

© The Author(s) 2024
A. Stewart Ibarra, A. D. LaBeaud (eds.), *Transforming Global Health Partnerships*, Sustainable Development Goals Series, https://doi.org/10.1007/978-3-031-53793-6_7

**Key Tenets**

1. Disrupt the Funder-Implementer Model: Local partners must be involved in strategic decision-making from the beginning about how to allocate, reallocate and utilize resources throughout the lifespan of the program.
2. Create Opportunities for People to Speak for Themselves and for Those in Power to Listen: Creating opportunities for people to speak for themselves, directly to those mandated to serve them, can strengthen global health planning outcomes.
3. Build Strong Relationships to Foster Trust and Strengthen Programs: Valuing different perspectives shaped by different experiences as part of one's methodology and program design will strengthen programs, interventions and outcomes
4. Move Beyond Binary Thinking: Rather than a North vs. South model, global health and international development would benefit from a 'sharing lessons learned' model across regions, economies and perspectives.
5. Diversity is a Strength: Diverse and even unlikely partnerships can lead to programmatic innovations, new resources, and greater impact.
6. Learning is a Critical Component of Successful Partnerships: Different experiences and perspectives result in different expertise that create opportunities for rich learning within partnerships of diverse stakeholders. This mutual learning can enhance the partnership to be greater than the sum of its parts.
7. This chapter addresses the following SDGs: 5: Gender Equality (cross-cutting and necessary for the achievement of all the other goals); 1: No poverty; 3: Good health and wellbeing; 4: Quality education; 6: Clean water and sanitation; 8: Decent work and economic growth; 10: Reduced inequalities; 16: Peace, justice, and strong institutions; 17: Partnerships for the goals

# 1    Background

This chapter provides an overview of lessons learned through diverse, and sometimes unlikely, partnerships jointly facilitated and navigated by the 3D Program for Girls and Women[1] and Mahila Sarvangeen Utkarsh Mandal (MASUM)[2] in rural Pune District, India, from 2017 to 2021. It includes insights we gained during a process of mutual learning as we:

- Facilitated and navigated our own North-South partnership and multi-sectoral partnerships;
- Advanced gender equality by putting girls and women at the center of partnerships and decision-making at the community level;
- Held those in power accountable to protect the rights of women and girls;
- Adapted through the COVID-19 pandemic; and
- Worked together intentionally on different 'sides' of our partnership.

We explore power and trust within our own partnership and in the other partnerships we jointly facilitated as we designed and implemented programs to address social determinants of health and advance gender equality.[3] We also highlight how different priorities and needs among stakeholders enriched the process when power differentials were managed in a spirit of trust and camaraderie, within a process of identifying and working towards shared commitments. Based on this analysis, we share the lessons that we learned and key tenets for global health and international development partnerships. Our insights and perspectives are informed primarily by our experiences, which we see as relevant to current and emerging frameworks and discourse on decolonization of international development and global health (see Chapter "Colonialism,

---

[1] For more information about the 3D Program for Girls and Women, see https://the3dprogram.org/

[2] For more information about Mahila Sarvangeen Utkarsh Mandal (MASUM), see https://www.masum-india.org.in/

[3] Throughout this chapter, '3D Program programs and interventions' refers to programs that were initiated and funded by the 3D Program and jointly designed and implemented with MASUM and other partners.

Decolonization, and Global Health"), feminist ways of working, and localization and community-based development (see Glossary for Key Terms and Frameworks).

The 3D Program for Girls and Women was founded in 2017 to advance gender equality and girls' and women's empowerment. From 2017 to 2021, the 3D Program worked in Pune District, Maharashtra State, India, demonstrating a multisectoral program model designed to help local governments work more efficiently across departments, and with civil society and the private sector, while strengthening women's voices and platforms to hold government accountable. MASUM, a key strategic and implementing partner in rural Pune, was founded in 1987 to strengthen women's self-reliance and consciousness of human and constitutional rights; empower women to put pressure on the State to fulfill its obligations towards its people; nurture women's physical and emotional health; provide vocational training and credit facilities to advance women's economic empowerment; create a sustainable and humane mode of development through people's active involvement; create a progressive space in society for all subordinated groups; and resist casteism, sexism, religious chauvinism, homo/transphobia and able-bodied hegemony.

Within India, Pune District and Maharashtra State rank high on economic development indicators and both have well-established, well-resourced local government bodies (Government of India 2021; India Development Review 2020). However, the status of girls and women remains low, as evidenced by indicators on sex ratio, early marriage, contraceptive choice, gender-based violence (GBV), digital access, and representation of women in the formal work force (International Institute for Population Sciences 2019; Woetzel et al. 2015). Building on these strengths and shortcomings, the 3D Program focused our programs in Pune on good governance, strengthening links between women's collectives and local government, increasing women's participation in local governance, and creating feedback loops to increase accountability (3D Program for Girls and Women 2018).

The 3D Program, MASUM and other implementing partners[4] used a feminist, pragmatic approach that prioritized girls and women, while engaging local government as a key stakeholder to increase accountability and reach girls and women at scale. We approached our work from a feminist perspective, ensuring that program decisions were informed by girls' and women's realities and priorities, and our work processes reflected mutual respect across all levels of our organizations.

At the same time, we sought out partnerships with government officials and worked to embed our approach in local government systems. We did this because government has both the reach and obligation to impact a large number of girls and women, and while difficult to change, has the systems in which to embed and sustain programs, policies and processes.

Reflecting shared priorities of both women's organizations and government, we addressed health, gender-based violence (GBV) in public spaces, education, and economic empowerment. MASUM's expertise and experience of community-based initiatives and advocacy to strengthen public health, demand comprehensive health rights, and focus on the social determinants of health were invaluable to the design and implementation of 3D Program interventions (see Box 1. for 3D Program Principles and Approaches).

---

**Box 1: 3D Program for Girls & Women: Principles and Approaches**

The 3D Program for Girls and Women was created to address the needs of girls and women wholistically, understanding that the lives of girls and women are multi-dimensional

(continued)

---

[4]Other 3D Program rural partners included the non-governmental organizations Chaitanya, the International Center for Research on Women (ICRW) Asia and Sangini. Urban partners included the Pune City waste pickers cooperative SWaCH and union Kagad Kach Patra Kashtakari Panchayat (KKPKP) and the Centre for Environment Education (CEE). The 3D Program was hosted in Washington DC by our partner the United Nations Foundation, and was funded by the Bill & Melinda Gates Foundation.

**Box 1** (continued)

and do not reflect the siloed nature of government and other programs. More specifically, the 3D Program was created to:

**Document:**

- Global, national and local evidence on what works to address complex, inter-related issues such as women's economic empowerment and public safety.
- Evidence on the status of girls and women, existing programs, resources, actors, opportunities and challenges in our program sites.
- Evidence and experiences on what drives stakeholders and sectors to work together.
- Our story on diverse platforms to assess and share lessons learned.

**Drive:**

- Key government departments, including health, education, rural development and women and child development, to work together.
- Stakeholders across government, civil society and the private sector to strategically align programming.
- Community collectives to strengthen girls' and women's voices in holding government accountable for effective solutions.
- Resources to fund and support sustained convergent action.

**Deliver:**

- Convergent district and municipal plans and programs with improved capacity to serve girls and women.
- Processes for girls and women to participate in and monitor government programs.
- Commitments by stakeholders across sectors to ensure sustainability.
- Better outcomes for girls and women in health, education, economic empowerment and public safety.

In 2020, after 3 years of implementation, the U.S.-based 3D Program conducted an internal assessment of the financial and operational impact of COVID-19 (see Box 2 for details on the impact of COVID-19). In consultation with our partners, and in accordance with social justice movements challenging traditional development and global health models, we decided to close U.S. operations, reallocate a significant portion of the remaining program budget, and transfer ownership of the program to partners in India, including MASUM, in 2021 (Nowrojee 2021a). The findings in this chapter include our joint reflections on our partnership and programs, as well as the transition of ownership of the program from a team in the Global North to partners in the Global South.

**Box 2: The Impact of the COVID-19 Pandemic**

Like other international development and global health programs, the 3D Program, MASUM and other partners were impacted by the COVID-19 pandemic. 3D Program sites in Pune District were within the first epicenter of the pandemic in India.

Globally, the pandemic exacerbated the impact of gender inequality and revealed weaknesses in government systems in delivering basic, emergency, and last-mile services. While the need for strong public health services was highlighted, so was the need for well-resourced, nimble education systems, along with inclusive housing policies, quickly activated financial safety nets, rights-based policing, far-reaching communications infrastructure, and effective and inclusive emergency responses.

The pandemic confirmed the need for convergence across sectors and between government, civil society, and the private sector to leverage an optimal combination of systems and reach, expertise and innovation, and resources. 3D Program platforms, which were designed to address disparities,

(continued)

inequalities, and barriers to access in a convergent way before COVID-19, proved effective in facilitating COVID-19 relief, information, and responses. Our partners such as MASUM and our platforms pivoted to support essential workers and migrant workers, distribute rations and other essential goods (especially to vulnerable groups such as single women), provided prevention and vaccine information and education, and facilitated access to life-saving services and supplies. The crisis effectively validated key components of our approach, laying the foundation for a role in COVID-19 recovery and post-COVID-19 programs.

The 3D Program and MASUM worked together to overcome some of the constraints posed by the pandemic at the bureaucratic, policy and intervention levels. We also identified and leveraged opportunities. For example, we reallocated savings from travel budgets to meet the needs of underserved groups, including women. The suspension of state-run public transport during lockdown enabled us to access over 200 otherwise unoccupied staff members of the Maharashtra State Road Transport Corporation (MSRTC) in Purandar taluka, and provide them with gender training, which had a significant impact on the way in which bus drivers and conductors understood their responsibilities in protecting the right to public safety of women and girls.

COVID-19 disrupted 3D Program operations. It stalled travel between the U.S. and India, as well as travel within India. The pandemic also resulted in the erosion and reallocation of donor funds, with a focus on localization. In 2020, the 3D Program effectively adjusted to online platforms, and partners such as MASUM adjusted and led program implementation. Ultimately, the U.S.-based 3D Program team closed down our U.S. operations and transferred ownership of the program to MASUM and other partners in India.

## 2 Facilitating Transformative Partnerships

By design, partnerships were at the heart of the 3D Program's approach of bringing together diverse stakeholders to advance gender equality. This section describes some of the key processes and components within our own partnership, as well as other partnerships we facilitated to address girls and women's needs and priorities.

### 2.1 Our Own North-South Partnership

The 3D Program and MASUM teams leveraged our differences to serve as strengths in our partnership. We had a clear understanding of our relative advantages, respected our different perspectives and approaches, and maximized the resources we each brought to the table. The 3D Program team understood that community-based organizations like MASUM have critical knowledge and skills. From previously working in similar networks, we also knew that we were aligned in terms of our feminist approaches and values, and deliberately sought them out as partners. As other feminists working to intentionally create and maintain equal, honest and productive partnerships have noted, the partnership between the 3D Program and MASUM teams was rooted in shared priorities, deep respect, growing trust, and genuine friendship (Johnson and O'Malley 2021). This positioned us well for working together in new ways, communicating honestly, reconciling differences, and facing challenges.

In terms of the resources and knowledge we each brought to our partnership, the 3D team brought global program experience, financial resources and the opportunity to try something new to our partnership. MASUM brought deep connections to local communities, participatory program design and implementation expertise, and knowledge of local government systems. Leveraging these, we co-created our interventions based on priorities identified by girls and women, drawing on both local and global best practice and ideas, and created the space to make mistakes, learn and adapt.

MASUM is firmly located within the communities it serves and provided valuable local knowledge and direct access to women community leaders and ensured ground truthing. The 3D Program team often adjusted plans based on insights and challenges identified by the MASUM team, which highlighted how realities on the ground required different approaches and adaptations. For example, we initially focused on creating multi-sectoral interventions by engaging government officials at the district level, relying on stated commitments in policy documents or the cooperation of individual influential officials. With MASUM's advice, we shifted our focus to the village level, where convergence was then driven by the demand of girls and women and government officials were directly held to account. Similarly, the MASUM team shifted their typical way of working to include government bureaucracy as an essential, rather than a peripheral partner, a key component of the 3D Program approach, leading to new relationships and fruitful interactions between MASUM and government officials and departments.

Local knowledge has long been the primary source of wisdom for those of us working in feminist movements around the world. However, even when the focus is on local contexts, programs should also be attuned to global trends, pressures and resources that impact those contexts and ensure that local decisions and solutions inform the global space. This two-way flow of information and expertise is critical for global health and international development programs to remain relevant and effective (Shaw 2014). The 3D Program US-based team was uniquely positioned both by geography and experience to do this, as a program hosted at the United Nations Foundation[5] and as a Global Member of the Movement for Community-led Development,[6] and could provide unique opportunities to highlight our work and to engage in dialogue with other initiatives across the globe working on gender equality, community development, multi-sectoral interventions, and global health.

*"The 3D Program and MASUM worked well together, leveraging their relative advantages to design and then implement a different way for girls and women to hold their communities and government officials accountable. While they brought different strengths and resources to the table, they also brought a shared commitment to the empowerment of girls and women and a mutual respect to the partnership, which enabled them to try new things, make mistakes, and learn from each other, which strengthened the program."*

Ravi Verma, Director, International Center for Research on Women Asia, 3D Program partner.

More practically, as partners in different countries with different roles, we prioritized communication in our operations. We had weekly team calls, as well as program-specific calls, to strategize, brainstorm, seek and provide feedback, troubleshoot and when necessary, to course-correct. The 3D Program team traveled to India several times a year, with a large part of those visits focused on full-team strategy and connection. Documentation was produced collaboratively, with all partners providing inputs and feedback. Our approach to the program was both intentional and iterative, allowing for strategic and practical changes as needed. As the program developed, so did our mutual trust and our relationship.

Over the 4 years, the nature of our partnership, our relative advantages and our ways of working together enabled the 3D Program and MASUM teams to build and implement the program. When faced with the decision to close U.S.-based operations, they enabled a smooth transition of the program to the partners in India, with MASUM playing a strong role in that process (Nowrojee 2021a).

## 2.2  Unlikely Partnerships[7]

Multi-sectoral action or what the 3D Program called 'convergence' requires a shared vision and coordinated but differentiated action by diverse

---

[5] For more information, see: https://unfoundation.org/

[6] For more information, see: https://mcld.org/

[7] The program details in this section were previously described in Jain K, Aralkar S, Buke G, Kedia S, Gupte M, Kothari S, et al. From Vulnerability to Leadership: Lessons Learned from Collective and Collaborative Action for Rural Girls and Women in India. Washington, DC: 3D Program for Girls and Women; 2021.

stakeholders, based on the resources, perspectives and objectives they bring to the partnership. The approach combats the persistent limitations of development programs caused by working in silos, with limited data and evidence and without the active engagement of the people they serve (Gupta 2017; Nowrojee 2017).

The 3D Program looked to various models on how to facilitate convergence. Within India, government departments also use the term 'convergence' to describe their interventions, but often limit multi-sectoral initiatives to the more typical girl- and women-focused departments of health, education, and women and child development. We sought to expand that focus, with the understanding that girls and women have a stake in all sectors, including water and sanitation, community development, transportation, workforce development, and public safety. Additionally, while many government officials recognized the value and need to work across sectors, and even wanted to, implementation was a challenge for often overstretched bureaucrats (Jain et al. 2021).

*"Too often we are not seeing the big picture, busy with the day-to-day work of government. The result is that we work in silos and see limited impact and limited satisfaction. To truly serve girls and women effectively, we need to coordinate multiple inputs and provide them simultaneously. By talking to each other within the Zilla Parishad and sharing data, we will be able to jointly plan and implement programs more effectively. By working with partners in civil society and the corporate sector, who can provide technical and other inputs, we can fill gaps and benefit from new methodologies and additional resources."*
—Suraj Mandhare, Indian Administrative Service Officer and former CEO of the Zilla Parishad, (District Council), Pune, Maharashtra State.

The Collective Impact approach provided a useful model for a convergent strategy. However, it recommends the creation of a new, purpose-build organization to manage the relationships and processes of the partnerships. It also highlights equity among all partners as being key to the process (Kania and Kramer 2011). We adapted elements of Collective Impact, but the 3D Program played a facilitative (but not separate) role in our partnerships, and we prioritized two key stakeholders: women's collectives and local government officials.

## Collaboration Between Women's Collectives and Government Officials

A key strategy of the 3D Program was bringing together those in power with those most impacted or neglected by the decisions those in power make. So, despite considerable distrust between government and civil society, the lumbering size of the government bureaucracy, and consistent, disruptive administrative turnovers, the 3D Program insisted on prioritizing government as a critical partner to reach girls and women at scale in a sustainable way. To increase accountability in government business, we also prioritized women's collectives,[8] and with MASUM, created multi-sectoral rural women's village collectives called Village Convergence Planning Committees (VCPCs) that brought these two key stakeholders together.

The objective of the VCPCs was to facilitate coordination and formal collaboration throughout government departments across sectors, create opportunities for girls and women to engage directly with local government officials, and to increase accountability for improved access, quality, and choice within government programs. Where there were gaps in government services, the 3D Program and MASUM teams engaged corporate and NGO partners.

In the pilot phase of the program, VCPCs were created in five villages in rural Pune.[9] Membership included girls and women, and local village administrative and elected officials, such as the *Sarpanch* or head of the village *Panchayat* or governing body, the *Talathi* or Revenue Officer, and the lead officials for each department, including the Accredited Social Health Activist (*ASHA)* or community health worker, the *Anganwadi* or local childcare center worker, the local police constable, the school principal, and the local water and sanitation officer.

The VCPCs proved popular with both girls and women, and local front-line government

---

[8] For example, the waste pickers trade union Kagad Kach Patra Kashtakari Panchayat (KKPKP) and cooperative, SWaCH in Pune City. More information can be found at http://kkpkp-pune.org/ and https://swachcoop.com/

[9] This included Naigaon and Bhivari villages in Purandar *taluka* (administrative block) and Mandoshi, Kharoshi and Dehane villages in Khed *taluka*, Pune District.

workers and elected officials. There was no equivalent forum for girls and women to identify and solve problems collaboratively with each other, as well as with those in positions of power at the village level. The well-established self-help group (SHG) model for women, a mechanism for rural women to gain and leverage collective power, particularly for economic empowerment, is popular, well organized and supported across Pune district by civil society organizations and the government (Mehra and Shebi 2018). However, SHGs do not provide women with a direct way to influence local governance or political processes.

The only other forum for women to influence local governance is the *Mahila Gram Sabha* (MGS) or the women's general body meeting at the village level. India's *Panchayati Raj* or rural governance system includes a provision for MGSs to be held regularly, prior to the *Gram Sabha* or village general body meeting, to enable women to identify priorities and prepare for participation in the *Gram Sabha*. However, MGSs are rarely held on a regular basis. Government and local elected officials complain that even when MGSs are held, women do not participate, whereas women insist that they would attend if they were held regularly and were not controlled by powerful men. Finally, there is no mechanism for adolescent girls in rural areas to have their voices heard and for them to participate in local governance. The VCPCs filled these gaps left by the restricted mandate of the SHGs, the absence of MGSs, and the lack of platforms for adolescent girls to engage directly with their community and government officials.

> *"MASUM inculcates confidence among women of being equal and having entitlement to rights, and the belief that they can challenge power relationships in politics and the bureaucracy. When they get organized and question the powers that be, they dislodge one brick of oppressive structures at a time, creating a seismic impact. The VCPC is one such effective intervention that helps balance the power by bringing rural women and girls to the center of planning and decision-making."*
> —Kajal Jain and Shailaja Aralkar, 3D Program consultants

The VCPCs were successful not just in serving as an effective platform to converge the perspectives and resources of women with those of govern-

ment and elected officials, but they were also effective in solving problems and leading to concrete outcomes. These included improving basic village facilities; increasing girls and women's access to and enrollment in government programs; and addressing strategic issues, such as securing women's property rights. During the COVID-19 pandemic, VCPC members continued to meet via phone and members shared data with government officials on the specific impact of COVID-19 on girls and women, a focus that was generally ignored in government responses. Overall, VCPCs have been credited by girls and women and government officials with:

- Increasing women's participation in local governance and decision-making;
- Raising awareness of girls' and women's realities and priorities among local officials;
- Creating a bond between local officials and the communities they serve;
- Strengthening local governance and women-led accountability of government actions;
- Facilitating COVID-19 relief, disseminating prevention information, identifying vulnerable families and individuals, and distributing vital emergency supplies, such as food rations; and
- Facilitating concrete outcomes to meet girls' and women's needs and address their priorities (Jain et al. 2021).

The VCPCs demonstrated that it is possible to create pathways for girls and women to interact directly and effectively with government officials and hold them accountable to increase access and improve the quality of services and programs. MASUM is scaling up and replicating the VCPC model in 25 additional villages in Purandar *taluka*, Pune District, and it continues to play a critical role in strengthening government and other programs for girls and women.

## Innovative Multi-Sectoral Partnerships

The 3D Program also facilitated several partnerships between stakeholders who typically do not work together to test solutions to problems raised by girls and women in VCPC meetings. MASUM took the lead in these partnerships, identifying and liaising with partners, designing the interventions, overseeing implementation and documenting outcomes. These partnerships led to pilot programs to increase:

- Economic opportunities for young rural women by making job skills training programs more accessible to them (3D Program for Girls and Women 2020);
- The safety of girls and women in public transportation to prevent GBV and enable them to pursue educational, job and other opportunities; (3D Program for Girls and Women 2021); and
- Options for menstrual hygiene management (MHM).

Each of these partnerships led to innovative demonstration programs that resulted in concrete outcomes for girls and women and generated useful lessons about effectively working across sectors to advance gender equality (see Box 3. for details

**Box 3: Multi-sectoral Partnerships Facilitated by The 3D Program and MASUM[a]**

| Objective | Gap and Gender Issues Addressed | Partners and Roles across Sectors | Structure | Outcomes |
|---|---|---|---|---|
| To increase economic opportunities for young rural women to match their aspirations and delay marriage | – Most job skills and placement programs focus on urban youth. <br> – Gender norms and lack of mobility prevent rural young women from accessing job skills programs. <br> – Without access to job skills programs, young rural women are at risk of early marriage. | – **Civil Society:** MASUM provided outreach and support to young women and their parents, training on related gender issues, and job placement in Purandar block. <br> – **Academia:** Shreemati Nathibai Damodar Thackersey (SNDT) Women's University Pune provided dormitories, meals and classroom facilities, and instruction in English, IT, typing and office etiquette. <br> – **Private Sector:** Tech Mahindra Foundation provided vocational training and job placement support in Pune city. | – Adapted an urban, long-term evening-class job skills program to be a 3-week residential summer program. <br> – Training included two vocational programs (Office Administration and Goods and Services Tax and Accounting) and other skills (IT, English, typing, job interview skills) and issues (GBV, menstrual hygiene management, sexual harassment in the workplace). <br> – Job placement support tailored to include opportunities in Pune city and in Purandar block. <br> – Additional support included outreach to parents to secure participation, delay marriage, and provide support as participants adjusted to their new environment. | – 45 young women, aged 16–26, from 22 villages successfully completed the training, 36 in Office Administration and nine in GST Accounting. <br> – 21 women were placed in jobs after the course, although five dropped out, <br> – leaving 16 who are currently employed. <br> – The five who dropped out decided to continue their education, while also looking for another job. <br> – 22 young women chose to go back to school or college to complete their higher education. <br> – 13 remained in Pune city, either working (Gopaldas 2013) or in educational programs (Abimola and Pai 2020), including one at SNDT University. <br> – None of the participants were married during that season. |

(continued)

**Box 3** (continued)

| Objective | Gap and Gender Issues Addressed | Partners and Roles across Sectors | Structure | Outcomes |
|---|---|---|---|---|
| To increase the safety of girls and women on public transportation | – Girls and women feel unsafe in all public spaces, including public transportation due to violence.<br>– Safe transportation is critical for girls and women to access educational and economic opportunities and to fully participate as citizens.<br>– Most officials do not understand that they are accountable for preventing and addressing violence against women and girls (VAWG). | – **Civil Society:**<br>– MASUM and International Center for Research on Women Asia provided gender training expertise, trainers, facilities, COVID-19 safety plan and protocol.<br>– **Government:** Maharashtra State Road Transport Company (MSRTC) provided an endorsement and mandated officials and staff to attend. | – MASUM facilitated 11 one-day training sessions with approximately 20 participants each.<br>– Training sessions provided an overview of the scope and impact of VAWG, girls' and women's right to be in public spaces, the responsibility of public officials to prevent and respond to VAWG in public spaces, an overview of gender norms that facilitate VAWG, an overview of women's rights and relevant laws and policies, and the opportunity for participants to discuss challenges and commit to acting. | – 200 MSRTC officials and staff (drivers, conductors, depot staff) participated in training.<br>– Knowledge on gender norms and VAWG, accountability to address VAWG, and impact on quality of services increased significantly.<br>– MSRTC leadership and participants recognized value of the training and need to do more on VAWG in their facilities and services.<br>– Infrastructure failures and policy gaps were identified to increase accountability.<br>– Participants made firm commitments to prevent and respond to VAWG in their facilities and services.<br>– The training provided the foundation for future trainings with other MSRTC staff and public officials in other sectors, including the police and officials at schools and colleges. |

(continued)

**Box 3**  (continued)

| Objective | Gap and Gender Issues Addressed | Partners and Roles across Sectors | Structure | Outcomes |
|---|---|---|---|---|
| To increase understanding of women's experiences and needs related to menstrual hygiene management (MHM), provide MHM options during the COVID-19 pandemic, and test the acceptability of reusable cloth pads | – MHM is a critical dimension of women's sexual and reproductive health and rights.<br>– Women have few affordable, high quality options and facilities for MHM.<br>– MHM programs rarely listen to women or focus on quality and choice.<br>– -These challenges have been exacerbated by the COVID-19 pandemic. | – **Civil Society:** MASUM oversaw the research program and implemented the research in Purandar. ICRW Asia provided research expertise, training for the research team, Institutional Review Board (IRB) clearance, and assistance with the data collection and analysis. Chaitanya and Sangini served as implementation partners in Khed and Nashik respectively.<br>– **Private Sector:** Essity, a global health and hygiene private sector company provided funding.<br>– **Social Enterprise:** Allforasmile Foundation provided innovatively designed, reusable, absorbent cloth pads at a reduced price. | – A research study was implemented to determine the acceptability of reusable cloth pads, with a sample of 150 women aged 18–35 years from 15 villages and one urban slum in Purandar and Khed rural blocks and the city of Nashik.<br>– Each participant received a set of four reusable cloth pads.<br>– Participants were interviewed three times over 6 months, allowing for an average of four menstrual periods.<br>– Findings were documented and shared to improve government and non-governmental MHM programs. | – 150 women received disposable pads and a packet of 4 reusable pads free of charge.<br>– Findings were used to inform government and non-governmental MHM programs. |

[a]Detailed analysis and case studies are available on each of these interventions (Jain et al. 2021; 3D Program for Girls and Women 2020, 2021)

on the partners and outcomes in each intervention). Each intervention was designed based on the clear and stated needs of girls and women. We collectively engaged stakeholders with the resources and mandated responsibility to address those needs, even when they did not typically work together, providing opportunities for each partner to learn and grow together. For example, the job skills training program brought together six diverse stakeholders[10] to take on roles, respon-

sibilities and experiences none of them had undertaken before. As each partner adapted to their new role, challenges were faced and courses were corrected, and in the end, program participants benefited in multiple, sometimes unexpected ways.

*'Our parents must be grappling with predicaments:*
*"Can we hinder our girls now, after having traversed so far?"*
*…We will not burnout like lamps, merely as extensions of anyone's family line*
*But we'll cherish the flame that enlightens our own being.*
*Thus empowered, we will respond to our parents' dilemma.'*

—Excerpt from a poem by Reshma Khaladkar, Job skills program participant

---

[10]MASUM, the 3D Program, the corporate Tech Mahindra Foundation, Shreemati Nathibai Damodar Thackersey (SNDT) Women's University, and adolescent girls and their parents.

Similarly, the gender sensitization training of the state transportation staff in Purandar *taluka* we facilitated was the first ever in Maharashtra State. The program was designed based on the mapping of unsafe public places by girls and women, with a focus on increasing awareness and accountability of public service officials. With the support of the Maharashtra State Road Transportation Corporation, Pune Division, MASUM strategically leveraged the COVID-19 public transportation shutdown to engage and train public transport staff.

> *"We wouldn't respond differently to consensual relationships and sexual harassment until now, so we would sometimes blame the girl when she complained to us. We will actively apply the new perspective from today's training to make transport safe for girls and women."*
> —Balasaheb Ladkat, an MSRTC bus driver who participated in the MASUM-led gender training.

The MHM intervention brought together grassroots organizations, a research partner and a social enterprise to provide much-needed disposable and reusable menstrual products during COVID-19, address the stigma surrounding menstruation, provide opportunities for women to share their experiences via telephone interviews, surveys and menstrual diaries, and assess what women are willing to pay for reusable menstrual products until the demand for these to be distributed freely through the public health system is recognized. Findings will inform government and other programs, to help them move from simply distributing menstrual products to increasing the quality and choices girls and women have in MHM.

> *"The reusable pads are so convenient and unobtrusive, that travelling is no longer a problem! They don't need disposal or burning because they are washable and they dry fast. They should be made available with health workers at the village level so that women and girls can access them easily."*
> A young woman participant in the MHM study

These multi-sectoral partnerships demonstrate that it is possible to cross sectoral siloes and engage in sometimes unlikely partnerships to work in a different way towards a common goal. While there were challenges, the shared commitment to improve access to and the quality of services for girls and women was strong enough to overcome them across diverse sectors and implementing partners.

## 3    What We Learned from Our Partnerships

This section includes insights and lessons learned from our partnership, and based on our analysis of our experiences, key tenets for global health and international development partnerships (see Box 4).

---

**Box 4: Key Tenets for Global Health and International Development Partnerships**

Disrupt the Funder-Implementer Model: As donors are increasingly reviewing their funding models, the typical North-South/funder-implementer model will be disrupted. However, currently, even within the most equitable relationships, partners from the Global North should be cognizant of the reality that resources are skewed in favor of those who are located in geopolitically powerful locations and must seek ways to correct that imbalance. While partners in the Global North typically bring and control financial resources, local partners cannot simply be involved in implementation because that establishes a caste system which distinguishes who leads the intellectual and financial aspects of the project and who does the work of implementation. It is essential that local partners are involved in strategic decision-making from the beginning about how to allocate, reallocate and utilize resources throughout the lifespan of the program.

---

(continued)

Create Opportunities for People to Speak for Themselves and for Those in Power to Listen: Gathering and sharing evidence is a key pillar of global health practice to guide the development of policies, program design, resource allocation and advocacy. Creating opportunities for people to speak for themselves, directly to those mandated to serve them, can also be a powerful way to strengthen global health planning outcomes. While seemingly obvious, it does not happen enough. In addition to ensuring that local realities and expertise are considered and officials and institutions are held accountable, this approach provides an opportunity for global health practitioners to model the changes in power dynamics and resource control that many global health programs claim to want to impact.

Build Strong Relationships to Foster Trust and Strengthen Programs: Working across borders, issues and shared resources requires trust. Finding and committing to a shared vision is a critical anchor in building trust, as is investing in people and relationships by building in the time and space to connect with and learn from each other. Strong relationships built on mutual respect, equality and affection help everyone concerned to tide over differences because frank dialogue and collective learning are possible when camaraderie and friendships are secure and trustworthy. In that process, valuing different perspectives shaped by different experiences as part of one's methodology and program design will strengthen programs, interventions and outcomes.

Move Beyond Binary Thinking: Rather than a North vs. South model, global health and international development would benefit from a 'sharing lessons learned' model. Movements for social justice by diverse activists working on a range of issues, such as intergenerational advocacy on gender

equality and climate change and global advocacy on LGBTQI rights, and more recently, vaccine equity, are leading the way in this approach, growing and supporting each other across borders, regions, generations and issues, revealing the futility of simple, binary approaches to identity and advocacy.

Diversity is a Strength: The best outcomes can often come about when you converge diverse stakeholders and allow for different perspectives and interests. This can be challenging as each partner is pushed beyond their own comfort zone, sphere of influence, and expectations and may find themselves working with stakeholders they have previously chosen not to work with. However, within a broad shared vision, diverse and even unlikely partnerships can lead to programmatic innovations, new resources, and greater impact.

Learning is a Key Component of Successful Partnerships: Different experiences and perspectives result in different expertise. This creates opportunities for rich learning within partnerships of diverse stakeholders. By being open to this learning, each stakeholder can grow, the program will benefit, and the partnership will be greater than the sum of its parts.

**Shifting the Power** The 3D Program and MASUM teams shared the understanding that colonization created and exacerbated development problems in India. The depletion of resources, identity, self-esteem and local governance skills before independence, and the continued erosion of economic, social and political rights through neo-liberal policies has had a lasting adverse impact on the provision of basic needs such as health and education through privatization. The teams were careful not to replicate colonial models, legacies and dynamics by challenging conventional wisdom in international development that the Global South is simply the location of development problems and the Global

(continued)

North is the only source of resources and solutions.

The 3D Program strove to equalize power with its Indian partners, and in turn, the Indian partners challenged power equations at the local level. MASUM's core strategies include questioning unequal access to resources in both private and public domains, and challenging the backlash faced by women, especially members of minority and disadvantaged groups. MASUM also challenged the U.S.-based 3D Program team about how things should or should not be done in India. For example, they stressed the importance of not working through the most powerful members of village society, even if their voice or intervention could expedite the project. Being cognizant of caste dynamics and other vested interests of those who align with us was also highlighted by MASUM. This resulted in an increased understanding of how multiple systems of domination and exclusion operate in a community and how those systems impact programming and outcomes.

MASUM acknowledged the advantages of working with government agencies through the 3D Program, but also cautioned against letting interventions becoming too 'state-dependent' and relying on the individual commitments of ever-changing officials. Securing orders from high-level bureaucrats might increase the cooperation of local officials, but the process of people demanding accountability from the state is essential to strengthen and sustain grassroots democracy. MASUM also stressed the need to maintain the autonomy of women's collectives from government interventions, rather than fully integrating them into the state machinery.

The 3D Program team secured and provided the funding for the program. However, Indian partners were involved in strategic decision-making from the beginning about how to allocate (or reallocate) and utilize resources. Additionally, the 3D Program team encouraged sometimes difficult conversations about resource allocation and were open to changes based on the experience gained through the different interventions and realities on the ground. This intentional process helped 3D Program and MASUM build the necessary trust to respond effectively to the COVID-19 crisis and to focus on issues that were not being adequately focused on either by the public health system or by local communities, such as GBV, preventing early marriages during the pandemic, and addressing the needs of migrants and displaced people. The 3D Program team, in discussions with our donor, reallocated funds originally earmarked for travel and staff salaries, to these interventions.

The 3D Program and MASUM partnership challenged the model of typical North-South partnerships because it explicitly included trusting the decisions of local partners to make changes in the project plan and practicing transparency about financial (re)allocations. Additionally, the dynamic process of learning (and unlearning) through the partnership was possible because of the honesty of the MASUM team and the genuine willingness of the US-based 3D Program team to listen, and our shared commitment to sharing and decentralizing power at all levels.

**Power and Influence in 'Insider'/'Outsider' Relationships** People from the outside cannot resolve issues for local communities. This reality guided the 3D Program and MASUM partnership and our program design and implementation at different levels. At the most local level, only women and girls can bring about a change in their lives. On the other side of the equation, government and organizations serving girls and women must be held accountable to listen to them and effectively address their needs, however time- or human resource-intensive that process may be. To this end, the 3D Program and MASUM linked girls and women directly with those mandated to serve them, creating platforms, programs and feedback loops to facilitate transparent communication and participatory decision-making.

As facilitators at the local and national levels, MASUM and other Indian partners used their platforms and expertise to influence processes and government officials at the village, district and state level, and advised and challenged the 3D Program team. As an external partner based at an international organization, the 3D Program team played an important facilitative role, linking stakeholders across sectors, providing opportunities to amplify the voices of rural women and their advocates, and identifying and securing the necessary support and resources to make those collaborations work. Rather than primarily engendering mistrust, being outsiders with no prior history with the actors in the district, worked to our advantage. The 3D Program team was able to leverage our outsider status to start with a clean slate and help stakeholders who previously may not have chosen to work together to find common ground. This included MASUM working more closely with the district level government officials and was also evident in the multi-sectoral partnerships facilitated for the demonstration programs. The team understood that the technical expertise, in-depth knowledge of the local context, and prioritization of activities lay with the local partners and rural communities, and that each partner had their own unique strength and capability. The 3D Program team was also uniquely positioned to maximize impact by catalyzing or reinvigorating partnerships, resources and opportunities, using their presence and resources to get state and district level senior bureaucrats to listen and providing additional global platforms through which to share findings and lessons learned with a broader audience.

**Complexities in Decolonizing Global Health and International Development** The awareness that local knowledge is the best starting point is dominating discussions on localization and decolonization of global health and international development. The 2020 wave of social justice movements put the spotlight on structural racism and power imbalances, leading to a global reckoning in global health and international development. Traditional development and aid models are being critically examined. Questions that have long been asked by grassroots activists, particularly feminists, are now being asked at board meetings and are reshaping institutional criteria and decisions (Nowrojee 2021b; FP2030

2022). Who leads programs? Where does decision-making power lie? How do you measure impact? Who has access to and controls resources? These questions have led many international NGOs and donors to contend with issues related to equity and inclusion and helped the 3D Program team intentionally examine and transform the structure of the program.

At the same time, our partnerships revealed a key limitation of these conversations. Generally, approaches to what are being referred to as 'decolonization' and 'localization' have the starting point of an *us vs. them* model, a simple North-South dichotomy. The global North and South are facing similar development trends that disenfranchise excluded and subordinated groups and individuals even further. While global geopolitical power imbalances persist, inequalities and human rights violations are in focus everywhere. In the U.S., the spark for both injustice and advocacy has been race, and in India, it has been caste, class, gender and religion. COVID-19 further revealed how public systems are failing everywhere. For example, the U.S. was ill-prepared to deal with the pervasive deep mistrust of public systems and the challenges of widespread COVID-19 testing and mass vaccinations. India applied global recommendations, such as lockdowns, social and physical distancing, handwashing and travel bans, with little assessment of how local realities made those recommendations difficult and often impossible to follow. In both countries, hospitals struggled to provide beds, oxygen and ventilators in the face of COVID-19 spikes. Civil society organizations stepped in to fill vital gaps in services and supply chains and to demand accountability from both public and private systems.

Additionally, many of us working in international development and global health, including 3D Program staff members, exist in 'the spaces in-between'. We are neither from the North nor the South, and in the 3D Program's case, team members had roots in India. Increasingly, with globalization and immigration, many of us bring multiple social identities to our work, as well as knowledge of a range of cultures, languages and places. This itself is challenging and strengthening the fields of international development and global health, enriching them with diverse perspectives and increasing accountability both within organizations and across geographies.

**Multi-sectoral Partnerships Require a Shared Vision and Allowing for Differences** The multisectoral partnerships we facilitated helped each stakeholder grow through the agreement of a shared vision. Trust was cultivated through the difficult process of negotiating power dynamics and different priorities. The collaborations that worked best, such as the partnership with the State Transportation Corporation, were built on a shared commitment to the goal of the project. Like us, transportation senior officials believed that the gender sensitization training would benefit girls and women customers, as well as the public transportation system itself. However, we also saw positive outcomes when we had to navigate differences among partners. For example, our corporate partner in the job skills training program defined success quantitatively (job placement and retention). The 3D Program and MASUM had more nuanced measures of success, based on the full range of girls' aspirations (job placement, continued education, starting a business, and delaying marriage). In the end, the outcomes for girls and young women were successful by most measures.

## 4    Conclusion

Through our partnership, the 3D Program and MASUM teams intentionally created ways of working together that challenged traditional North-South development and global health partnership norms. With a focus on mutual respect and building relationships, we were able to jointly develop and implement a programmatic model that allowed us to move outside our comfort zones and dare to think of new strategies. We challenged our implementing partners to work together in different ways to create unlikely partnerships and to prioritize spaces through which girls and women could speak for themselves and

hold government officials and partner staff accountable. While each partner brought different resources and perspectives to the program, at the core of those partnerships was the shared stated commitment of making programs work better for girls and women.

More personally, when the 3D Program and MASUM teams embarked on our partnership, also based on our shared commitment to gender equality and conviction that we could all do better by girls and women, we learned about ourselves and each other, and what it meant to work together intentionally and honestly. Through the negotiation of our partnership, navigation of power dynamics, and the process of jointly designing and implementing interventions to advance that shared commitment, we came to understand that learning is a critical part of successful partnerships.

**Acknowledgements** This chapter reflects the collective learning of the 3D Program and MASUM teams and other partners through the implementation of the 3D Program in rural Pune from 2017-2021. The authors thank the following for their insights and support: Geeta Rao Gupta, Shailaja Aralkar, Vanessa Coello and Alisha Chopra of the 3D Program team; Kajal Jain and Ramesh Awasthi of MASUM; Ganga Buke, Sudha Kothari and Kalpana Pant of Chaitanya; and Sapna Kedia and Ravi Verma of the International Center for Research on Women (ICRW) Asia.

## Glossary

**Collective Impact:** An approach to social problem-solving based on the commitment of a group of important actors from different sectors to a common agenda. Collective impact initiatives involve a centralized infrastructure, a dedicated staff, and a structured process that leads to a common agenda, shared measurement, continuous communication, and mutually reinforcing activities among all participants (Kania and Kramer 2011).

**Community-led Development:** A development approach in which local community members work together to identify goals that are important to them, develop and implement plans to achieve those goals, and create collaborative relationships internally and with external actors—all while building on community strengths and local leadership. (CLD) is characterized by 11 attributes: participation and inclusion, voice, community assets, capacity development, sustainability, transformative capacity, collective planning and action, accountability, community leadership, adaptability, and collaboration (Veda et al. 2021).

**Convergence:** Bringing together diverse stakeholders to address a problem, by agreeing on a shared vision and coordinated but differentiated action based on the resources, perspectives and experiences each stakeholder brings to the partnership (Jain et al. 2021).

**Decolonization:** Most literally, decolonization is the process through which colonies become independent of a colonizing country. Within international development and global health, it has come to mean recognizing and removing all forms of supremacy within countries, between countries and at the global level (Abimola and Pai 2020; Büyüm et al. 2020).

**Feminism:** is a movement to end sexism, sexist exploitation, and oppression. Intersectionality, or the interactivity of social identity structures, such as race, class, caste and gender, in facilitating privilege or oppression, has shaped global feminism, allowing for the complexities of different contexts and identities (Hooks b 2000; UN Women 2020; Alok 2017; Gopaldas 2013).

**Global North:** The term 'Global North' has emerged as the counterpoint to the 'Global South', providing a philosophically aligned term that is an alternative to the terms 'First World' and the 'developed world'.

**Global South:** The term 'Global South' is a critical concept with different definitions. It has traditionally been used in international development and global health to refer to economically and politically disadvantaged nation-states and as an alternative to the terms 'Third World' and the 'developing world'. It has also been used to describe spaces and peoples negatively impacted by a shared experience of contemporary capitalist globalization and post-coloniality, regardless of physical geography (Mahler 2017).

**Localization:** The process through which traditional power structures are transformed in international development and global health to ensure that local and national communities and organizations set development objectives, lead the development process and control the allocation of resources, and international organizations and donors provide resources and, when needed, technical support. There are efforts to document what responsible localization looks like in international development, capturing cases where there have been fundamental changes in relationships and power dynamics as well as shifts in understandings of expertise and capacity (Renoir and Boone 2020).

**Power:** Power can be defined in different ways, all of which are accurate and can co-exist—as a resource that needs to be redistributed, as a source of domination which needs to be overcome, and as a source of empowerment that enables you to transform yourself, others, and the world (Allen 1999).

**Trust:** Firm belief in the reliability, truth, ability, or strength of someone or something (Oxford Learner's Dictionaries 2020).

# References

3D Program for Girls and Women. Good governance through convergent action, program brief. Washington, DC: 3D Program for Girls and Women; 2018. https://the3dprogram.org/content/uploads/2018/10/Good-Governance-through-Convergent-Action-September-2018.pdf

3D Program for Girls and Women. Dreaming the impossible: Insights from an innovative job skills training program for women in India, Case Studies in Convergence Series, no. 1. Washington, DC: 3D Program for Girls and Women; 2020. Available from: https://the3dprogram.org/content/uploads/2020/09/Case-study-no.-1-Job-skills-training-May-2020.pdf

3D Program for Girls and Women. Safe travels: Increasing girls' and women's safety on public transport, Case Studies in Convergence Series, no. 3. Washington, DC: 3D Program for Girls and Women; 2021. Available from: https://the3dprogram.org/content/uploads/2021/01/3D-Program-case-study-no.-3-MSRTC-Gender-training-January-2021.pdf

Abimola S, Pai M. Will global health survive its decolonisation? Lancet. 2020;396(10263):1627–8.

Allen A. The power of feminist theory: Domination, resistance, solidarity. New York: Routeledge; 1999.

Alok NP. Intersectional feminism 101: Why it's important and what we must remember. Feminism in India; 2017. Feb 13 [cited 2022 April 9]; Available from: https://feminisminindia.com/2017/02/13/indian-intersectional-feminism-101/

Büyüm A, Kenney C, Koris A, Mkumba L, Raveendran Y. Decolonising global health: If not now, when? BMJ Glob Health. 2020;5(8):e003394.

FP2030. Global FP2030 support network; 2022 March 28 [cited 2022 April 9]. Available from: https://fp2030.org/Building2030#:~:text=So%20far%2C%20three%20regional%20hubs,AmRef%20Africa%20in%20Nairobi%2C%20Kenya

Gopaldas A. Intersectionality 101. J Public Policy Mark. 2013;32:90–4.

Government of India. Ministry of Statistics and Programme Implementation. Indian states by GDP. 2021 March [cited 2022 March 30]; Available from: https://statisticstimes.com/economy/india/indian-states-gdp.php

Gupta GR. Putting together the pieces of the puzzle for gender equality. Blog. 3D Program for Girls and Women; 2017. https://the3dprogram.org/convergent-action-putting-together-the-pieces-of-the-puzzle-for-gender-equality/

Hooks b. Feminism is for everybody. Passionate politics. London: Pluto Press; 2000.

India Development Review. IDR explains: Local government in India. 2020 Jan 28 [cited 2022 April 9]; Available from: https://idronline.org/idr-explains-local-government-in-india/

International Institute for Population Sciences. National Family Health Survey. State Fact Sheet, Maharashtra; 2019–20. Available from: http://rchiips.org/nfhs/NFHS-5_FCTS/COMPENDIUM/Maharashtra.pdf

Jain K, Aralkar S, Buke G, Kedia S, Gupte M, Kothari S, et al. From Vulnerability to Leadership: Lessons Learned from Collective and Collaborative Action for Rural Girls and Women in India. Washington, DC: 3D Program for Girls and Women; 2021. Available from: https://the3dprogram.org/content/uploads/2021/07/FINAL_DIGITAL_3D-Program-Rural-report-From-Vulnerability-to-Leadership.pdf

Johnson R, O'Malley D. Feminist friendship as method: Experiences of re-organising power in philanthropy. Alliance Magazine; 2021.

Kania J, Kramer M. Collective Impact. Stanf Soc Innov Rev. 2011;9(1):36–41.

Mahler AG. Global South. Oxford bibliographies in literary and critical theory. New York: Oxford University Press; 2017.

Mehra R, Shebi K. Economic programs in India: What works for the empowerment of girls and women. Washington, DC: 3D Program For Girls and Women; 2018. Available from: https://the3dprogram.org/content/uploads/2018/10/3D-Economic-Empowerment-Report-August-2018.pdf

Nowrojee S. One thing at a time doesn't work for women. Blog. 3D Program for Girls and Women; 2017. https://the3dprogram.org/one-thing-at-a-time-isnt-the-reality-for-women/

Nowrojee S. Responsible transitions to local ownership: Reflections from the 3D Program for Girls and Women from Where I Stand: Unpacking "local" in aid. In CDA Virtual Learning Forum; 2021a. https://www.cdacollaborative.org/blog/responsible-transitions-to-local-ownership-reflections-from-the-3d-program-for-girls-and-women/

Nowrojee B. The Open Society Foundations move ahead on transformation. Voices, new approaches. Open Society Foundations; 2021b. [cited 2021 Nov 9]. Available from: https://www.opensocietyfoundations.org/voices/the-open-society-foundations-move-ahead-on-transformation

Oxford Learner's Dictionaries. Oxford Learner's Dictionaries. [Online]; 2020 [cited 2021 September 10]. Available from: https://www.oxfordlearnersdictionaries.com/us/definition/english/trust_2

Renoir M, Boone G, editors. What transformation takes: Evidence of responsible INGO transitions to locally led development around the world. London: Peace Direct; 2020.

Shaw J. 'Glocalization'? What is that? The global, the local, and health policy research. BioMed Central (BMC) Blog Network. On Health Blog, 9 June, 2014.

UN Women. Intersectional feminism: What it means and why it matters right now. 2020 July 1 [cited 2022 April 9]; Available from: https://www.unwomen.org/en/news/stories/2020/6/explainer-intersectional-feminism-what-it-means-and-why-it-matters

Veda G, Donohue C, Nicholls R, Cloete E, Trandafili H, Wright M, et al. Impact of Community-Led Development on Food Security (InCLuDE): A rapid realist review. The Movement for Community-Led Development & Charles Darwin University; 2021.

Woetzel J, Madgavkar A, Gupta R, Manyika J, Ellingrud K, Gupta S, et al. The power of parity: Advancing women's equality In India. McKinsey & Company; 2015.

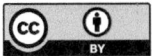

# Role of Social Science in Infectious Disease Research: A Case Study of Partnering with Communities in Vector Control in a Kenyan Village

Lydiah W. Kibe and A. Desiree LaBeaud [ORCID]

*He who masters the power formed by a group of people working together has within his grasp one of the greatest powers known to man.*

Idown Koyenikan

## Abstract

Partnering with communities is a vital component of public health research. Terms such as community participation, community engagement, and citizen participation have been used to denote community partnerships that aim to re-distribute power through negotiation between citizens and researchers and enable co-creative processes that bring non-researchers in as core partners. These citizen-researcher partnerships go beyond informed consent, voluntary participation, and intervention adherence but instead constitute a means by which shared planning, design, implementation, dissemination, and decision-making take place. In this case study, we describe our intervention study in coastal Kenya that included homeowners, schools, schoolchildren, and other stakeholders to increase people's awareness of vectors and vector-borne diseases and catalyze their participation in vector control. The partners for this work included researchers from local and international universities, social scientists, non-governmental organizations, officials from the ministries of health and education, and the community members themselves. We trialed new strategies to deeply engage adult and child community members to promote vector control activities at home and in the community. Strengthening community involvement and establishing prolonged interaction of community representatives with control services, municipalities, and other public actors were shown to be time-consuming and costly at the beginning but rewarding during the process and with excellent potential for sustainability. In this case study, we also investigate the concepts of *gender norms* and *patriarchy* and underscore how they interact with other forms of culture to impact decision-making processes, power imbalance and dominance, and vulnerability to ill health at our study site in Kenya. We highlight social science's contribution to enhancing a deeper understanding of

L. W. Kibe (✉)
Kenya Medical Research Institute, Eastern Southern Africa Centre of International Parasite Control, Nairobi, Kenya
e-mail: lkibe@kemri.go.ke

A. D. LaBeaud
Department of Pediatrics, Division of Infectious Diseases, Stanford University, Stanford, CA, USA
e-mail: dlabeaud@stanford.edu

the social constructs that underlie power structures and concepts of disease and health in the Kenyan village, thus fostering successful partnerships with the community and enhancing research outcomes. The key tenets from this case study are relevant to community-based research conducted in similar contexts.

### Keywords

Social science · Gender · Patriarchy · Community engagement · Vector-borne disease · Kenya

### Author Perspective

We are researchers and partners from diverse fields and backgrounds. Lydiah brings social science while Desiree brings medical and epidemiological perspectives to the chapter. We have partnered to conduct research on community prevention of mosquito borne diseases such as malaria, dengue fever, Rift valley fever, chikungunya, among others in Kenya for over 10 years. We have learned that our strength is our complementarity in skill and experience with community-based research. This has enabled us to support the development of innovative disease control interventions and overcome barriers while partnering with communities in the research process.

This chapter addresses the following SDGs: # 3—Good health and well-being, #16 Peace, Justice and Strong Institutions, and #17 Partnerships for the goals.

### Key Tenets

1. Social science brings an understanding of the social context, which can be used to bring attention to the human, social, and behavioral factors that facilitate or hinder communication between researchers and research participants. This can foster trust and confidence during research and in delivering public health interventions and clinical services.

2. Cultural norms and systems such as patriarchy and gender play critical roles in how power is shared, decisions are made, and resources are utilized for infectious disease control.

3. Interventions given and led by community members may reduce ambiguities brought about by community beliefs and perceptions about research, thus enhancing greater partnerships and sustainable collaborations in research.

4. Partnering with communities enhances co-learning and promotes trust. Understanding the local context, challenges, and opportunities helps shape health interventions and define practical solutions that are applicable, acceptable, and appropriate to the involved community.

5. Clear communication between the community and the research team fosters understanding, reduces rumors, suspicion, and misinformation, and enhances collaboration and willingness for communities to participate and innovate in co-creating new ideas and interventions.

## 1    Background

Vector-borne diseases, spread by arthropod vectors, continue to plague people worldwide. The World Health Organization estimates the following global annual impact: 300 million malaria cases (Malaria n.d.), 50–100 million symptomatic dengue cases (Dengue and dengue hemorrhagic fever n.d.), and 120 million filariasis cases (Lymphatic filariasis n.d.). Other vector-borne diseases like trypanosomiasis, leishmaniasis, Japanese encephalitis, Rift Valley fever virus, onchocerciasis, and yellow fever cause additional millions of disease cases each year (LaBeaud et al. 2011). Vector-borne diseases are estimated to represent 17% of the global disease burden due to all parasitic and infectious diseases recorded as disability-adjusted life years (Townson et al. 2005). In Kenya, mosquito-borne viral (arboviral) diseases such as dengue, chikungunya, and Zika occur along a spectrum from low levels of year-round endemic transmission to explosive outbreaks (Hortion et al. 2019). The result is a loss of economic productivity, school absenteeism, aggravation of poverty, high costs for health care, and a burden on public health services (Organization WH 2012). Even in places where communities are afflicted by multiple diseases (Rational Use of Personal Protective Equipment for Coronavirus Disease (COVID-19) n.d.), preventative vector control plays a key role in reducing and eliminating vector-borne diseases (Townson et al. 2005), reducing the use of drugs to treat the diseases and reducing the chances of pathogens becoming drug-resistant (Matthews 2009).

Many vector control programs are vertical (also known as stand-alone, categorical, or freestanding) where "the solution of a given health problem (in this case disease-carrying mosquitoes) [is addressed] through the application of specific measures through single-purpose machinery" (Msuya 2004). Consequently, many vector control programs lack substantial community involvement, even though engaging local communities and stakeholders is a key element for successfully implementing integrated vector management (IVM) (Mutero et al. 2012; Kibe et al. 2019). It has often been argued that human behavior and social, cultural, and economic contexts should inform research and intervention programs' design and implementation (Jones and Williams 2002). Social sciences can generate the data needed to understand the context in which diseases occur and factors that enhance or constrain the response of a population and the effectiveness of a public health intervention (Binka and Adongo 1997).

Infectious diseases occur within the context of human lives fraught with complexity. For any given disease, who gets it, when, why, the duration, the severity, the outcome, and the sequelae, are bound by a complex interplay of factors related as much to the individual as to interconnected physical, social, cultural, political, and economic systems. Furthermore, these factors are dynamic, evolving as they interact (see chapter "A Holistic Systems Approach to Global Health Research, Practice, and Partnerships"). Simple solutions to infectious diseases are, therefore, rarely sustainable solutions. Sustainability requires the development of interdisciplinary and transdisciplinary sciences that acknowledge, understand, and address the elements of complex interacting systems rather than relying solely on traditional biomedical disciplinary models that reduce disease management to simple paradigms. Community engagement aims to create a sense of trust, identify extra resources, apply sound communication, and enhance the overall result as a better program with sustainable collaborations (Gopalan et al. 2021).

This chapter focuses on a case study of a community-based intervention implemented in a Kenyan village in Kwale County by scientists from Stanford University, the Kenya Medical Research Institute (KEMRI), and the Technical University of Mombasa (TUM). In 2016, we came together to address the issue of vector-borne diseases in Kenyan villages. Social science was identified as a pillar of this work. In this chapter, we share examples from an intervention aimed at partnering with school children as change agents in controlling *Aedes aegypti* mosquitoes to prevent dengue fever in the community (Ngugi et al. 2017).

## 2  The Intervention: School—Household Based Dengue Control

A community-based dengue control intervention was carried out in the coastal town of Msambweni in Kwale County, Kenya, located approximately 60 kilometers south of Mombasa and 50 kilometers north of the Kenya-Tanzania border (4°28′0.0114″S, 39°28′0.12″E). The annual mean temperatures range from 23–34 °C with average relative humidity between 60–80%. Precipitation varies throughout the year: February is the driest month, with an average of 18 mm of rain, and May is the wettest month, with an average of

347 mm. The seasons are classified based on precipitation levels, with the long dry season between January–March, the long rainy season between April–June, the short dry season between July–September, and the short rainy season between October–December. With low population densities of 460 people/km2, central water systems transporting piped water to households are lacking. As a result, residents obtain water for domestic purposes from rainfall in the wet months and wells and boreholes in the dry months. Fishing and subsistence farming are the primary livelihoods among residents. Islam is the dominant religion. The area was selected based on dengue virus (DENV) transmission evidence. In 2000–2003 dengue fever exposures were over 50% reported in pregnant women in Msambweni location (Sutherland et al. 2011). More recent data from this area reported dengue prevalence of between 20% and 50% in children (Hortion et al. 2019; Vu et al. 2017a, b; Shah et al. 2020).

Ten public primary schools participated in the study. Out of these, five schools received the intervention, and five schools were controls (the control schools received the curriculum after the end of the study). Social scientists at KEMRI and researchers from the Technical University of Mombasa and Stanford University complemented each other in developing and implementing a school-based community intervention curriculum on vector behavior and household larval source reduction. This was done by engaging community members to improve household management of outdoor water containers and reduce the risk of mosquito infestation in rural coastal Kenya. Others, such as teachers, scientists, local non—governmental organizations, and public health specialists from the Ministry of Health, participated in developing the curriculum. Some topics and methods used in the school-based curriculum included mosquito biology, mosquito lifecycle, potential breeding areas, diseases transmitted, and control options. The knowledge gained by the school children stimulated discussions in their homes and subsequently led to increased community engagement and uptake of positive actions to control mosquitoes in their homes.

To enhance community engagement, participatory techniques were delivered innovatively, such as demonstrations of a mosquito life cycle using real objects, pictures of different mosquito species, role playing, stories, and experiential sharing. During these activities, men and women—young and old—were encouraged to participate because the Kenyan village context and its social norms influenced the interactions and decision-making processes of the household (see Fig. 1 below). All family members were encouraged to participate, especially during the clean-up exercises and the mosquito awareness sessions. With the realization of the inherent social norms, including *patriarchy* and *gender roles*, efforts were made to involve everyone, especially men and elderly parents, who are perceived to be key decision-makers in the households' resources. Despite having access to resources and participating in water management and waste disposal, women had little control over these resources. This is a major challenge since men must permit research activities to be conducted in their homes. This power dynamic in the family and society had the potential to derail planned activities; however, having a social scientist on the research team helped in understanding the societal challenges and determining the best strategies to overcome them. In this regard, consultations were held using house tours (door -to - door visitations) to identify the best time for visiting the household to perform study activities. As a result, we (the study team and the participants) agreed on what needed to be done, by whom, when, and the resources required. The best approaches to dealing with water management and waste disposal were agreed upon with consideration of gender roles, uses of water, and purposes of dumped containers. For example, household owners devised simple and sustainable interventions such as covering water containers, cleaning water containers regularly, and discarding/selling unused containers to scrap dealers. In instances where an action required specialized intervention such as covering an open well or any other community water sources, stakeholders' meetings were held to sensitize them on the progress and challenges and issues that required their

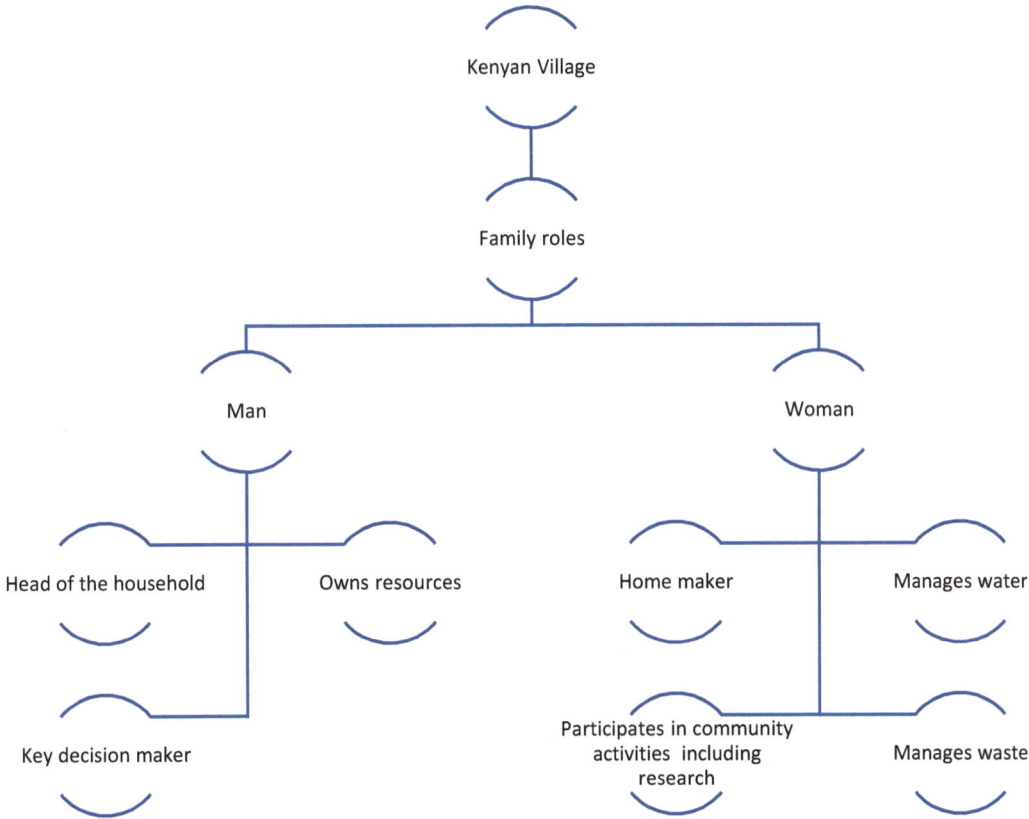

**Fig. 1** An illustration of the family roles relevant to vector-borne disease research and control in a Kenyan Village

support (see Fig. 2 below). The intervention faced some barriers, including stigma, *gender roles*, patriarchy, and differing beliefs about disease causation. However, a number of the facilitators sustained the intervention, including the history of a previous engagement, shared common goals, and integration of social science to enhance community engagement, as shown in Fig. 3 below.

**Personal History**

Lydiah Kibe's journey as a social scientist in vector-borne disease studies started in the year 2000 during her visit to the Kenya Medical Research Institute (KEMRI) in Kilifi. This led her to the "Kenyan Village," where she was able to support public health research and practice using social science skills. Her three-year term with the Aga-Khan Community Health Services as a training officer was coming to an end, and she was hoping for an opportunity to join the KEMRI—Vector Control Unit. Malaria was ranked number one as the leading cause of death in the community and responsible for 30% of hospital admissions. Many residents had misconceptions about public health interventions. These misconceptions were contributing to poor health. Mosquito nets treated with long-lasting insecticides were being distributed for free in the community. Still, residents refused to use them under the guise that the nets were "talking" and, therefore, associated them with evil spirits (Mayoyo 2006). Some residents returned the nets to the distributors, others burned

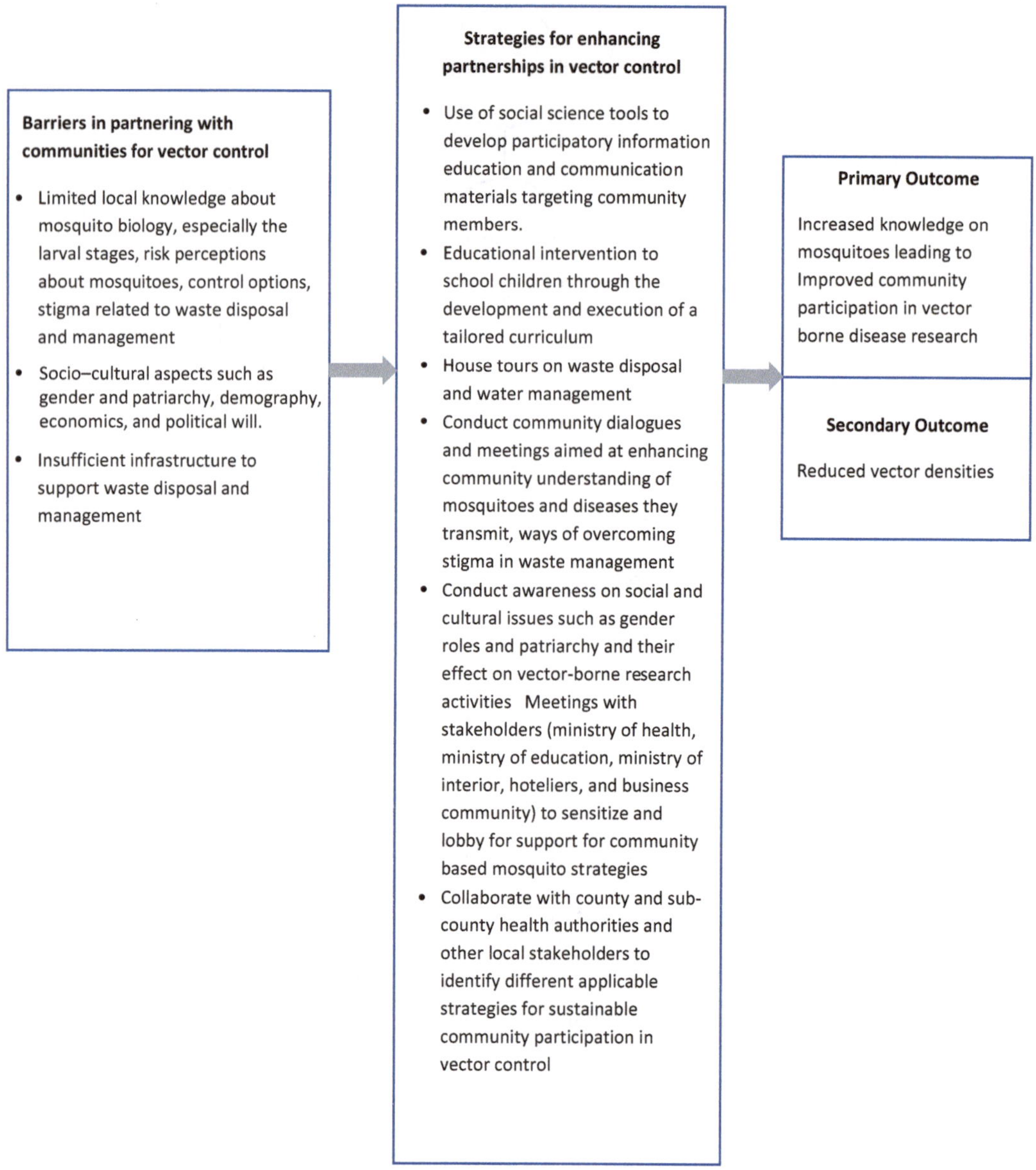

**Barriers in partnering with communities for vector control**

- Limited local knowledge about mosquito biology, especially the larval stages, risk perceptions about mosquitoes, control options, stigma related to waste disposal and management
- Socio–cultural aspects such as gender and patriarchy, demography, economics, and political will.
- Insufficient infrastructure to support waste disposal and management

**Strategies for enhancing partnerships in vector control**

- Use of social science tools to develop participatory information education and communication materials targeting community members.
- Educational intervention to school children through the development and execution of a tailored curriculum
- House tours on waste disposal and water management
- Conduct community dialogues and meetings aimed at enhancing community understanding of mosquitoes and diseases they transmit, ways of overcoming stigma in waste management
- Conduct awareness on social and cultural issues such as gender roles and patriarchy and their effect on vector-borne research activities   Meetings with stakeholders (ministry of health, ministry of education, ministry of interior, hoteliers, and business community) to sensitize and lobby for support for community based mosquito strategies
- Collaborate with county and sub-county health authorities and other local stakeholders to identify different applicable strategies for sustainable community participation in vector control

**Primary Outcome**

Increased knowledge on mosquitoes leading to Improved community participation in vector borne disease research

**Secondary Outcome**

Reduced vector densities

**Fig. 2** An Illustration of the process of partnering with communities for vector control in Kenya

them, and others threw them on the streets. These nets were nicknamed "the talking nets." At this time, elephantiasis was said to be caused by witchcraft or drinking too much mnazi (traditional brew or palm wine) and malaria was thought to be caused by eating too many unripe mangoes. Children with seizures due to cere-bral malaria were believed to have been "watched by a big bird in the sky." Research studies were frequently con-fused with treatment for disease (Marsh et al. 2008). Amidst these ambiguities, myths, misinformation, and misconceptions, she joined KEMRI in Kilifi as a social behavioral scientist.

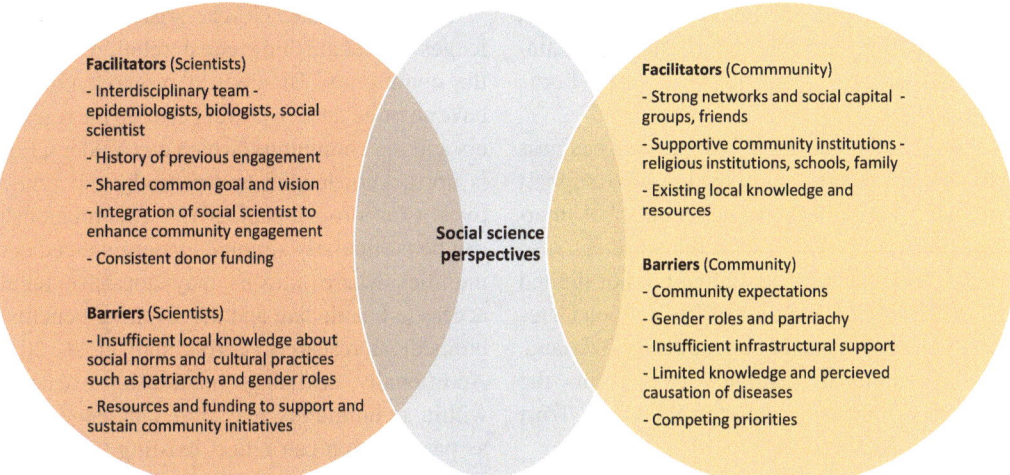

**Fig. 3** Facilitators and barriers to research and implementation of vector control strategies when partnering with communities in Kenya

Her experience working in KEMRI with the vector control department enhanced her capacity as a social scientist. She was responsible for social science studies and community and stakeholder engagement. She also led the training of community health volunteers, mosquito scouts, and school children in integrated vector management.

## 3    Description of the Partnerships

In this case study, the main partners derived from a local university (Technical University of Mombasa-TUM), an offsite university (Stanford University-SU), a leading governmental research institute- Kenya Medical Research Institute (KEMRI), and a local non-profit organization (NGO e.g. SCOPE) for their experience in community-based initiatives in the area. Researchers from TUM and SU had worked together previously in other vector-borne disease projects. They recognized the need to fully engage the community for this community-led intervention program through engagement with a

social scientist. Researchers at TUM had previously worked with a social scientist at KEMRI and invited her to the study team to lead community engagement. The social scientist from KEMRI had also previously worked with a local NGO during a bed-net distribution campaign and invited SCOPE to collaborate in the intervention.

In addition, community residents were vital partners in this research, including household owners, particularly women and children, in school health and mosquito clubs. The continued presence of a social scientist within our project ensured the identification and well-timed engagement of existing interest groups, county government representatives, and local environmental groups.

Critical research infrastructure also supported this work. At the heart of infectious disease research was the Ministry of Health at the national and county governments, providing curative and preventive services. Today, every Kenyan County has a research department where clearance for research in their areas is reviewed and granted. The National Council for Science, Technology, and Innovation (NACOSTI) regulates research carried out in the country and dispenses National Research Funds (NRF). An excellent collaboration exists between the

International Centre of Insect Physiology and Ecology (ICIPE) and KEMRI to support sustainable community control of vector-borne diseases.

Other stakeholders included the local business community, hoteliers, and banks, who support community-based initiatives. A number of international institutions who fund the work can also be considered partners, including but not limited to the Global Fund and the Bill & Melinda Gates Foundation, Bio-Vision Foundation, Switzerland, the U.S. National Institutes of Health, the European Commission, and the Wellcome Trust (Head et al. 2017).

# 4 Principles of Broader Understanding

Our vector-borne disease interventions were successful because we adopted a Community Engagement (CE) strategy through close partnering with social scientists and community members. Dickert and Sugarman (2005) have proposed four main goals of CE: enhanced protection, enhanced benefits, legitimacy, and shared responsibility (Dickert and Sugarman 2005). Relationships are important to CE and research conduct because they allow researchers to understand a community's priorities, needs, and context (Yarborough et al. 2013; Ahmed and Palermo 2010). The relationships between the community and the research program influenced the community members' perception of the research study and their willingness to participate (Gikonyo et al. 2008). CE also helped us mitigate challenges faced during our partnership with the community in the biomedical research (Muia et al. 2019). CE requires both time and resources and social science researchers who are competent and capable of establishing equitable relationships with the community (Fregonese 2018). CE activities can address and reduce public mistrust towards biomedical research by demonstrating respect for the communities involved in the research program (Holzer et al. 2014; Moreno-John et al. 2004).

Some barriers to CE can arise from the challenges of establishing equal relationships with the community. Biomedical research programs have an imbalance in power between the researchers and the community, which can hinder CE if it is not acknowledged transparently and productively (Yarborough et al. 2013). This relationship can be particularly strained in marginalized communities where citizens may not have regular access to health care and the resulting benefits of biomedical research (Yarborough et al. 2013). Additionally, existing relationship structures within a community may pose challenges in CE as participation can reflect existing "social hierarchies and economic or political divisions" (McCoy et al. 2012). In addition to the potential benefits of CE, a review of evidence conducted by Attree et al. highlighted the potential for unintended negative impacts (Attree et al. 2011), including physical and mental exhaustion from the requirements of engagement that may not always outweigh the expected benefits (Attree et al. 2011) as well as further entrenching existing inequalities influenced by power and resource prioritization (McCoy et al. 2012).

To succeed, many CE activities rely on mutually beneficial relationships and high levels of trust between the research program and the community (Gikonyo et al. 2008; Lavery et al. 2010). Trust is crucial but contextual: citizens' experiences of specific interventions and perceptions of the institutions delivering them are shaped by social, political, and economic structures and historical trajectories (see chapter "Collective Learning: Power and Trust in Partnerships in the 3D Program for Girls and Women in Rural Pune District, India") (Dhillon and Kelly 2015; Enria et al. 2016). At the same time, trust is not static: it can be built or lost throughout the response or program. Research during the 2014–2016 West African Ebola outbreak, for example, showed how local responders employed varied "technologies of trust," such as openness, accountability, and reflexivity, to respond to on-the-ground realities and build confidence in the measures implemented to contain the epidemic (Ryan et al. 2019). To develop trust with the community, a study on the informed consent practices of a vaccine trial in Kenya used external technical experts and local field assistants who were known to the community to communicate information about a trial before it began (Gikonyo et al. 2008). As risk communication and community engagement become increasingly recognized as central to global epidemic response strategies, understanding the dynamics of mistrust and the factors influencing the message's legitimacy is crucial. Communication plays an important role in community engagement (See chapter "Foundations and Future Directions of Global Health Communication"). It must ensure that crucial information (who, what, when, where, why, and how) is both delivered and understood by community members.

## 5    Conclusion

Unwrapping the complex social relationships among all involved in research in the Kenyan village is a process of communication and compromise. Integrating social scientists and community members into research teams can improve equity, communication, and social mobilization of the community, thus creating an environment that improves cohesiveness and mutual understanding by all. Cultural norms such as *gender roles* and *patriarchy* play a key role in decisions at the household level in global health research. Disease control messages must be clear, address a specific problem, be delivered within a specific time when the target group is available (Kibe et al. 2022), and be disseminated by trusted individuals (see chapter "Foundations and Future Directions of Global Health Communication") (Forsyth et al. 2022; Mutero et al. 2015). In our case study, community members served as equal team members. They were the trusted sources of new information in our intervention, which allowed us to overcome some of the barriers we faced. Interventions given and led by community members may reduce ambiguities brought about by community beliefs and perceptions about research, thus enhancing greater partnerships and sustainable collaborations in research. This has

consequently reinforced community awareness of research conduct, increased public education on disease causation (e.g., for malaria, dengue fever, lymphatic filariasis), and increased the use and uptake of interventions such as long-lasting insecticide-treated nets, drugs, and vaccines. In addition, we, the researchers, have gained a greater understanding of community perceptions, beliefs, and relations which have taught us to listen to and uplift the community voices, identifying and co-creating workable solutions that benefit the community and the research.

## References

Ahmed SM, Palermo A-GS. Community engagement in research: frameworks for education and peer review. Am J Public Health. 2010;100(8):1380–7.

Attree P, French B, Milton B, Povall S, Whitehead M, Popay J. The experience of community engagement for individuals: a rapid review of evidence. Health Soc Care Community. 2011;19(3):250–60.

Binka FN, Adongo P. Acceptability and use of insecticide impregnated bednets in northern Ghana. Trop Med Int Health. 1997;2:499–507.

Dengue and dengue hemorrhagic fever. https://www.who.int/news-room/fact-sheets

Dhillon RS, Kelly JD. Community trust and the Ebola endgame. N Engl J Med. 2015;373(9):787–9.

Dickert N, Sugarman J. Ethical goals of community consultation in research. Am J Public Health. 2005;95(7):1123–7.    https://doi.org/10.2105/AJPH.2004.058933

Enria L, Lees S, Smout E, Mooney T, Tengbeh AF, Leigh B, Greenwood B, Watson-Jones D, Larson H. Power, fairness and trust: understanding and engaging with vaccine trial participants and communities in the setting up the EBOVAC-Salone vaccine trial in Sierra Leone. BMC Public Health. 2016;16(1):1–10.

Forsyth JE, Kempinsky A, Pitchik HO, Alberts CJ, Mutuku FM, Kibe L, Ardoin NM, LaBeaud AD. Larval source reduction with a purpose: designing and evaluating a household-and school-based intervention in coastal Kenya. PLoS Negl Trop Dis. 2022;16(4):e0010199.

Fregonese F. Community involvement in biomedical research conducted in the global health context; what can be done to make it really matter? BMC Med Ethics. 2018;19(1):39–47.

Gikonyo C, Bejon P, Marsh V, Molyneux S. Taking social relationships seriously: lessons learned from the informed consent practices of a vaccine trial on the Kenyan Coast. Soc Sci Med. 2008;67(5):708–20.

Gopalan RB, Babu BV, Sugunan AP, Murali A, Ma MS, Balasubramanian R, Philip S. Community engagement to control dengue and other vector-borne diseases in Alappuzha municipality, Kerala, India. Pathog Glob Health. 2021;115(4):258–66.

Head MG, Goss S, Gelister Y, Alegana V, Brown RJ, Clarke SC, Fitchett JR, Atun R, Scott JAG, Newell M-L. Global funding trends for malaria research in sub-Saharan Africa: a systematic analysis. Lancet Glob Health. 2017;5(8):e772–81.

Holzer JK, Ellis L, Merritt MW. Why we need community engagement in medical research. J Investig Med. 2014;62(6):851–5.

Hortion J, Mutuku FM, Eyherabide AL, Vu DM, Boothroyd DB, Grossi-Soyster EN, King CH, Ndenga BA, LaBeaud AD. Acute flavivirus and alphavirus infections among children in two different areas of Kenya, 2015. Am J Trop Med Hyg. 2019;100(1):170.

Jones C, Williams HA. Social science in malaria control. Trends Parasitol. 2002;18:195–6.

Kibe L, Habluetzel A, Kamau A, Gachigi J, Mwangangi J, Mutero C, Mbogo C. Low awareness and misconceptions of immature mosquito stages hinders community participation in integrated vector management in Malindi, Kenya. 2019.

Kibe LW, Kimani BW, Okoyo C, Omondi WP, Sultani HM, Njomo DW. Towards elimination of Lymphatic Filariasis in Kenya: improving advocacy, communication and social mobilization activities for mass drug administration, a qualitative study. Trop Dis Travel Med Vaccines. 2022;8(1):1–13.

LaBeaud A, Bashir F, King CH. Measuring the burden of arboviral diseases: the spectrum of morbidity and mortality from four prevalent infections. Popul Health Metrics. 2011;9(1):1–11.

Lavery JV, Tinadana PO, Scott TW, Harrington LC, Ramsey JM, Ytuarte-Nuñez C, James AA. Towards a framework for community engagement in global health research. Trends Parasitol. 2010;26(6):279–83.

Lymphatic filariasis. WHO Fact Sheet No. 102. https://www.who.int/news-room/fact-sheets

Malaria. WHO Fact Sheet No. 94. https://www.who.int/news-room/fact-sheets

Marsh V, Kamuya D, Rowa Y, Gikonyo C, Molyneux S. Beginning community engagement at a busy biomedical research programme: experiences from the KEMRI CGMRC-Wellcome Trust Research Programme, Kilifi, Kenya. Soc Sci Med. 2008;67(5):721–33.

Matthews A. A mathematical model for anti-malarial drug resistance. 2009.

Mayoyo P. Why I rejected mosquito nets In: Nation Newspaper. Edited by allAfrica.com. Kenya; 2006.

McCoy DC, Hall JA, Ridge M. A systematic review of the literature for evidence on health facility committees in low-and middle-income countries. Health Policy Plan. 2012;27(6):449–66.

Moreno-John G, Gachie A, Fleming CM, Napoles-Springer A, Mutran E, Manson SM, Pérez-Stable EJ. Ethnic minority older adults participating in clinical research. J Aging Health. 2004;16(5_suppl):93S–123S.

Msuya J. Horizontal and vertical delivery of health services: what are the tradeoffs. Background paper for the World Development Report. 2004.

Muia D, Kamau A, Kibe L. Community health workers volunteerism and task-shifting: lessons from malaria control and prevention implementation research in Malindi, Kenya. Am J Sociol Res. 2019;9(1):1–8.

Mutero CM, Schlodder D, Kabatereine N, Kramer R. Integrated vector management for malaria control in Uganda: knowledge, perceptions and policy development. Malar J. 2012;11(1):1–10.

Mutero CM, Mbogo C, Mwangangi J, Imbahale S, Kibe L, Orindi B, Girma M, Njui A, Lwande W, Affognon H. An assessment of participatory integrated vector management for malaria control in Kenya. Environ Health Perspect. 2015;123(11):1145–51.

Ngugi HN, Mutuku FM, Ndenga BA, Musunzaji PS, Mbakaya JO, Aswani P, Irungu LW, Mukoko D, Vulule J, Kitron U. Characterization and productivity profiles of Aedes aegypti (L.) breeding habitats across rural and urban landscapes in western and coastal Kenya. Parasit Vectors. 2017;10(1):1–12.

Organization WH: Global strategy for dengue prevention and control 2012–2020. 2012.

Rational Use of Personal Protective Equipment for Coronavirus Disease (COVID-19).: Interim Guidance.

Ryan MJ, Giles-Vernick T, Graham JE. Technologies of trust in epidemic response: openness, reflexivity and accountability during the 2014–2016 Ebola outbreak in West Africa. BMJ Glob Health. 2019;4(1):e001272.

Shah MM, Ndenga BA, Mutuku FM, Vu DM, Grossi-Soyster EN, Okuta V, Ronga CO, Chebii PK, Maina P, Jembe Z. High dengue burden and circulation of 4 virus serotypes among children with undifferentiated fever, Kenya, 2014–2017. Emerg Infect Dis. 2020;26(11):2638.

Sutherland LJ, Cash AA, Huang Y-JS, Sang RC, Malhotra I, Moormann AM, King CL, Weaver SC, King CH, LaBeaud AD. Serologic evidence of arboviral infections among humans in Kenya. Am J Trop Med Hyg. 2011;85(1):158.

Townson H, Nathan M, Zaim M, Guillet P, Manga L, Bos R, Kindhauser M. Exploiting the potential of vector control for disease prevention. Bull World Health Organ. 2005;83:942–7.

Vu DM, Banda T, Teng CY, Heimbaugh C, Muchiri EM, Mungai PL, Mutuku FM, Brichard J, Gildengorin G, Borland EM. Dengue and West Nile virus transmission in children and adults in coastal Kenya. Am J Trop Med Hyg. 2017a;96(1):141.

Vu DM, Mutai N, Heath CJ, Vulule JM, Mutuku FM, Ndenga BA, LaBeaud AD. Unrecognized dengue virus infections in children, western Kenya, 2014–2015. Emerg Infect Dis. 2017b;23(11):1915.

Yarborough M, Edwards K, Espinoza P, Geller G, Sarwal A, Sharp R, Spicer P. Relationships hold the key to trustworthy and productive translational science: recommendations for expanding community engagement in biomedical research. Clin Transl Sci. 2013;6(4):310.

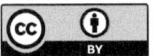

# Partnership-Based Approach to Infectious Disease Research in Papua New Guinea

Annie Dori, Rachael Farquhar, Trevor Kelebi, Enoch Waipeli, Zebedee Kerry, Shazia Ruybal-Pesántez, Diana Timbi, Samuel McEwen, Leo Makita, Moses Laman, and Leanne Robinson

*Partnerships in Papua New Guinea are the door into technical work and research activities across the country.*

NMCP Program Manager & Project Partnership Manager

## Abstract

Infectious disease research requires expertise from multiple diverse backgrounds. In Papua New Guinea (PNG), relationships are an integral part of the culture, both historically and today, and play a critical role in conducting infectious disease research activities across the country. Research efforts on vector-borne diseases (VBDs), such as malaria and dengue, run parallel to rigorous implementation research to reduce the burden of other neglected tropical diseases and combat growing anti-microbial resistance in the country. This chapter will highlight the history of collaborative research in Papua New Guinea and specifically, how the partnership-based approach to implementation research has been adopted to conduct infectious disease research at different levels of the health system. In PNG, genuine trust-based relationships have been established over time by incorporating a set of guiding principles into daily practice and focusing on principles such as authenticity, courage, equality, equity, mutual benefit, and transparency throughout the research cycle. This chapter showcases key learnings across multiple

A. Dori (✉)
Burnet Institute, Port Moresby, Papua New Guinea
e-mail: annie.dori@burnet.edu.au

R. Farquhar (✉) · S. McEwen
Burnet Institute, Melbourne, VIC, Australia
e-mail: rachael.farquhar@burnet.edu.au; samuel.mcewen@burnet.edu.au

T. Kelebi · E. Waipeli
West Sepik Provincial Health Authority,
Vanimo, Sandaun, Papua New Guinea

Z. Kerry · D. Timbi · M. Laman
PNG Institute of Medical Research,
Goroka, Papua New Guinea
e-mail: zebedee.kerry@pngimr.org.pg; diana.timbi@pngimr.org.pg; moses.laman@pngimr.org.pg

S. Ruybal-Pesántez
Burnet Institute, Melbourne, VIC, Australia

School of Public Health – Faculty of Medicine,
Imperial College, London, UK
e-mail: ruybal.s@wehi.edu.au

L. Makita
National Malaria Control Program, NDoH,
Port Moresby, Papua New Guinea

L. Robinson
Burnet Institute, Melbourne, VIC, Australia

Walter and Eliza Hall Institute,
Parkville, VIC, Australia
e-mail: leanne.robinson@burnet.edu.au

© The Author(s) 2024
A. Stewart Ibarra, A. D. LaBeaud (eds.), *Transforming Global Health Partnerships*, Sustainable
Development Goals Series, https://doi.org/10.1007/978-3-031-53793-6_9

133

and interconnected levels of the health system. It also sheds light on nuanced approaches to partnerships which harness local knowledge and empower champions to enable meaningful research and systemic change.

## Keywords

Implementation research · Vector borne diseases · Localisation · Principles-based research · Partnerships

**Author Perspective**

The authors represent a multi-disciplinary background. Many of the authors have worked together for more than 15 years conducting health research in Papua New Guinea bringing with them expertise in policy, malaria epidemiology, implementation research, clinical medicine, health systems research and partnership brokering. The authors have Papua New Guinean, Australian and Ecuadorian cultural backgrounds and work for Medical Research Institutes, Departments of Health (National & Provincial) and International Government Organisations.

**Key Tenets**

1. Expertise from multiple diverse backgrounds and perspectives is required to solve complex problems.
2. As efforts towards evidence-based policy and service delivery models accelerate in resource-constrained settings, it is critical to recognise the broader societal and economic benefits of partnerships, such as shared visions and objectives, local ownership, and resource sharing.
3. The ways in which research partners engage needs to be context-specific, depending on culture, location, and pre-existing relationships.
4. Opportunities for engagement are crucial to continue establishing and building strong and robust partnerships

between researchers and decision-makers, underpinned by a set of guiding principles.
5. Research partnerships are about reciprocal trust and understanding.
6. This chapter addresses the following SDGs: #3: Ensure healthy lives and promote well-being for all at all ages; #10: Reduced inequalities; #16: Promote peaceful and inclusive societies for sustainable development, provide access to justice for all, and build effective, accountable and inclusive institutions at all levels; #17: Partnerships for the goals.

# 1 Introduction

Expertise from multiple backgrounds and perspectives is required to solve complex global health problems (Chambers and Azrin 2013). There is a growing movement to strengthen evidence-based policies and service delivery to drive sustainable changes in public health systems (Fransman and Newman 2019). The long-term sustainability of health programs and activities leverages the strengths and resources of partners. It embeds values and principles into practice to ensure equitable partnerships that work towards improved health outcomes. This partnership-based approach facilitates mutual learning and capacity strengthening amongst all involved to generate meaningful research data relevant to contexts, communities, and stakeholders (Brown et al. 2012).

Prior studies have highlighted clear benefits to partnerships between academics, development practitioners, communities, policymakers and the medical faculty (Fransman and Newman 2019). Social and economic benefits of partnerships, including co-development of shared visions and objectives, local ownership, and resource sharing, supports efforts towards evidence-based policy making and sustainable systemic change. However, to date, most of these studies have focused on international development partnerships centred around improving the lives of individual worldwide in areas such as education, democracy, health, sustainability and economics rather than research partnerships focussed on advancing the field of study, research and practise that places a priority on achieving equity in health for all people.

This case study highlights the history of collaborative research in Papua New Guinea (PNG) and, specifically, how a partnership-based approach to implementation research has been adopted to conduct infectious disease research at different levels of the health system. We will draw on experiences at an individual learning level (public health practitioners, researchers, partnership brokers) and also from an organisational perspective.

Relationships have always been an integral part of PNG's culture. When navigating the initial stages of building the independent state of PNG in the 1970s, national leaders capitalized on the innate wisdom from their forefathers, that dialogue and consensus were essential (Committee PNGNP, Somare MT 1974). The unification of a country with more than 800 languages, and a vast diversity of both beliefs and cultural practices meant questioning and understanding both *"what would bring people together"* and *"how to bring them together"* (Narokobi and Inc 2010). These key questions were integral catalysts to ensure that the work towards the country's development was established in a way that allowed leaders to capitalize on their relationships with other prominent leaders. Though there have been many challenges and learnings throughout this journey, there are many success stories that indicate the benefit of utilising an approach that resonates with people's beliefs, cultures and way of living (Chilisa 2019). Papua New Guineans have experienced the importance of genuine partnerships, bringing people together from different places with diverse strengths and challenges (Somare 1975). It is said by the Alliance for Health Policy and Systems Research, that "learning in health systems occurs by making the link between past actions, the effectiveness of those actions and future actions" (Sheikh et al. 2021). As we work towards better health outcomes through infectious disease research, adopting the same sentiment of 'genuine trust-based partnerships' is of the utmost importance to enable meaningful research and systemic change.

## 2    Impact of Infectious Diseases in PNG

Infectious diseases are a growing concern in PNG. Research on vector-borne diseases (VBDs) such as malaria and dengue runs parallel to rigorous implementation research to reduce the burden of other neglected tropical diseases, such as lymphatic filariasis and soil-transmitted helminths. PNG has the highest transmission of malaria in the Western Pacific Region, where it accounted for 80% of the reported confirmed cases in 2018 (Kattenberg et al. 2020). Considerable progress has been made toward controlling malaria and vector-borne diseases in PNG (Cleary et al. 2021).

However, COVID-19 stretched the health system, rediverting resources towards the COVID-19 response nationwide. As of 27th November 2022, PNG had recorded a cumulative total of 46,068 COVID-19 cases and 668 COVID-19 deaths. Localised community transmission is occurring and continues to strain the health system.

Additionally, since 2016 there has been a significant focus on strengthening the capacity of public health laboratories to monitor Antimicrobial Resistance (AMR) across the country. The rise of AMR is reversing the gains made in modern medicine and endangering the lives of people and animals in PNG (Kase et al. 2019).

PNG's health system is decentralised. Responsibility for the management and organization of health care is divided between central (NDoH) and local (Provincial Health Authority) governments (Grundy et al. 2019). Research partnerships at the National, Provincial, District, and community levels have been established and fostered over decades of work to support evidence-based interventions to reduce the burden of infectious diseases. Below are several experiences and examples of how the partnership-based approach has been adopted and utilised at different levels of the health system in PNG. These experiences highlight how the research teams have overcome systemic challenges to conduct innovative and locally-relevant VBD implementation research that has changed global and local public health policies.

## 3 What Do We Mean by 'Partnership'?

Before we share our experiences, it's important to highlight what we mean by the term 'partnership.' The term 'partnership' is used widely to describe many different relationships and arrangements (Tennyson and Mundy 2018). Throughout our experiences working with partners across levels of the health system, we acknowledge that our definition of partnership changes. For those of us from the team in PNG, the word partnership means 'a way of working' that promotes local and cultural contextualization of activities. Despite calling the 'way of working' a partnership, we have found that it is the relationships that are built, nurtured, and established behind the scenes that give significant meaning to the word 'partnership.' Relationships are perceived as valuable and considered an asset. From a local PNG context, it's these relationships that strengthen the partnership and enable broader teams to overcome barriers, bottlenecks, and challenges.

Furthermore, it is important to recognise that we use the term 'partnership' to signal 'fit-for-purpose engagement.' At times, we have experienced partners that need to shift their relationship or engagement towards a more 'collaborative' approach when activities are centered around health systems strengthening. At other times partners are engaged in a more transactional/service-delivery model. These shifts in the partnership are all dependent on the partnership's evolving aims (becoming more ambitious or less), changes in their operating environment (responding to opportunities or barriers), or even internal changes (less or more time, less or more permission space for risk etc). The examples below showcase how *fit-for-purpose engagement* is needed at different points in the *partnership* to undertake implementation research in PNG.

## 4 A Principles-Based Approach to Research in Papua New Guinea

The explicit use of the partnership-based approach in infectious disease research in PNG was first adopted by the Trilateral Malaria Project; Australia-China-PNG Pilot Cooperation on Malaria Control in 2016 (Hombhanje et al. 2018). However, upon reflection with lead researchers from several organisations, it was identified that principles-based research was central in all activities, even before the Trilateral Malaria Project.

> *Just as health systems are rooted in society and in people, learning in health systems is people-centered and therefore must be informed by values such as equity, justice and solidarity.*
> (Sheikh et al. 2021)

Genuine trust-based relationships have been established over time by incorporating co-developed guiding principles into daily practice and focussing on these principles throughout the entire research cycle—remembering that "the little things matter." These guiding principles were initially co-developed by PNG, Chinese, and Australian Technical Directors on the Trilateral Malaria Project. Over time, as the individual VBD projects came and went, the guiding principles remained the same. However, as new projects begin, partners are asked to describe what these guiding principles mean to them in practise and how they will 'live' by them in the project. This highly collaborative activity, attaching a descriptive set of behaviours to principles, sets the tone and foundation for the partnership moving forward. These guiding principles include:

- Authenticity
- Courage
- Equality
- Equity
- Mutual Benefit
- Transparency

Whilst 'walking the talk' of all these guiding principles remains critical, for research activities in PNG, principles such as 'authenticity' and 'mutual benefit' are *"expected [by PNG Partners] and very important"* for meaningful engagement and research across the country, as expressed by a malaria research program director. Below we highlight key learnings across multiple interconnected levels of the health system, shedding light on how we have embedded the guiding principles into practise.

## 5  Forging Partnerships at the National Level Between Government Agencies

The introduction of partnership brokering, referred to as *"the essential intermediary function that enables partners to work together well (equitably) and ensure the maximum effectiveness of their partnership"* (Mundy and Tennyson 2019), has been a gradual yet effective way of bringing together National organisations in PNG. "Health systems informed by experience, stakeholder deliberations, reliable information and evidence and ready to recognise and adjust past mistakes are in a better position to adapt and tailor actions to meet contextual changes" (Sheikh et al. 2021). With a growing portfolio of work under the leadership of the National Malaria Control Program (NMCP), there is now a team of partnership brokers from PNG, New Zealand, and Australia, who work together to streamline information management, partnership engagement, and ensure strategic alignment with NMCP strategies and policies to support evidence-based decision making amongst PNG research and government organisations. Over time, with support from an accredited partnership broker, profes-

sional working relationships have been built and established between the VBD Program at the Papua New Guinea Institute of Medical Research (PNGIMR) and NMCP at the National Department of Health, providing linkages and opportunities to collaborate, improve and strengthen existing and new programs of work.

However, opportunities for engagement are not to be taken lightly.

> We are really privileged to have the relationship with the NMCP. For other programs of work [at PNGIMR], there have been many challenges however we have worked really hard for the relationship and to establish trust and we cannot take this for granted.
> —PNGIMR Deputy Director

During the initial stages of forging the relationship, there were several factors that contributed to meaningful engagement. Despite not being explicitly spoken, they were implicitly applied. As the PNG Project Partnership Manager reflects—*"in PNG, your actions speak louder than your words. The demonstration of how you work is enough to establish a really good working relationship"*. Reflections from during this time of engagement from the PNGIMR VBD Director and NCMP Manager include;

- Using guiding principles in daily practice; *Demonstrating respect and that partnerships are not just about 'working together' but 'how' to work together well.*
- Reflecting honestly about the motivations for engagement: what are the *shared and individual agendas*? Where did we align? Where did we agree? Where are there differences? What brought us both to the table?
- Contributions and shared resourcing: How could we draw on each other's strengths— what was the mutual benefit?

These key factors were the first steps toward shifting the way of thinking. A shift from *"just working together, to then actually demonstrating the respect and defining joint-decision making. It was important to let the path emerge instead of set the path below us,"* as indicated by a Malaria Research Program Director.

Prior to this partnership approach, colonial ways of working dominated various sections of the health system, often resulting in research that was unaligned with government priorities, over-powered government processes, and led to a lack of mutual benefit. The research was often one-sided, with the questions, objectives, and out-comes were developed and led by research organisations or international partners, with little benefit or even consultation given to PNG gov-ernment organisations. This unbalanced and colonial way of working created a culture of power imbalance and exacerbated an existing lack of trust.

Trust takes time to build, and with a change in leadership within PNGIMR, an opportunity to shift the pendulum and work in a way that dem-onstrated that partnerships based on guiding prin-ciples was possible. Today, these partnerships have been reflected across several key projects that are guided by the NMCP and implemented by the PNGIMR, including Trilateral Malaria Project,[1] STRIVE PNG,[2] NATNAT[3] & PAVE PNG.[4] These opportunities for engagement have been crucial to continue establishing and build-ing strong and robust partnerships between research and decision-makers underpinned by a set of guiding principles (Farquhar et al. 2021).

---

[1]The *Australia-China-Papua New Guinea Trilateral Collaboration on Malaria and Health Security Malaria Project* commenced in January 2020. It is a four-year project that contributes to a longer-term, 10-year collabo-ration between the three countries.

[2]STRIVE PNG aims to strengthen Papua New Guinea's vector-borne disease (VBD) surveillance and outbreak response capacity. Through piloting a real-time integrated sentinel surveillance system, the project is generating evi-dence to enable the implementation of rapid-response strategies for surveillance of malaria and other VBDs

[3]The NATNAT project aims to strengthen capacity to assess and adopt new vector control tools to combat VBD transmission in Papua New Guinea.

[4]PAVE PNG is a partnership between the PNG National Department of Health, PNG Institute of Medical Research and Burnet Institute to determine the operational feasibil-ity and cost-effectiveness of improved case management for Plasmodium vivax (*P. vivax*), the most prevalent form of recurring malaria and a risk to an estimated 2.5 billion people worldwide

## 6 Leadership and Local Champions: Tailoring the Partnership Approach for Provincial and District Engagement

Given PNG's decentralised health system, gov-ernance, leadership, and management of health centres, rural hospitals, and aid posts is the responsibility of the Provincial Health Authorities (Grundy et al. 2019). In some Provinces, where provincial health teams have been resourced sufficiently, well-established processes, sub-governance structures, and struc-tured activities exist. However, in other prov-inces, where provincial and district teams face challenging working environments, high turn-over of leadership roles, and resource challenges, there is an added complexity to partnering and working within the province or district. Over the past 15 years, a nuanced partnership-based approach to research within provinces has been utilised to strengthen engagement between Provincial Health Authorities (PHA) and research health facilities for several different VBD research programs. This includes working closely with individuals that support different roles to find the 'local champions' such as *Provincial Malaria Control Supervisor, District Disease Control Officer, Health Information Manager.* This also includes supporting capac-ity-strengthening activities that may not always fall within the realm of 'malaria activities' such as Provincial Health Monitoring and Evaluation. The team has also learned to be flexible and adaptive to local environments, for example, by modifying their schedules to better suit local staff or by supporting provincial staff in the work that is most pressing or important to them. That being said, across all work programs, the role of local leaders has been essential for 'initiating, championing and creating an environment that favours learning' within the province (Sheikh et al. 2021). Below we share examples of how the team has tailored its engagement with local leaders based on individual relationships and a partnership mindset to validate new ways to learn and to generate knowledge.

## STRIVE PNG

The STRIVE PNG Program is piloting a real-time integrated sentinel surveillance system across eight provinces in PNG to generate evidence to enable the implementation of rapid-response strategies for the surveillance of malaria and other VBDs. STRIVE has adopted the Tupaia platform to link febrile illness surveillance data with diagnostic test results, parasite genomic data, mosquito abundance and insecticide resistance data, and available resources (including diagnostic and treatment consumables). This platform will support provincial, district, and national health authorities in their investigation and public health interventions. The STRIVE Program has established four new sentinel sites since the commencement of the project in 2018.

For provincial engagement, STRIVE's internal partnership broker uses the analogy of entering a 'home' or 'house' as working within a province (Farquhar et al. 2021). As a visitor to the province, it's essential to allow space for the host or *'homeowners'* to take the lead in serving you as an act of *respect* towards the home [province]. Indirectly this *builds trust* and is conducive to an environment of teamwork, cooperation, and readiness for new ideas, appreciating the differences and ensuring the inclusivity of provincial teams. This approach differs from other research, where a program of work and study protocol is developed. Formal approval is sought from a sub-national ethics committee or a formal letter from the Director of the Provincial Health Authority to allow the research to continue in the province from a research team [who typically do not reside in that province]. Whilst this approach might be appropriate in some circumstances, it often misses the opportunity to promote leadership and ownership of the program by the province and includes local priorities, losing foresight of the mutual benefit to both the research team and provincial health authority by working together in genuine partnership.

## 6.1 Establishment of Monfort Clinic, Kiunga, Western Province—Walking the Talk of the Guiding Principles

The establishment of the Kiunga sentinel site was a staged process. Kiunga, located in the North Fly District of Western Province, was a new sentinel site for the STRIVE team. Engagement with critical partners in Kiunga happened over three different provincial visits, a scoping visit, the establishment of the sentinel site, and a further visit to socialise and build relationships. It has been critical for the team to invest time into building relationships with the *right* people. By this, we don't mean the most 'influential,' 'senior,' or 'experienced.' What we do mean is the partners that are in it for the reasons that align with the partnership's values. Finding these critical local champions has not always been straightforward, and in some instances, we have not gotten it right. However, through the team's existing networks (professional and personal), we have been able to capitalise on existing relationships to engage with critical partners in provincial sites.

In Papua New Guinea, the Wantok System[5] is integral to how local communities organise themselves and how local customs are employed in intra and inter-group relationships (Nanau 2011). On the one hand, it provides a platform to unblock challenges in specific communities and encourages local ownership and genuine partnership at the community level. However, as mentioned by one of the Program Directors, the influence of the system, if misused, *"enables nepotism, corruption and poor outcomes."* The Wantok system *"is a double-edged sword, so the leaders on the ground must know how to use it well,"* and thus, it's

---

[5]Wantok is a concept associated with networks of district tribal, ethnic, linguistic and geographic groupings in Melanesia. It is a term used to express patterns of relationships and networks that link people in families and regional localities and is also a reference to provincial, national and sub-regional identities.

essential to acknowledge the influence of the Wantok system in implementation research partnerships. The cultural systems allow partners to call for support from others when needed, facilitate conversations with other provinces where the teams have family linkages, and unite locally through reciprocal gestures and goodwill (Nanau 2011). However, where the systems are fragmented, the Wantok system 'presents potential challenges, as it can lead to the misallocation of national and provincial resources undermining the laws, excluding people outside social networks, leading to various forms of corruption that inhibit reliable and impartial service delivery' (Walton and Jackson 2020). For the STRIVE team, these networks have expanded sentinel sites to provinces, such as Western Province, Kiunga, where PNGIMR has previously conducted fewer research activities.

In setting up sentinel sites, it has been essential that the team is flexible, adaptive, and lean on existing relationships. There are no straightforward steps! In a complex setting like PNG, where challenges are inevitable, relationships and guiding principles become even more important to navigate the roadblocks that arise. Personal trusted relationships enable a focal point and project champion within respective provinces who acts as the ambassador for the project, socialising the project through their internal networks. For Kiunga, engagement with the Catholic Church Diocese Health Manager for the Health facility was critical to the establishment and ongoing sustainability of project activities. Responsibility for recruitment, engagement with subsequent district and provincial partners for the signing of a memorandum of understanding (MOUs), and discussion around activity plans was led by the District Health Manager. Localisation of activities and genuine partnerships have been essential to promoting ownership, equity, and leadership for the STRIVE team.

## 6.2 Prior Practises and Beliefs: Snapshot from West Sepik Province, Director of Public Health—Provincial Health Authority

Communication and consensus in PNG have been a part of the culture and community since before PNG was declared independent in 1975 (Matane 1992). The same approach is applied today. Constant dialogue between Provincial Health Authorities, national government agencies (NMCP, PNGIMR), and research institutes (international and local) has provided transparency. As reflected by the West Sepik Director of Public Health.

> One thing about working in a setting like PNG is that over time, you can start working out what is genuine and what is not. This is not to say that there are criteria that guide you to pick what is genuine and what is not. However, the behaviour that partners present usually outlines the agendas that various partners bring to either the PHA or institution.

Open dialogue has enabled the team to create an environment that allows the recipient party to understand what is being brought into the Province (no hidden agendas exist). It allows the Province to direct or advise if the task or project will work in their settings and how it can best be implemented to maximise outcomes—an example of mutual benefit, transparency, and authenticity in practice. In addition, in a culture where relationships are critical to everyday activities,

> Who you know also influences the decisions. Reputation and track records enables Provincial partners an opportunity to decide if Projects or Programs coming in are genuine, and there are no hidden agendas that may have implications on the Provinces.
>
> (Provincial Director of Public Health)

Fit-for-purpose engagement is not a one-way street that falls in the hands of researchers. Provinces or Districts similarly reflect on the opportunity to establish a 'genuine partnership' with researchers or 'approve or disapprove' a research request for their setting. When the focus is on changing health systems, partnerships are critical. For this reason, the STRIVE team has invested significant time and effort into identifying local champions to support and advocate for the team's collaboration in the province and subsequent activities. As mentioned by one of the STRIVE PNG program directors,

> *In PNG, if you want things to move, you must belong to a tribe, a group of colleagues, and a church. If you belong to these three groups, you can make things happen. In the province, we were able to set up sentinel sites because our staff is long-term, committed members and contributors in all three of these social arenas.*

Forming genuine relationships beyond the work arena has been critical to working with provinces where Provincial health teams are well established, and, more importantly, in areas where provincial health teams experience additional challenges.

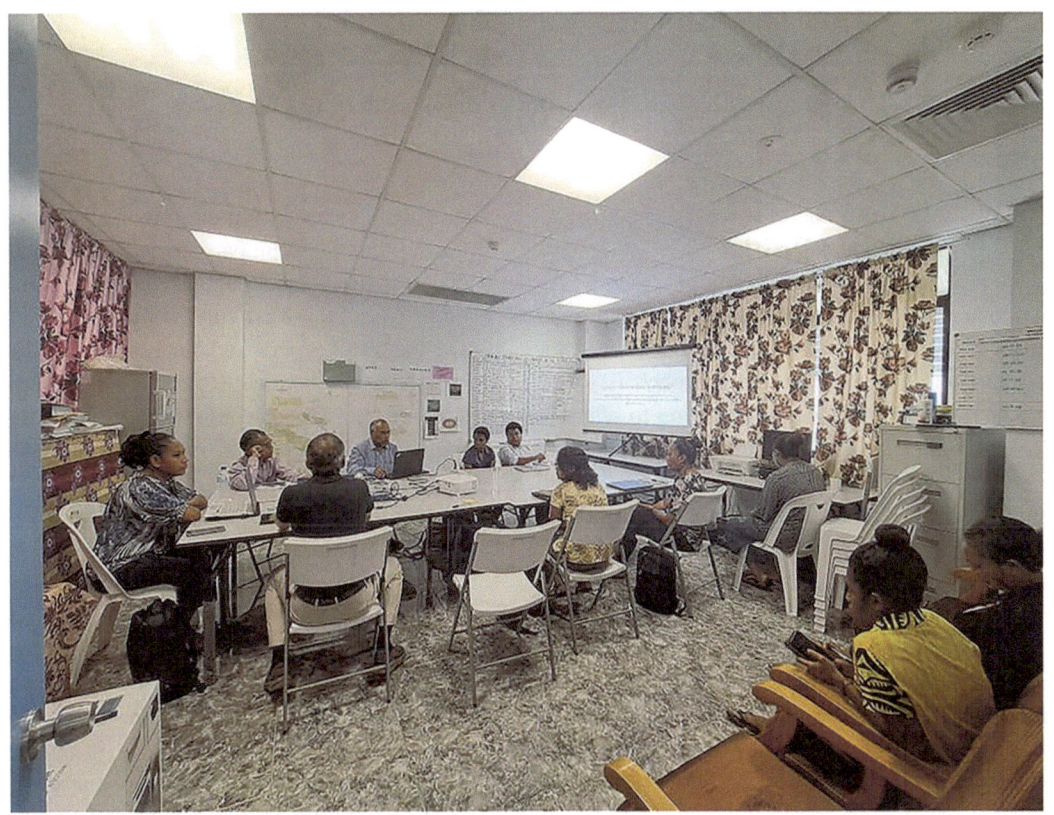

**West Sepik Provincial Health Authority & partners from STRIVE PNG & Trilateral Malaria Project**

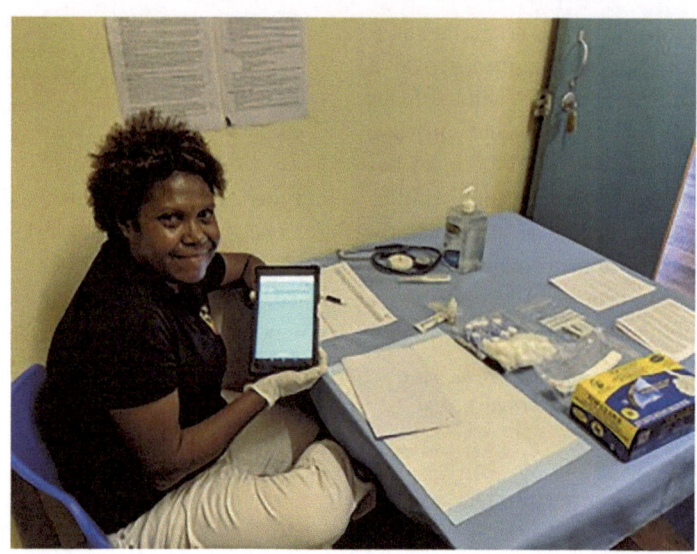

**Marlyn Yakam, Research Nursing Officer, Baro Health Facility West Sepik**

### 6.2.1 Take Hom.e Messages: Provincial & District Engagement

Implementation research activities require a nuanced approach to provincial and district-level partnership engagement. This approach is gaining momentum, and we are beginning to see and feel the added value of working in a partnership. However, it depends heavily on establishing strong working relationships between key individuals and, therefore, takes considerable effort to develop and nurture the partnership throughout the project journey (Tennyson and Mundy 2018). In addition to the significant time required, we found that balancing the technical research priorities of a project whilst forming a robust partnership took much work. Our take-home messages for provincial & district engagement are:

(a) **The importance of local leadership and champions:** A functional Provincial Health Authority (PHA) often has a well-established governance structure that takes the lead in ensuring the delivery of essential primary health care services within their setting. The outcome of health care is reflected through their input. Whilst having an established governance body in place is one indicator of

good leadership within the province, it's not the defining factor in partnering with provincial or district stakeholders. The local champions within these provinces or communities are the gatekeepers and guardians and are critical to the project's success. They can support and advocate for the project, highlight mutual benefits in meetings, and lead the activities as they progress.

(b) **'Don't be tied down to what's on paper:'** Systems in PNG are fragmented, so having a flexible mindset is essential. Across the country, there are the 'same' standard systems for PHAs. However, every province is unique and has its own set of challenges. What works in West Sepik Province may not work well in Western Province. Therefore, flexibility and adaptiveness are vital in working in a complex setting like PNG, where systems are not straightforward.

(c) **Provincial and District Contexts are crucial:** Culture, beliefs, and localisation resonate with partners. Embedding ways of working that ensure trust, respect, and ownership in the hands of the provinces can lead to meaningful engagement and systemic change.

# 7 Community Partners in Research

Genuinely engaging with communities to build and maintain trust-based relationships has been a critically important philosophy underpinning PNGIMR's approach to conducting community-based infectious diseases research over the last 50 years (Reeder and Taime 2003). This starts with a fundamental recognition that engagement needs to be different (context-specific) depending on where you are and the pre-existing relationships. Equally important has been to closely monitor the relationship throughout project cycles, addressing community concerns openly and honestly as they arise and finding opportunities within the research project to ensure mutual benefit and a common goal.

Recruitment of local staff is critical to embed the research within the community. This increases the likelihood that the community's interests are protected, and concerns are quickly and frankly addressed from trusted sources. There is also an obvious economic benefit to the community from the training and employment of village-based workers. In the critical long-term VBD research sites of Maprik, Dreikikir, and north-coast Madang, involving the community as research staff, community reporters, and mosquito collectors have been an essential part of the long-term partnership.

Appropriately managing the flow of information to the community through different layers of authority and decision-making is also essential. This needs to be a phased process whereby the village leaders and broader community first consent to be involved in the program of work. Then, individuals provide informed consent to participate in the research. Community information sessions are a significant opportunity for the reciprocal sharing of perspectives and priorities about the proposed work. They are a chance for the community to openly share concerns and question the research investigators in front of the whole community. This can reduce situations where mistruths can seed and spread unchecked, jeopardising the relationship and the study.

PNGIMR and partners also ensure staff is well trained in conducting robust but sensitive informed consent, per ICH Good Clinical Practice E6 (R2) (see chapter "Ethical Challenges in Global Health Research"). Research staff is trained to perform the informed consent process in ways that avoid the generation of fear and mistruth. Equally important is ensuring timely and vital feedback to the community on the results of previous studies and any ongoing preliminary findings during longitudinal studies. There is an example from Dreikikir near Maprik. One of IMR's long-term collaborators on lymphatic filariasis research engaged with a remote community on a study and told people that feedback would be provided after the study. More than 15–20 years later, when working on a subsequent study in the area, the researcher was approached by an older man who said that he remembered him and still wanted to receive feedback from the previous study. This experience highlights the importance of and the challenges of maintaining strong engagement with communities during and between studies that span many years. In particular, there is a critical need to respect the trust built. Research partnerships are about reciprocal trust and understanding.

Partnering with communities on long-term research programs involves developing a shared understanding of the problem, the relevance of the findings to the local community, and how the research can inform measures that improve health, quality of life, and opportunities. This is achieved in numerous ways, from extensive awareness, consultation, and discussion of preliminary and final research findings, to ensuring that participation provides immediate beneficial knowledge. Examples of helpful knowledge include information about infection and anaemia status (if rapid diagnostic tests are used), the types of mosquitoes transmitting VBDs locally, and actions people can take to reduce their risk of exposure to the disease.

It is essential that the team not over-promise or extend into areas beyond the reach of the health research project. Community development projects, such as water and sanitation, are often a high priority for communities and can offer numerous mutual benefits for vector control, reducing exposure and disease. However, these infrastructure projects are typically beyond the scope and reach of the research program being implemented. In our experience, helping communities connect with NGOs and government programs explicitly designed to support community development programs has been an appropriate way to support the implementation of research partnerships.

---

**Case Study of Impact: Partnerships at all health system levels—from nuanced community mobilisation toglobal policy change (King et al. 2018; Weil et al. 2019; Organization WH 2017)**

The lymphatic filariasis research (LF) program in PNG that led to the current mass drug administration and LF elimination efforts in New Ireland and East New Britain Provinces was first initiated in the Dreikikir District of East Sepik Province. The Dreikikir study showed the superior efficacy of a triple-drug therapy (Ivermectin, Albendazole, and Diethylcarbamazine) in clearing microfilaraemia (Reeder and Taime 2003). This led to strong advocacy for this regimen, prompting the World Health Organisation (WHO) to request a more extensive multi-country safety study. In PNG, additional studies were conducted in Madang Province in response to the WHO request as part of a global consortium, and these studies showed the regimen to be safe and effective (King et al. 2018). This paved the way for the WHO to change its international guidelines to the triple-drug regimen for Mass Drug Administration in LF-elimination endemic countries (Weil et al. 2019). The recommendation also led to the drug company Merck Inc. increasing their donation of ivermectin to 100 million additional doses per year for seven years to support the rollout of the triple drug therapy in LF endemic countries worldwide.

In PNG, East New Britain Province was one of the first Provinces to benefit from this donation and embark upon a new pro-gram of MDA with the triple-drug regimen as a result of the strong PHA leadership and established relationships between PNG and overseas Institutions who had partnered together in the initial trials in Dreikikir and Madang. The ENB PHA-led elimination effort resulted in administering the triple-drug regimen to over 308,000 out of the 376,000 eligible individuals in ENB Province.

This again highlights the importance of partnerships/relationships when conducting research or delivering health services in PNG. The workaround LF in ENB, Madang, and ESP provinces leveraged the community networks and relationships that were already in place. For example, in ENB, the ENB PHA used its networks to mobilise community participation. In Madang and Dreikikir, the well-established relationship between PNG IMR and the surrounding communities ensured that this globally impactful research could be successfully conducted.

---

## 8    Conclusion

Principles-based partnerships, local champions, and strong country-based leadership are crucial to meaningful and sustainable implementation research activities. Partnering at the National, Provincial, District, and Community levels enables new ways of working together that build on the diversity of interests, skills, and contributions each partner can bring. In our experience, every partnership is unique. In some cases, the partnership has been built from scratch. In contrast, in other cases, the partnership has been able to lean on existing cultural systems to grow to achieve mutual benefit and positive outcomes. What has become abundantly clear throughout all these experiences of conducting infectious disease research in PNG is that each partnership is highly context-specific and varies depending on how they work and what the team hopes to achieve jointly. Genuine partnerships in infectious disease research provide opportunities for local ownership, promote and harness diversity across individuals and strengthen systems for sustainable change. Although the partnership-based approach has only recently been explicitly discussed in PNG, it's been the 'way of working' for several decades. Guiding principles have underpinned activities from the past and will continue to do so into the future. Investing in the partnership-based approach is crucial to continue meaningful infectious disease research by empowering communities, local leaders, and governments to improve health outcomes for all.

# References

Brown CH, Kellam SG, Kaupert S, Muthén BO, Wang W, Muthén LK, et al. Partnerships for the design, conduct, and analysis of effectiveness, and implementation research: experiences of the prevention science and methodology group. Adm Policy Ment Health Ment Health Serv Res. 2012;39(4):301–16.

Chambers DA, Azrin ST. Research and services partnerships: partnership: a fundamental component of dissemination and implementation research (1557–9700 (Electronic)). Psychiatr Serv. 2013;64(6):509–11.

Chilisa B. Indigenous research methodologies. Sage Publications; 2019.

Cleary E, Hetzel MW, Siba PM, Lau CL, Clements ACA. Spatial prediction of malaria prevalence in Papua New Guinea: a comparison of Bayesian decision network and multivariate regression modelling approaches for improved accuracy in prevalence prediction. Malar J. 2021;20(1):269.

Committee PNGNP, Somare MT. Strategies for nationhood: policies and issues, December 1974. National Planning Committee of Cabinet; 1974.

Farquhar R, Dori A, MacCana S, Tefuarani N, Lavu E, Barry A, et al. STRIVE PNG: using a partnership-based approach in implementation research to strengthen surveillance and health systems in Papua New Guinea. BMC Health Research Policy and Systems; 2021.

Fransman J, Newman K. Rethinking research partnerships: evidence and the politics of participation in research partnerships for international development. J Int Dev. 2019;31(7):523–44.

Grundy J, Dakulala P, Wai K, Maalsen A, Whittaker M. Papua New Guinea health system review. 2019;9:1.

Hombhanje F, Yan G, Roggero R, Kelly L. Mid-term review of the Australia China Papua New Guinea Pilot Cooperation on Malaria control. 2018.

Kase P, Kombuk DO, Joku G, Alu J. National Action Plan on Antimicrobial Resistance (AMR) 2019-2023. In: National Department of Health, Department of Agriculture & Livestock, Conservation and Environment Protection Authority, Authority NAQI, editors; 2019.

Kattenberg JH, Gumal DL, Ome-Kaius M, Kiniboro B, Philip M, Jally S, et al. The epidemiology of Plasmodium falciparum and Plasmodium vivax in East Sepik Province, Papua New Guinea, pre- and post-implementation of national malaria control efforts. Malar J. 2020;19(1):198.

King CL, Suamani J, Sanuku N, Cheng Y-C, Satofan S, Mancuso B, et al. A trial of a triple-drug treatment for lymphatic Filariasis. N Engl J Med. 2018;379(19):1801–10.

Matane P. To serve with love. Dellasta Pacific; 1992.

Mundy J, Tennyson R. Brokering better partnerships handbook (2 edn). Association PB, editor; 2019.

Nanau G. The Wantok system as a socio-economic and political network in Melanesia. OMNES. 2011;2:31–55.

Narokobi B, Inc BNF. Foundations for nationhood. University of Papua New Guinea Press and Bookshop; 2010.

Organization WH. Guideline: alternative mass drug administration regimens to eliminate lymphatic filariasis. World Health Organization; 2017.

Reeder JC, Taime J. Engaging the community in research: lessons learned from the malaria vaccine trial. Trends Parasitol. 2003;19(6):281–2.

Sheikh K, Abimbola S, Organization WH. Learning health systems: pathways to progress: flagship report of the Alliance for Health Policy and Systems Research; 2021.

Somare MT. Sana: an autobiography of Michael Somare. Niugini Press; 1975.

Tennyson R, Mundy J. Partnership brokers in action. Skills, tools, approaches. 2nd ed. Partnership Brokers Association; 2018.

Walton G, Jackson D. Reciprocity networks, service delivery, and corruption: the wantok system in Papua New Guinea. U4; 2020.

Weil GJ, Bogus J, Christian M, Dubray C, Djuardi Y, Fischer PU, et al. The safety of double- and triple-drug community mass drug administration for lymphatic filariasis: a multicenter, open-label, cluster-randomized study. PLoS Med. 2019;16(6):e1002839.

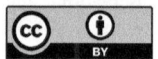

# Partnerships to Improve Access to Healthcare for Refugees and Immigrants in Philadelphia

Jessica Deffler (iD), Chelsea Salas-Tam, Jenna Gosnay, and Marc Altshuler

*It is the obligation of every person born in a safer room to open the door when someone in danger knocks.*

Dina Nayeri

## Abstract

The United States has welcomed refugees since World War II. Currently, the world is experiencing an unparalleled refugee crisis that calls for action by nations across the globe. There are over 82 million people who are forcibly displaced from their homes today (UNHCR Global Trends, Forced displacement in 2020. [cited 2021 Sep 28]. Available from: https://www.unhcr.org/flagship-reports/globaltrends/). Over the last decade, Philadelphia has become home to hundreds of refugees from countries in Southeast and Central Asia, Africa, the Middle East, as well as many others. For newly arrived refugees, finding stable housing, medical care, and employment is difficult due to cultural, language, and socioeconomic barriers. To provide comprehensive care to refugees in Philadelphia, a network of medical providers and social services was formed in 2010. Through the Philadelphia Refugee Health Collaborative, refugees access medical care and refugee resettlement services upon arrival. More recently, inspired by the need for a patient-centered medical home with collocated medical and social services, the Hansjorg Wyss Wellness Center opened in 2021 and serves both refugees and immigrants in the community. This case study explores the partnership journey to serve refugees and immigrants in Philadelphia.

## Keywords

Refugee (health) · Immigrant (health) · Newcomer (health) · Care navigation · Primary care

## Author Perspective

The authors belong to a multidisciplinary medical team that cares for newcomer populations in Philadelphia, Pennsylvania. One provider has worked with refugees in Philadelphia for over fifteen years and was instrumental to bringing comprehensive refugee health care to the city. Together this team provides comprehensive medical care and social work support to newcomers.

J. Deffler (✉) · C. Salas-Tam · J. Gosnay · M. Altshuler
Department of Family and Community Medicine, Thomas Jefferson University Hospital, Philadelphia, PA, USA
e-mail: jessica.deffler@jefferson.edu

© The Author(s) 2024
A. Stewart Ibarra, A. D. LaBeaud (eds.), *Transforming Global Health Partnerships*, Sustainable Development Goals Series, https://doi.org/10.1007/978-3-031-53793-6_10

147

**Key Tenets**

1. Culturally comprehensive and competent care informed by community members is key to the successful resettlement and ongoing health of newcomer populations.
2. Prioritizing the social, financial, and medical needs of newcomers through multidisciplinary collaboration helps to overcome socioeconomic barriers.
3. Medical providers play an important role in compassionate advocacy and social justice for refugees and immigrants.
4. This chapter addresses the following SDGs: 3: Good Health and Wellbeing; 10: Reduced Inequalities; 16: Peace, Justice, and Strong Institutions

# 1 Introduction

**Definitions**

1. Newcomer: Includes refugees, immigrants, displaced persons, and asylum seekers, and others recently arrived to live in a country other than their country of origin.
2. Refugee: Someone who is unable or unwilling to return to their country of origin owing to a well-founded fear of being persecuted for reasons of race, religion, nationality, membership of a particular social group, or political opinion (United Nations High Commissioner for Refugees). Refugee status is typically obtained while the individual is in a country other than their home country (known as the first asylum country).
3. Asylum Seeker: An individual who is seeking international protection and meets criteria for refugee status. This person petitions for legal status as asylee after they arrive in the country where they plan to resettle.
4. Immigrant: A person living in a country other than their country of origin.

There were 82.4 million forcibly displaced people in the world in 2020, an increase from 68.5 million in 2018 (UNHCR Global Trends 2021). This number includes refugees, asylum seekers, and other displaced persons who are survivors of war, violence, persecution, and natural disasters. In 2020, a total of 9.8 million new displacements occurred. Most of these displaced individuals were from Syria, due to ongoing conflict in their country since the start of the civil war in 2011. Large numbers were also displaced from Afghanistan, Sudan, Myanmar (Burma), the Democratic Republic of Congo, and Venezuela.

In the United States, refugee resettlement began after World War II with the Displaced Persons Act of 1948, permitting the admission of some European refugees (Tran 2020). In the years following the end of the Vietnam War in 1975, the U.S. began accepting refugees from Vietnam and Southeast Asia. In the early 1990s, the collapse of the Soviet Union led to a wave of Eastern European and Central Asian refugees. The early 2000s saw the arrival of a wave of African refugees primarily from Sudan, Somalia, and Eritrea. In more recent years, there have been influxes of refugees from Burma, Bhutan, Iraq, and Afghanistan, as well as continued arrivals from Syria.

Philadelphia, with a population of 1.5 million, is one of many large cities in the United States that accepts refugee arrivals. From 2002–2016, the largest numbers of arrivals to Philadelphia were from Bhutan, Liberia, Myanmar, and Iraq. In 2016, a total of 794 refugees were settled in the city, most from Syria (Gammage 2021). In 2017, the government under President Trump dramatically reduced refugee resettlement by banning travel from Muslim countries, suspending resettlement for Syrian refugees, and decreasing the quota on the number of resettled refugees (Pierce and Meissner 2017). Only 444 refugees resettled in Philadelphia in 2020, reflecting this political climate.

Across the globe, refugee health providers seek to provide quality, comprehensive medical care to refugees—care that not only prevents the spread of infectious disease, but also addresses chronic disease, preventive health services, and mental health. This is a large task, and the work of refugee health providers is only successful in collaboration with resettlement agencies and social services teams. These partners help newly arrived persons to the United States navigate the complex medical system, obtain affordable housing, enroll children in school, and find employment. In a collaborative environment, both healthcare and social services providers are continuously learning how to provide culturally competent care to changing newcomer populations and dynamic communities.

This chapter describes the Philadelphia Refugee Health Collaborative (PRHC) that was developed in 2010. This collaborative, patient-centered model coordinates the work of medical providers, refugee resettlement agencies, and other social services partners to ensure that every refugee arriving in Philadelphia has access to comprehensive medical care. In addition, we will discuss how the collaboration's mission recently expanded to include care for immigrants, another often underserved population living in Philadelphia. Our goal is to inspire other practitioners of medicine, allied sciences, and social work to work together in creating sustainable networks that provide quality care to newcomers.

## 2 Nationalities Services Center and the Creation of the Philadelphia Refugee Health Collaborative

Partnerships with community organizations play an integral role in refugee health. Typically, during a twenty-minute visit with a healthcare provider, patients are given a diagnosis, expected to understand that diagnosis, ask any immediate questions, and leave with a new treatment plan to follow at home. But what if that patient is non-English speaking? What if the patient is given written follow up instructions in their preferred language, but they cannot read? What if the patient is uninsurable and needs close follow up, but cannot afford the out-of-pocket cost of subsequent visits?

Each of these barriers require time that is not accounted for during medical appointments. It is not unusual for refugee and immigrant populations to experience one if not all of these barriers when navigating the healthcare system. Access for newcomers to additional community resources and partnering with agencies who cater specifically to these needs is an essential part of ensuring well rounded care. Fortunately, the refugee and immigrant populations of Philadelphia have access to several agencies whose mission includes filling in those gaps.

One of the most important aspects of building and maintaining productive partnerships with community organizations is the idea of a shared mission and values. While the approach and methods of each organization might differ, the end goal is typically shared: to provide quality care to ensure the overall wellbeing of the clients, and to empower them to become thriving members of society.

The United States spent a total of 2.14 billion dollars to fund refugee resettlement services in 2017 (DiVito et al. 2016). Resettlement agencies are responsible for sponsoring new refugee arrivals in the United States and providing the services that each refugee needs, including access to quality medical care. These agencies must ensure that refugees receive a domestic medical screening exam within 30 days of arrival, although they are not legally obligated to ensure that they establish a relationship with a primary care provider for longitudinal care. The Nationalities Service Center (NSC) was founded in 1921 and is the largest refugee resettlement agency in Philadelphia.

Prior to 2007, new refugee arrivals in Philadelphia had difficulty accessing healthcare for their immediate and long-term healthcare needs (Pierce and Meissner 2017). To obtain their domestic medical screening, they were responsible for seeking care on their own, and most sought care in already crowded health centers (Fig. 1). For many refugees, it could take up to 120 days after arrival to access health care, leading to significant delays in the diagnosis and treatment of acute and chronic health conditions.

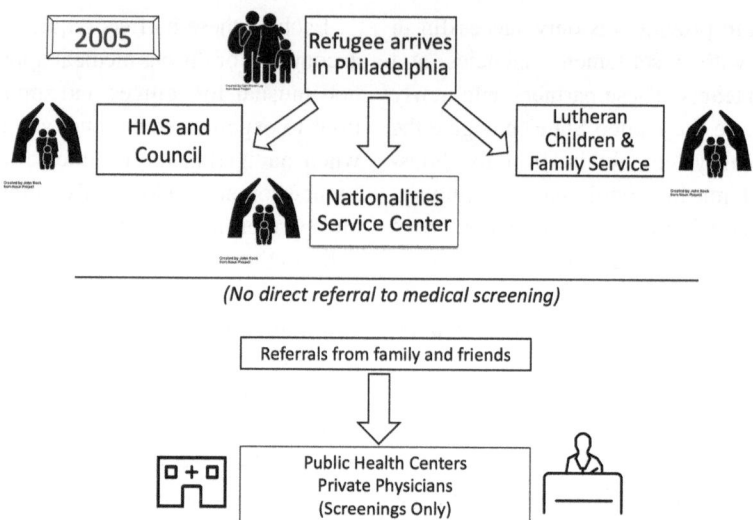

**Fig. 1** Each refugee approved for admission into the United States is sponsored by a non-profit resettlement agency. Prior to the creation of the Philadelphia Refugee Health Collaborative (PRHC), the three refugee resettlement agencies did not collaborate amongst each other or with medical centers. Upon arrival, refugees were responsible for obtaining domestic medical screening exams on their own, and often relied on word of mouth from family and friends. Furthermore, refugees were not assisted in making follow up appointments, such as those for preventative health screenings or specialist consults. *HIAS Hebrew Immigrant Aid Society. (Figures: thenounproject. com)

During this time, it was not uncommon for children to enter the public school system prior to their domestic medical exam, bypassing tuberculosis screening and necessary vaccinations and posing a public health risk.

Gretchen Shanfeld, who served as the senior director for NSC until 2023, began her career as a clinic liaison in 2008, helping clients navigate their domestic medical exam and arranging follow up care. In this role she quickly learned of the language and systems barriers that refugees face when navigating the medical system. One in four of the clients served by NSC had extensive medical needs that required additional evaluation by specialist providers and long-term follow up for chronic health conditions. Recognizing that patients would benefit from a medical home rather than fragmented care, Gretchen contributed to early discussions at NSC to explore the establishment of a partnership between their resettlement agency and medical providers. NSC sought to establish a collaboration with the Department of Family and Community Medicine (DFCM) at Thomas Jefferson University in 2007, recognizing the department's commitment to underserved populations in the city.

In 2007, DFCM partnered with NSC to create the first refugee medical home in Philadelphia. The need quickly grew over the first few years of the partnership, prompting an expansion to other clinical sites throughout the city, and leading to the creation of the Philadelphia Refugee Health Collaborative (PRHC) in 2010. The PRHC is a collaborative model of care that includes three resettlement agencies and eight academic medical centers, harmonizing their efforts to promote health equity and continuity of care for all refugees in the city (Fig. 2). Prior to the creation of the PRHC, new refugee arrival visits occurred on average 80–90 days after arrival. After its creation, this time was reduced to just 20 days, facilitating initial health screenings for all refugees prior to entering school or the workforce. Prompt access to care and a robust network of providers

**Fig. 2** In the PRHC, any of the three resettlement agencies can access care for their clients at any medical center, creating a patient-centered model and prompt access to care. The PRHC also set up a network of patient care navigators to accompany them to their appointments and assist with scheduling follow up, such as specialist appointments, dental visits, imaging and cancer screenings. (Figures: thenounproject.com)

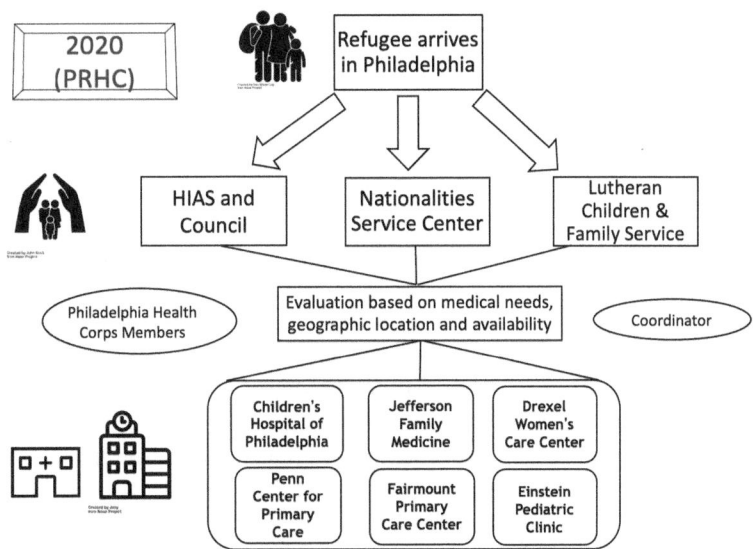

allowed NSC to accept refugees with high level medical needs, such as patients with end stage renal disease requiring hospital admission for dialysis within 24 hours of arrival. NSC was recognized nationally as being able to handle the most medically complex refugees who were eligible for resettlement to the United States, and the organization has never had to turn down a refugee resettlement request. Of note, NSC and the other resettlement agencies in the PRHC did not receive any additional funding for this collaboration. They proactively applied for grants to cover the costs of the increased staffing and time required to support care navigation.

## 3    The Role of Research

With an established relationship with NSC since 2007, DFCM at Jefferson became a medical home for refugees and established the Jefferson Center for Refugee Health (CRH) in 2008, led by Dr. Marc Altshuler. Recognizing the opportunity to collect health data on refugees to improve quality of care, Dr. Altshuler and colleagues worked to create a data set which captured the medical history for every refugee patient screened

by the CRH providers. After receiving institutional IRB approval, the team collected deidentified data on numerous ongoing data points. The CRH database expanded over time, and captured data that could answer numerous research questions, including, but not limited to, latent tuberculosis treatment completion rates, incidence of chronic health conditions by country of birth, and specialist provider and emergency department utilization. Jefferson partnered with other clinical leaders across the country to share similar data with the Centers of Disease Control (CDC) through a 5-year comprehensive surveillance program grant (2010–2015). Research from this group was published in numerous peer-reviewed journals and presented at national and international conferences.

In 2015, Jefferson received ongoing funding through CDC as a designated Center of Excellence (COE) in Refugee Health Care (Rahman 2021). In addition to being tasked with ongoing research collection, the COE has also been responsible for creating an online interactive refugee screening tool for healthcare providers, in addition to updating the CDC's Refugee Health Provider Guidelines (Centers Of Excellence Guidelines 2021).

## 4 Building a More Comprehensive Medical Home for Refugees and Immigrants

The PRHC dramatically improved access to care for newly arrived refugees. However, after the 90 days resettlement period, refugees may no longer be eligible for resettlement services and often lose contact with their agency. Many refugees lose medical insurance if they do not apply for Medicaid or live in a state without Medicaid expansion, leaving 40–50% of refugees uninsured at eight months post-arrival (Refugee Health Guidance | Immigrant and Refugee Health | CDC 2021; Kumar et al. 2021). Without access to patient care navigators, they may struggle to get to appointments because of barriers of transportation, language, and health literacy. Refugee populations have a high burden of chronic disease (20–25%), greater than non-refugee immigrants in the U.S. For these now resettled refugees, there was a need to provide accessible, longitudinal care for chronic conditions such as diabetes, obesity, hypertension, heart disease, as well as address their social needs. Hence began the vision to create a permanent refugee medical home in Philadelphia, which would continue to provide primary care and integrated social services to refugees long after resettlement.

In early discussions about the vision for the medical home, it was clear that one other group in Philadelphia was in similar need of a medical home—many immigrant communities in Philadelphia struggle to access medical care. Since the 1990s, the immigrant population in Philadelphia has grown significantly. Philadelphia is a growing diverse city with a majority of its immigrants from China and Southeast Asia, the Dominican Republic, Jamaica, India, Haiti, and Mexico, with different groups settling in different parts of the city (Yun et al. 2012). This growth has a profound impact on the economics, culture, and health of the city. In fact, immigrants and their children are largely responsible for the growth of the city since 2006, representing more than a quarter of the city's population (approximately 390,000 people) in 2018 (Philadelphia's

Immigrants 2021). Like refugees, immigrants may face pre-, peri-, and post-immigration trauma that influence their health and wellbeing in the country in which they have settled (The State of Immigrants in Philadelphia 2019). Often disadvantaged in healthcare due to documentation status and ineligibility for insurance, immigrants underutilize preventative health care services and often rely on emergency care. They have high rates of chronic disease including obesity, hypertension, and diabetes. Because more immigrants are staying longer in the US, there is an aging undocumented population, which increases the likelihood of more complex care needs (Perreira and Ornelas 2013). The need for expanded access to care for immigrants inspired the idea to include immigrants, regardless of insurance status, in the vision for the medical home.

In 2016, Dr. Altshuler began exploring this idea of a medical home that would be accessible to both refugees and immigrants, with the vision to bring healthcare into the community. After reviewing numerous community needs assessments and speaking with public health leaders throughout the city, Dr. Altshuler and his colleagues recognized a South Philadelphia neighborhood that served a large immigrant community. The surrounding neighborhood is a melting pot of diverse groups of refugees and immigrants, including large numbers from the Southeast Asian, Mexican, Central American, and West African immigrant community. While traditionally the neighborhood was home to primarily Italian immigrants, today, over twenty languages are spoken at one local elementary school, row-homes house multigenerational and multilingual families, the streets are lined with Mexican, Indonesian, and Cambodian restaurants, and parks are used for community cultural events.

The vision for the Center developed into a hub for clinical and educational outreach activities, a shared space for medical providers and community partners that serve the larger immigrant community. After a successful fundraising campaign, the Wyss Wellness Center was born, in partnership between Jefferson and SEAMAAC (Southeast Asian Mutual Assistance Association

Coalition)—the largest community agency serving the immigrant community in this area. SEAMAAC is a community organization that has advocated for immigrants in Philadelphia for over thirty years. The community in which they work is home to many Southeast Asian immigrants and refugees. Southeast Asians are one of the most prominent Asian immigrant groups in Philadelphia and have built a thriving and resilient neighborhood, mostly residing in South Philadelphia. Since the 1970s, refugees from Vietnam, Cambodia and Laos have left their homes and resettled in the U.S. The SEAMAAC team provides assistance to their clients with basic needs, housing, employment and vocational training, and literacy.

Prior to construction of the Center, Dr. Altshuler and his colleagues from Jefferson and SEAMAAC met with twelve different cultural representatives from the community in focus groups, to gain input on community needs and how to create a welcoming medical home and community center. The doors of the Wyss Center opened in March 2021. Today, the Wyss Center provides both medical care through Jefferson and access to social services through SEAMAAC, in addition to partnering with other medical leaders and community members to offer free vision screening, breast cancer screening, and a COVID-19 vaccine clinic.

The Wyss Center is the first Jefferson Health clinic created specifically to serve patients regardless of insurance status. Large academic health centers often do not prioritize providing care for uninsured patients or patients with government medical assistance. Estimates from a neighborhood analysis were that 20% of patients would be uninsured; unexpectedly, in the first six months, almost 60% were uninsured. If focused only on short term financial goals and profit, opening the vision of the Center may not have come to fruition, especially during the COVID-19 pandemic. Fortunately, Jefferson and SEAMAAC leadership were able to look beyond the potential for short term losses and prioritize the mission of the Center and potential benefits that it would have for the community served. Through the generous philanthropy of numerous donors, we were

able to not only design and open the Wyss Wellness Center, but also support a team of providers and staff to carry out our mission. In the near future the Center will apply to become a Federally-Qualified Health Center (FQHC), and if successful, this will bring in additional financial resources to provide ongoing care to our community.

By bringing healthcare into the community, we can expand preventative services for the underserved, promote earlier cancer detection, reduce emergency room utilization by increasing access to outpatient care, and help offload crowded hospitals. Leaders were willing to see the potential for these long-term goals and investments in the future of the health of the community. One of the ways in which the construction of the Center showed its value in community public health was by increasing vaccination rates during the COVID-19 pandemic, as we will discuss below.

## 5    Immigrants in Philadelphia and the COVID Pandemic

### 5.1    Case Example

*Luis\* is 53 years old and works as a dishwasher in a restaurant in South Philadelphia. He came to the United States over twenty years ago to support his wife and three daughters in Mexico, and he has not seen his family since. He lives in an apartment with his brother and another roommate, who are also in their fifties and restaurant workers. Luis started feeling ill one day in March 2020 with chills and a headache, and after a week of his illness he developed a cough and shortness of breath. He attributed his symptoms to catching pneumonia from a coworker. He called his nephew, who speaks better English, to make him a doctor's appointment. "I need antibiotics," he told him. Unfortunately, the clinic wouldn't see him without a COVID test. When his condition worsened, his nephew*

---

\**Name has been changed to protect this individual's identity.*

*took him to the emergency room where he has a 103.5 fever and slightly low oxygen. His COVID test was positive, and he was discharged with cough medicine. He did not understand why he wasn't treated with antibiotics and attributed it to his lack of insurance and his citizenship status. He continued to have a cough and fever for several days. Luis says, when his symptoms were worsening, he was afraid he was going to die. He avoided going to the hospital because of fear of lack of insurance, and because he had heard of others dying in the hospital. He was afraid he would never see his family again. Fortunately, Luis recovered. Despite his efforts to quarantine at home, both his brother and his roommate, who share a bedroom and a bathroom, were also infected. His brother stayed home from work and quarantined, but his cousin continued to work through his illness, feeling pressure that they wouldn't be able to pay the rent if all three were out of work. Luis borrowed 500 dollars from his nephew to help pay the rent.*

In Philadelphia, immigrants, in addition to African Americans, were disproportionately affected by COVID-19, with higher rates of hospitalizations and mortality. In the U.S. and other countries, more immigrants work in jobs that were impacted most by the pandemic, and have less access to paid leave, unemployment insurance, and government assistance. The pandemic exacerbated the already existent healthcare disparities for immigrants (Wiltz 2018). Among those affected were Latin American immigrants, who represent approximately 15% of the population in Philadelphia (Lazo et al. 2021). Approximately 32% of Latino workers are essential workers, and undocumented immigrants are disproportionately employed in jobs with greater COVID transmission risk, such as restaurant work and cleaning services. 37% of Latinos in Philadelphia live in poverty, and they are likely to live in crowded housing, making quarantine difficult. Most utilize transportation or ride shares to commute to work. Undocumented immigrants

also have limited access to government relief funds, increasing the pressure to work despite potential COVID symptoms.

During the COVID pandemic, recognizing the barriers that immigrants face to access health care, such as language and citizenship status, the Philadelphia Health Department called for a response to increase vaccine access to all communities. There was a need for increased outreach to non-English speaking communities and translated public health materials given the prevalence of misinformation in certain communities, for example in social media posts or videos aimed at certain immigrant groups, including Spanish speakers (U.S. Census Bureau QuickFacts 2021). Other communities lacked any media coverage of the vaccine, and information was spread primarily by word of mouth. There was also a need for community vaccination and testing sites. The large central Convention Center building in downtown Philadelphia was one of the first sites to provide vaccines to the public but was not easily accessible to patients living away from downtown or those with limited English proficiency. The Wyss Wellness Center was proposed as a community vaccine site given its location in a culturally diverse neighborhood. Jefferson implemented a vaccine campaign that included translated messaging, as well as collaboration with SEAMAAC to recruit community leaders. Building on community trust and the strong "word of mouth" networks in certain communities, SEAMAAC encouraged community leaders and elders to promote vaccines. Over 5000 individuals were vaccinated at the Wyss Center since the Jefferson Mobile Vaccine Clinic started bringing vaccines into the community in May, 2021. Due to this effort, the culturally and linguistically diverse neighborhood surrounding the vaccine clinic, previously deemed a "vaccine desert," became one of the highest vaccinated areas in the city.

Below are some of the facilitators and challenges to our team providing quality care to refugees and immigrants at the Wyss Center:

| Facilitators | Notes |
|---|---|
| Clinic Location | In a neighborhood in which many of our patients live, work, and go to school. Reduces transportation barriers, improves no-show rates, builds community trust |
| Design | We were able to design a clinic "from scratch" that is welcoming and accessible, incorporating voices from the community |
| Refugee Health Champion | Dr. Altshuler is an expert on refugee health and has years of experience providing care to refugees; he serves as a mentor to other providers and learners |
| Learners | Ability to schedule longer appointments for more complex patients in resident clinic |
| Culturally Competent Team | Providers and social work staff have experience providing culturally competent care, and can access appropriate training resources for staff training |
| Language Access | We have immediately available interpreter services |
| Services | Labs and vaccines on site, regardless of insurance status. The Philadelphia Department of Health funds vaccines for uninsured children and adults |
| Collaborations | We have a strong partnership with resettlement agencies through the PRHC |
| Support | We have on site case management and social work through SEAMAAC |

| Challenges | Notes |
|---|---|
| Insurance Barriers | Staff were not initially familiar with billing and collection practices for the uninsured. In addition, some services are not easily accessible for uninsured patients, such as specialist visits and advanced imaging. We recommend early discussions about logistics of care for the uninsured. |
| Complexity of Patients | Many patients, due to insurance, language, and cultural barriers have not seen a doctor in several years and present with poorly controlled disease. This is particularly a challenge for uninsured patients. |
| Language Capabilities | While we prioritize hiring bilingual staff, it can be a challenge to find candidates, particularly behavioral health providers. |

**Vignette: Patient Teachers (Jessica Deffler MD; Medical Director, Hansjorg Wyss Wellness Center)**

Working with refugees, immigrants, and other newcomers, I have realized that cultural competence is not about memorizing the characteristics of each cultural group I see. It is important to acknowledge the cultural, political, and religious contexts from which our patients and clients come to us. But for me, the real learning arises from my interactions with patients themselves. Cultural competency is a skill that requires training and practice over years, possibly never to be fully achieved. It is a reminder to practice self-awareness, think critically, and question my biases. It is also an opportunity to hone my listening and communication skills.

Since I started caring for newcomers, I have learned more from my patients than from didactics or country profile fact sheets. On a given day in clinic, I might see individuals from five to seven different countries. Many of the challenges they experience are ones that I solve only with the help of our social worker and community health worker. For example, on one day I see a man from Eritrea, in his fifties, who comes in with a gout flare. During the visit, he asks me if the clinic can offer him a job as a janitor. In his country, he was a retired nurse. Next, a Swahili speaking woman from Sudan*, pregnant with her eighth child, would like to have a tubal ligation but worries that her husband will not approve. At 34 weeks pregnant, she is looking for work because their family of nine is behind on rent. I see a six-month-old baby, born in Guatemala* who arrived in the U.S. two weeks ago, chubby and healthy, here for vaccines. A middle-aged

---

*Demographic information has been changed in order to protect identity of individuals.

(continued)

woman who has a chronically disfigured limb from an accident with a rice plow in Cambodia* thirty years ago, asks if anything can be done to fix it; she is not eligible for Medicaid insurance. A Burmese woman in her 60 s comes in after noticing a hard breast lump; she has never had a mammogram and has not been to a doctor for twenty years. I know what can be done medically for these patients, and in some cases, what cannot. What I don't know about the medicine, I can find by researching in a medical journal or by consulting colleagues. Finding the skills to navigate cultural differences with patients is not so easily attainable, and requires more self-awareness and practice. Each of these patient interactions is practice in developing cultural competence.

Seventy percent of our patients at the Wyss Wellness Center have emerging English proficiency and require an interpreter for their visits. I find I am much more self-aware during visits with these patients that require a third presence in the room. I am more conscious of my words, choosing them carefully to avoid overburdening or confusing the interpreter or patient. I am more observant of patients and their body language and expressions. Some patients may laugh when they are nervous, others seem detached or distracted. Some patients make eye contact while others limit it. Instead of judging behavior, I'm curious about it.

When I became the medical director of the Wyss Wellness Center, I knew that cultural competence would have to be something we continually address. When things get stressful and staff are overwhelmed, even those who value cultural competence can cut corners. There have been times when a patient isn't offered an interpreter at the front desk, because four other patients are waiting behind them, and the phone is ringing. Cultural competence, like other processes we implement in our clinic, is dynamic and needs to be continuously assessed and improved. It also needs to be prioritized or it might get ignored when we are more focused on outcomes data or financial sustainability. While tempting to say that we have achieved the goal of a "culturally competent" medical home, this is much more exhibited by daily actions than by words on our website.

It's not easy for providers or social services staff to see twenty patients a day, when many of them speak a foreign language, or are ineligible for insurance, or live in fear that they won't make this month's rent. Like other refugee and immigrant health providers, I went into this work with certain ideals. When things get tough, I remember that this is not a reflection of shortcomings of our patients, but of faulty systems. The gratitude of our patients is a large part of what keeps me going. Burn out and compassion fatigue threaten the well-being of our providers. I am grateful to have a team that shares a vision for equitable care for all of our patients, and our mission is what keeps us whole. During long weeks when we are all feeling the exhaustion, when we are focused on the numbers—wait times, no-show rates, etc.—it's helpful to remind ourselves and our staff of our mission and values, and the opportunities we have to exhibit that mission every day. Our patients teach us to keep going, to be patient, to have hope. They also need us to advocate for them and help them find their voice.

(continued)

### Vignette: Time, Patience, and Perseverance (Jenna Gosnay, MSW LSW, Wyss Wellness Center)

My role as a social worker engaging with refugee and immigrant communities relies heavily on the partnerships with other community organizations who share similar missions; to empower the clients we serve to be healthy, independent individuals who can be thriving members of society. Working in a healthcare facility, I serve as a broker connecting the patients I encounter with the community resources they need. At Wyss, we are fortunate enough to partner with SEAMAAC and Nationalities Service Center (NSC) to address the concerns and the barriers our clients face that may go beyond the scope of a healthcare facility. As each organization has different structures and purposes, it's impractical to think that one organization alone could be a one-stop-shop for every patient or client, as much as we'd like them to be. The components of refugee health, such as fulfilling basic needs, healthcare, and social services are interdependent. Addressing just one of those components may alleviate some of the symptoms of another, but each requires sufficient consideration. And each community organization brings different invaluable skills and resources to the table to begin to address those needs

While many of the struggles and needs of the refugee community of Philadelphia are like those of the average American citizen, the systems and the policies in place make finding the solutions much more difficult. Much of my work involves screening patients to determine eligibility for public benefits. On a good day, I'm able to work with eligible patients to complete applications and submit supplemental documents to be reviewed. However, afterward, those patients often receive a letter in the mail, in English, requesting additional documents

before the application can be processed. A patient may call their county assistance office for an application status update, but he or she is not understood on the phone and is not offered an interpreter. Often, these patients and their applications fall through the cracks. The systems in place are not easy to navigate for refugee and immigrant populations in Philadelphia, and barriers such as language and low literacy levels often prevent individuals from being able to take full ownership in their care.

The work we do within the refugee and immigrant communities takes time, patience, and perseverance. Time spent monitoring applications online, so the patients don't have to. Patience to say the same thing three different ways to an interpreter because it didn't translate well the first two times in the patient's dialect. And persistence when collecting documents from an illiterate patient for applications for public benefits. It's truly a team effort to advocate on behalf of our patients as they encounter these barriers.

Through all of this, I've learned to ask for help from community partners when the services at the Wyss Center don't meet all the patients' needs. I've learned not to take 'no' for an answer, at least not the first time around. And I've learned that despite these barriers and outdated systems, the patients we have the honor to work with every day are incredibly strong and resilient people. I find that I have to remind myself that the fact that these individuals arrived to the United States at all speaks for itself. The question is not whether the refugees of Philadelphia are capable of being empowered, independent members of society—it is—what is getting in their way, and how do we make it a more realistic obstacle to overcome? I'm truly grateful to the patients we serve for trusting us quite literally with their lives, and for the partnerships with community organizations who continue to work to fulfill this mission.

(continued)

# 6 Closing

Participating in the lives of refugees and immigrants is a privilege. We want to thank our patients for sharing their stories; we do this work for them. In addition, we owe so much to our collaborators, especially the Nationalities Services Center, without whom we would not be able to provide quality care to our patients. We complete this chapter as the world experiences a crisis in Afghanistan, and we are privileged to work with such dedicated resettlement agency that has resettled over 750 Afghan newcomers in Philadelphia since October 2021.

We also want to thank the SEAMAAC staff, who always lead from the heart, and who never think twice about doing what's needed for their clients. We are grateful to be able to work with others who share our mission to serve the marginalized and underserved in our communities. As the authors of this chapter, we hope that our story serves as a guide to inspire providers to open their clinic doors to the immigrant and refugee community or assist current refugee health providers who are looking to expand their services and create new partnerships with community agencies.

# References

Centers Of Excellence Guidelines | CDC. 2021 [cited 2021 Sep 28]. Available from: https://www.cdc.gov/immigrantrefugeehealth/guidelines/centers-of-excellence.html

DiVito B, Payton C, Shanfeld G, Altshuler M, Scott K. A collaborative approach to promoting continuing care for refugees: Philadelphia's strategies and lessons learned. Harv Public Health Rev. 2016;9:1–12.

Gammage J. Philly readies for new neighbors, part of Biden's plan to resettle more of the world's most vulnerable people. https://www.inquirer.com. [cited 2021 Sep 28]. Available from: https://www.inquirer.com/news/refugees-resettlement-nationalities-service-center-hias-pa-biden-trump-20210221.html

Kumar GS, Beeler JA, Seagle EE, Jentes ES. Long-term physical health outcomes of resettled refugee populations in the United States: a scoping review. J Immigr Minor Health. 2021;23(4):813–23.

Lazo M, Bilal U, Correa C, Furukawa A, Martinez-Donate A, Zumaeta-Castillo C. The impact of COVID-19 in Latino Communities in Philadelphia | Drexel Urban Health Collaborative | Drexel University. Drexel University Urban Health Collaborative. 2021 [cited 2021 Sep 28]. Available from: https://drexel.edu/uhc/resources/briefs/Latino%20Covid-19%20in%20Context/

Perreira KM, Ornelas I. Painful passages: traumatic experiences and post-traumatic stress among immigrant Latino adolescents and their primary caregivers. Int Migr Rev. 2013;47(4):976–1005. https://doi.org/10.1111/imre.12050.

Philadelphia's Immigrants. [cited 2021 Sep 28]. Available from: https://pew.org/2swfWPw

Pierce S, Meissner D. Trump executive order on refugees and Ttravel ban: a brief review. 2017, February [cited 2023 April 14]. Policy Briefs. Migrationpolicyinstitute.org

Rahman N. Edition 30 – An economic analysis of refugee health policy and a structural comparison of the Philadelphia Refugee Health Collaborative with Colorado, Kentucky, and Minnesota – Harvard Public Health Review: A Student-Run Peer-Reviewed Journal. [cited 2021 Sep 28]. Available from: https://hphr.org/30-article-rahman/

Refugee Health Guidance | Immigrant and Refugee Health | CDC. 2021 [cited 2021 Sep 28]. Available from: https://www.cdc.gov/immigrantrefugeehealth/guidelines/refugee-guidelines.html

The State of Immigrants in Philadelphia. 2019 [cited 2021 Sep 28]. Available from: https://pew.org/2WeyHUg

Tran L-G. A new beginning: early refugee integration in the United States. RSF Russell Sage Found J Soc Sci. 2020;6(3):117.

U.S. Census Bureau QuickFacts: Philadelphia County, Pennsylvania. [cited 2021 Sep 28]. Available from: https://www.census.gov/quickfacts/philadelphiacountypennsylvania

UNHCR Global Trends - Forced displacement in 2020. [cited 2021 Sep 28]. Available from: https://www.unhcr.org/flagship-reports/globaltrends/

Wiltz T. Aging, undocumented and uninsured immigrants challenge cities and states. [cited 2020 Aug 3]; 2018. Available from: https://www.pewtrusts.org/en/research-and-analysis/blogs/stateline/2018/01/03/aging-undocumented-and-uninsured-immigrants-challenge-cities-and-states

Yun K, Fuentes-Afflick E, Desai MM. Prevalence of chronic disease and insurance coverage among refugees in the United States. J Immigr Minor Health. 2012;14(6):933–40.

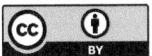

# Building Partnership Through Malaria Research in Thailand

## Michele Spring and Krisada Jongsakul

*We ourselves feel that what we are doing is just a drop in the ocean. But if that drop was not in the ocean, I think the ocean would be less because of that missing drop.*

—Mother Teresa

## Abstract

The Armed Forces Research Institute of Medical Sciences (AFRIMS) is a US Department of Defense (DoD) institution under the US Embassy in Bangkok, Thailand. In partnership with the Royal Thai Army, AFRIMS has conducted in-depth malaria research for the past 60 years, with a specific focus on anti-malarial product development as well as monitoring and surveillance of product effectiveness and signs of anti-malarial drug resistance. While the primary mission is DoD-sponsored medical research to protect armed services personnel, developments and accomplishments are shared with the community at large. Conducting malaria research, particularly human clinical studies, requires investments in time, resources, and people, as well as dedicated partnerships. This commitment to medical research by its very nature does not provide rapid responses to epidemics or outbreaks. However, through its long-term collaborations and relationships, AFRIMS has been asked to assist with outbreaks in infectious diseases such as malaria, diarrhea, avian influenza and Zika. As a research lab, AFRIMS cannot readily provide diagnostic testing or clinical care, requiring regulatory and ethical approvals to engage in such. The time it takes to meet all logistical requirements may exceed the time interval for which interventions are urgently needed. In this chapter, the AFRIMS response to a malaria outbreak in Thailand is described, outlining the strengths and hurdles encountered. While steps can be taken to facilitate AFRIMS' involvement in epidemic responses, ultimately it will need to be better incorporated, and planned for, within the primary "interepidemic" research mission.

M. Spring (✉)
Department of Microbiology and Immunology, State University of New York (SUNY) Upstate Medical University, Syracuse, NY, USA

Armed Forces Research Institute of Medical Sciences (AFRIMS), Bangkok, Thailand
e-mail: sprinmic@upstate.edu

K. Jongsakul
Contractor, Royal Thai Army, based at US Armed Forces Research Institute of Medical Sciences (AFRIMS), Bangkok, Thailand

## Keywords

Partnerships (government National local) · Malaria · Clinical field research · Surveillance · Drug resistance · Outbreak response · Outbreak planning · Thailand

**Author Perspective**

The authors are both civilian physicians, one American and one Thai, working within a US Department of Defense research organization to conduct malaria clinical trials with the Thai Ministry of Public Health. Both have found that over the years maintaining partnership between two government organizations (often with outside institutions in the mix) requires investments in people/time beyond the logistics of execution. Government organizations often have high turnover, and the job position of the authors has enabled them to provide continuity in the research and the relationships, both of which are underpinnings in success of planned (and unplanned) infectious disease threats.

**Key Tenets**

1. The team is what will get you far. Everyone should feel equally important to a project's success.
2. Understanding and working within the local system will usually facilitate your progress, rather than arriving with and applying your previous mindset.
3. Engage with those who are as determined as you to succeed in infectious disease research but who also see the tangential opportunities to collaborate and help others in order to achieve benefits for all.
4. This chapter addresses SDG #3 Good Health and Well-Being.

# 1    Introduction

First formed as the Southeast Asia Treaty Organization (SEATO) Lab following the 1956–1958 cholera pandemic in Thailand, the Armed Forces Research Institute of Medical Sciences (AFRIMS) is a research collaboration between the US Department of Defense (DoD), under the direction of the US Embassy, and the

Royal Thai Army (RTA). The US Army Medical Directorate (USAMD-AFRIMS) is a special foreign activity of the Walter Reed Army Institute of Research (WRAIR) whose mission is to conduct biomedical research that is responsive to DoD and US Army requirements and sustains the force health protection of soldiers. With special foreign activity research institutions disbursed worldwide, each program can focus on regional health threats encountered by local and deployed service personnel.

At AFRIMS, this translates to surveillance and development/evaluation of medical products (drugs, vaccines, diagnostics) for infectious disease threats such as malaria, diarrheal disease, dengue, chikungunya, other arboviral illnesses, scrub typhus, human immunodeficiency virus (HIV), and multidrug-resistant organisms (MDROs) responsible for wound infections. AFRIMS headquarters is located in Bangkok, with over 40 field sites in Thailand, Nepal, Philippines, Cambodia, Vietnam, Laos, and Bangladesh. About 90% of the approximately 400 staff are Thai scientists and technicians, complemented by US military and contractor personnel.

## 1.1    Background on Malaria

Malaria is a parasitic disease transmitted by *Anopheles spp.* of mosquitoes. There are four main human species: *Plasmodium falciparum, P. vivax, P. ovale, P. malariae.* Several simian malarias which can cross over and infect humans, two of which have been found in Thailand: *P. knowlesi* and *P. cynomolgi* (Thailand Malaria Elimination Program, Ministry of Public health, Thailand 2022; Sai-Ngam et al. 2022). The *Anopheles* mosquitoes in Southeast Asia are largely forest-dwelling which results in malaria being concentrated in the mountainous/forested border regions of the country, as opposed to Bangkok or the low-lying plains of central Thailand.

Until recent years, malaria was widely endemic in Southeast Asia, with stable and moderate levels (30,000–40,000 cases per year) in Thailand. In the late 1970s/early 1980s, prevalence rose dramatically, peaking to over 400,000 cases/year (Thailand Malaria Elimination Program, Ministry of Public Health, Thailand 2022; Konchom et al. 2005), largely attributed to influx of Cambodians into Thailand as the Khmer Rouge government left power. Ten years later, yearly cases had re-stabilized to several tens of thousands, but in 2014, prevalence began a steady decrease, and by 2021 only an estimated 3211 cases were reported (Thailand Malaria Elimination Program, Ministry of Public Health, Thailand 2022). The proportions of *P. falciparum* and *P. vivax* infections each hovered around 50% until 2014 when *P. vivax* became the dominant species (95% in 2021). Malaria cases tend to peak at the start of the rainy season, May through July, and continue with occasional lower peaks November through January, as the dry season commences.

The Thai government began to recommend artemisinin combination therapies (ACTs) in 1995 for treatment of *P. falciparum*. Since then, treatment regimens have been changed in accordance with documented resistance patterns (Chaisatit et al. 2021). *P. vivax* infections remain susceptible to chloroquine, with primaquine, and as of 2024, tafenoquine, recommended for radical cure.

in malaria clinical research blossomed, motivating me to return to Bangkok and undertake further graduate study (DTM&H, and M.Sc. degrees) at Mahidol University. As an academic instructor, I began to collaborate with the Thai Ministry of Public Health (MoPH), and, in 1991, I was able to bring these collaborations to my position at the US DoD Armed Forces Research Institute of Medical Sciences (AFRIMS).

During the past 28 years at AFRIMS, I have overseen execution of clinical research studies all over Thailand, working in partnership with MoPH staff from the national to the village level. By fostering these relationships, building up mutual trust and respect with each new project or site, it has permitted us to apply research practices to real world situations while aligning with Thailand's public health strategies. Finally retiring in 2019, I remained at AFRIMS with the Defense Medical Assistance Program (DMAP), a DoD funding agency, which allows me to continue to engage with MoPH partners in infectious disease operations research as well as help mentor junior researchers in Thailand.

**Vignette Dr. Krisada Jongsakul**

As a medical student in Thailand, it was not uncommon to see patients with tropical diseases such as dengue, malaria, scrub typhus, etc. It was not until I was an attending physician at Thongphaphum District Hospital along the Thai-Myanmar border, working alongside clinical researchers from Mahidol University (Thailand) and Hawaii University (USA), that my interest

**Vignette: Dr. Michele Spring**

My interest in tropical medicine started with an undergraduate class in parasitology, but it was not until I enrolled in a master's program in parasitology at Tulane University School of Public Health and met career parasitologists that I began to see how this interest could become a vocation. Each step afterwards, Peace Corps, medical and infectious disease training, overseas electives and consultancies, introduced me to tropical medicine and global health mentors who exposed me to different ways a tropical medicine career could manifest, and who assisted me along my own path. After meeting US Army malaria researchers from Walter Reed Army Institute of Research (WRAIR) while in Kenya, I took a (planned) short-term position at WRAIR to learn how to conduct human clinical trials for the evaluation and advancement of malaria vaccines and therapeutics. This "stepping-stone" lasted 18 years.

Product development is a team sport. Through my position at WRAIR and its overseas component, Armed Forces Research Institute of Medical Sciences (AFRIMS), I have learned how to partner with pharmaceutical companies, funding agencies, Ministries of Public Health and local government clinics, non-governmental organizations, and malaria patients, all who have the same goal of reducing malaria burden, whether globally or locally. Conducting clinical translational research in malaria while within a DoD institution necessitates looking outward toward our partnerships to understand better what will help succeed in the fight against malaria.

## 2 AFRIMS Malaria Research

Since its inception, AFRIMS has focused on clinical development and evaluation of anti-malarials and characterization of any drug resistance thereof, in order to ensure safe, effective malaria chemoprophylaxis and treatment. Most AFRIMS research studies are not US Food and Drug Administration (FDA)-regulated (unless part of a licensure package), but all are conducted under ethical and regulatory supervision of Institutional Review Boards (IRBs) from the United States (WRAIR) and the Thai Ministry of Public Health (MoPH) and/or RTA. These studies can consist of samples collected for surveillance and requiring a very minimal footprint, or involve a greater than minimal risk (GTMR) human clinical trial, requiring AFRIMS to set up forward lab capabili-

ties for assays that need to be run while in the field or processed before shipping back to Bangkok or the US.

The clinical field research teams consist of physicians, clinical research coordinators (CRCs), and lab technicians who travel from Bangkok to the local field site, rotating on a regular schedule while the study is executed. The team is mobile, and as such, is able to travel to the presenting malaria patient if needed versus being fixed at one clinic or hospital. Malaria clinics, posts and village health workers are under the purview of the Thai MoPH or RTA. Thus studies and protocols must be planned and coordinated not only through AFRIMS, but with local, regional and national involvement and/or support. The benefit of having on-site AFRIMS mobile teams allows for studies with complex schedules and specific regulatory procedures to be run without disturbing the regular workload of local staff. The current group of Thai physicians and CRCs at AFRIMS have been running these studies for more than 20 years and are familiar with the US, Thai, and local clinical trial ethical and regulatory processes that need to be maintained. This continuity also helps bridge the changes of continually rotating US military and contract staff. Limitations of this AFRIMS clinical field team approach include less local ownership of a project and higher costs of staffing the study with a team from Bangkok.

Depending on the procedures of a particular malaria study, the clinical field team can perform blood smears for malaria diagnosis, as well as complete blood counts (CBCs), liver and renal function tests, and quantitative testing for glucose 6-phosphate dehydrogenase (G6PD) deficiency, a condition which can affect whether it is safe to receive primaquine for latent *P. vivax* infections. Sample processing is also conducted for pharmacokinetic testing, antimalarial drug susceptibility, molecular marker identification (polymerase chain reaction or genomic sequencing), immunology measurements, etc., as the study requires.

While the results from these tests can be used for decision-making within the context of a research clinical study, results cannot be provided as a clinical diagnosis. In this context, assays would need to be run under Clinical Laboratory Improvement Amendments (CLIA) standards. There are a limited number of AFRIMS labs with this certification, such as those that measure HIV viral load. The malaria field technicians do undergo microscopy proficiency certification by the World Health Organization (WHO), and recently the WRAIR IRB agreed that malaria smear results from AFRIMS WHO-certified microscopists can be provided directly to the general public and used for treatment decisions.

## 3    Description of Partnerships

Because of the longstanding cooperation between AFRIMS and the Thai government, AFRIMS is known as a reliable partner for assessments of infectious disease threats if the need arises. These kinds of requests first pass through official US and Thai government channels. Despite its role as a research institute, AFRIMS has been able to successfully divert from an "inter-epidemic" clinical research focus to an acute, epidemic or outbreak response over the years. In an article reviewing AFRIMS activities over the first 50 years, Brown et al., describe how AFRIMS was able to assist US Embassy and USAID efforts to diagnose infectious disease outbreaks in Cambodian refugee camps set up on the Thai-Cambodian border in late 1970s and 1980s (Brown and Nitayaphan 2011). In the days after the catastrophic 2004 tsunami, the Thai MoPH and US Embassy requested AFRIMS and US CDC staff to travel from Bangkok to six southern provinces to determine the condition of health centers and availability of supplies, assess medical and mental health needs, and set up infectious diseases active surveillance systems for reporting to the MoPH (Guerena-Burgueno et al. 2006). This role then allowed AFRIMS investigators to analyze malaria data in the years post-tsunami when cases were expected to increase (Jongsakul et al. 2006). This data analysis built upon the initial outbreak role, a humanitarian mission at the behest of the US Embassy, and was supported

through a DoD-funded malaria surveillance protocol under the purview of WRAIR and Thai MoPH IRB-supervised research.

A more recent request for outbreak assistance was in 2017, when malaria cases in the northeast of Thailand, along the Thailand-Cambodia border in Sisaket Province, began to increase rapidly. Initially, in April and May, the outbreak was investigated by MoPH staff from multiple levels. By June, four malaria-related deaths were reported, an unusual circumstance for Thailand. By July, without an obvious focus responsible for the outbreak, the MoPH coordinated a 3-day blanket investigation of the three most affected districts in Sisaket Province along the Cambodian border. AFRIMS had no ongoing research projects in the province. However, in 2016, Dr. Krisada had developed working relationships with the MoPH's Vector Borne Disease Unit (VBDU) of northeastern Thailand (which covered Sisaket, Ubon Ratchathani and three other provinces) during a short, minimal-risk AFRIMS malaria study. Dr. Krisada also had professional relationships with a Provincial Health Officer (PHO) of northeast Thailand and the MoPH malaria subject matter expert consultant, both of whom were involved in the outbreak response. He was invited to attend a meeting to establish an Emergency Operations Center (EOC) to address the outbreak as well as to review potential contributing factors in the malaria deaths.

With other MoPH officials present at the meeting, discussions were initiated on the support that AFRIMS could bring and necessary next steps to take to engage the assistance of a medical research organization. Similar to past humanitarian missions, a formal letter requesting participation would be required, this time from the Thai MoPH, and a scope of work (SOW) developed. AFRIMS would provide support for the ongoing Thai MoPH public health response by augmenting diagnostic capacity in the field with AFRIMS microscopists, and assess any role of anti-malarial drug resistance by conducting molecular marker testing at AFRIMS on dried blood spots (DBS) obtained by fingerstick.

The AFRIMS team, consisting of a clinical field team plus US military leadership from the malaria department did an advance trip to Sisaket to meet with Thai government officials and map out the best course of action for this collaboration. It was agreed that AFRIMS would use already instituted MoPH malaria surveillance and data collection forms which had been developed as part of the National Malaria Elimination Operational Plan (NMEOP) for 2017–2021 (Bureau of Vector Borne Disease 2016). AFRIMS would also assist on an upcoming Thai MoPH/University of California-San Francisco (UCSF) collaboration to assess the outbreak cause.

However, to officially join the malaria outbreak investigation, AFRIMS also needed a WRAIR IRB determination to ensure the role was commensurate with a US DoD research organization assisting with Thai public health activities. One mechanism was through AFRIMS' designation as a World Health Organization (WHO) Collaborating Center for Diagnostic Reference, Training and Investigation of Emerging Infectious Diseases. This provides a policy framework upon which AFRIMS can participate in testing for public health, and join in interventions if the crisis is deemed "potentially dangerous to humans". The AFRIMS Scope of Work (SOW) would thus serve as a research "protocol" to be submitted to the WRAIR IRB for approval, along with the MoPH request. Non-research determination and approval was received in October 2017.

In November 2017, AFRIMS sent a team of twelve people including two physicians (the authors), four nurses, and eight lab technicians, to spend 10 days embedded with local and national level Thai MoPH teams to conduct a mass blood smear survey. The objective was to find any malaria cases or foci in the three affected districts of Sisaket Province, focusing on the areas along the Cambodian border.

Every day, the group of approximately 50 people split up into three groups, each group covering a specific region of the province. Certain towns and district centers were set up to call in all residents for aural temperature check, fingerstick for blood smears and DBS, and to have a short travel and malaria history taken using the Thai MoPH NMEOP forms (Fig. 1). In addition to

town foci, teams traveled to rubber plantations, took boats across reservoirs and visited students in schools, in an attempt to reach all residents, including those in remote areas and likely most at risk. The blood smears were all read in real-time during the survey, and the DBS transported to AFRIMS (Bangkok) and the VBDU in Ubon Ratchathani.

The number of outbreak cases did begin to decrease in August 2017 and, by the onset of the malaria season in 2018, cases were in the expected range with no rebound or continued increase. The AFRIMS/MoPH outbreak activity performed blood smears in almost 4000 individuals, and the investigations by UCSF/MoPH and AFRIMS into the causes and risk factors have been published (Roh et al. 2021). In 2019, AFRIMS opened a DoD-funded malaria surveillance study in Ubon Ratchathani and Sisaket Provinces which further strengthened the successful partnerships with MoPH and RTA teams in the region.

In late September 2017, while the preparations were being made for the AFRIMS SOW and mass blood survey, the Thai MoPH convened an emergency meeting in Bangkok to review, and possibly change, Thailand's national malaria treatment policy. Select research organizations in Thailand, including AFRIMS, were invited to present data obtained from clinical studies. AFRIMS presented a comprehensive set of malaria drug resistance data from two IRB-approved AFRIMS malaria studies conducted over three years (2013–2015) just prior to the outbreak.

One was a *P. falciparum* malaria surveillance protocol with the RTA, drawing samples from the soldiers stationed along the Thai/Cambodia border in Sisaket Province. This data was particularly pertinent since a significant proportion of the outbreak cases appeared to occur in RTA personnel, and most other research institutions do not work with or have access to local military personnel for malaria studies.

The second trial was a *P. falciparum* therapeutic efficacy study in Kanchanburi Province along the Thai-Myanmar border. The molecular markers of drug resistance and *in vitro* anti-

**Fig. 1** Sisaket Outbreak response team. (AFRIMS team members assist in mass blood smear surveys in Sisaket province in 2017)

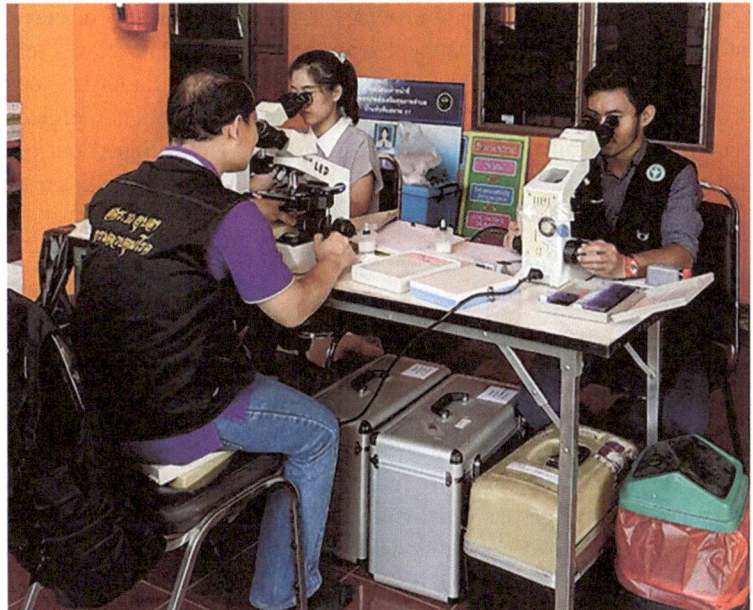

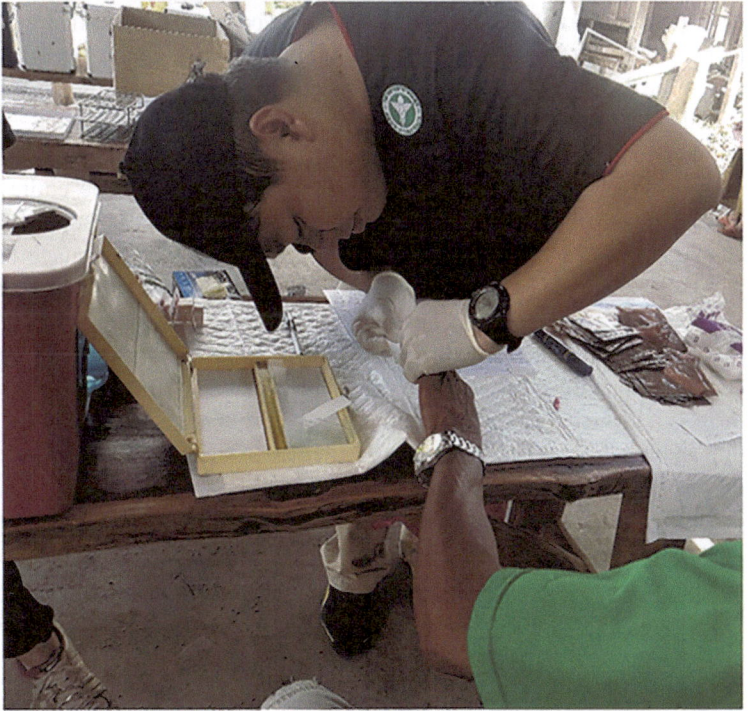

malarial drug sensitivity testing were shown to be strictly region specific, with Sisaket having increasing evidence of drug resistance, and Kanchanaburi with 100% clinical efficacy and a much lower frequency of molecular markers of resistance.

The summary of lab and clinical data from USAMD-AFRIMS and others in Thailand led to a consensus that revision of Thailand malaria drug policy was likely to be needed. The Thai MoPH took the bold initiative to revise the *P. falciparum* treatment policy, although only for only

Sisaket and Ubon Ratchathani Provinces. At the sites near Myanmar, the treatment regimen had remained effective. The outbreak data and DBS highlight how long-term malaria research projects can be dovetailed into planning/response for a short-term outbreak.

## 4    Discussion

AFRIMS did have a framework and plan for public health outbreak activities, but there was a time lag to implement it; a time lag which may have missed the opportunity to intervene. As mentioned earlier, malaria cases rise most quickly at the start of rainy seasons, predominately May–July, then begin to decrease slowly. The 2017 outbreak also followed this general trend, with case numbers in April/May greater than two standard deviations above the previous year. The early MoPH action likely played a significant role in the decrease in cases, and the expansion to include all levels of MoPH staff reflects its commitment to the containment of malaria transmission. In the several months it took for AFRIMS to become aware of the outbreak and then to obtain all approvals in order to deploy to the field, cases had largely already been brought under control. With malaria elimination on Thailand's horizon, it is likely that malaria outbreaks in Southeast Asia will generally be easier to contain. However, there is a chance that future outbreaks are more dire and require a rapid response. In anticipation of this scenario, AFRIMS and WRAIR could develop streamlined procedures to allow for more facile actions.

Funding for this AFRIMS outbreak project (travel and supplies) was also not without difficulties, as non-research public health activities may not be covered by DoD funds directed to research and development. There are DoD funding sources designated for operational research, although even if obtained, the funds have expiry dates and would need to be obtained on a regular schedule to ensure availability when needed. In addition, this outbreak response activity occurred at the transition of fiscal years, when most funds have already been allocated and new fiscal year funds may or may not have yet arrived. Funding ultimately was obtained through the Defense Malaria Assistance Program which specialized in operational projects. As this organization has transitioned out of malaria work, other funding sources will be needed to respond to future outbreaks.

The success of the 10-day mass blood smear campaign, while perhaps not resulting in a large decrease in outbreak cases, was due to teamwork. The outbreak response team was comprised of district, provincial and national Thai MoPH personnel, RTA soldiers and AFRIMS staff, and included public health workers, physicians, nurses, lab technicians, entomologists, scientists, government functionaries and drivers. All were considered equal parts of the team, and all in Sisaket worked for one purpose. AFRIMS staff did not act as external consultants, but rather were enmeshed within the mobile groups, trying to diagnose every case and characterize the extent of the outbreak. While each team member may not have had the same skill set, the teams blanketed the three districts in Sisaket Province, working the entire day, side by side. With the majority of the AFRIMS team being Thai, there was no language barrier, and being part of the MoPH project enabled AFRIMS staff to move easily into the villages and call the population for testing.

The project esprit de corps was further bolstered by the sense of team developed outside of working hours. The Thai culture is to eat together, whether at home or at work. Meals are often family-style with many dishes presented so that each may be shared. The AFRIMS staff, sometimes joined by other outbreak team members, ate together at the end of each day, either stopping at a local restaurant or an MoPH or RTA team member's house (Fig. 2). This hour-long meal did much to engender a sense of cohesiveness. American culture tends to focus more on working hours during projects, and while there may be an initial "kick-off" dinner and then a concluding "congratulatory" meal at the end of the mission, often the end of a workday means to separate individually or into small groups. Bonds and trust were

**Fig. 2** Meals and Teamwork: Sisaket outbreak teams, November 2017

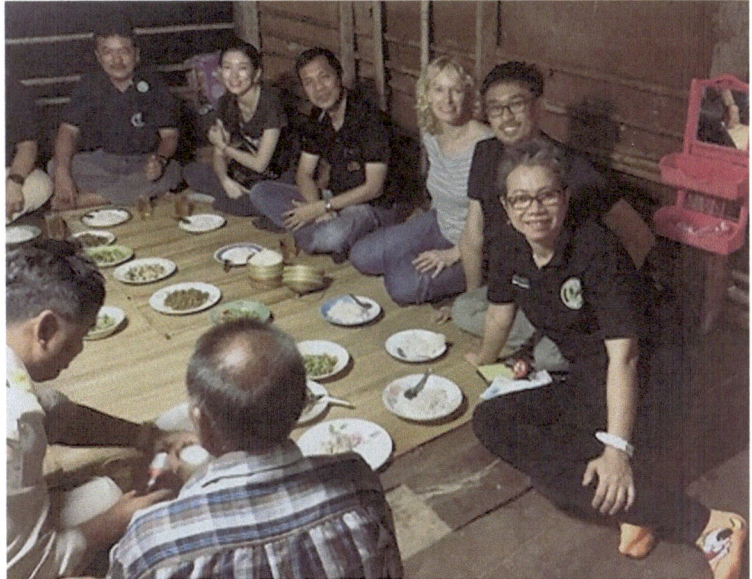

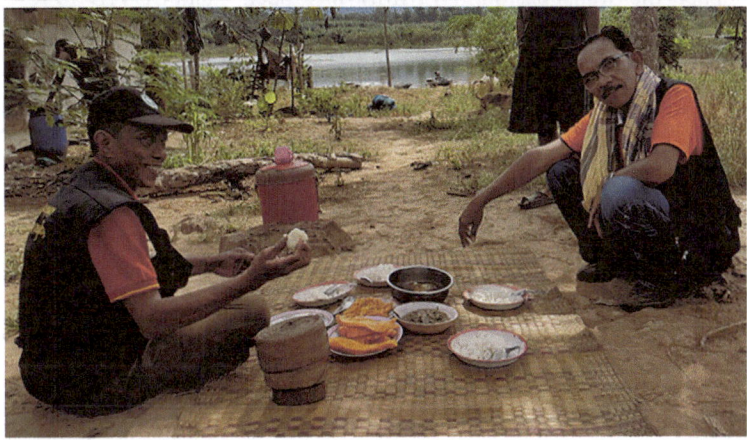

strengthened during those 10 days in Sisaket, getting to know team members and sharing the stories of the day's activities, of meeting local families, teachers, and farmers and of experiences of traveling to remote places over dirt road terrain. Meals play a similar role AFRIMS field staff when conducting malaria clinical trials. It serves as an opportunity to teach new team members informally about malaria, AFRIMS or MoPH frameworks, and team roles as well as to share the many experiences the clinical field staff have had over the years. Eating together at small local restaurants at field sites is also an informal way to learn about the community in which one is working and to introduce the AFRIMS team.

Cases of malaria have plummeted in Sisaket Province since that outbreak in 2017. The MoPH has tirelessly worked to implement an effective vertical malaria control program. However, the impact of reaching out to communities and visiting small towns and farms with a more personalized message about the risk of and protection against malaria should not be discounted.

The invitation to AFRIMS to assist in the outbreak investigation was a testament to its long-term presence in Thailand and the benefits its research has brought to populations in both the US and Southeast Asia. It was also evidence of the professional relationships developed, particularly by the Thai physicians and scientists. The general Thai public may not be familiar with medical research conducted by the US DoD, since AFRIMS is a free-standing research institution with no US military bases in Thailand. There may also be a lack of awareness of how the research accomplishments from Thailand contribute to the larger global community. US military scientists regularly rotate through AFRIMS, and those in Thai MoPH positions often do not remain there long-term. So it is the AFRIMS Thai researchers who are the continuity within the institution and can share the past work and current mission of AFRIMS with the scientific community in Thailand. They are a valuable asset to the frequently changing US staff and provide insights into the endemic tropical diseases of Thailand and cultural practices and lifestyles that may impact the transmission. AFRIMS has been lucky to have longstanding employees to bridge staffing changes and develop a depth of professional experience, a major factor in the institution's success over the years. Yet this also means collaborations may be too relationship-dependent and affected by interpersonal relationships. More codified involvement in Thai MoPH or RTA government committees could assist in maintaining formal lines of communications and keeping AFRIMS abreast of outbreaks when it can be of service.

## 5    Global Health Partnerships

For many of us who work in global infectious disease research, the desire to help understand or mitigate a disease threat is within the very nature of our profession. Outbreaks and epidemics are inherently not amenable to regularly scheduled stakeholder meetings and multi-step memorandums. Organizations primarily focused on rapid mobilization and deployment thus may be best suited in responding to outbreaks. However, there still may be a place for involving long-term, trusted research partners, such as AFRIMS, in these efforts to immediately reduce the disease threat and to collect data that can inform future interventions.

The COVID-19 pandemic was quite different from AFRIMS' past outbreak experiences, perhaps because it was so widespread, long-lasting and disruptive. From the outset of the pandemic in March 2020, the Thai government established strong policies regarding COVID-19 control and medical management, and requests to conduct studies required the highest level of MoPH approval. Unlike for malaria, the novelty and the unknowns of SARS CoV-2 also may have contributed to the desire of the Thai government to be the primary entity responsible for research in this area. Public health measures such as quarantine, travel restrictions, mask mandates and curfews were implemented quickly and with much less politicization than seen in the US. While there has not been much overlap between malaria and COVID-19 research, others at AFRIMS have engaged with the Thai MoPH in research projects focused on COVID-19. These are clinical research studies, capitalizing on the strengths and roles by which AFRIMS can assist in disease epidemics.

It is unclear whether AFRIMS can maintain a major role in epidemic responses while maintaining long-term "inter-epidemic" research. It pits the positives of its extensive and multifaceted research program against the regulatory and funding limitations a US government research organization may encounter in rapid-response efforts. AFRIMS by design is not an aid organization. Other US institutions may be able to give funding, donate mosquito nets or other prevention tools, or act in humanitarian crises, but these are not part of the AFRIMS mission. US government research funding mechanisms are fairly regimented, and DoD funding sources may shift disease threat priorities, aligning with medical conditions currently expected to be encountered on the present-day battlefield. It is sure that if called upon, such as in the 2004 tsunami response, AFRIMS will jump to serve. Hopefully, such disasters will be rare. In the meantime, for smaller events such as the Sisaket malaria outbreak and others, moving the machinery of a public health response project, while not agile, remains feasible.

**Acknowledgments** The authors would like to thank COL (Ret.) Arthur Brown and Dr. Deb Yourick for their critical reading of this chapter. Material has been reviewed by the Walter Reed Army Institute of Research and The Henry M. Jackson Foundation for the Advancement of Military Medicine, Inc. There is no objection to its presentation and/or publication. The opinions or assertions contained herein are the private views of the author, and are not to be construed as official, or as reflecting true views of the Department of the Army, the Department of Defense or The Henry M. Jackson Foundation for the Advancement of Military Medicine, Inc. The investigators have adhered to the policies for protection of human subjects as prescribed in AR 70–25.

# References

Brown A, Nitayaphan S. The Armed Forces Research Institute of Medical Sciences: five decades of collaborative medical research. Southeast Asian J Trop Med Public Health. 2011;42:477–90.

Bureau of Vector Borne Disease. National Malaria Elimination Strategy, Thailand 2017–2026. Ministry of Public Health; 2016.

Chaisatit C, et al. Molecular detection of mutation in the propeller domain of K13 and pfmdr1 copy number variation in *Plasmodium falciparum* isolates from Thailand collected from 2002 to 2007. Am J Trop Med Hyg. 2021:tpmd210303.

Guerena-Burgueno F, et al. Rapid assessment of health needs and medical response after the tsunami in Thailand, 2004-2005. Military Med. 2006;171:8–11.

Jongsakul K, et al. Malaria incidence before and after the December 2004 tsunami in Phang Nga province, Thailand. Poster presentation at annual meeting of American Society of Tropical Medicine and Hygiene; 2006.

Konchom S, et al. Chronical of malaria epidemics in Thailand, 1980-2000. Southeast Asian J Trop Med Public Health. 2005;36:64–7.

Roh ME, et al. Civilian-military malaria outbreak response in Thailand: an example of multi-stakeholder engagement for malaria elimination. Malar J. 2021;20:458.

Sai-Ngam P, et al. Case series of three malaria patients from Thailand infected with the simian parasite, *Plasmodium cynomolgi*. Malar J. 2022;21:142.

Thailand Malaria Elimination Program, Ministry of Public health, Thailand. http://malaria.ddc/ma.moph.go.th/malariar10/index_newversion.php. Accessed 31 Jan 2022.

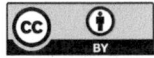

# Building Partnerships and Confronting Challenges: Implementation of an Ebola Virus Vaccine Clinical Study During an Outbreak in the Democratic Republic of the Congo

Daniel G. Bausch, Hugo Kavunga-Membo, Rebecca F. Grais, Nathalie Imbault, Natalie Roberts, Robert Kanwagi, Deborah Watson-Jones, Jean-Jacques Muyembe Tamfum, and on behalf of the DRC-EB-001-JnJ Ebola Vaccine Study (TUJIOKOWE) Team

*With rare exceptions, all of your most important achievements on this planet will come from working with others—or, in a word, partnership.*

Paul Farmer

## Abstract

Research, especially clinical trials, during outbreaks often poses enormous challenges, and up until very recent times was often con-

The original version of the chapter has been revised. A correction to this chapter can be found at https://doi.org/10.1007/978-3-031-53793-6_28

See full list of TUJIOKOWE team members at the end of the manuscript.

D. G. Bausch (✉) · D. Watson-Jones
London School of Hygiene and Tropical Medicine, London, UK
e-mail: Daniel.Bausch@FINDdx.org

H. Kavunga-Membo · J.-J. M. Tamfum
National Institute for Biomedical Research, Kinshasa, Democratic Republic of the Congo

R. F. Grais
Epicentre, Paris, France

sidered almost impossible. However, for diseases such as Ebola virus disease, which are seen almost exclusively in outbreak form, outbreaks are the only opportunity to perform studies and accrue knowledge. Here, we discuss our experiences and lessons learned implementing a clinical study of an Ebola virus vaccine during an outbreak of that disease in 2018–20 in eastern Democratic Republic of the Congo. Keys to success is these settings include forging partnerships

N. Imbault
The Coalition for Epidemic Preparedness Innovations, Oslo, Norway

N. Roberts
MSF-France, Paris, France

R. Kanwagi
World Vision, Dublin, Ireland

© The Author(s) 2024, Corrected Publication 2025
A. Stewart Ibarra, A. D. LaBeaud (eds.), *Transforming Global Health Partnerships*, Sustainable Development Goals Series, https://doi.org/10.1007/978-3-031-53793-6_12

with diverse and complementary experience and skills, working out clear roles and responsibilities, communicating and engaging with the community as an essential partner, and maintaining flexibility to adapt to unexpected events. Progress in these complex settings requires both quick action to implement studies as soon as possible, coupled with patience, realizing that results often come with a sequential long-term approach across outbreaks as opportunities arise. Despite the many challenges, where the political will is there and the right team assembled, significant progress can be made, contributing both to control of the present outbreak and prevention or enhanced control of the next one.

### Keywords

Ebola virus disease · Vaccine · Clinical trial · Outbreak · Partnership · Democratic Republic of the Congo

## Author Perspective

The authors are scientists, healthcare providers, and public health workers with diverse training and skills from a consortium of governmental, non-governmental, academic, industry, and foundation partners. They come from at least 15 different countries and five continents. Together they offer decades of complementary expertise in clinical trials, field research, and emergency response in complex humanitarian settings, in particular on Ebola virus and other emerging pathogens in Africa.

### Key Tenets

1. Although research, especially clinical trials, during outbreaks often poses enormous challenges, for diseases such as Ebola virus disease, which are seen almost exclusively in outbreak form, outbreaks are the only opportunity to perform studies and accrue knowledge.
2. Keys to success for research during outbreaks include forging partnerships with diverse and complementary experience and skills, working out clear roles and responsibilities, communicating and engaging with the community as an essential partner, and maintaining flexibility to adapt to unexpected events.
3. The approach must find the balance between sound scientific methodology and humanitarian response, integrating the study into the local outbreak response efforts as much as possible while respecting the autonomy and jurisdiction of the country and region where the study takes place.
4. Research during outbreaks must often be considered as longitudinal multicenter trials, recognizing that clear conclusions may not come after a single study during a single outbreak. Flexibility and a "no regrets" policy, i.e. an approach that provides a net benefit in response to a crisis, even if a worst case scenario is never realized, are essential.
5. Where the political will is there and the right team assembled, significant progress can be made, contributing both to control of the present outbreak and prevention or enhanced control of the next one, while contributing to health systems strengthening.
6. This chapter addresses SDG #3, Good Health and Well-Being, and SDG #17 on implementation and revitalization of global partnerships for sustainable development.

## 1 Ebola Virus Disease

Ebola virus is one of the most lethal and feared pathogens on the planet, with case fatalities sometimes approaching 90 percent (Bausch and Crozier 2018). Outbreaks of Ebola virus disease (EVD) appear sporadically in Central and West Africa, usually starting in remote and often impoverished areas. Bats are believed to be the natural reservoir, with primary introduction into humans thought to occur through direct contact with body fluids of bats or a number of intermediate animal hosts through hunting as a food source or via indirect contact through food preparation or contaminated food. Large outbreaks occur almost exclusively through secondary human-to-human transmission through contact with infected body fluids of sick persons, often fueled by nosocomial transmission due to substandard infection prevention and control measures in care settings. In some EVD survivors, delayed virus clearance in immunologically privileged body sites, especially the male gonads, can result in sexual transmission and renewed outbreaks.

Control of EVD outbreaks has historically relied on the classic public health measures of rapid case identification for isolation and treatment, thorough contact tracing, and implementation of infection prevention and control measures in both the community and healthcare facilities. In recent years, vaccines have become an important addition to the armamentarium against EVD (see below). Virtually all EVD outbreak response measures are predicated on community participation—i.e. the willingness of community members to self-identify as cases or contacts and accept isolation and care if sick, be regularly monitored if a contact, and to accept vaccination. Given the fear and stigma often associated with EVD, and the fact that outbreaks often occur in areas with weak public health infrastructure, poor access to affordable and quality healthcare, and where there is a generalized distrust of state authorities, this essential cooperation of the community to help control outbreaks is not always certain.

## 2 The 2018–20 Outbreak in the Democratic Republic of the Congo

On August 1, 2018, the Ministry of Health of the Democratic Republic of the Congo (DRC) reported an outbreak of EVD in North Kivu

Province in eastern DRC (Fig. 1). It would ultimately prove to be the second largest EVD outbreak on record, with 3481 cases (3323 confirmed, 158 probable) and 2299 deaths (case fatality 66%) (World Health Organization Regional Office for Africa 2018). The response to the outbreak was impeded by a weak health system, initially ineffective messaging and community engagement, and civil insecurity. The presence of over 100 different armed groups in the region with varied economic and political interests posed a constant specter of violence (Roberts 2021).

In this challenging and complex socio-cultural and political environment, community participation proved a formidable challenge. Rumor, and at times intentional misinformation, from suspicious communities and individuals, sometimes fueled by political and financial motivations, led to people denying or hiding disease or status as a contact, sometimes even resulting in violent armed resistance. Fatal attacks on EVD response workers from militias or angry civilians occurred (Roberts 2021).

During much of the outbreak, epidemiologic data showed that a considerable proportion of cases, often half or more, were not previously recognized contacts, with estimates from statistical modeling that perhaps 25% of daily cases were going undetected (World Health Organization Regional Office for Africa 2019). Furthermore, roughly a third of detected daily EVD cases were community deaths. These were likely highly infectious persons, with ample opportunity for community transmission prior to death. Faced with these challenges, and despite tremendous efforts on the part of the DRC Ministry of Health and its primary research institution, the Institut National de Recherche Biomédicale (INRB), the World Health Organization (WHO), and a host of national and international partners, the outbreak persisted for almost two years.

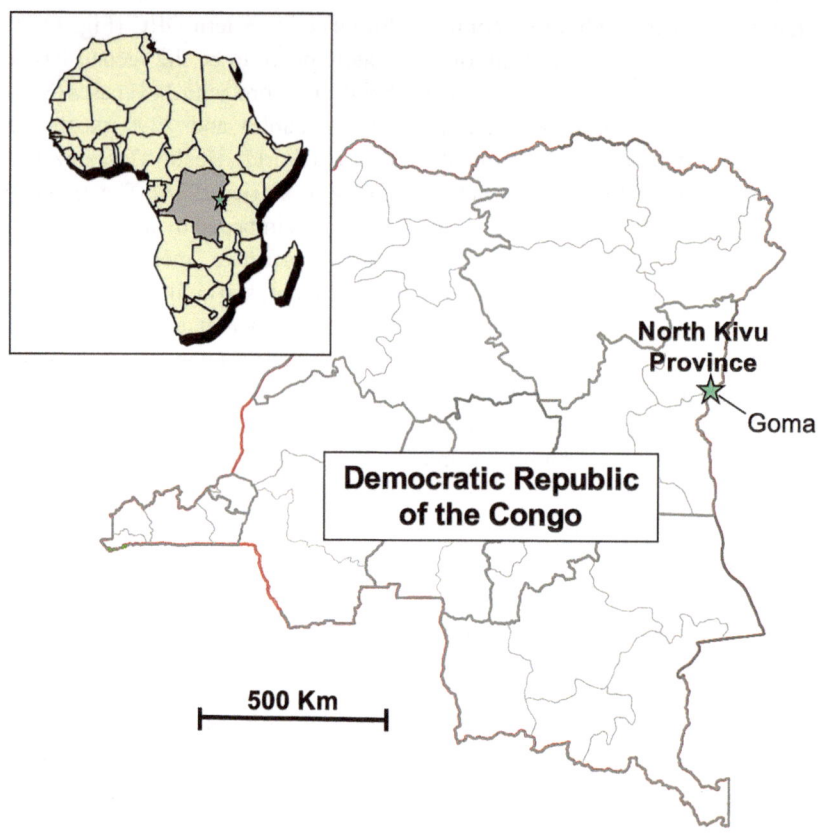

**Fig. 1** Map showing the area of the 2018–2020 outbreak of Ebola virus disease in the Democratic Republic of the Congo and Goma, the site of the Tujiokowe Study

## 3    Vaccines for Ebola Virus DISEASE and Their Application in Eastern DRC

Two EVD vaccines have now received regulatory approval—a single dose vaccine, rVSV-ZEBOV (Merck & Co, Inc., Darmstadt, Germany), approved by the U.S. Food and Drug Administration and European Medicines Agency in 2019, and a heterologous two-dose (days 0 and 56) vaccine, Ad26.ZEBOV/MVA-BN-Filo (Janssen Vaccines and Prevention B.V., Leiden, The Netherlands), approved by the European Medicines Agency in 2020.

Both of these vaccines were in the experimental phases during most of the 2018–20 outbreak in eastern DRC. rVSV-ZEBOV was further along in its development, having undergone a Phase III trial during the large 2013–16 West Africa EVD

outbreak, with reported efficacy of 100% (Henao-Restrepo et al. 2017) (although this number has been questioned (Metzger and Vivas-Martínez 2018)). The vaccine was being used extensively in the eastern DRC outbreak under an expanded use protocol generally employing a ring vaccination approach (i.e., vaccinating contacts and contacts of contacts of persons with EVD) as well as healthcare and other frontline workers (World Health Organization 2018). Nevertheless, despite its high efficacy and widespread use, with ultimately over 300,000 people vaccinated, the outbreak in eastern DRC smoldered on, with new cases repeatedly popping up in areas where transmission had been thought to be extinguished.

Most experts believed that the effectiveness of ring vaccination was tempered by the inability to consistently and rapidly identify cases and contacts, as noted above. Furthermore, feedback from the community indicated that, while most were in favor of vaccination, the ring vaccination approach, which limits eligibility to a relatively small group, was not always understood and accepted. If there was a vaccine, why not offer it to everyone? The outlook in late 2018 seemed dire, prompting WHO and others to consider what new approaches and tools were necessary.

In January 2019, WHO held a meeting in London to discuss possible use of a second vaccine in DRC. Why a second vaccine if you already had the highly efficacious rVSV-ZEBOV? There were multiple justifications, some directly related to the situation in DRC and others with a broader long-term perspective, including:

1. Uncertainty regarding the supply of rVSV-ZEBOV, especially if the outbreak should escalate and/or persist for months or even years (as many predicted, and unfortunately came true). The lead time for further production of rVSV-ZEBOV was often estimated at one year, and there were numerous issues with Merck's production facilities in the United States and Germany,

2. The need to have diverse products in the pipeline, each with distinct features with regard to cold chain requirement, coverage of different species of Ebola virus, anticipated adverse effects and duration of immunity, and ease of manufacturing and administration (Lévy et al. 2018). It is never wise to rely on one product, especially when it is new (one example is the Rotashield™ vaccine for rotavirus, for which an increased incidence of intussusception in children was observed only post-marketing, eventually forcing the vaccine off the market and regulatory approvals to be withdrawn) (Bines et al. 2009).

3. The need to evaluate the safety of EVD vaccines for pregnant and lactating women, as well as other immunocompromised persons, who were eligible for rVSV-ZEBOV vaccination in the North Kivu outbreak due to their high-risk of severe disease if infected, but for whom the safety of the live virus rVSV-ZEBOV vaccine has not been tested,

4. The need to provide opportunities for field trials of products for emerging infectious diseases to encourage the pharmaceutical industry to stay engaged in their development, and

5. The need to develop EVD vaccines for preventive use, as opposed to reactive use once an outbreak is declared. Deployment and trial of a second experimental vaccine for EVD was also recommended by the WHO Strategic Advisory Group of Experts on Immunization (World Health Organization 2019).

Following the January meeting, WHO convened an independent group of experts to evaluate the existing experimental vaccines for EVD and prioritize products for a potential trial based on existing pre-clinical and early stage clinical data. Ad26.ZEBOV/MVA-BN-Filo scored highest based on immunobridging data (i.e. immunogenicity, assessed by antibody titers, on par with rVSV-ZEBOV, which had already been shown to be protective)(Roozendaal et al. 2020), having demonstrated 100% protective efficacy in non-human primate studies and shown to be well tolerated and immunogenic in extensive Phase I-II trials (Callendret et al. 2018; Anywaine et al. 2022; Barry et al. 2021; Ishola et al. 2022; Afolabi et al. 2022; Pollard et al. 2021).[1] In addition to ongoing studies of this vaccine in Sierra Leone, a Phase II trial in frontline workers was underway in Uganda and a large demonstration project was planned for Rwanda in order to pre-emptively protect the population living across the border (Nyombayire et al. 2023). Janssen pledged 500,000 vaccine regimens for DRC, with another million available if needed, free of charge. There was now consensus that Ad26.ZEBOV/MVA-BN-Filo was the next EVD vaccine to be put into the field, and a promise of ample supply, but the question remained—how to deploy it effectively and safely in DRC?

---

[1] Most of the cited publications came after the 2019 meeting, but much of the data were communicated informally at the time.

## 4  Study Partners

A consortium gradually emerged to lead the study, still of undefined design, led by INRB, with the London School of Hygiene & Tropical Medicine (LSHTM), which had been engaged extensively in previous clinical trials of both rVSV-ZEBOV and Ad26.ZEBOV/MVA-BN-Filo, as the study sponsor. Other key partners at the onset were Epicentre, MSF-France (which later withdrew—see below) and Janssen, with WHO as an observer. All of the partners have extensive experience with clinical trials, and many specifically on EVD vaccines. The Coalition for Epidemic Preparedness Innovations (CEPI) played a critical role as a convener to provide organizational and funding support to the implementing partners. Additional funders ultimately included the Wellcome Trust; UK Foreign, Commonwealth & Development Office; European Union; and Paul G. Allen Family Foundation. To streamline processes and financial management, it was agreed early on that all donor funding for the study would be funneled through CEPI, with LSHTM contracted as the study sponsor to manage funds through subcontracts with the other partners. A Study Steering Committee was created with a representative from each consortium technical partner, with CEPI and the Wellcome Trust representing the donors. The team eventually settled upon the name "Tujiokowe" for the study, roughly translated as "save or take action for yourself" in Swahili.

## 5  Alignment on Objectives and Study Design

The next step was a meeting in Kinshasa of the partners and various stakeholders, which took place in March 2019. As always happens when one contemplates clinical trials in an outbreak setting, it is necessary to find an appropriate balance of robust science to evaluate a still unproven and unlicensed product, and the desire to use that product for maximal public health impact—in the case of a vaccine, to limit transmission and

stop an outbreak. Understandably, there are often initially almost diametrically opposed expectations, and this diversity of opinion was on full display at the Kinshasa meeting; clinical trialists and members of regulatory agencies will demand the tightest trial designs to achieve the soundest evidence of efficacy, while public health officials with an outbreak on their hands will want a large vaccination campaign to halt transmission. A middle ground must be sought, but it will never satisfy all perspectives. The ultimate decision must be made by the authorities in the place where the outbreak is occurring and the study is to take place, in this case authorities of the DRC.

After hashing out some basic principles in Kinshasa, a protocol writing team was established, led by LSHTM. After much debate, and given the worsening outbreak, the team eventually settled upon a test-negative design that held the potential to yield effectiveness data but also to have a greater public health impact through a strategy that targeted greater numbers than the more restrictive ring vaccination with rVSV-ZEBOV. rVSV-ZEBOV vaccination would be continued but complemented, in a still undefined approach and region, by Ad26.ZEBOV/MVA-BN-Filo (Watson-Jones et al. 2022). The test-negative design was also among those proposed at the January WHO meeting.

However, this was not the end of the matter; eventually all consortium partners agreed to move forward with a study, with one major exception—the DRC Minister of Health. At the time the DRC was going through a transition, with newly elected President Félix Tshisekedi ascending to the presidency. Tshisekedi had not yet established his cabinet, including who would be the new Minister of Health. Meanwhile, the incumbent Minister, Oly Ilunga Kalenga, in contrast to INRB, firmly opposed introduction of a second vaccine, an opinion often shared by many at WHO (Roberts 2021). Leaving aside controversies over Minister Ilunga himself, (Cohen 2019)[2] a major and legitimate concern was that

---

[2]Minister Ilunga later resigned his post and was subsequently arrested and sentenced to five years of prison for misuse of $4.3 M in funds allocated by the United States

introduction of a second vaccine, especially one with a different regimen and approach than rVSV-ZEBOV, would confuse an already hesitant and beleaguered population, potentially undermining acceptance of rVSV-ZEBOV which, despite the aforementioned challenges, was clearly a vital tool keeping the outbreak in check.

The matter was eventually solved when President Tshisekedi appointed a new Minister of Health and INRB, whose director was firmly in favor of conducting a study on Ad26.ZEBOV/MVA-BN-Filo, as the lead institution to manage the outbreak response. Many WHO colleagues nevertheless remained reserved, with what seemed a fluctuating view—supportive when the epidemiologic picture looked grim, forcing the thought that maybe another vaccine *was* needed, but enthusiasm quickly waning if the epidemiological data looked more favorable the following week. Although WHO had only observer status for the planned Ad26.ZEBOV/MVA-BN-Filo study, there were concerns about conflicts of interest, considering WHO's prominent sponsorship and involvement in competitive research, including the use of rVSV-ZEBOV in the DRC, while issuing policy on research done by others.

# 6    Getting Started

With political hurdles cleared and a design and protocol in place, the major question was where precisely to conduct the study. It was eventually decided to pilot it in high-risk areas of North Kivu's capital and major city, Goma, in which Ebola virus was not circulating at the time but whose population of over one million was considered highly vulnerable, especially since there was frequent travel to Goma from the epicenter of the epidemic to the north. Indeed, a few imported cases of EVD from the epicenter to Goma had already occurred, fortunately with no secondary transmission. The plan was to get started in Goma, learn from and resolve any early obstacles, and then move closer to the epicenter

---

for the EVD outbreak response

in a second phase, guided by the latest epidemiologic data and prognostic modeling.

An extensive recruitment and communication plan was developed and implemented by MSF-France, Epicentre and INRB in advance of any vaccination in Goma. This consisted of door-to-door visits, radio and television spots, and SMS automatic messaging. Rapid Knowledge, Attitudes, and Practices studies were conducted to publicize the vaccine study and help communities understand its rationale and structure. Six vaccination sites in Goma were established, and participant enrollment began in November 2019.

# 7    Implementation Challenges

Implementing a study in a remote, politically and socio-culturally complex area with ongoing conflict and frequent movement of displaced people in the middle of an EVD outbreak is an extraordinarily challenging undertaking. At times it seemed like a new challenge every day, like an unrealistic movie where everything that could happen did. The risk register maintained for the study reflects these frequent challenges (Table 1). Below we summarize some of the most formidable implementation challenges and efforts at resolution or mitigation. While some challenges may have been specific to this study, time and circumstance, they may nevertheless be illustrative for those engaged in field work elsewhere. The key message: Be prepared, flexible, and expect the unexpected!

## 7.1    Alignment on Roles and Responsibilities

In the early stages we experienced "growing pains" while trying to define and streamline roles and responsibilities and reporting structures between partner institutions with diverse histories and objectives. Our consortium included partners from government (INRB and MOH), academia (LSHTM), non-governmental organizations (MSF-France and Epicentre), founda-

**Table 1** Risks noted in the study Risk Register over the course of the project

| Date (month-year) | Risk or Event Cited | Details | Consequences |
|---|---|---|---|
| Dec-2019 | Theft of vehicle, computers, and photo equipment | A vehicle containing 14 laptop computers and photo cameras used daily at the vaccination sites was stolen by a driver employed by the consortium. | The study sites were temporarily closed while investigation took place. Police were notified and eventually apprehended the driver. The incident was immediately reported to the LSHTM Data Protection Officer, who determined that it did not constitute a data breach because (1) Data are not stored on the computers, but rather downloaded to a server at the end of each day (the theft occurred in the morning, prior to starting that day's work), (2) The computers are doubly password protected and the data are encrypted, (3) The computers were used only for temporary data storage, not for email or other messaging, and (4) The camaras were of the type to instantly print a study participant's photo and with no storage of image media. |
| Mar-2020 | Study suspension due to COVID-19 pandemic | The pandemic led to the suspension of in-person study activities for the protection of both participants and staff. The study was paused from 10 April until 15 September 2020. | Delays in the study and additional risk of more participants lost-to-follow-up. |
| Jun-2020 | End of the EVD outbreak in eastern DRC and forcing change in program objectives | The EVD outbreak was declared over on 24 June 2020, making evaluation of vaccine protective efficacy impossible. Following discussions with Janssen, it was agreed that there was nevertheless a need to collect immunogenicity data, particularly for children, and safety data in pregnant women. In August 2020, the protocol was amended to incorporate these objectives and the study continued. | This new objective added additional costs to support blood sample acquisition, storage, shipment and analysis for antibody testing at Q2 Solutions in the United States. The budget was reprofiled to accommodate these costs. |
| Jul-2020 | MSF-France leaves the consortium | In May 2020, during the study suspension due to the COVID-19 pandemic, MSF-France informed that they would withdraw from the consortium after handover of their activities to other partners, which occurred and was completed in July 2020. | MSF-France's roles and responsibilities were adjusted across the remaining partners and World Vision joined the consortium to take on community engagement activities, with funding provided from another source. The budget was reprofiled accordingly. |
| Nov-2020 | Loss of a vaccine shipment in Brussels airport for over 48 hours | The MSF/Epicentre logistics team could confirm that the shipment was picked up in Brussels on 13 November and was due to depart on a Lufthansa flight to Kigali the next day. However, 48 hours passed in which Lufthansa could not locate the shipment. It was subsequently located in the Brussels airport, where it had been put in a secure and refrigerated location. | Vaccine eventually shipped safely to DRC, but with the consequence of much worry and energy expenditure. |

(continued)

**Table 1** (continued)

| Date (month-year) | Risk or Event Cited | Details | Consequences |
|---|---|---|---|
| Mar-2021 | Fire in data storage site | On 10 March 2021, the OVH facility in Strasbourg, France, in which the study database was kept, took fire. | The study data management team had to reconstruct some of the database using prior audit trails, resulting in delays in data analysis. There were fortunately no major cost implications, other than time spent by study staff. |
| Apr-2021 | Difficulty in shipping samples out of Goma | With transport options out of Goma limited, especially during the COVID-19 pandemic, the study team struggled to find suitable options to ship samples for antibody testing to the Q2 Solutions laboratory in the USA. Eventually a company was found, but the first shipment was delayed when an airline employee noticed vapor emanating from the cold box and removed if from the plane. After communications to explain that this was normal, the company added more ice in Goma and proceeded with shipment on the first leg to Kinshasa. However, there were additional cold chain concerns as the samples were changed to a new box in Kinshasa before onward shipment to the USA via Istanbul. | Fortunately, despite concerns, the samples arrived in good condition with little temperature variation. |
| May-2021 | Volcano eruption | Mount Nyiragongo erupted on 22 May 2021, causing disruption across Goma. The project house was closed and some staff had to evacuate the city. | Project incurred security costs of evacuation, potential additional loss to follow-up due to disruption caused, and delays in various project activities, in addition to possible detrimental mental health impact. |
| Nov-2021 | Need for Study Data Tabulation Model data conversion | Janssen colleagues informed the consortium that study data would need to be converted to the Study Data Tabulation Model format. However, this was not foreseen nor budgeted, posing a challenge on how to achieve this work near the very end of the project with limited resources remaining. | Additional cost to the project, which was added at the No-Cost-Extension stage. Fortunately, existing funds were sufficient. |
| Feb-2022 | Technical problem at Q2 Solutions | Q2 Solutions informed the consortium of a technical problem (increase in ZEBOV/Ebola IgG ELISA plate failure) forcing suspension of testing while the problem was investigated and resolved. | Significant delay in sample testing and provision of results causing delays in statistical analysis and publication. |

*DRC* Democratic Republic of the Congo; *EVD* Ebola virus disease

tions (CEPI and Wellcome Trust) and the private sector (Janssen). The challenges were less about power dynamics than building trust and communications to overcome institutional cultural differences and traditional ways of working. For example, most MSF-France staff usually focus on humanitarian response and pragmatic service provision and are accustomed to nimble *ad hoc* adaptation to obstacles encountered in the field. While this makes sense for MSF-France's usual field missions, it did not always mesh with the requirements of international standards of Good Clinical Practice (GCP) for a clinical trial, which require methodical systematic rigor, including sometimes painstakingly detailed procedures and documentation in order to have valid data suitable for eventual submission to regulatory agencies to apply for product licensure. High staff turnover in MSF also posed a challenge, with new team members sometimes unaware of procedural agreements made by their predecessors. In contrast, some personnel from academic partners like LSHTM and industry partners like Janssen were less experienced regarding the realities of program implementation on the ground in emergency settings such as an EVD outbreak, although both LSHTM and Janssen did benefit from previous collaborations on EVD vaccine trials in West Africa and elsewhere.

To solve this, after having several meetings of all partners and virtually all personnel to discuss expected roles, we created workstreams for each study component –e.g. one each for safety, data management, quality management—with a named lead and separate weekly call for each workstream (Table 2). The leads then reported progress to the Principal Investigators and whole team on a weekly teleconference.

Another challenging aspect at times was the dual role of CEPI—a global organization that provides funding but also technical and logistic support for vaccine development. While CEPI's technical expertise proved to be essential, especially in establishing some of the early essential training of in-country personal in matters such as GCP, the dual role of funder and technical partner at times created tensions when disagreements developed.

**Table 2** Workstreams created for the Tujiokowe study

| Workstream | Lead organization | Weekly meeting lead person |
|---|---|---|
| Study Steering Committee | LSHTM | Principal and Co-Principal Investigators |
| Consortium General | LSHTM | Senior Project Manager |
| Logistics/Pharmacy | Epicentre | Logistics Lead |
| Pharmacovigilance | LSHTM | Study Coordinator |
| Sponsorship | LSHTM | Co-Principal Investigators |
| Finance Management | LSHTM | Senior Project Manager |
| Data Management | LSHTM | Data Systems Coordinator |
| Test Negative Analysis | Epicentre | Data Scientist |
| Immunogenicity | LSHTM | Study Coordinator |
| Social Sciences | LSHTM | Research Fellow |
| Quality Management | LSHTM | Quality Manager |
| Internal Monitoring | Epicentre | Coordinator |
| Vaccination Team | Epicentre | Coordinator |
| Community Engagement and Informed Consent Process | World Vision | Program coordinator |

*LSTHM* London School of Hygiene and Tropical Medicine

## 7.2 Effective Communications

While frequent and reiterative communications through weekly teleconferences were essential, we learned that you can have *too* much communication (see chapter "Foundations and Future Directions of Global Health Communication"). With so many partners and personnel, copying everyone on every email resulted in a daily accumulation with which it was impossible to keep up. It took time to find the balance—streamlining communications to those who needed to know to address needed actions but not inundating those who did not need to know regarding a particular aspect of the project. The workstreams as described above helped focus these communications.

## 7.3    Language Barriers

The official national language of the DRC is French, with Swahili and various other local languages commonly spoken in Goma. However, the primary language of some of the consortium partners and personnel is English, and most documents were originally produced in English. Hence, formal translation of all official study documents from English to French was required. Furthermore, materials meant to interface directly with the community had to also be translated into Swahili. These processes were time consuming and costly. Languages also presented challenges in day-to-day operations, with most meetings needing to be conducted in both English and French. What helped tremendously in overcoming these challenges was hiring multilingual and local staff who could help bridge the language gap. Bilingual program managers who could run meetings in English or French as required were especially helpful. Furthermore, the principal investigator spoke both French and English, as did one of the co-principal investigators, while the other co-principal investigator spoke both English and Swahili.

## 7.4    Training

Conducting a clinical trial requires a cadre of personnel with the appropriate training, including in GCP. No such trained cadre existed in Goma. Therefore, an early step was to identify personnel in the Goma region with the right biomedical background and interest in participating in the study and to train them in GCP and Good Clinical Laboratory Practice. CEPI had experience in organizing this sort of training and was particularly instrumental in this regard. Data management trainings were also conducted by Epicentre.

## 7.5    Trial Monitoring

Monitoring is an essential part of any clinical trial or study and is often accomplished via a contract research organization. For this study, the investigators felt that it was essential to find an African-based organization who would be accustomed to the context and practical realities of implementing a trial in this setting, which require flexibility with regard to plans and proposed study sites. A research organization based in Kenya that had worked with LSHTM and Janssen on earlier vaccine trials, with personnel who could speak both English and Swahili, was ultimately selected. Nevertheless, trial monitors' lack of French fluency still led to delays in the monitoring activities on occasion.

## 7.6    How to Plan and Budget for a Dynamic and Unpredictable Event?

As discussed above, the original plan was to begin the study in Goma and then, based on the most recent epidemiologic data and prognostic modeling, move to areas closer to the epicenter to maximize the public health impact. While logical, the uncertainty inherent in this plan created considerable challenges and consternation. Where is the next vaccination site after Goma? How do we ensure that we have the required personnel and security and allocate the required budget if we don't know where it is? How long will it take to set up in the next site and complete site initiation activities? And after we decide, what happens if the outbreak ends before we can get set up at the next site?

Due to this uncertainty, the budgeting processes often seemed protracted and everchanging, requiring numerous rounds of reprofiling. In May 2020 MSF-France, citing uncertainties about the budget and competing commitments with regard to humanitarian response, announced that they would withdraw from the project, and did so in July 2020 (Roberts 2021). Their roles and responsibilities were transferred to INRB, Epicentre, and a new partner already on site—the non-governmental organization World Vision. Fortunately, by the time MSF-France withdrew, the other partners, especially Epicentre and INRB, were well versed in the functions MSF-France had been covering and were able to assume them without undue challenge or delay, with World Vision's added contribution.

The large budget dedicated to the international outbreak response in eastern DRC—ultimately measured in billions of dollars—was a sensitive issue, often criticized, justly or unjustly, as "Ebola business," i.e., a problem introduced or made up by government authorities, international agitators or local power-brokers with nefarious economic and/or political motivations. Understandably, a population living in a situation of poverty, violence and massive inequality was aggrieved by an enormous investment in something that was not always perceived as a major problem, if it indeed existed at all. While efforts to be transparent and inclusive were admirable, the budget, including the tens of millions of dollars for our vaccine trial, became major topics of discussion and rumor, sometimes aggravating local political sensitivities, particularly when it was not made clear what the local population would get out of it, i.e. possible access to a probably-effective vaccine.

## 7.7    Insecurity

Throughout the study, which ran for over two years, there were periodic security alerts in Goma, including strikes and protests, at times turning violent. None of these were specifically related to our study or EVD vaccination, but rather most often to the population's perception that the Unite Nations' Mission in eastern DRC was failing to keep them safe from the many armed groups present in the region. Despite early concerns that our vaccination activities would be targets of community retaliation (as seen in the EVD response further north), the study was well accepted and did not become a flashpoint for protest, a result perhaps attributable to our proactive community engagement and communication campaigns. Nevertheless, on numerous occasions, protests on other issues forced suspension of activities to ensure the safety of study participants and staff, in addition

to the logistical challenges that the protests posed in simply navigating crowded streets jammed with protestors in order to arrive at study sites.

## 7.8    COVID-19

The arrival of the COVID-19 pandemic brought major concerns for the safety of both study participants and staff. The congregation of people at enrollment and vaccination sites, which were relatively small buildings with cramped quarters, had the potential to facilitate transmission and even become super-spreader events. Assessing the risk of COVID-19 in the region was difficult since little was known about the SARS-CoV-2 virus at the time and surveillance capacity in Goma was limited. In April 2021, the Steering Committee decided that the most prudent decision was to suspend the study. This decision was communicated to all study participants as well as to the community at large by radio, telephone and SMS text. Weekly meetings of the study team were held to review the epidemiologic situation and risks and benefits of resumption of activities. However, decisions could be based on little more than best guesses, since there was still no systematic surveillance data for COVID-19. As the months wore on, sporadic cases continued to be reported, usually related to importation by humanitarian aid workers coming from Europe or North America, but there were no reports of major spikes of respiratory disease or inundated healthcare centers in Goma.

As with the world over, the pandemic's impact reached far beyond the daily activities on the ground. Reduced flight routes and travel restrictions posed challenges in transporting vaccine from the Janssen production facilities in Europe to Goma (in the confusion of the pandemic, one shipment was lost for more than 48 hours in Brussels airport) and severely curtailed visits from international staff. These included supervisory visits from the Principal Investigators, who were based in Kinshasa; Mwanza, Tanzania; and London, and from quality control monitors. Most of these functions were forced to be conducted remotely for the remainder of the study.

In August 2021, the decision was made to cautiously resume the study, initially limiting daily participant numbers at each site and implementing measures such as physical distancing to prevent SARS-CoV-2 virus transmission. Although certainly there must have been participants and staff who became infected in the community, no cases of COVID-19 were ever attributed to study activities or the contacts at the study sites. Nevertheless, delays due to the COVID-19 pandemic and the other obstacles cited here ultimately necessitated prolongation of the study by four months and a corresponding no-cost extension of funding.

While the precise impact of new participant enrollment due to the COVID-19 pandemic is hard to quantify, the five month suspension certainly had an impact on receipt of the second dose of the vaccine regimen, delaying it in half of the participants, with some receiving the second dose up to a year after the first one. Since, prior to the pandemic, the study team consistently emphasized to participants the importance of timely return to receive the second dose at day 56, the delay caused by the pandemic created considerable anxiety among some participants, who were unsure whether it was still beneficial to receive a late second dose. Not all participants returned to receive their second dose and the retention rate suffered. In addition to the logistic impediments, vaccine hesitancy and misinformation may have played a role in adherence since, when the team resumed activities, rumors circulated, countered by our community engagement team, that the EVD vaccine was actually a vaccine against COVID-19 (James et al. 2023).

## 7.9 Volcano Eruption and Earthquakes

In May 2021, the Nyiragongo Volcano on the outskirts of Goma erupted. Lava flow and volcanic ash followed by a series of earthquakes affected more than 400,000 people in the city, killing at least 31. The events forced thousands of people to flee to neighboring Rwanda, including numerous study staff. Fortunately, all staff survived without injury or major loss of property. Nevertheless the event forced suspension of the study for approximately one month while geological perturbations settled and staff could make their way back to Goma and reestablish normal activities. Upon return, large cracks were noted in the study headquarters building, raising concerns regarding its structural integrity and the safety of allowing staff to re-enter. It took over four weeks to arrange a formal evaluation of the building, during which time staff worked from home or hotel rooms. The fortunate final conclusion was that the damage was largely cosmetic, and staff could return to work.

## 7.10 Fire at Data Storage Site

On 10 March 2021, the OVHcloud Data Center in Strasbourg, France, in which the study databases were kept, took fire. After weeks of uncertainty and investigation, it was revealed that both the main and back-up servers for the study data, located in the same room, were both destroyed, with resultant loss of study data and audit trails. The study data management team had to reconstruct some of the database using prior audit trails, resulting in delays in data analysis. There were fortunately no major cost implications, other than time spent by study staff.

## 8 Lessons Learned

At the time of this writing, the study has concluded, albeit with considerable extension due to the aforementioned challenges and delays. Data are being analyzed and manuscripts prepared (Table 3). While the welcome cessation of transmission and end of the outbreak precluded any evaluation of vaccine efficacy, we nevertheless anticipate valuable findings and perspectives important to not only to Ad26. ZEBOV/MVA-BN-Filo and EVD, but also to field studies in general. Below we summarize key take home messages and lessons learned

**Table 3** List of planned publications from the Tujiokowe study which is periodically reviewed and updated

| |
| --- |
| Vaccination uptake, coverage and safety in adults and children |
| Immunogenicity subset |
| Social science—decision-making |
| Vaccination card manuscript |
| Pregnancy/birth outcomes and neonatal outcomes |
| Systematic review on birth outcomes in North Kivu |
| Retention within the cohort & factors associated with failure to complete the vaccine course |
| A detailed data management paper |
| Clinical paper: incidence rates of different conditions in this population |
| Book chapter on partnerships (i.e. what you are reading now) |

that we hope will be of value to those undertaking field research, especially in the context of outbreaks and other complex humanitarian emergencies.

## 8.1 Partnerships: Assembling your Team

• *Include diverse and complementary experience and skills.* Implementation of research in the midst of complex humanitarian emergencies is inevitably challenging and requires partners with diverse skill sets, including experience and knowledge with protocol methodology, setting up research sites during complex emergencies, data analysis, resource mobilization, program management, logistics, and field implementation. Soft skills, such as speaking multiple languages and having experience with the political geography and culture of the region of study, should not be overlooked. It would be the rare institution that offers all these capabilities; thus, partnerships are essential. In our study, it was especially helpful to have partners such as INRB and Epicentre, who were conversant in both the practical implementation of field research and the demands of clinical trials, often serving as a bridge between the different partners to facilitate communication and understanding, as well as speaking the languages in both the area of study and of many of the collaborators.

Beyond providing all the necessary skill sets for trial implementation, partnerships can ensure that diverse viewpoints are incorporated to bring additional uptake to respond to patient, population and scientific needs; provide visibility, legitimacy, and quality to the trial to enhance future use and endorsement; and provide opportunities for new and innovative ways of working.

• *Be conscious of power imbalances and work to correct them.* Successful partnerships in global health research must take into account much more than high level science and competent scientists. Equally important are the partners' ability to manage all of the operational processes and international regulations surrounding research, including financial management and good practices, plans for professional development, and expertise in contracting and negotiation. There are often unequal research management capacities between partners that must be recognized, requiring a commitment to providing knowledge transfer and support to help build sustainable capacity. We must also recognize the inherent difficulty of conducting research in low- and middle-income countries with partners from high income countries, who typically provide most of the funding. This creates an inherent power imbalance that favors the wealthiest and best-equipped organizations who have disproportionate power in competitiveness for research funding and in exercising control over the goals and terms of partnerships. A core commitment to strive for equity is essential.

• *Work out roles and responsibilities at the onset, and revisit and revise periodically to ensure that they are still fit-for-purpose.* Diverse partners will inevitably come with their own diverse institutional viewpoints and ways of working, which may at times cause friction. Early discussions on roles and responsibilities and ways of working are essential to bring and keep the team together. These should be periodically revisited and reaffirmed or adapted as the project and team evolve, including consideration of mid-term meetings specifically dedicated to the topic. Especially for longer studies, partner organizations with high turnover must ensure that previously agreed roles and responsibilities are passed on and respected by successive generations of staff.

- *Engage the community as an essential partner.* The most important partner is the community where the study takes place, and thus local engagement right from the start is essential. Strategies using diverse modalities should be established for proactive two-way dialogue, participant representation, and feedback. Early Knowledge, Attitudes and Practices studies can be a useful tool, but do not entirely capture complexity and diversity of experiences and concerns. Specific strategies to deal with areas of civil unrest may be needed. In our study, dialogue was critical, with answering questions posed during the process perhaps even more important than the prescribed messages.

- *Consider the full range of possible conflicts of interest.* While evaluation and declaration of conflicts of interest is, of course, the norm, with guidelines and procedures in place, not all conflicts of interest are necessarily rooted in conventional concerns regarding financial profit. Conflicts, perceived or real, may also exist between nonprofit partners, who may be involved in possibly competing research projects, engaged in research as well as providing public health guidance on the same question or domain, or hold positions at institutions that make both financial and technical contributions to a research endeavor. While such situations do not automatically exclude a given person from participation in a study, their role, and appropriate firewalls, should be thoroughly considered at the onset.

## 8.2    Approach

- *Find the balance between sound scientific methodology and humanitarian response.* Clinical trials of emerging infectious diseases that are generally seen only in outbreak form pose particular challenges. For large outbreaks, there may be pressure from international attention, with considerable influx of international resources and expectation of rapid results. A balance must be found and compromises made between the ideal scientific methodology, the speed of implementation, and the recognition that communities are suffering and in urgent need beyond the longer-term benefits that research may provide. Of course we want to implement rapidly, but we must be cautious to not select rapid designs so filled with compromise that no definitive conclusions can be made at the end of the study. Pre-positioning generic protocols, contractual and legal frameworks as much as possible ahead of outbreaks can help streamline and speed the process.

- *As much as possible, integrate the study into the local outbreak response efforts.* In these complex humanitarian settings, scientific studies should be integrated into the local response as much as possible to avoid competition for human and financial resources. When full integration is not possible, external resources and personnel must be procured for the research so that it does not detract from the public health response to the outbreak, which must remain the priority to curtail transmission and save lives. In order to achieve this, considerable advance planning is required, including forming and structuring teams dedicated to research. WHO's recent addition of "Research" as a named and dedicated pillar of outbreak response is a step forward.

- *Respect the autonomy and jurisdiction of the country and region where the study takes place and engage and invest locally.* It is important that the principle research institution and principal investigator are from the country where the study is taking place, as was the case with INRB, whose contribution and critical role were essential in our study. The majority of staff should be hired locally, with a shared goal of capacity development and mutual learning. International standards for research partnerships have been proposed (Research Fairness Initiative n.d.).

- *Adopt a no regrets approach to research in outbreak settings.* Just as the policy for outbreak response must be one of "no regrets" (i.e. one that provides a net benefit in response to a crisis, even if a worst case scenario is never realized), so must we take this same approach to research during outbreaks. As we were preparing this study many people would skeptically caution us, saying "This is going to be an extremely difficult thing to implement." Undoubtedly true, but what choice is there? There is no way to conduct field trials on EVD and other diseases that are seen only in outbreaks other than during the outbreak itself, and these often occur in the setting of complex humanitarian emergencies. There may be trial and error, but the error should never be to avoid engaging in research in these situations, which would prevent evaluation of many new tools to prevent or ameliorate future outbreaks.

- **Avoid preconceived notions that may hinder a study from the outset.** Many assumed that a two-dose vaccine as used in our study could not be administered in such a difficult setting—that few would return for the second dose. However, with proper follow-up, and despite the challenges of insecurity, a COVID-19 pandemic, and a volcanic eruption, among many others, over 75 percent of participants eventually returned for dose 2, albeit often delayed beyond the prescribed day 56 due to the aforementioned obstacles. This finding has clear implications for future assumptions about vaccine administration schedules and uptake. In addition, while unintended, the delay in administering the second dose allowed the team to study immunogenicity outside the prescribed dosing window.

- *Flexibility is essential.* Even when things do not go as planned, there are still usually important questions to ask and evidence and experience to gather. Revising and amending our study to investigate immunogenicity and safety in pregnancy are examples. There may also be collateral benefits for other diseases. For example, the knowledge gained from ours and other studies involving the Janssen adenovirus platform has been useful in the development of Janssen's COVID-19 vaccine.

## 8.3 Logistics

- **Budget for dynamic projects and account for uncertainty.** Fixed budgets and cumbersome reprofiling processes may pose challenges when dealing with the near-inevitable uncertainty of research during outbreaks, which is inherently dynamic and unpredictable. While of course total budgets for a study are always fixed and accountability must be maintained, as much as possible, thinking through and creating flexible budgeting processes and contingencies for reprofiling when necessary can improve project efficiency and relieve stress.

- *Work out anticipated publications at the outset and agree on divisions of labor and authorship.* Research will inevitably lead to scientific publications. Agreement on data ownership and authorship should be pursued from the beginning. We developed a publications policy agreement at the beginning of the study, and as the study progressed, a dynamic database of planned manuscripts and lead persons (Table 3). Beyond the more formal data, take the time to have an after-action review meeting, and communicate internally and externally the findings, experiences and lessons learned that may be valuable to the local population; local, regional and national health authorities; and other investigators.

- *Ensure safe data storage.* Although this might seem obvious, assure that there are redundant systems for data storage and retrieval, and that they are not co-located physically or linked in a vulnerable manner through the internet (i.e. ensure cyber-security).

## 8.4    Long-Term Impact

- *Consider research during outbreaks as longitudinal multicenter trials.* There is always a risk that the trial conducted during an outbreak will not get fully and optimally implemented before the outbreak ends, or that it there will not be a sufficient number of study participants to reach the statistical endpoints to make definitive conclusions. Implementation may be impeded by a long list of practical field obstacles, but that must not prevent research teams from preparing and engaging. Given the inevitable uncertainty regarding when and where an outbreak will occur and how long it will last, it is important to take a pragmatic approach to clinical trials, effectively considering them as longitudinal multicenter studies that may, when necessary, span across outbreaks. Much has been learned, for example, from successive EVD vaccine trials across outbreaks in West and Central Africa that has informed vaccine trials for COVID-19. The "false starts," or incomplete studies, nevertheless help us get there, both in terms of collecting early data and learning what works and what does not in terms of practical implementation, including getting interested collaborators together, working through mundane but important issues like import permits and data management policies, and figuring out supply and cold chain issues in austere environments. Indeed, recent success in developing vaccines and therapeutics for EVD has come from the cumulative field research efforts starting with the 2013–16 outbreak in West Africa (if not before) and continuing into subsequent outbreaks in the DRC, as well as other safety, immunogenicity and demonstration studies in Burkina Faso, Cote d'Ivoire, DRC, Guinea, Kenya, Mali, Rwanda, Sierra Leone, Tanzania, and Uganda.
- *Use research during outbreaks as an opportunity to strengthen health systems.* Outbreak response and research during outbreaks pres-

ent opportunities for strengthening health systems, with the potential for long-term positive impact (Durski et al. 2020). For example, the response and research oriented toward the EVD outbreak in eastern DRC contributed to the establishment of a high-performing INRB laboratory in Goma (Fig. 2), advanced training in GCP, and provided valuable field experience for a large cadre of Congolese scientists and healthcare workers, enhancing capacity to conduct future clinical trials and other studies on EVD and beyond. Still more concretely, with the licensure of the Ad26.ZEBOV/MVA-BN-Filo in 2019, INRB, Janssen and partners conducted a preventive vaccination campaign in the Equateur Province of DRC, an area where repeated EVD outbreaks have been recorded and considered endemic for the disease. Ad26. ZEBOV/MVA-BN-Filo has also been used in preventive campaigns in neighboring Rwanda and on the periphery of EVD outbreaks in West Africa (Nyombayire et al. 2023).

## 9    Future Challenges

Although our study has now conclude, many challenges for long-term impact remain; how to keep the created infrastructure and team intact, including many trained and skilled healthcare workers, for continued vaccine administration and monitoring (from the study and post-marketing) to address any clinical consequences? Still more broadly, how do we ensure institutional memory so that the lessons learned and practical knowledge accumulated will not be lost, that we will not start anew for the next outbreak and clinical trial? Lastly, and perhaps most importantly, how can we ensure that the knowledge gained through clinical trials translates to impact—to policies and actions that saves lives? How can we use the two approved EVD vaccines to not only effectively respond to outbreaks when they occur but, even better, to prevent them from occurring in the first place through vaccination of populations at risk, including frontline health profes-

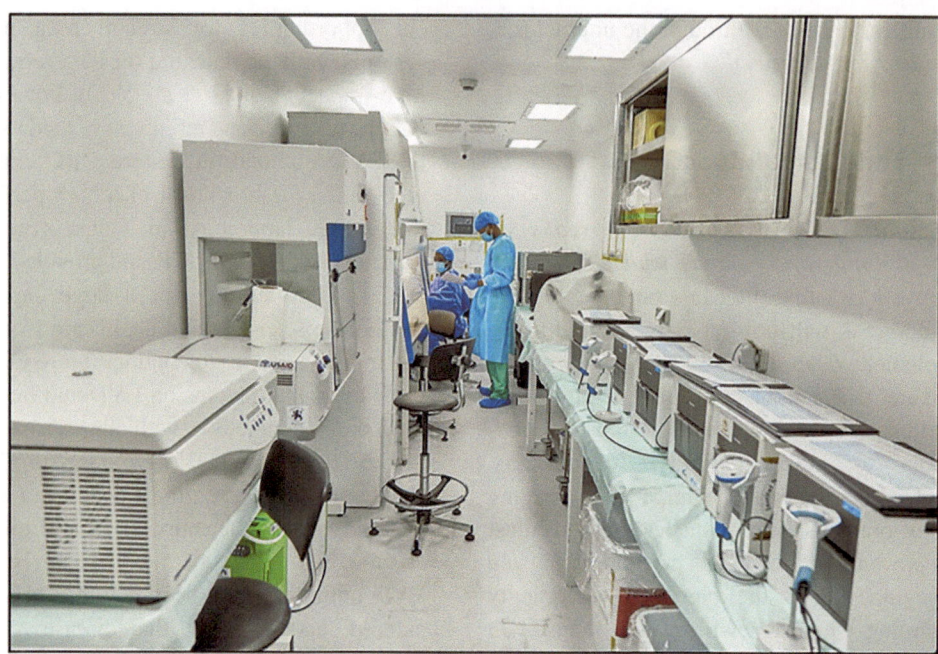

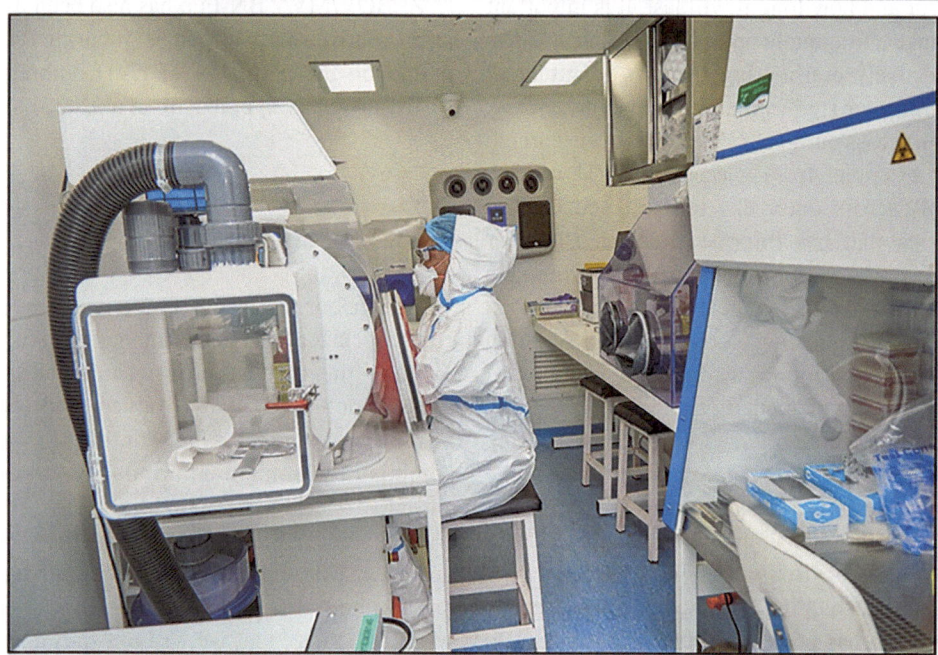

**Fig. 2** The new Institut National de Recherche Biomédicale laboratory in Goma, whose establishment was partly in response to the public health and research needs highlighted by the 2018–2020 outbreak of Ebola virus diseases in eastern Democratic Republic of the Congo

sionals? (Bausch 2021) While laudable, the aforementioned preventive vaccination campaign in DRC's Equateur Province represents only a small fraction of the population at risk for EVD. Guidance and discussions on how best to use both Ad26.ZEBOV/MVA-BN-Filo and rVSV-ZEBOV for broader prevention and response to EVD outbreaks across the regions at risk in Africa are ongoing (Bausch 2021; World Health Organization 2021).

# 10    Conclusions

Clinical trials in outbreak settings pose diverse and often enormous challenges, and up until very recent times have often been considered almost impossible. However, the gravity of the 2013–16 West Africa EVD outbreak galvanized support for such endeavors, despite the difficulty, and clinical trials have been at least under consideration during every EVD outbreak since and have now been extensively performed for COVID-19 vaccines. These have achieved considerable success, including data showing efficacy and leading to regulatory approval of the Merck and Janssen EVD vaccines, as well as two therapeutics for EVD Mulangu et al. (2019). This can only be achieved with political will to push forward with trials in these difficult settings, and the commitments and partnerships of diverse organizations offering diverse capacities and skill sets. The study presented here represents the progress made in assembling a team of experts form previous studies, with significant new partners. The success is a testament to the drive and determination of study sponsors, implementors, and participants. The key message: If the will is there, it can be done!

**Acknowledgments** The authors thank the following:

- All study participants, their families and communities
- Macaya Douoguih, Dirk Gille, Dirk Heerwegh, Adriana Hollenstein, Babajide Keshinro, Maarten Leyssen, Kerstin Luhn, Jos Noben, Valerie Oriol-mathieu, Helga Pissens, Cynthia Robinson, Paul Stoffels, Johan Van Hoof and Saskia Wilken at Janssen Vaccines & Prevention B. V. for their fervent material and logistic support
- Yazdan Yazdanpanah, Ebunoluwa Adejuyigbe, Matthias Egger, Benoit Kebela Ilunga, Florian Marks, Marie Akatshi Onyamboko, Tamara Giles-Vernick, and Oumou Younoussa Bah Sow for their contribution as members of the Data Safety and Monitoring Board, chaired at Inserm, Paris, France
- Ana Maria Henao-Restrepo and Mike Ryan at WHO

**Authors' Contributions** Daniel G. Bausch wrote the first draft of the manuscript, which all authors then reviewed and gave feedback.

**Conflict of Interest Statements** In addition to participating in the study of Ad26.ZEBOV/MVA-BN-Filo vaccine described here, many of the authors and institutions have also taken part in previous studies on both Ad26.ZEBOV/MVA-BN-Filo and rVSV-ZEBOV.

**Role of Funding Source** No funding required.

**Ethics Committee Approval** None required for this manuscript.

**Disclaimer** The views expressed in this publication are those of the authors and not necessarily those of LSHTM, INRB, Epicentre, the DRC Ministry of Health, CEPI, World Vision, Janssen Vaccines & Prevention B. V., MSF-France or Wellcome Trust.

**The DRC-EB-001-JnJ Ebola Vaccine Study (TUJIOKOWE) Team**[3] *National Institute for Biomedical Research, Kinshasa, Democratic Republic of the Congo.* Jean-Jacques Muyembe, Hugo Kavunga-Membo, Steve Ahuka, Zephirin Mossoko, Pierre Mukadi.

*Ministry of Health, Kinshasa and Goma, Kinshasa, Democratic Republic of the Congo.* Sylvain Yuma, Stephane Hans Bateyi Mustafa.

*London School of Hygiene and Tropical Medicine, London, United Kingdom.* Daniel G. Bausch, Deborah Watson, Edward Choi, Kambale Kasonia, Hannah Brindle, Jennifer Brown, Badara Cissé, Nicolas Connor, John

---

[3]Personnel from Janssen Vaccines and Prevention B.V. elected to be mentioned in the acknowledgements rather than as co-authors.

Edmunds, Tansey Edwards, Myfanwy James, Brian Greenwood, Kelly Howard, Camille Le Baron, Shelly Lees, Daniela Manno, Peter Piot, Chrissy H. Roberts, Mateus Kambale Sahani, Peter Smith, Darius Tetsa Tata.

*Epicentre, Paris, France.* Rebecca F. Grais, Soumah Aboubakar, Jonas Bahati, Benith Balingene, Anton Camacho, Soazic Gardais, Michel Kakule, Rockyiath Makarimi, Grace Mambula, Esther Kaningu Mapendo, Oumar Toure.

*The Coalition for Epidemic Preparedness Innovations, Oslo, Norway.* Nathalie Imbault, Richard Hatchett, Joseph Simmonds-Issler, Gerald Voss.

*Wellcome Trust, London, United Kingdom.* Jeremy Farrar, Josie Golding, Mark Whittaker.

*MSF-France, Paris, France.* Nathalie Roberts, Isabelle Defourny, John Johnson, Clair Mills.

*World Vision, Dublin, Ireland.* Robert Kanwagi.

# References

Afolabi MO, Ishola D, Manno D, Keshinro B, Bockstal V, Rogers B, et al. Safety and immunogenicity of the two-dose heterologous Ad26.ZEBOV and MVA-BN-Filo Ebola vaccine regimen in children in Sierra Leone: a randomised, double-blind, controlled trial. Lancet Infect Dis. 2022;22(1):110–22.

Anywaine Z, Barry H, Anzala O, Mutua G, Sirima SB, Eholie S, et al. Safety and immunogenicity of 2-dose heterologous Ad26.ZEBOV, MVA-BN-Filo Ebola vaccination in children and adolescents in Africa: a randomised, placebo-controlled, multicentre Phase II clinical trial. PLoS Med. 2022;19(1):e1003865.

Barry H, Mutua G, Kibuuka H, Anywaine Z, Sirima SB, Meda N, et al. Safety and immunogenicity of 2-dose heterologous Ad26.ZEBOV, MVA-BN-Filo Ebola vaccination in healthy and HIV-infected adults: a randomised, placebo-controlled Phase II clinical trial in Africa. PLoS Med. 2021;18(10):e1003813.

Bausch DG. The need for a new strategy for Ebola vaccination. Nat Med. 2021;27(4):580–1.

Bausch DG, Crozier I. Ebola and Marburg viruses. In: Ryan ET, Hill DR, Solomon T, editors. Hunter's tropical medicine and emerging infectious disease. 10th ed. Philadelphia: Saunders Elsevier Publishing; 2018.

Bines JE, Patel M, Parashar U. Assessment of postlicensure safety of rotavirus vaccines, with emphasis on intussusception. J Infect Dis. 2009;200(Suppl 1):S282–90.

Callendret B, Vellinga J, Wunderlich K, Rodriguez A, Steigerwald R, Dirmeier U, et al. A prophylactic multivalent vaccine against different filovirus species is immunogenic and provides protection from lethal infections with Ebolavirus and Marburgvirus species in non-human primates. PLoS One. 2018;13(2):e0192312.

Cohen J. Congo arrests former health minister for alleged misuse of Ebola funds 2019. Available from: https://www.science.org/content/article/congo-arrests-former-health-minister-alleged-misuse-ebola-funds

Durski KN, Osterholm M, Majumdar SS, Nilles E, Bausch DG, Atun R. Shifting the paradigm: using disease outbreaks to build resilient health systems. BMJ Global Health. 2020;5(5)

Henao-Restrepo AM, Camacho A, Longini IM, Watson CH, Edmunds WJ, Egger M, et al. Efficacy and effectiveness of an rVSV-vectored vaccine in preventing Ebola virus disease: final results from the Guinea ring vaccination, open-label, cluster-randomised trial (Ebola Ça Suffit!). Lancet. 2017;389(10068):505–18.

Ishola D, Manno D, Afolabi MO, Keshinro B, Bockstal V, Rogers B, et al. Safety and long-term immunogenicity of the two-dose heterologous Ad26.ZEBOV and MVA-BN-Flo Ebola vaccine regimen in adults in Sierra Leone: a combined open-label, non-randomised stage 1, and a randomised, double-blind, controlled stage 2 trial. Lancet Infect Dis. 2022;22(1):97–109.

James M, Kasereka JG, Kasiwa B, Kavunga-Membo H, Kambale K, Grais R, et al. Protection, health seeking, or a laissez-passer: Participants' decision-making in an EVD vaccine trial in the eastern Democratic Republic of the Congo. Soc Sci Med. 2023;323:115833.

Lévy Y, Lane C, Piot P, Beavogui AH, Kieh M, Leigh B, et al. Prevention of Ebola virus disease through vaccination: where we are in 2018. Lancet. 2018;392(10149):787–90.

Metzger WG, Vivas-Martínez S. Questionable efficacy of the rVSV-ZEBOV Ebola vaccine. Lancet. 2018;391(10125):1021.

Mulangu et al. A Randomized, Controlled Trial of Ebola Virus Disease Therapeutics. PubMed (nih.gov): N Engl J Med. 2019;381(24):2293–2303. https://doi.org/10.1056/NEJMoa1910993. Epub 2019 Nov 27.

Nyombayire J, Ingabire R, Magod B, Mazzei A, Mazarati JB, Noben J, et al. Monitoring of adverse events in recipients of the 2-Dose Ebola vaccine regimen of Ad26.ZEBOV followed by MVA-BN-Filo in the UMURINZI Ebola vaccination campaign. J Infect Dis. 2023;227(2):268–77.

Pollard AJ, Launay O, Lelievre JD, Lacabaratz C, Grande S, Goldstein N, et al. Safety and immunogenicity of a two-dose heterologous Ad26.ZEBOV and MVA-BN-Filo Ebola vaccine regimen in adults in Europe (EBOVAC2): a randomised, observer-blind, participant-blind, placebo-controlled, phase 2 trial. Lancet Infect Dis. 2021;21(4):493–506.

Research Fairness Initiative. n.d. Research Fairness Initiative. Available from: https://rfi.cohred.org/

Roberts N. MSF and Ebola in Nord Kivu: positioning, politics and pertinence. J Human Affairs. 2021;3:14–24.

Roozendaal R, Hendriks J, van Effelterre T, Spiessens B, Dekking L, Solforosi L, et al. Nonhuman primate to human immunobridging to infer the protective effect of an Ebola virus vaccine candidate. npj Vaccines. 2020;5(1):112.

Watson-Jones D, Kavunga-Membo H, Grais RF, Ahuka S, Roberts N, Edmunds WJ, et al. Protocol for a phase 3 trial to evaluate the effectiveness and safety of a heterologous, two-dose vaccine for Ebola virus disease in The Democratic Republic of the Congo. BMJ Open. 2022;12(3):e055596.

World Health Organization. Ebola virus disease Democratic Republic of Congo: External Situation Report 21. Brazzaville: World Health Organization Regional Office for Africa; 2018.

World Health Organization. SAGE Interim Recommendations on Vaccination against Ebola Virus Disease (EVD), February 20, 2019. World Health Organization; 2019.

World Health Organization. Wkly Epidemiol Rec. 2021;96(22):197–216.

World Health Organization Regional Office for Africa. Ebola virus disease Democratic Republic of Congo: external Situation Report 1. World Health Organization. Regional Office for Africa; 2018.

World Health Organization Regional Office for Africa. Ebola Virus Disease Democratic Republic of Congo: external Situation Report 64 / 2019. Brazzaville: World Health Organization. Regional Office for Africa; 2019.

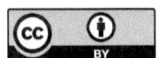

# Community-Based Approaches to Respond to Epidemics and Natural Disasters in Coastal Ecuador

Avriel Díaz, Andrew Jeffery, Ismelda Cedeño,
Yessenia Pallaroso, Gloria Jaramillo,
Blas Mera Rodriguez, Breana Wonsey,
Margarita Zambrano, and David Cedeño Rodriguez

*Y así, aunque el miedo nos haga temblar, caminamos hacia el futuro, hacia la luz que alumbra nuestro camino.*
*And so, although fear makes us tremble, we walk towards the future, towards the light that illuminates our path.*

—Jorge Carrera Andrade

## Abstract

Effective disaster response starts well before the disaster strikes. International aid, research, and recovery work must involve collaborations in which partners are working together at every stage to co-develop and co-create research that can help inform decision-making and establish sustainable programming and prevention initiatives. These partnerships require consistent engagement with community leaders, collaboration across levels of government, and comprehensive team training. Established channels for fundraising are essential for an organization to succeed in the face of chaotic disaster conditions. In this case study, we share our experience with Walking Palms Global Health (WPGH), a non-profit organization serving the communities of Bahía de Caráquez, Ecuador. Through WPGH, we continue to navigate disaster relief and recovery and foment well-being in our community. Our team has worked in the field during two emerging disease outbreaks, extreme weather events, and natural disasters, leading emergency relief efforts, and collaborating with local stakeholders and international institutions to implement holistic, long-term public health research and programming alongside partner communities.

A. Díaz (✉)
Walking Palms Global Health, Bahía de Caráquez, Manabí, Ecuador

International Research Institute for Climate and Society (IRI), Columbia University, Palisades, New York, USA

Department of Earth and Environmental Science, Columbia University, New York, New York, USA
e-mail: avriel@walkingpalms.org;
info@walkingpalms.org
https://www.walkingpalms.org

A. Jeffery · I. Cedeño · Y. Pallaroso · G. Jaramillo · B. Mera Rodriguez · B. Wonsey · M. Zambrano · D. Cedeño Rodriguez
Walking Palms Global Health, Bahía de Caráquez, Manabí, Ecuador

© The Author(s) 2024
A. Stewart Ibarra, A. D. LaBeaud (eds.), *Transforming Global Health Partnerships*, Sustainable Development Goals Series, https://doi.org/10.1007/978-3-031-53793-6_13

**Keywords**

Community health · Partnerships · Disaster
recovery · Climate and health

**Author Perspective**
We are authors representing Walking Palms Global
Health (WPGH), a community-based nonprofit
organization in Bahía de Caráquez, Ecuador. Our
team comprises individuals from different backgrounds, including scientists, community leaders,
non-profit directors, advocates, nurses, musicians,
and students. This chapter highlights our use of
community-based approaches in responding to a
range of disasters, such as the Zika epidemic,
earthquake, and the COVID-19 pandemic. Our
experiences and insights demonstrate the efficacy
of community-driven responses in times of crisis.

**Key Tenets**

1. Pre-disaster planning: Effective disaster
   response begins well before a disaster
   strikes. It is essential to plan and prepare
   for emergencies to ensure that communities and organizations can respond effectively when disasters occur.
2. Collaboration and partnerships:
   International aid, research, and recovery
   work must involve collaborations in
   which partners are working together at
   every stage to co-develop and co-create
   research that can help inform decision-
   making and establish sustainable programming and prevention initiatives.
   These partnerships require consistent
   engagement with community leaders,
   collaboration across levels of government, and comprehensive team training.
3. Established channels for fundraising:
   Established channels for fundraising are
   essential for an organization to succeed in
   the face of chaotic disaster conditions.
   Adequate funding is crucial to providing
   effective disaster relief and recovery efforts.
4. Long-term planning and implementation:
   Effective disaster response requires a
   long-term planning and implementation
   approach. Holistic, long-term public
   health research and programming must be
   implemented alongside partner communities to establish sustainable prevention
   initiatives and ensure that communities
   can build resilience to future disasters.
5. This chapter addresses the following
   SDGs: #3: good health and well-being,
   #5: gender equality, #10: reduced inequalities, #17: partnerships for the goals.

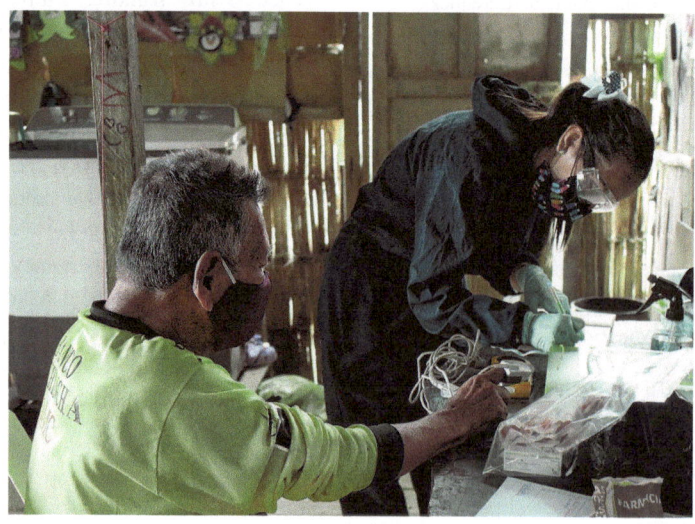

Pictured here: WPGH Nurse and Community Health Program Coordinator Gloria Jaramillo conducting at home patient
checkups and testing.

# 1    Introduction: Our Motivation

Situated on the Pacific coast of Ecuador, an hour's drive south of the equator, at the mouth of the Chone River, Bahía de Caráquez, or Bahía, is home to approximately 20,000 residents. Local economic activities focus on fishing, shrimp farming, agriculture, and tourism. With its location at the juncture of the Nazca and South American tectonic plates, Bahía and Ecuador have a long history of strong seismic activity. The low-lying region is also strongly impacted by the El Niño Southern Oscillation, resulting in heavy rainfall and flooding during El Niño events that occur every 3–7 years.

In addition to the threat of earthquakes and flooding, local residents contend with acute health challenges stemming from mosquito-borne diseases (e.g., dengue fever), and infectious and chronic diseases resulting from inadequate access to clean drinking water, inconsistent medical services, contaminated rivers, and local crops heavily treated with chemical pesticides. Like many small towns in the developing world with struggling economies, Bahía faces heightened risks from natural disasters due to inadequate public health services, inconsistent delivery of electricity and water, and a vulnerable supply chain infrastructure.

On April 16, 2016, a devastating 7.8 earthquake struck the north-central coast of Ecuador.

> *Right in front of us houses began to fall in front of our eyes. We ran to the highest point in our community, searching for our families. We grabbed our little dog, it was one of the longest nights of our lives, we thought it would never end. Screams, blood from people injured from their homes falling on them. It started raining, it was cold, and none of us were worried about eating dinner, just being with our families. Everyone was scared; we didn't know what would happen.*
> – Community President, Bahía

Due to substandard construction standards and unstable soil, Bahía became a disaster zone in minutes. Buildings collapsed, including schools and the local hospital, killing and trapping hundreds of loved ones in our small town. In the aftermath, electricity, phone, and internet services were severed, and emergency responders contended with unrelenting aftershocks and dangerous rescue conditions.

Residents were forced to collect and store their water, which in conjunction with the strongest El Niño event on record, brought high temperatures and increased rainfall, spurring a Zika outbreak along with the co-circulation of other *Aedes aeygpti mosquito-transmitted* diseases such as dengue (Sorensen et al. 2017).

The immediate impact of the earthquake reached over 700,000 people in our region, with 660 lives lost, 4650 injuries and 9750 buildings destroyed (National Sub-Secretary for Public Health Surveillance 2017). Months after the earthquake, living conditions were tenuous as government agencies struggled to repair and remove damaged infrastructure and structures. Thousands of people left Bahía, crippling the local economy, and those who remained struggled to rebuild the city while grappling with mental health scars from the earthquake and the subsequent months of strong aftershocks. Our experience in the wake of the 2016 earthquake was not unique or surprising. Natural disasters damage housing and health care facilities, inhibit sanitation services, force overcrowding and cut off utility service - especially in resource-limited settings. Increases in morbidity and mortality from infectious diseases have often been observed in their wake (Waring and Brown 2005; Kouadio et al. 2012).

And just as our recovery was picking up in 2020, the COVID-19 pandemic knocked us back down.

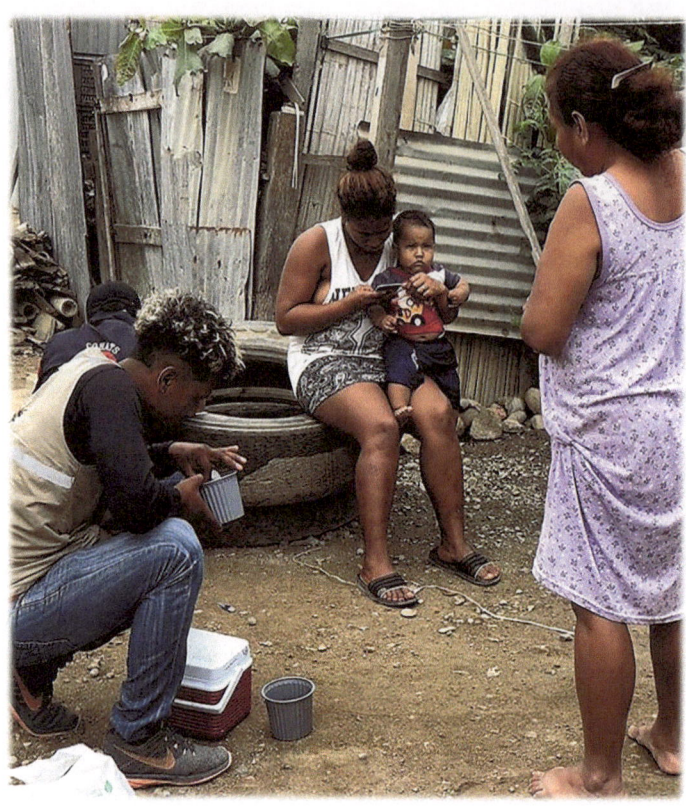

Pictured here: WPGH vector research team receiving training from Universidad Técnica de Machala to learn how to use ovitraps for mosquito egg detection.

With our hospital destroyed in the earthquake and not yet rebuilt, public health facilities were operating at limited capacity heading into the pandemic. During the lockdowns in the spring and summer of 2020 our food supply chain broke down, and suspended public transportation service meant thousands in our communities could not access basic food requirements. The co-circulation of the dengue virus complicated disease identification and treatment protocols. Residents faced limited access to medications and reduced treatment options.

Yet even after six grueling years, our community members remain remarkably resilient. This relentless optimism in the face of repeated disaster drives our team to continue to collaborate and serve. In this spirit of partnership, we have found the mission of Walking Palms Global Health (WPGH). With the alliances we have formed and nurtured, our work is possible.

**Personal history: [1]** *Avriel Diaz, Co-Founder & President WPGH, Ph.D. Candidate in Climate and Health.*

I grew up in New York City and am a first-generation Ph. D. student studying Climate and Health in Latin America and the Caribbean. I am a LatinX woman in science and believe that we can drive deep changes in the field of global health through inclusion, diversity and listening.

In the months before the April 2016 earthquake, I was invited to join the State University of New York (SUNY) Upstate Medical University's Ecuadorian research group based in southern coastal Ecuador. I had planned to work as a volunteer intern

(continued)

on an ongoing surveillance study focused on the new outbreak of the Zika virus in the urban periphery of the city. When the 2016 earthquake hit, I was reassigned to support disaster relief and research efforts in Bahía de Caráquez.

I worked alongside other volunteers from SUNY Upstate, local school administrators, social workers, and numerous local, national, and international medical volunteers who formed community medical brigades. SUNY conducted a study with the provincial Ministry of Health (MOH) and local communities to assess the prevalence of psychological distress and Zika/ dengue infections, and I assisted with this study. This was my first time engaging in on-the-ground global health work. The research was eye opening and heartbreaking.

I spent much time simply listening to community members, not only to stories about their current situation and trauma from the earthquake but also about the beauty of the city before the destruction. This experience taught me the need to adapt in the field to respond to local needs and uncertain conditions. Collaborating with the local MOH, doctors, and volunteers paved the way for future projects, which would not have been possible had we not already developed these key relationships.

My initial volunteer commitment turned into a months-long immersion into disaster response work, during which my connections with strong community leaders showed me just how much work was left to do. After falling in love with the city and the people, I relocated permanently in 2017 and became one of the co-founders of WPGH. I have spent the last six years co-creating and co-developing local to international transdisciplinary partnerships to strengthen community resilience on the front lines of climate hazards and environmental degradation. More over, I have committed to implementing strategies that

(continued)

dismantle and de-colonize traditional NGO savior complexes and focus on building true equitable international partnerships. Today, we have formed our local sister organization SOSi Ecuador - Somos Salud Integral, Ecuador, which gives us even more flexibility and support for local staff and beneficiaries.

## 2    Our Partnerships

Disaster recovery focusing on mitigating the impact of infectious diseases relies on partnerships with key local stakeholders and often international organizations and individuals. This type of consortium, typically comprised of individuals from diverse backgrounds often and with varied motivations and incentives, is challenging to assemble and manage. In Ecuador, we have found that the essential component of our work is close relationship with community leaders.

These strong individuals offer some obvious benefits, like contacts within the community and understanding of the specific needs of their constituents, but also more nuanced ones, like access to hard-to-secure facilities and local credibility, which is essential when building consensus with government agencies. We have identified these leaders through traditional networking, finding and developing genuine bonds with community members who can offer warm introductions to their leaders.

In the aftermath of the 2016 earthquake, a community of local and international volunteer health professionals began to self-organize. This community worked with the local MOH, schools, and other trusted partners to assess which parts of Bahia most needed medicine, supplies, mental health services, housing, etc. The WPGH team (before WPGH was formally born) supported these efforts by convening meeting spaces where leaders from high-risk, marginalized communities could come and express their specific needs. Community leaders identified the exact types of aid needed in their communities. This informa-

**Box 1: Perspective from community leaders who are authors of this chapter, on how to begin research or projects in a new community**

- Always meet with a community leader before starting a project.
- Identify, with community leaders and members, their top priorities for research.
- Always have a translator if the researcher does not speak the language.
- Collect research data with someone well known and respected in the community.
- Communicate with community members about objectives, rationale, and goals.
- Discuss the process to follow up with the results from the project's onset.

tion and the legitimacy granted to us by entering the community with the blessing of the local leader and local authorities allowed us to make much more efficient use of our limited human resources to make a more significant impact at that crucial time.

Those first relationships were set up with care. The interactions between volunteers and community leaders seeded long-term partnerships. When we launched WPGH, we invited the community leaders to form part of the organization and to use WPGH as a platform to increase their voices, voices that had too often been silenced or ignored.

Not only do local leaders offer access and trust within the community, but research requires approval from and collaboration with local government agencies, who want to know that ties are established within the communities where the study will take place.

Three months after the earthquake, WPGH worked with SUNY Upstate Medical University Ecuador and the local MOH to better understand the aftermath of the earthquake. In collaboration with the MOH and community leaders, we investigated the level of destruction, status and categories of stress, the presence of suspected arbovirus infections, and comorbidities. The study strengthened the partnerships, and the findings informed further community relief efforts, including the beginning of the WPGH long-term recovery plan.

Two years after the earthquake, WPGH again worked with community leaders and the MOH to conduct genetic surveillance research to determine whether the Zika virus was circulating. This project also involved collaboration with international (Columbia University, USA) and national (Pontificia Universidad Católica, Ecuador) academic partners.

Local governments are often overwhelmed with critical demands and under-resourced during and after disasters, making collaboration efforts challenging. Communication channels between government agencies and local community leaders can break down, leading to confusion and frustration on both sides. As an NGO, it has been essential that we engage closely with government and communities, acting as a bridge at times, even if it seems easier to work directly with community leaders. In our experience, forging strong bonds with community leaders was essential to building trust and giving our programs a chance to succeed. Community leadership tends to be more enduring than formal government representatives, with high turnover rates.

While we didn't know it then, the teams and partnerships we built after the earthquake prepared us for the COVID-19 pandemic in 2020. Had it not been for these relationships, and the trust we had fostered at the community, governmental and international levels, our work during the most acute phases of the pandemic would not have been possible.

In the first months of the country-wide lockdowns of spring and summer of 2020, we identified a need for emergency food and medical supply deliveries to remote and low-income communities that could not access local markets. We mobilized our donor network to fund the "More Than Food" program, which delivered over 40,000 pounds of supplies to hundreds of families in our hardest-hit communities. Transportation of these deliveries was a significant challenge with strict movement restrictions in place.

Colleagues at the MOH contributed vehicles and approvals, which at the time would not have been possible through purely civilian channels. We are currently analyzing the impact of this program on food security and stress to inform future disaster response strategies.

encing the event, with persistent avoidance of factors associated with the event and negative thoughts/feelings after the trauma [25]. Anxiety, depression and suicidal ideation have also been noted to severely impact the lives of earthquake survivors (Chen et al. 2001; Goenjian et al. 2000).

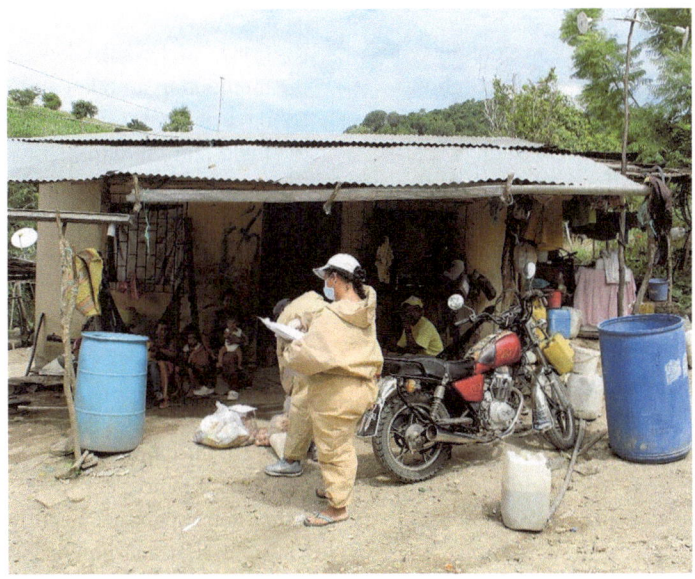

Pictured here: Community Leaders Ismelda Cedeno & Blas Mera collecting data for More Than Food C O V I D - 1 9 program.

## 3    Barriers and Opportunities

While overcoming the on-the-ground logistical challenges of disaster relief is formidable, personal and cultural situations are often greater barriers to achieving your service goals. These dynamics however, when properly understood and appreciated, can become your greatest ally as a global health professional. Here we will share some reflections about barriers and opportunities related to mental health and gender dynamics.

WPGH has placed a focus on mental health care and awareness. Populations affected by natural disasters may experience psychological morbidity (Zhang et al. 2011; Chen et al. 2001; Galea et al. 2005). Earthquake survivors commonly suffer from post-traumatic stress disorder (PTSD) (Goenjian et al. 2000; Zhang et al. 2014; Farooqui et al. 2017), characterized by re-experi-

We have witnessed the importance of considering the nexus of mental health and infectious diseases in disaster response planning, as seen with the Zika outbreak in the aftermath of the earthquake (Diaz and Stewart-Ibarra 2018). Acute and chronic stress may affect immune system function, cortisol levels, and susceptibility to arboviral infections (Vega Ocasio et al. 2021; Stewart-Ibarra et al. 2017). Other studies found that cortisol levels were associated with more severe DENV infections. However, additional research is needed to better understand these complex interactions.

In our studies and programs, we are careful to ensure that we are not re-traumatizing the people we are speaking with (whether that is for research or program development). We engage local and international specialists to train our field staff in emergency psychological preparedness and response. However, mental health is a taboo subject for many people who we serve. This is even harder when mental health providers come from outside of the community. Providers are trained to listen, adapt, and self-reflect to avoid forcing imported cultural views.

### Compassionate Listening

In 2016 after the earthquake, we conducted mosquito surveillance, visiting neighborhoods that were severely damaged. During the home visits, people were keen to participate in the surveillance study but also wanted to share stories about how they lost their home and were displaced to new areas with more mosquitoes. We listened and connected with those people, holding space for their grief. This part of research is not often taught. It is through compassion that we forge the human bonds necessary to effect lasting change in the communities we serve. Moreover, after field work was over, we held team debriefing sessions and engaged psychologists to support our staff through the heavy issues we encountered on a daily basis.

Beyond mental health issues within the communities we serve, it has been important to care for the wellbeing of our team. We stress the importance of self-care to prevent burnout, since global health field work can be stressful and traumatizing. We offer free therapy sessions to staff members and hold monthly group debriefing sessions to ensure that our team members are empowered to voice their opinions and provide feedback to one another and to directors.

Another barrier we have encountered in our work in Ecuador is the challenges that women face in making their voices heard (also see chapter "Gender Equity in African Academia: An Implementation Science Evaluation of the Kenya Context" and several case studies). Even long-

**Box 2: Key points for conducting community-based research from the perspective of field workers, who are authors of this chapter**

- Field staff should receive full training ahead of time to be well versed on study topics.
- Field staff should be able to ask questions, make mistakes, and learn new methods in an open and safe workplace environment.
- Field staff should receive personal protective equipment (not just in times of COVID-19) to feel safe in the field.
- Field staff should feel support from directors that their safety is the top priority.

standing women community leaders can struggle to be heard during times when their communities needs them the most.

One such experience occurred in the years following the 2016 earthquake, WPGH had grown close to an experienced leader of a rural community who was a longstanding advocate for people living with HIV/AIDS. She had been unable to convince local authorities to address water insecurity in her community during the most acute period of the COVID-19 pandemic. The trust we had established with local health authorities and our standing as an international organization helped elevate the community's needs and ultimately played a role in getting water service restored.

While we were grateful to be of service, this experience exposed the reality that local advocates face significant challenges if they are (1) a woman, (2) an advocate for people living with stigmatized diseases (e.g., HIV/AIDS), (3) from a rural area, and (4) from a lower socio-economic status. WPGH ensures that community leaders are always involved in project decision making as they represent the voice of their community and are experts in their own needs and solutions.

# 4    Lessons Learned

## 4.1    Engaging with Community Leaders

Given the importance of connecting with community leaders, we learned the hard way that there can be a big difference between a community *President* and a community *Leader*. In a community that has a true leader, the members of the community listen, follow, unite with a common vision, and work together to overcome a problem. True leaders set an example for other communities, motivating all to work together, to solve problems, and improve the issue at hand.

Presidents on the other hand, are elected as the official representative of a community. Many times, these Presidents are also strong leaders, but there are often situations where elected Presidents do not fulfill their role. In these cases, there will sometimes be a Leader and a President residing in the community. This can become difficult to navigate.

This lesson was illustrated by an issue that arose during the pandemic. A private donor, with good intentions but poor planning, entered a local community to donate food rations during the COVID-19 pandemic. The food rations were dropped off to the President with no understanding of the political dynamics in the community. The President did not distribute the rations fairly or timely, resulting in spoiled produce that was unusable. This caused even more stress in the community and more work for the community Leader. This also eroded the trust that we had built, as the community became wary of outside groups promising help. This emphasizes the critical need to understand the social and political dynamics of a community before conducting any research or other work.

# 5    Nimble Fundraising

Another critical lesson for effective disaster relief relates to fundraising for projects that arise quickly and change often. Raising money for

> **Box 3: The profile of true community leaders, as identified by community leaders, who are authors of this chapter**
> - Committed to unifying each family amidst crisis.
> - Capable of positively influencing and motivating members to help their neighbors.
> - Participates and is actively involved in community projects.
> - Committed to listening to the needs of others.
> - Organized and knowledgeable of their community members' situations.
> - Motivated and nurtures the achievement of common goals.

disaster relief often relies on real-time, grass-roots fundraising efforts and the creative use of existing funds. For example, in April 2020, to launch *More Than Food*, our COVID-19 emergency food relief delivery program, we worked with an existing donor to reallocate previously donated funds for this immediate need. Leveraging this initial "seed" donation, we then launched a broader fundraising campaign that leaned on the early success of the program funded by the seed money. Having demonstrated our ability to execute at a small scale, we showed donors that with their financial support, we could dramatically expand the program.

# 6    Coordination to Address Medical Supply Shortages

We have also learned about the need to anticipate medical supply shortages. Medical and field supplies are critical for global infectious disease research and aid. In Bahía, there are constant shortages due, in part, to limited supply chains. This means that medications that are normally provided freely by the public health system can become limited or nonexistent, especially during a crisis.

Our city experienced medical supply shortages (e.g., insulin) during the earthquake and the pandemic's beginning. During the pandemic it was very challenging for people in rural areas to access medications, as public transportation was shut down and delivery services were limited or too expensive to many people. For this reason, we work with our international partners to secure critical donations for our program participants (e.g., low-income senior citizens) to deliver life-saving medical supplies to their homes.

Normally, transporting these donations is a smooth process, however, during the pandemic we ran into some issues. We had transported medical donations with the same MOH paperwork for roughly five years, and we anticipated that the international shipment would arrive smoothly. We contacted the MOH ahead of time, received the proper documents and were assured that the rest of the paperwork would be handed to customs. However, when we arrived in Ecuador with the medical supplies, we were detained for several hours and the supplies were put in holding. What we later learned was that our paperwork had been received but not entered into the national customs computer system. Luckily, we were able to clear up the situation and strengthen our relationship with the customs agency. We learned the importance of clear communication and coordination across the multiple agencies that we were working with. During the pandemic it was especially important to be kind and patient, recognizing that everyone in the health sector was working double time.

## 7 Importance of Co-authored Research and Data Ownership

When wanting to produce an article for a scientific journal, we have learned that it is essential to include as co-authors the partners who were essential to the research planning, implementation, or analysis aspect of the study. In Ecuador, for example, language and funding constraints are barriers for publishing in reputable scientific journals. This is extremely problematic; important community health data, information and research findings thus become unavailable for entire geographic regions. The lack of local scientific evidence also increases the likelihood that misinformation can spread more quickly. Additionally, local partners are unable to showcase their critical work and expertise, which limits their chance of securing funding for future work, since funders look at a researcher's track record of publications in evaluating which projects to support.

Researchers from high-income regions who want to work in low and middle-income countries should not do this work without local collaboration. The collaboration should be well defined from the outset. Clear data acquisition, data ownership, and informed consent processes must be outlined before the initiation of a project. Permissions should be secured prior to study start from the national and local MOH, other regulatory agencies, community leaders and other community members.

Researchers from outside the community must understand that without these collaborators, there would be no study.

## 8 Adopting New Communication Tools

Partnerships of all kinds rely on high quality communication and regular follow up. Disasters and infectious disease outbreaks disrupt traditional communication patterns. This distance—even if we are still physically close to our collaborators—can decay multi-year efforts to establish trust with local community members.

The importance of these partnerships means that we, as global health workers, must adapt to changing conditions on the ground to maintain these key relationships. For example, we found that WhatsApp and other messaging applications, video conferencing, and other communication methods that seemed impersonal before the pandemic became a lifeline for those who embraced them, and a barrier for those who could not access them.

New communication tools, like social media, offer ways for global health organizations to build community trust (see chapter "Foundations and Future Directions of Global Health Communication"). By sharing updates from field work and health programs on Instagram, Facebook, Twitter and others, we built a presence through repetition, visibility and brand awareness. This has helped WPGH gain more acceptance in the communities we serve and has led to new partnerships with local and international organizations.

## 9 Addressing Colonial Legacies

Our experience in the field in Ecuador has led to several observations on how to break down colonial models of international aid and research (see chapter "Colonialism, Decolonization, and Global Health"). First, explicit discussion of the white saviorism complex is essential for global health professionals from high-income countries who want to work in low-income settings. At WPGH, we stress to our students and volunteers that their primary objective is to learn from local experts, and that they will be receiving far more than they are contributing during their 10-day stay.

Within low-income and high-income countries, students from diverse backgrounds have traditionally been left out of international education opportunities and global health careers, due to the high cost of these training programs (see chapter "Learning from the Past to Inform the Future: Perspectives on Future Directions in International Health and Research"). Additional scholarships and recruitment efforts could increase the diversity of students, allowing for the exchange of trainees between organizations in the Global North and South. WPGH is working with corporate sponsors to provide scholarships to our student research fellows.

Similarly, travel and associated training opportunities within the country or internationally are typically cost-prohibitive for local health workers. Institutions from the Global North should offer more funding opportunities for local partners to travel to international conferences, workshops, and team meetings. Visa challenges are an immediate concern in this area, requiring close collaboration with the host country embassies. WPGH has successfully advocated for this type of travel and our funding partners have graciously collaborated with positive results. Supporting local leaders is an essential pathway to empowering local communities.

## 10 Transforming Gender Roles

We have also witnessed the importance of transforming traditional gender roles in the Global South, combatting the "machismo" culture with a concerted effort to support women (see chapter "Gender Equity in African Academia: An Implementation Science Evaluation of the Kenya Context"). This support not only comes in the form of women and girl-centered health and wellness programs, but also in supporting and training strong women in community leadership positions. Women in Ecuador face high mortality rates due to domestic violence. It can also be challenging for women to participate in community health programs due to childcare responsibilities and controlling male spouses and partners who do not grant them permission to participate.

We have also seen the importance of community programs that support men in feeling more comfortable in non-traditional roles (such as childcare) and being more open about their emotions. Working with men and women creates an environment where the entire family can benefit from the community health programs.

## 11    Local Leadership for Sustainable Change

Lastly, we have found that programs co-created and co-managed by local staff is an essential piece of our work. Not only are our programs better received and attended when led by locals, but having local leaders cultivate the next generation of leaders is the best way to ensure that our efforts have a sustainable impact on improving the health and wellbeing of the communities that we serve.

## 12    Conclusion

Disaster recovery is inherently challenging and chaotic, with stressful and changing conditions on the ground, the breakdown of communication, and high levels of emotional distress. Effective planning, training, and preparation are essential to implement community-based health programs that reduce the impacts of disasters. These goals can be difficult to execute in regions with resource challenges and a limited history of collaboration with trusted partners.

In our experience, effective disaster response starts well before the disaster strikes. Co-creation and co-delivery of all projects need true partnerships which involve consistent engagement with community leaders, collaboration with local government, comprehensive team training and established channels for fundraising. Here in Bahía, we at WPGH are proud of our work over the past seven years, and we realize that there is much left to be done. We strive to be a model for other organizations in our region and around the world, and feel blessed to be part of this wonderful community in Ecuador.

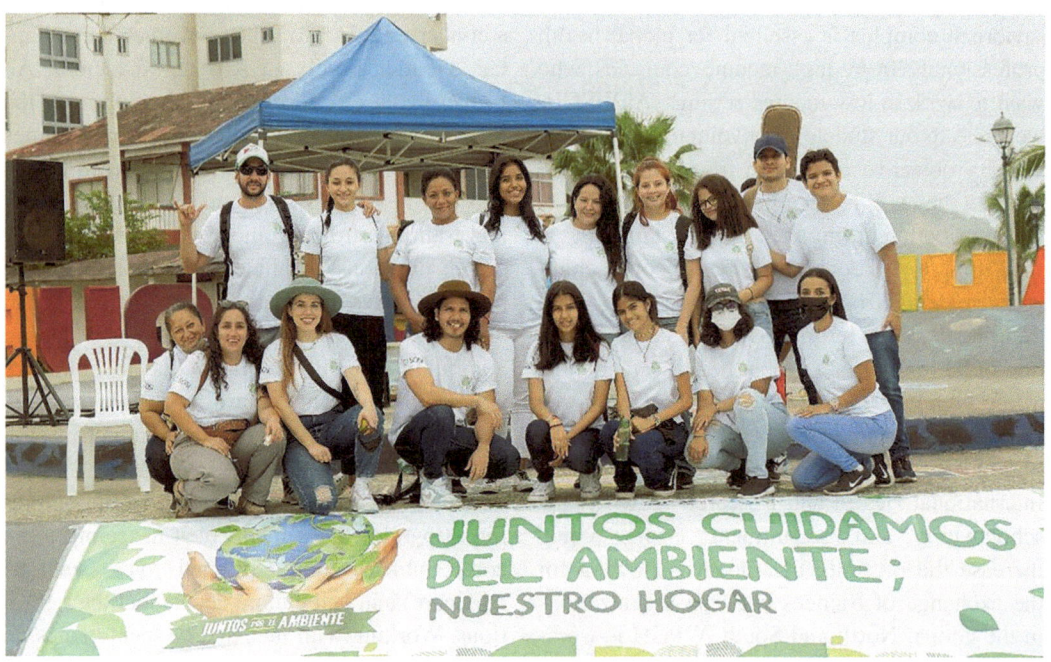

Team Photo with volunteers at a community event that WPGH hosted.

# References

Chen C-C, Yeh T-L, Yang YK, Chen S-J, Lee IH, Fu LS, Yeh CY, Hsu HC, Tsai WL, Cheng SH, et al. Psychiatric morbidity and post-traumatic symptoms among survivors in the early stage following the 1999 earthquake in Taiwan. Psychiatry Res. 2001;105:13–22.

Diaz A, Stewart-Ibarra AM. Zika virus infections and psychological distress following natural disasters. J Fut Med. 2018;

Farooqui M, Quadri SA, Suriya SS, Khan MA, Ovais M, Sohail Z, Shoaib S, Tohid H, Hassan M. Posttraumatic stress disorder: a serious post-earthquake complication. Trends Psychiatry Psychother. 2017;39:135–43. [CrossRef] [PubMed].

Galea S, Nandi A, Vlahov D. The epidemiology of posttraumatic stress disorder after disasters. Epidemiol Rev. 2005;27:78–91. [CrossRef] [PubMed].

Goenjian AK, Steinberg AM, Najarian LM, Fairbanks LA, Tashjian M, Pynoos RS. Prospective study of posttraumatic stress, anxiety and depressive reactions after earthquake and political violence. Am J Psychiatry. 2000;157:911. [CrossRef] [PubMed].

Kouadio IK, Aljunid S, Kamigaki T, Hammad K, Oshitani H. Infectious diseases following natural disasters: prevention and control measures. Expert Rev Anti Infect Ther. 2012;10:95–104. [PubMed].

National Sub-Secretary for Public Health Surveillance. Zika Gazette SE 38-2017; Ministry of Health of Ecuador: Quito, Ecuador; 2017. Available online: http://www.salud.gob.ec/wp-content/uploads/2015/12/vvGACETA-ZIKA_SE-38.pdf. Accessed 9 Oct 2017.

Sorensen CJ, Borbor-Cordova MJ, Calvello-Hynes E, Diaz A, Lemery J, Stewart-Ibarra AM. Climate variability, vulnerability, and natural disasters: a case study of Zika virus in Manabi, Ecuador following the 2016 earthquake. GeoHealth. 2017;1(8):298–304.

Stewart-Ibarra AM, Hargrave A, Diaz A, Kenneson A, Madden D, Romero MM, Molina JP, Macias Saltos D. Psychological distress and Zika, Dengue and Chikungunya symptoms following the 2016 earthquake in Bahía de Caráquez, Ecuador. Int J Environ Res Public Health. 2017;14(12):1516.

Vega Ocasio D, Stewart-Ibarra AM, Sippy R, Li C, McCue K, Bendinskas KG, et al. Social stressors, arboviral infection, and immune dysregulation in the coastal lowland region of Ecuador: a mixed methods approach in ecological perspective. Am J Trop Med Hyg. 2021;

Waring SC, Brown BJ. The threat of communicable diseases following natural disasters: a public health response. Disaster Manag Response. 2005;3:41–7. [CrossRef] [PubMed].

Zhang Z, Shi Z, Wang L, Liu M. One year later: mental health problems among survivors in hard-hit areas of the Wenchuan earthquake. Public Health. 2011;125:293–300. [PubMed].

Zhang W, Liu H, Jiang X, Wu D, Tian Y. A longitudinal study of posttraumatic stress disorder symptoms and its relationship with coping skill and locus of control in adolescents after an earthquake in China. PLoS One. 2014;9:e88263. [PubMed].

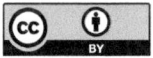

# Nipah Outbreak Investigation in Bangladesh, 2007: A Case Study of One Health Partnership and Intersectoral Coordination

Mahmudur Rahman, Nadia Ali Rimi,
Rebeca Sultana, Nusrat Homaira,
Jonathan H. Epstein, and Stephen P. Luby

*....(this illness) which we considered as 'asmani bala' (crisis/hard time given by Allah), you (the research team) call it virus. Now we have to agree that virus is the 'bala' (crisis to us) and 'bala' is the virus (to the team).*

Parveen, S., et al. BMC Public Health (2016)

## Abstract

One Health is increasingly recognized for its value in addressing emerging infectious disease threats. In Bangladesh, the integration of One Health approaches into outbreak investigation and response can be traced back to the advent of outbreaks of Nipah and avian influenza viruses. Through accounts from epidemiological, anthropological, ecological, and animal health investigations, this chapter narrates a case study of partnership among the government, development partners, and research organizations in Nipah virus outbreak management. It depicts how persuadable, collaborative and problem-solving leadership, cooperative approaches, common goals and mutual support could result in strong partnerships among different individuals and organizations towards building a One Health platform to achieve common goals.

## Keywords

One Health partnership · Nipah virus · Outbreak investigation · Multidisciplinary approach · Bangladesh

The original version of the chapter has been revised. A correction to this chapter can be found at https://doi.org/10.1007/978-3-031-53793-6_27

M. Rahman (✉)
Global Health Development/EMPHNET,
Dhaka, Bangladesh

N. A. Rimi
icddr,b, Dhaka, Bangladesh

R. Sultana
icddr,b, Dhaka, Bangladesh

University of Copenhagen, Copenhagen, Denmark

Institute of Health Economics, University of Dhaka, Dhaka, Bangladesh

N. Homaira
University of New South Wales (UNSW), Sydney, NSW, Australia

J. H. Epstein
EcoHealth Alliance, New York, NY, USA

S. P. Luby
Infectious Diseases and Geographic Medicine, Stanford University, Stanford, CA, USA

**Author Perspective**

The authors represent a group of collaborators from Bangladesh and the US who have worked together for several years to advance the understanding of Nipah virus in Bangladesh. We come from a variety of professional backgrounds—human and veterinary medicine, epidemiology, wildlife ecology and anthropology. We represent different institutions including the Government of Bangladesh, the US Government, and nongovernment organizations in the US and in Bangladesh. Although we often had to address conflicting perspectives in our collaboration, we recognized that we were much more likely to develop a sound public health response to Nipah outbreaks by working together.

**Key Tenets for Global Health Partnerships**
1. Expertise from multiple diverse backgrounds and perspectives is required to solve complex problems
2. Successful engagements require sensitivity to local conditions and pre-existing relationships.
3. Strong and robust partnerships between researchers and decision-makers are developed by mutual respect and working together on related issues over time
4. This chapter addresses the following SDGs: 3: Good Health and Wellbeing; 17: Partnerships for the Goals: Strengthen the means of implementation and revitalize the global partnership for sustainable development.

# 1   Introduction

One Health—an approach that considers the interconnections among the health of humans, animals, and the environment in disease prevention and control measures—is increasingly recognized for its value in addressing emerging infectious disease threats, such as Ebola, severe acute respiratory syndrome (SARS), avian influenza and Nipah (see chapter "A Holistic Systems Approach to Global Health Research, Practice, and Partnerships"). In Bangladesh, with recurrent outbreaks of emerging and re-emerging zoonotic infectious diseases, such as Nipah, anthrax, rabies and avian influenza, a One Health approach and partnership have been an integral part of outbreak investigations since 2007. Although efforts to formalize this approach started with the establishment of One Health Bangladesh in 2008 (Strategic framework for One Health approach to infectious diseases in Bangladesh n.d.), integration of One Health approaches and partnerships into outbreak investigation and response can be traced back to the advent of outbreaks of Nipah (first reported in 2001) and avian influenza viruses (first reported in poultry in 2007). This chapter narrates a case study of how partnership among three parties—the government, development partners, and research organizations—in Nipah virus outbreak management have strengthened the integration of a One Health approach in the health systems of Bangladesh.

Nipah virus (NiV) is an emerging zoonotic paramyxovirus that has repeatedly spilled over from bats to cause outbreaks in people and livestock with high case fatality rates. NiV was first identified in Nipah village of Malaysia in 1998 (Chua et al. 1999). *Pteropus* fruit bats are the apparent natural reservoir for the virus (Middleton et al. 2007). To date, human NiV infections have been identified in India, Bangladesh, Malaysia, Singapore, and the Philippines (Chadha et al. 2006; Hsu et al. 2004; Chua et al. 2000; Paton et al. 1999; Ching et al. 2015) causing repeated outbreaks in Bangladesh and India, with a mean case fatality rate greater than 70% (Chadha et al. 2006; Luby et al. 2009; Morbidity and mortality due to Nipah or Nipah-like virus encephalitis in WHO South-East Asia Region 2001-2018).

## 1.1   NiV Outbreak Investigations from 2001 to 2006 in Bangladesh

NiV has caused a total of 38 recognized outbreaks in Bangladesh from 2001 through 2021 (unpublished data, IEDCR). 'Drinking raw date palm sap' contaminated by NiV infected fruit bats (*Pteropus medius*)' and 'close contact with bodily secretions of highly infectious NiV patients' have been identified as the two most common pathways of NiV transmission to humans in Bangladesh (Chadha et al. 2006).

In 2004, the Institute of Epidemiology Disease Control and Research (IEDCR), the government department responsible for outbreak instigation for human health, initiated the journey of Nipah investigation during an outbreak investigation in Faridpur, Bangladesh. At the same time, icddr,b, an international health research institute, with support from US Centers for Disease Control and Prevention (CDC) also sent a team separately to investigate the same outbreak. NiV was first confirmed during this investigation, which provided evidence for person-to-person transmission of NiV. Anthropologists were included in the outbreak investigation for the first time in Bangladesh (Blum et al. 2009). However, the route of transmission for the index/primary case could not be determined. The outbreak continued for more than 2 months and the chain of transmission involved five generations (Blum et al. 2009). Conducted after the 2004 outbreak revelation, a retrospective investigation of two outbreaks in 2001 and 2003 also confirmed NiV infection (Hsu et al. 2004).

After the Nipah investigations in 2004, there was a change in leadership both at the government human health department (i.e., IEDCR) and the research organization (i.e., icddr,b). During the investigation of Tangail Nipah outbreak in 2005, the then-Director of IEDCR visited the field together with the Head of Program for Infectious Diseases and Vaccine Science (PIDVS), icddr,b (and also the US CDC Bangladesh Country Director) and others. In this joint investigation, which was also supported by anthropological exploration, raw date palm sap consumption was significantly associated ($P < 0.01$) with NiV infection for the first time (Luby et al. 2006a). It was this investigation that first led to the hypothesis that *P. medius* feeding on date palm sap likely contaminated the sap with saliva containing NiV (Luby et al. 2006b).

## 1.2 Other Initiatives Strengthening Multisectoral Collaboration

In 2005, the government human health department, together with Department of Livestock Services (DLS), Bangladesh Forest Department and development partners developed the first National Avian and Pandemic Influenza Preparedness and Response Plan (Government of Bangladesh 2006). In 2006, a hospital-based surveillance system was established to detect NiV infection and a laboratory was established at IEDCR in collaboration with icddr,b with technical support from US CDC. Formal organizational collaboration was established to investigate NiV and avian influenza between the government human health department and the research organization through MoUs in 2007. To strengthen the partnership, the research organization seconded (temporarily re-assigned) outbreak investigator officers at the government human health department with financial support from the US CDC.

**How it Started...**

When I joined IEDCR as the director in October, 2004, Dr. Steve Luby joined icddr,b as the Head of PIDVS and US CDC Bangladesh Country Director about the same time. We met in a rooftop dinner party at icddr,b and started communicating. During the investigation of Tangail NiV outbreak in January 2005, Steve and I went together to the field with the Director General of Health Services and others. However, at that time icddr,b was investigating the outbreak separately. Steve and I discussed, and decided to work together as a single combined investigation team. We formed collaborative multidisciplinary rapid response teams from IEDCR and icddr,b. In 2006, we decided to establish the surveillance system and do the laboratory tests in Bangladesh. The IEDCR, icddr,b and CDC collaboratively contrib-

(continued)

uted to the establishment of both the surveillance system and the laboratory. Then during the NiV outbreak in 2007, we, IEDCR and icddr,b, moved to the field together for the first time. Lessons learned from the 2004 outbreak helped to foster our collaboration. Early detection was possible due to the establishment of the surveillance system. Early diagnosis was possible due to the laboratory set up. There was enough preparedness for the NiV outbreak detection and response. Since then, IEDCR and icddr,b have collaboratively and successfully investigated several outbreaks. In my perspective, there were three major contributing factors behind the successful collaboration: first and foremost—the leadership, second—the division of labor to minimize overlaps and conflicts, and last but not the least—continuous exchange of ideas and discussion during and after the outbreak investigations, particularly during unknown outbreaks.

—*Prof Mahmudur Rahman, Medical Epidemiologist*

## 1.3    Investigation of NiV Outbreak in Thakurgaon District of Bangladesh, 2007

The initiatives described above laid the base for a successful partnership among the government human health department, the research organization, US CDC and EcoHealth Alliance (a science-based NGO focused on understanding the ecology and emergence of zoonotic pathogens, including NiV) during the outbreak investigation of 2007 NiV. This investigation is perhaps one of the best examples of a comprehensive and multidisciplinary approach in coordinated human and animal investigations (e.g. a 'One Health' approach) to understanding its spillover ecology and epidemiology. On 9 February 2007, a physician (surveillance focal point) at Rangpur Medical College Hospital of Bangladesh, one of

10 hospitals involved in active encephalitis surveillance in Bangladesh (Naser et al. 2015), reported to the Director of IEDCR the occurrence of a cluster of fatal encephalitis of unknown origin in a sub-district of Thakurgaon District.

A collaborative outbreak investigation team was assembled including medical epidemiologists, anthropologists, veterinarians (including wildlife and domestic animal expertise) and laboratory technicians from the three organizations. The investigation team reached the outbreak site and began field investigation with the objectives of identifying the cause of the outbreak and implementing control measures. While in the field, the investigation team had daily debriefing meetings with the local health officials and with the Director of the government human health department to provide situational updates on the outbreak. An initial investigation report was prepared within 3 days of completion of the epidemiological investigation and shared with the local health officials, the government human health department, the research organization and the Director General of Health Services (DGHS), Bangladesh. A designated media contact person from the government human health department also provided media releases about the progress of the outbreak. The investigation was supported by the IEDCR/Government of Bangladesh (GoB), organization icddr,b/US CDC, World Health Organization (WHO) and EcoHealth Alliance (formerly the Consortium for Conservation Medicine, Wildlife Trust).

---

**How We Managed Some of the Tensions That Commonly Bedevil Collaborations**

There was a tension between IEDCR having the mandate for outbreak investigation, yet other partners having key capacities to aid an effective investigation, including diagnostic capacity from CDC and support for epidemiologic, anthropological and veterinary field investigation from icddr,b. This tension is common, both in lower income as well as in higher income coun-

(continued)

tries. I consistently told my icddr,b and CDC colleagues that IEDCR was the Government of Bangladesh authority for surveillance and outbreak investigation; our job was to support this effort. I explicitly prohibited anyone on the Nipah investigation team from talking to the press. I turned down all requests from the press to comment on Nipah investigations. I felt it important that IEDCR be the spokesperson for these outbreaks. I did hear grumbling from some members of the investigative team, both from icddr,b and IEDCR, but I'm gratified that we maintained a productive and professional collaboration. Our friendship and mutual respect strengthened our working relationship. Seconding icddr,b investigators into IEDCR did build capacity and strengthen collaboration, and we consistently included IEDCR collaborators as coinvestigators on scientific publications.

—*Stephen P. Luby, Medical Epidemiologist*

## 2 Epidemiological Investigation

Epidemiological investigation contributed to developing case definition, searching for additional cases, line listing, contact tracing, contact follow-up, post-outbreak surveillance, and designing and implementing the case-control study. The investigation team met with the Civil Surgeon, the local health authority and other relevant local health administrators and collected a list of all suspected cases from the local health office (Fig. 1). The team then visited the local hospital in order to identify suspected case-patients, and investigated all the deaths in the outbreak village between January and February 2007. The team recorded detailed information on an epidemiological case sheet, collecting information about date of onset of signs and symptoms, history of exposure, movement, and other relevant data (Homaira et al. 2010).

Initial discussion with community residents (Fig. 2) indicated that there could be thirteen suspected cases (individuals with illness) who met case definition. After the epidemiological investigation, the team identified seven suspected case-

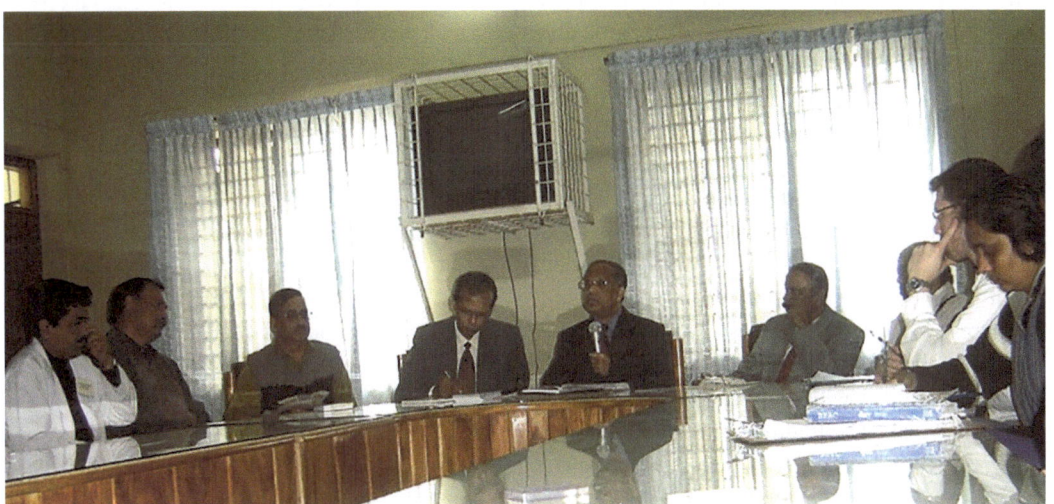

**Fig. 1** Meeting at the office of Civil Surgeon, Thakurgaon

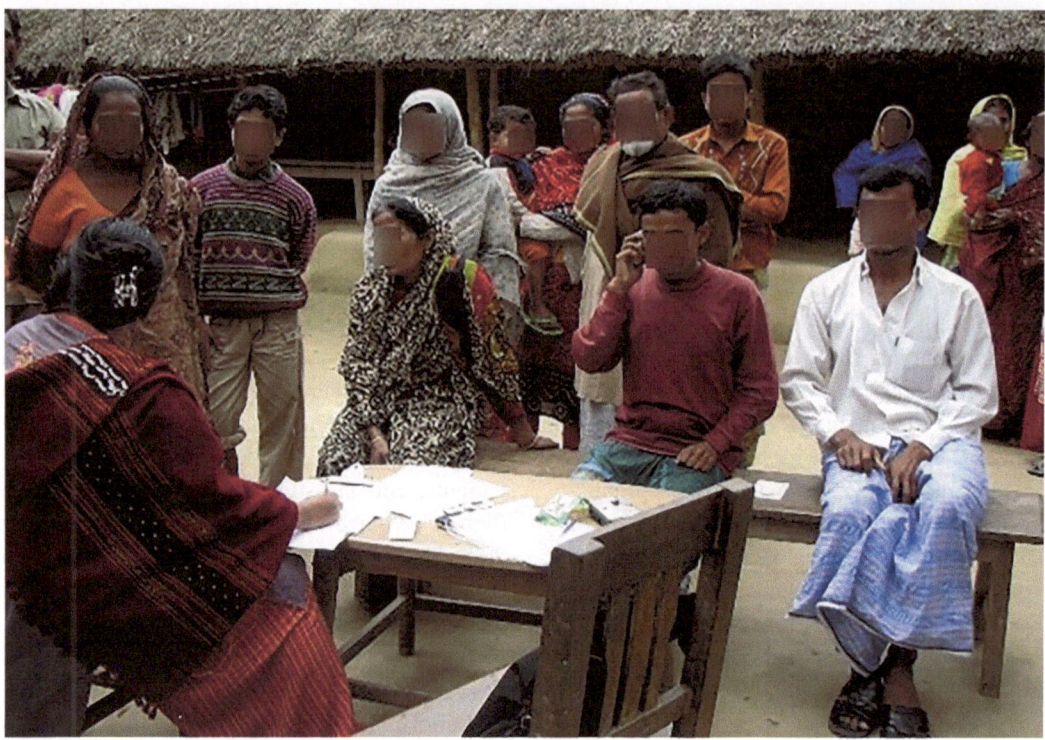

**Fig. 2** Outbreak investigation team collecting data from the community

patients, who were thought to be linked to the same cluster. Three of them died. Five of them were later confirmed positive by laboratory tests, and two case-patients who died before a sample could be collected were classified as probable cases. The cases were all clustered in time and place and were all related to each other.

An isolation unit was set up within the infectious disease wing at Rangpur Medical College Hospital. All suspected case-patients were advised to be transferred and isolated in the isolation ward. Healthcare workers were informed about the need for enhanced infection control measures within the hospital. Subsequently, a case control study was conducted to identify risk factors associated with acquiring NiV infection in this outbreak. The findings of the case control study suggested that NiV case-patients were more likely to have consumed raw date palm sap than controls (29% in case-patients vs. 0% in controls, OR undefined, $p = 0.056$) (Homaira et al. 2010).

**My Journey as an Outbreak Investigator**

When we are taught about outbreak investigation in epidemiology courses, it classically entails the ten steps of outbreak investigation which are clean, defined, and structured. Real-life outbreak investigation is just the opposite — it's messy, chaotic, exhausting and extremely challenging. It's also very rewarding.

I was seconded from icddr,b to IEDCR as an outbreak investigator on 3rd January 2007 and on 11th February 2007 was deployed to conduct field investigation of the Thakurgaon outbreak. Before that day, my only exposure to outbreak investigation was through the movie 'Outbreak' and those ten steps taught to me in the epidemiology course during my Master of Public Health program. The Thakurgaon outbreak investigation was the first of some 34 out-

(continued)

break investigations that I was involved in as the lead field outbreak investigator.

The field investigation team went to Thakurgaon not knowing it was a Nipah outbreak. It was reported as an outbreak of unknown origin with a cluster of deaths, which meant that everything was urgent. The Thankurgaon outbreak investigation was a sharp learning curve in my career as a field epidemiologist. The rapid deaths and high case fatality ratio taught me the importance of active case finding using probable case definition, isolation to contain the transmission, early clinical sample collection from 'hot cases' and laboratory testing of samples to determine etiology and rapid implementation of containment measures. The most important lesson was that all these actions needed to happen simultaneously and not one after another. The Thakurgaon NiV outbreak investigation can also be looked at as a 'poster child' example of successful multidisciplinary collaboration in outbreak investigation. The strong collaborative framework that developed between epidemiologists, anthropologists, clinicians, veterinarians, policymakers and community members through the Thakurgaon NiV outbreak investigation paved the pathway for successful outbreak investigations in the years to come.

—Dr. Nusrat Homaira, Medical Respiratory Epidemiologist

## 3    Anthropological Investigation

Anthropological investigation has complemented epidemiological (exposure, transmission pattern, and identification of appropriate proxy respondent) and clinical investigations (elaborate sign and symptoms, and contact pattern with case), and supported risk communication and stigma minimization in the community. The in-depth exploration using an anthropological approach captured detailed information, which facilitated further investigation to understand the epidemiology of the disease. The exploration also contributed in developing hypotheses and developing and modifying context-appropriate language for the case-control investigation.

The team conducted in-depth interviews and group discussions with the deceased cases' family members, who had spent the most time with the cases and/or provided care during the illness episodes, and neighbors and relatives, who gathered in the house premises. During in-depth interviews, the team explored information using a daily routine approach through a participatory rapid appraisal method (Chambers 1994). The information gathered included exposure, sign and symptoms, progression of severity of illness, and interactions with different individuals (family members, friends, neighbors, healthcare providers) at the different stages of symptoms and disease severity (Parveen et al. 2013).

***Partnership with the community*** An important element of a successful outbreak investigation is building partnership with the community. The team attempted to achieve this through social mapping and cautious interaction for building rapport and risk communication. The anthropologists conducted social mapping in a mass gathering with more than 50 participants in the nearest local market, where the index case had his shop and worked all day long. The mapping created a visual description of the outbreak area to explore the distribution of the cases in relation to different probable risk factors and exposures, including locations of a large bat roost, date palm trees, and other important landmarks (Fig. 3). During the mapping, the team, for the first time, heard information about selling of raw date palm sap (Fig. 4), which was consumed as a delicacy during the winter months (December–February), in that local market, *Jadurani Bazar*.

Based on the findings of social mapping, the team started exploring with index case's friends, colleagues, and adjacent shop owners using a snowball approach. They found that on a morning during the week before disease onset, the

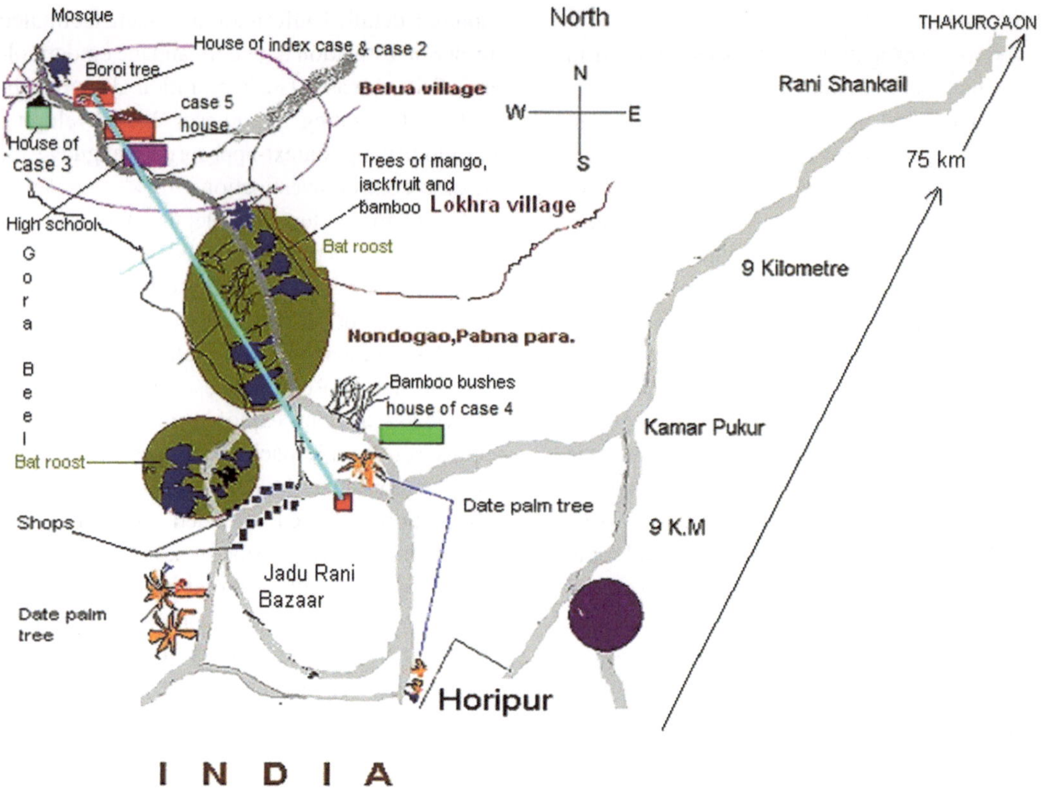

Mosque

House of index case & case 2

Boroi tree

**Belua village**

case 5
house

House of
case 3

Trees of mango,
jackfruit and
bamboo **Lokhra village**

High school

Bat roost

G
o
r
a

B
e
e
l

**Nondogao,Pabna para.**

Bamboo bushes
house of case 4

Bat roost

Date palm tree

Shops

Jadu Rani
Bazaar

Date palm
tree

Horipur

**I N D I A**

North

N

W          E

S

THAKURGAON

Rani Shankail

75 km

9 Kilometre

Kamar Pukur

9 K.M

**Fig. 3** Map of the outbreak areas from social mapping

**Fig. 4** A date palm sap
seller selling raw sap in
the outbreak community

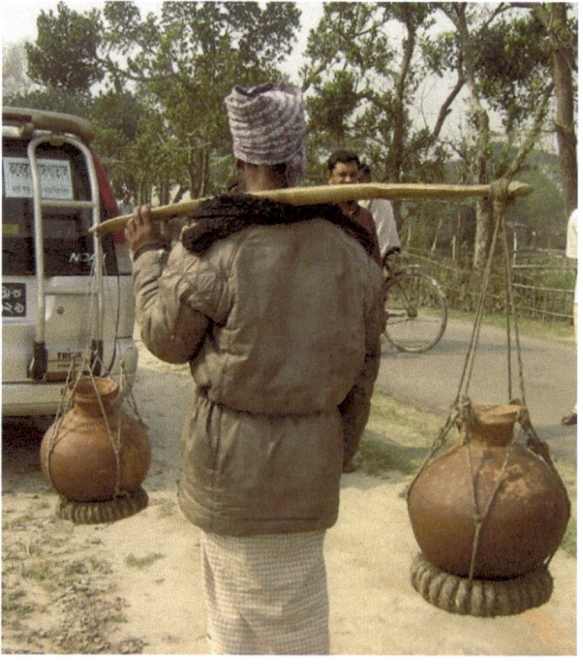

**Fig. 5** Children wearing blessed string *(shuta bandha)* around their necks as protection from the disease

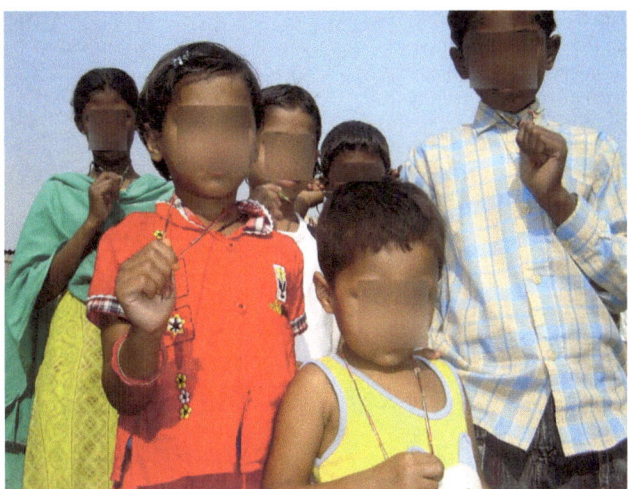

index case and a friend together drank date palm sap in that market. The social mapping (Fig. 3) aided in presenting the findings from the anthropological and epidemiological investigation in the post-investigation meeting with all partners by adding a visual context of the community.

The death of three community member cases and illness in several others within a very short time interval, initial communication by the local health authorities with the community, and heightened media attention and rumours about the source of the outbreak precipitated considerable fear and anxiety within the outbreak-affected community (Parveen et al. 2013). Additionally, repeated visits to the outbreak area by the investigation team who wore personal protective equipment, including N95 respirators, fuelled concerns about the nature of the outbreak. This resulted in isolation, fear, breaking of social relations, and stigmatizing and abandoning the families of the infected people within the outbreak community, and the villagers of case villages in the local markets. People started taking different precautions to protect their family members from this disease, for example, taking blessed water (*pani pora*) and wearing blessed string *(shuta bandha)* around their necks (Fig. 5). The investigation team had to be extremely cautious and ensure active engagement with the community residents at all steps of the investigation, which subsided fear, reinstated faith in the health system, and allowed for a comprehensive investigation. The team arranged dissemination sessions for the local people in nearby schools and elaborately described possible disease exposure, transmission routes, and preventive health messages.

**The Journey, as an Anthropologist, Has Not Always Been Smooth…**

There is a well-established disciplinary dominance of epidemiology in public health research, and outbreak investigation is no exception. The epidemiologist usually follows 'reductionistic' and 'positivistic' epistemology, whereas anthropology is 'holistic' and 'humanistic'. In other words, epidemiology is seen as highly 'scientific', offering broad 'scientific' extrapolation but does not go beyond identification of behaviours, whereas anthropology attempts culturally meaningful explanations and contextualization of those behaviours as well as generating rich information that can influence context-appropriate policy development. This difference results in a view that undermines the actual contribution of anthropology in public health research. Back in 2007, anthropological methods had recently been introduced in outbreak investigations of emerging infections in Bangladesh. We can, perhaps, say that we

(continued)

**Fig. 6** Temporary set up for sample collection from bats and pigs in a local government facility

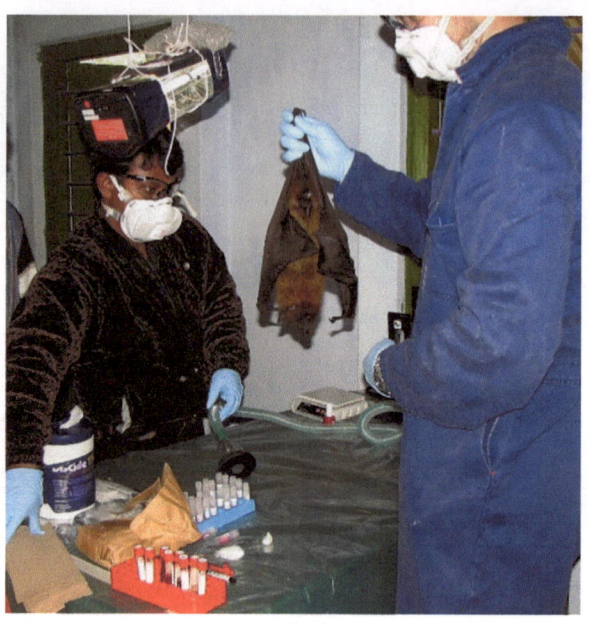

were among the pioneer anthropologists in this domain, and naturally the journey to establish our standpoint was not always smooth. The strong leadership of the team, through their comprehensive and progressive vision, guided us to minimize these tensions and overcome the challenges arising from interdisciplinary differences.

—*Rebeca Sultana, Anthropologist*

Community members also informed that 20–30 goats had died in the nearby areas, but there was no history of deaths in domestic or wild poultry. The investigation of bats in Thakurgaon provided evidence that NiV was, indeed, circulating in local bat populations. About half of the bats had antibodies against NiV and three pooled samples of oropharyngeal swabs tested positive for NiV RNA by PCR, suggesting that this bat population was likely the source of infection (Homaira et al. 2010; Epstein et al. 2020). Nothing was found in pig samples.

## 4 Ecological/Animal Health Investigation

A few weeks after the human team conducted its investigation, an animal team consisting of veterinarians with expertise in bat capture and sampling was deployed to the village to sample *Pteropus medius* (Fig. 6) and domestic animals.

Their objective was to determine whether NiV was circulating in the bats most closely associated with the case cluster, and to see whether domestic animals in the village had been infected as well. In this case, there were pigs being raised in the village, and samples were collected.

**Animal Investigation: Not an Integral Part of Outbreak investigations in Bangladesh Until 2007**

At the time of the outbreak investigation in 2007, the inclusion of bat and domestic animal surveillance was a novel component of Bangladesh's response to NiV outbreaks. During the Thakurgaon outbreak, little was known about the extent to which NiV was circulating in bats in Bangladesh. There had

(continued)

been a small number of outbreaks since NiV was first recognized in the region in 2001. It was also unclear to what extent livestock played a role in zoonotic transmission in Bangladesh. An earlier outbreak of NiV had identified contact with a sick cow as a risk factor for infection, though evidence was accumulating that date palm sap consumption was a major source of infection in many of the reported outbreaks. In the Thakurgaon investigation, the gap in time between the index case being infected and bat sampling was more than a month, which potentially limited our rate of detection in the bats. Ideally, animal investigations should occur contemporaneously with human outbreak investigations, and as soon as possible following the detection of an initial human case. Since the Thakurgaon outbreak, EcoHealth Alliance has maintained a collaborative partnership with IEDCR, building capacity within the organization and directly supporting bat and other animal sampling as part of NiV outbreak investigations. The Government of Bangladesh continues to respond to annual NiV outbreaks, and IEDCR consistently deploys an animal team as part of its initial investigation.

—*Jonathan H. Epstein, Veterinarian and Epidemiologist*

## 4.1 Outcome of the Partnership in NiV Investigations Over Two Decades

The greatest contribution of the partnership, involving a multidisciplinary team of experts in these outbreak investigations perhaps, was the introduction of a One Health approach in research, intervention, control and mitigation of emerging zoonotic infections, and development of strategies and policies. Although anthropologists were included along with medical epidemiologists since 2004, veterinarians, including wildlife experts, were first included in 2007. Later, the team was expanded to include other disciplinary experts relevant to specific outbreaks. This laid the basis for the formation of One Health Bangladesh, a civil society One Health forum, and the subsequent institutionalization of One Health Secretariat, which represents three ministries of the GoB.

Other outcomes from this collaboration included the following:

- *Global priority:* NiV has been identified by WHO as one of the pandemic potential pathogens. Data from Bangladesh was considered when formulating vaccination strategies on NiV (Nikolay et al. 2021).
- *Policy/advocacy:* The GoB circulated messages prohibiting the drinking of date palm sap in the country since 2009. A docudrama with the message, "Do not drink raw date palm sap," was broadcast on the national television channel (BTV) in 2015–16 through the Health Education Bureau of GoB.
- *Capacity building:* NiV investigations have built the One Health capacity of the country through training of medical, veterinary and wildlife officers and laboratory technicians, and development of NiV management guidelines, NiV surveillance protocol and NiV testing protocol.
- *Opportunities for new research:* NiV outbreak investigations instigated numerous new research projects to generate epidemiological data and develop interventions to prevent NiV infections. For example, the feeding behavior of bats was observed using infrared cameras at date palm sap trees (Khan et al. 2010, 2012). A community intervention trial was conducted in 2012–14 to assess behavioral change strategies to reduce the risk of NiV spillover by reducing the consumption date palm sap (Nahar et al. 2017).

## 4.2 Factors Contributing to Strengthening Partnerships in One Health Approach

Leadership: One Health partnerships not only need diverse disciplinary experts from the field of public health research, but also successful application of leadership skills and competencies in managing One Health challenges, leading to effective teams and multi-disciplinary collaborations (Stephen and Stemshorn 2016). Both leaders from the government human health department and the research organization displayed 'persuadability, the genuine willingness and ability to change one's mind in the face of new evidence,' which is a key leadership trait. This included recognizing counter-evidence, updating one's believes, avoiding binary default by thinking probabilistically, and taking the perspective of others (Pittampalli 2016). This led to effective team building in One Health research and outbreak investigations in both organizations within a short period of time.

> Dr. Luby always understood that icddr,b or CDC would have to support the government. He was always helpful and supportive, both in terms of technical and knowledge support. He used to listen to us and the arguments, and had the open mind to understand others' perspectives. He used to respond immediately to our invitations to knowledge sharing or training, and shared expertise even out of his scope. His temperament, understanding, depth of knowledge and supportive attitude contributed greatly to our partnership and mutual respect. During 2009 H1N1 outbreak, we used to sit together to discuss and plan our next steps. We maintained our partnership even in terms of social relationship and communication, inviting each other on many occasions, even to our homes.
> —*Prof Mahmudur Rahman, Medical Epidemiologist*

> While working with the former IEDCR Director, Prof. Rahman, I found his personal management style included providing opportunities for people under his charge and a remarkable willingness to be persuaded by various stakeholders. This contributed greatly to our collaborative productivity. I also think that his background as a professor contributed to his thoughtful reflection on the situations he faced and an interest to deploy sound methods to generate credible guidance.
> —*Stephen P. Luby, Medical Epidemiologist*

Partnership: Bringing 'stakeholders together to identify shared interests and reach consensus about actions to address grand challenges' is a primary role of the One Health leaders (Herrmann and Johnson-Walker 2018). The government human health department leadership approach focused on balancing between traditional attitudes and power practices within the government system and actively engaging external resources. The icddr,b/CDC leadership approach offered openness to acknowledge government ownership and readiness to provide support—financial, logistics and expertise—coupled with responsiveness in reporting and information sharing. This shared leadership built the trust needed for a long-term relationship, which survived beyond the investigation of a NiV outbreak, extending to investigate and mitigate many other outbreaks, including outbreaks of unknown causes. Consequently, the research organization became involved in the rapid response team of the GoB.

Common goal and mutual support: Setting collaborative goals, and transparent and explicit expectations that matched the partners' capacities, was critical to effective partnering. Similar understanding, temperament, and attitude towards achieving a common goal resulted in a strong partnership between the leaders from IEDCR and

(continued)

icddr,b/CDC. While government partners required technical and logistic support to achieve the goal, non-government research organizations and development partners also had the desire to work with the government for greater impact, policy implications, and endorsement. Such collaboration also existed in other areas. For example, HIV serosurveillance was a joint effort by the government of Bangladesh and icddr,b. For cholera, icddr,b researched the disease but the outbreak investigation was a responsibility of the government human health department. The partnership among the government human health department, the research organization, the development partner and the wildlife ecology institute was further strengthened by supporting each other and sharing resources including: training, technology transfer (NiV testing), setting up and operating the surveillance and laboratory, sharing reagents, expertise, funding, secondment, and division of labor. The government human health department lacked expertise in the field of veterinary and anthropological research, two essential components of One Health team, which was complemented by icddr,b and EcoHealth Alliance, and substantiated by global expertise.

This chapter provides a vivid account of how collaborative, problem-solving and cooperative leaderships, which are seen as critical aspects of One Health leadership (Pelican et al. 2021), can result in strong partnerships among different individuals and organizations towards building a One Health platform to achieve common goals. The area of work of IEDCR, icddr,b, US CDC and EcoHealth Alliance included a common objective—preventing and mitigating emerging zoonotic infections, which brought these partners together to complement each other's work. The partnership focused on complementing the government partner in their capacity building to achieve public health goals for the country, while pursuing individual organizational targets.

# References

Blum LS, Khan R, Nahar N, Breiman RF. In-depth assessment of an outbreak of Nipah encephalitis with person-to-person transmission in Bangladesh: implications for prevention and control strategies. Am J Trop Med Hyg. 2009;80(1):96–102.

Chadha MS, Comer JA, Lowe L, Rota PA, Rollin PE, Bellini WJ, Ksiazek TG, Mishra A. Nipah virus-associated encephalitis outbreak, Siliguri, India. Emerg Infect Dis. 2006;12(2):235–40.

Chambers R. The origins and practice of participatory rural appraisal. World Dev. 1994;22(7):953–69.

Ching PK, de los Reyes VC, Sucaldito MN, Tayag E, Columna-Vingno AB, Malbas FF Jr, Bolo GC Jr, Sejvar JJ, Eagles D, Playford G, et al. Outbreak of henipavirus infection, Philippines, 2014. Emerg Infect Dis. 2015;21(2):328–31.

Chua KB, Goh KJ, Wong KT, Kamarulzaman A, Tan PSK, Ksiazek TG, Zaki SR, Paul G, Lam SK, Tan CT. Fatal encephalitis due to Nipah virus among pig-farmers in Malaysia. Lancet. 1999;354(9186):1257–9.

Chua KB, Bellini WJ, Rota PA, Tamin A, Lam SK, Ksiazek TG, Rollin PE, Zaki SR, Shieh W, et al. Nipah virus: a recently emergent deadly paramyxovirus. Science. 2000;288(5470):1432–5.

Epstein JH, Anthony SJ, Islam A, Kilpatrick AM, Ali Khan S, Balkey MD, Ross N, Smith I, Zambrana-Torrelio C, Tao Y, et al. Nipah virus dynamics in bats and implications for spillover to humans. Proc Natl Acad Sci USA. 2020;117(46):29190–201.

Government of Bangladesh. National avian influenza and human pandemic influenza preparedness and response plan Bangladesh. In: Edited by Directorate General of Health services; 2006.

Herrmann JA, Johnson-Walker YJ. Beyond One Health: from recognition to results. 1st ed. Hoboken: Wiley Blackwell; 2018.

Homaira N, Rahman M, Hossain MJ, Epstein JH, Sultana R, Khan M, Podder G, Nahar K, Ahmed B, Gurley ES. Nipah virus outbreak with person-to-person transmission in a district of Bangladesh, 2007. Epidemiol Infect. 2010;138(11):1630–6.

Hsu VP, Hossain MJ, Parashar UD, Ali MM, Ksiazek TG, Kuzmin I, Niezgoda M, Rupprecht C, Bresee J, Breiman RF. Nipah virus encephalitis reemergence, Bangladesh. Emerg Infect Dis. 2004;10(12):2082–7.

Khan MSU, Hossain J, Gurley ES, Nahar N, Sultana R, Luby SP. Use of infrared camera to understand bats' access to date palm sap: implications for preventing Nipah virus transmission. EcoHealth. 2010;7(4):517–25.

Khan SU, Gurley ES, Hossain MJ, Nahar N, Sharker MA, Luby SP. A randomized controlled trial of interventions to impede date palm sap contamination by bats to prevent nipah virus transmission in Bangladesh. PLoS One. 2012;7(8):e42689.

Luby SP, Rahman M, Hossain MJ, Blum LS, Husain MM, Gurley E, Khan R, Ahmed BN, Rahman S, Nahar N, et al. Foodborne transmission of Nipah Virus, Bangladesh. Emerg Infect Dis. 2006a;12(12):1888–94.

Luby S, Rahman M, Hossain MJ, Blum LS, Husain NM, Gurley E, Khan R, Rahmin S, Nahar N, Kenah E, et al. Foodborne transmission of Nipah Virus, Bangladesh. Emerg Infect Dis. 2006b; 12(12).

Luby SP, Hossain MJ, Gurley ES, Ahmed BN, Banu S, Khan SU, Homaira N, Rota PA, Rollin PE, Comer JA, et al. Recurrent zoonotic transmission of Nipah virus into humans, Bangladesh, 2001-2007. Emerg Infect Dis. 2009;15(8):1229–35.

Middleton DJ, Morrissy CJ, van der Heide BM, Russell GM, Braun MA, Westbury HA, Halpin K, Daniels PW. Experimental Nipah virus infection in pteropid bats (Pteropus poliocephalus). J Comp Pathol. 2007;136(4):266–72.

Morbidity and mortality due to Nipah or Nipah-like virus encephalitis in WHO South-East Asia Region, 2001-2018 [http://www.searo.who.int/entity/emerging_diseases/links/morbidity-and-mortality-nipah-sear-2001-2018.pdf?ua=1].

Nahar N, Paul RC, Sultana R, Sumon SA, Banik KC, Abedin J, Asaduzzaman M, Garcia F, Zimicki S, Rahman M, et al. A controlled trial to reduce the risk of human Nipah virus exposure in Bangladesh. EcoHealth. 2017;14(3):501–17.

Naser A, Hossain M, Sazzad H, Homaira N, Gurley E, Podder G, Afroj S, Banu S, Rollin P, Daszak P. Integrated cluster-and case-based surveillance for detecting stage III zoonotic pathogens: an example of Nipah virus surveillance in Bangladesh. Epidemiol Infect. 2015;143(9):1922–30.

Nikolay B, Dos Santos GR, Lipsitch M, Rahman M, Luby SP, Salje H, Gurley ES, Cauchemez S. Assessing the feasibility of Nipah vaccine efficacy trials based on previous outbreaks in Bangladesh. Vaccine. 2021;39:5600–6.

Parveen S, Sultana R, Luby SP, Gurley ES. Anthropological approaches to outbreak investigations in Bangladesh. In: Banwell C, Ulijakzek S, Dixon J, editors. In when culture impacts health. edn ed. London/Waltham/San Diego: Academic Press; 2013. p. 215–24.

Paton NI, Leo YS, Zaki SR, Auchus AP, Lee KE, Ling AE, Chew SK, Ang B, Rollin PE, Umapathi T. Outbreak of Nipah-virus infection among abattoir workers in Singapore. Lancet. 1999;354(9186):1253–6.

Pelican K, Blair B, Adisasmito W, Allen I, Amir V, Bazeyo W, Errecaborde K, Le Thi H, Mahero M, Wanzala S, Bender J. One health leadership and team building training. In: Zinsstag J, Schelling E, Crump L, Whittaker M, Tanner M, Stephen C, editors. One Health: the theory and practice of integrated health approaches. UK: CABI; 2021.

Pittampalli A. Persuadable: how great leaders change their minds to change the world. HarperCollins Publishers; 2016.

Stephen C, Stemshorn B. Leadership, governance and partnerships are essential One Health competencies. One Health. 2016;2:161–3.

Strategic framework for One Health approach to infectious diseases in Bangladesh. n.d. [https://www.google.com/url?sa=t&rct=j&q=&esrc=s&source=web&cd=&cad=rja&uact=8&ved=2ahUKEwjPkNC9uuv1AhU7SGwGHV3ACyoQFnoECAQQAw&url=https%3A%2F%2Fwww.iedcr.org%2Fpdf%2FFfiles%2FOne%2520Health%2FStrategic_framework_for_One_Health_Bangladesh-26%2520Jan.pdf&usg=AOvVaw3XjxOVVjHVOlC67Mp_jjFY].

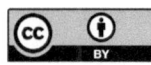

# Addressing Sexual and HIV-Related Stigma in Haiti: Need for Societal Engagement

## Willy Dunbar and Yves Coppieters

*Stigma and discrimination against LGBTI people violate human rights, deepening inequalities, and acts as a critical barrier to ending AIDS as a public health threat by 2030. Let human rights prevail!*

Winnie Byanyima, Executive Director of The Joint United Nations Programme on HIV/AIDS (UNAIDS)

## Abstract

As the world has entered the fourth decade of the AIDS epidemic, Men who have sex with men (MSM) continue to be disproportionately affected by HIV and victims of stigma, prejudice, and discrimination in the Caribbean and Haiti. Using a mixed-methods realist design, we have engaged with MSM communities, healthcare providers, policymakers, and members of civil society to analyze the impact of stigma on the linkages across the continuum of HIV services through engagement, linkage, and retention. Findings showed that from the social construction of heteronormativity to Christian religious and political influences, several factors lie behind sexual and HIV-related stigma, resulting in loss to follow-up and failure to realize the health benefits of proper treatment fully. However, societal engagement and partnerships, multi-level and contextual-based interventions can produce stigma mitigation through personal, health systems' and contextual mechanisms for better engagement, adherence, and retention in healthcare.

## Keywords

Stigma · Men who have sex with men · HIV · Haiti

## Author Perspective

The authors are global health researchers, physicians, and minority intervention specialists. For decades, they have been working to improve outcomes for those who have yet to fully benefit from public health and intervention strategies in Africa, Latin America, and the Caribbean.

## Key Tenets

1. As a well-documented global health barrier, Stigma is a dreadful, dehumanizing shaming and blaming process which impacts health-seeking behavior, engagement, and retention in healthcare services across various health conditions.
2. Due to social constructions and cultural factors, multi-level theoretical frameworks are critical to guide intervention development, measurement, research, and policy.
3. To intervene to mitigate the harmful consequences of the stigma associated with social, behavioral, and health conditions,

W. Dunbar (✉) · Y. Coppieters
Health Systems and Policies – International Health Research Centre, School of Public Health, Université libre de Bruxelles (ULB), Brussels, Belgium
e-mail: willy.junior.dunbar@ulb.be

A. Stewart Ibarra, A. D. LaBeaud (eds.), *Transforming Global Health Partnerships*, Sustainable Development Goals Series, https://doi.org/10.1007/978-3-031-53793-6_15

strong partnerships among affected populations, healthcare providers, policy stakeholders, and government bodies are essential to building multi-level, contextual-based, and socially accountable strategies.

4. This chapter addresses the following SDGs: 3: Good health and well-being; 10: Reduced inequalities.

# 1 Stigma, HIV and Men Who Have Sex with Men in Haiti: From Concepts to Contexts

HIV first emerged in Haiti in the late 1970s. But, by 1982, the US Centers for Disease Control (CDC) named four groups as "risk factors" for HIV infection: homosexuals, heroin addicts, hemophiliacs, and Haitians. The stigma conferred by the new disease on all these groups—designated in the popular press as "the 4H Club"—was immediate and severe (Rouzier et al. 2014).

In 2019, approximately 160.000 people were living with HIV in Haiti (prevalence of 2.2%). Although the exact number of Men who have sex with men (MSM) is not estimated due to disclosure issues, HIV prevalence was 18.2% in 2017, according to UNAIDS. In efforts of the Joint United Nations Program on HIV/AIDS (UNAIDS) to reach the ambitious goals of diagnosing 95% of all HIV-positive individuals, providing ART for 95% of those diagnosed, and achieving viral suppression for 95% of those treated by 2030 of by 2030, MSM is a high priority (UNAIDS 2019). Tracking progress toward the 90-90-90 goals, in 2019, of the 160,000 People living with HIV (PLHIV): 72% knew their HIV status, 71% were accessing antiretroviral therapy (ART), and 56% were virally suppressed (UNAIDS 2018).

Worldwide, MSM are among the community populations most affected by HIV. They continue to be one of the groups most vulnerable to infection and death related to HIV. Due to biological, behavioral, and social factors, MSM are 27 times more at risk for HIV. The 2020 data showed they accounted for 23% of new infections (Lieb et al. 2009; Aho et al. 2014; UNAIDS 2017).

*"I didn't know I had to use condoms because I don't have sex with women. After the training sessions, the trainer explained how we can get infected with HIV... He explained how it is easy for gays to be infected. At that moment, I realized I'd been at risk without knowing. This is why I am now a trainer, to help others understand that and participate in community meetings."*

[IDIMSM0004]

PLHIV are often victims of adverse behavior about their status. A despised label is therefore attributed, making them victims, sometimes unconsciously (Judgeo and Moalusi 2014). These same attitudes are also found towards sexual orientations that differ from what society, political, and religious norms describe as "normal." Hence, MSMs infected with HIV are "double victims" (Dunbar et al. 2021). These reactions have been described as *stigmatization*. According to Erving Goffman, *stigma* is defined as "any characteristic of the individual which, if known, discredits him in the eyes of others or makes him appear to be a person of lesser status" (Alvarez-Jimenez et al. 2011).

Haiti has the highest number of people living with HIV in the Caribbean and is the poorest country in the Western hemisphere. The Caribbean has the second highest prevalence rates globally, following Africa (Dunbar et al. 2021; Pape et al. 2014; Daniels 2019). Despite many public health interventions nationwide in the region, PLHIV in Haiti are vulnerable to stigmatization, particularly sexual minorities. The latter suffer considerable ostracism, which prevents access to care. Extreme marginalization also affects the social, emotional, and relational aspects of their lives. In addition, new prevention and treatment opportunities are likely unavailable for many MSM in Haiti, who are ignored, stigmatized, and persecuted by a new law prohibiting same-sex marriage and the promotion of homosexuality (Castro and Farmer 2005; Dunbar et al. 2020a).

In August 2017, the Haitian Senate passed a law prohibiting marriage between same-sex couples. While this measure is not new—as the national civil code recognizes only the unions between men and women—the vote reflects a growing intolerance towards the MSM community. It aims to prohibit any display of homosexuality in public spaces. In addition, there is no anti-hate crime law explicitly addresses the discrimination and harassment experienced by MSM because of their sexual orientation or gender identity. Homosexuality is considered taboo by Haitians, whom Christianity primarily influences. Weaknesses in government and legal structures—including the penal system—also contribute to stigmatizing and discriminating against people living with HIV. A proposal in December 2011 of a law to the Haitian Parliament to better protect people living with HIV against stigma and discrimination has not been considered. No other propositions have been introduced (Albert-Hope et al. 2016; Pape et al. 2011; Dunbar et al. 2020b; Surkan et al. 2010).

A national survey conducted by Population Services International in Haiti (PSI-Haiti) at 12 centers between October and December 2011 identified 54,700 MSM, 82.5% single. Almost half considered themselves homosexual, and almost half identified as bisexual. The average number of sexual partners per year was estimated at 7. Only one-third could demonstrate adequate use of condoms. Nearly one in five had a history of STI, increasing the risk of HIV infection. Data from the national program reported in 2019 that the number of identified MSM is 30,900 (Dube 2012). The discrepancy in MSM population data reveals a lack of accurate national and subnational MSM population estimates. These data are critical to inform national strategies around resource allocation, intervention planning, and program evaluation.

Christian religious communities continue to be homophobic and harm education and testing activities, a significant challenge. MSM refuse to participate because of the insults sometimes inflicted on them, even by healthcare providers. In addition, among MSM, several sub-groups are identified: assumed and known homosexuals, hidden homosexuals, and bisexuals (Dunbar et al. 2020a, 2021). Even between these subgroups, there is a lot of discrimination and stigmatization. Not only do socioeconomic vulnerability and structural barriers increase HIV risk, but they also affect care retention and quality of life for MSM

living with HIV. Recent findings from the region suggest that inability to pay for care, lack of food and shelter, and depression due to lack of employment opportunities conspire to interrupt HIV care and adversely affect their health (Koenig et al. 2010).

Our goal through this project was to analyze the impact of stigma on the continuum of HIV

**Personal Motivation**

Addressing health disparities is a priority while planning the global health of tomorrow. In the time of the Sustainable Development Goals with the motto "Leave no one behind," we can no longer keep unchecked the invisibility of marginalized and minority populations. Therefore, the academic and professional community urgently needs to join forces in working towards innovation-based, evidence-driven, tailored, and socially responsible public health systems while adopting intersectionality approaches. However, these goals cannot be reached without emphasizing social agreement between academic health entities, policymakers, and the territory they serve. These prior reflections were central in motivating us to work with Men who have sex with Men (MSM) in Haiti. We strongly believe that preserving the human dignity of individuals who may be subjected to multiple social identities will not be achieved without societal engagement and partnership. Throughout our careers, we have worked at various levels to explore individual-level and structural barriers and develop behaviorally and culturally adapted interventions toward the most underserved minority populations. We have gained significant insights navigating the complex inter-institutional relationships in designing, implementing, and evaluating health systems research and programs to analyze health practices, knowledge, and perceptions within the MSM communities and various stakeholders better to address gaps, service uptake, and acceptance.

services for MSM in Haiti to ascertain why, how and under which circumstances MSM are engaged, linked, and retained along the continuum of care from engagement to viral suppression. The research process, from scientific proposal development to final findings, has included the following:

- Overall context exploration;
- Identification of gatekeepers;
- Participant observations;
- Engagement with MSM communities to explore their perceptions and experiences and to assess needs and priorities;
- Engagement with practitioners and policymakers to assess their attitudes and to explore suggestions of opportunities;
- Data collection, analysis, and scientific writing.

## 2 Haiti HIV National Responses Through Public, Private Sectors, and International Partnership

Even in this non-favorable environment, several international funding programs such as The President's Emergency Plan for AIDS Relief (PEPFAR), the Global Fund to fight AIDS, and the USAID have economically supported the country. In partnership with national institutions, they have also launched specific initiatives to expand MSM's access to and retention in HIV services. There is also a strong presence of civil society organizations and community-led networks. Civil society has been instrumental in the country's HIV response and human rights activism.

To control the HIV epidemic, MSM patients and those at risk must flow efficiently, consistently, and sustainably through the entire HIV continuum of prevention, care, and treatment services (Castro and Farmer 2005). This seamless integration of interventions requires strong linkages among program components so that HIV

transmission is reduced and people diagnosed with HIV obtain early access to antiretroviral treatment and other social supports (Jones et al. 2019). The Pan American Health Organization (PAHO) has also advocated for combination prevention programs as rights-, evidence-, and community-based programs that promote a combination of biomedical, behavioral, and structural interventions designed to meet the HIV prevention needs of specific people and communities (Dunbar et al. 2021).

## 3 Factors Underlying the HIV Epidemic and Persistent Challenges Despite Strong Responses

Several factors influence the epidemic among MSM in Haiti. However, stigma and discrimination underlie the social vulnerability in driving the HIV epidemic and play a central role in (Dunbar et al. 2021; Castro and Farmer 2005).

## 4 The Social Construction of Heteronormativity

The social construction of *heteronormativity* is central to the stigmatization of MSM and the transmission of HIV. *Heteronormativity* can be defined as the institutions, structures, practices, identities, and understanding that legitimize and hierarchize heterosexuality as the standard, natural, and only socially and morally acceptable form of sexuality. This means that any other form of sexual orientation outside the norm (heterosexual) is seen as a deviant act. This situation reinforces the rejection, ostracism, and discrimination of MSM. Homophobia and stigma toward MSM are the key factors in what is considered socially acceptable in being a man. The "heteropatriarchy concept" defines the existing social and political organization in different Caribbean countries, including Haiti, shaped by a history of slavery, colonialism, and post-emancipation nationalism. Thus, a heteronormative and hegemonic model of masculinity is essential to the socialization process and cultural identity (Dunbar et al. 2021; Sharma 2009; Knight et al. 2013).

Cultural constructions of masculinity impose obligations and restrictions leading to risky sexual practices. Highly stigmatized by both religious and social norms, homosexual practices are driven underground. Nevertheless, some men are involved with male and female sexual partners, and sometimes they appear to adopt a socially acceptable heterosexual lifestyle. Marrying women and fathering children are, for some, a strategy to avoid the negative consequences of public disclosure of homosexuality and can be used to help dispel doubts about masculinity. By having female sexual partners, MSM fulfil the traditional gender roles and respect the heteronormative and hegemonic model of masculinity (Dunbar et al. 2020a; Surkan et al. 2010; Pape et al. 1986). In this way, structural factors are interconnected and converge to increased individual risk practices, thus increasing both social and other individual drivers of HIV vulnerability.

Another factor is violence towards MSM, which is not only perpetuated at a community level but also overlooked by police forces. The lack of legal protections contributes to insecurity, including poverty and homelessness for rejected people. This elevates HIV vulnerability and decreases access to sexual and HIV information, testing, prevention, and care (Figueroa et al. 2013; Figueroa 2014).

*"It is difficult to take the medications and come to appointments when everyone at your house and neighborhood doesn't accept that you are gay."*
[IDIMSM0014]

## 5 Barriers to Healthcare and Bias in Medical Education

Access to prevention, counseling, testing, care, and treatment remains difficult for MSM. Fear of non-voluntary disclosure and a lack of confidentiality and privacy aggravate the limited access to healthcare. MSM perceives medical providers as judgmental and unable to respect confidentiality. Barriers to HIV testing include healthcare provider mistreatment, confidentiality breaches, and HIV-related stigma. Healthcare provider discrimination and judgment in the provision of HIV testing present barriers to accessing HIV services and result in participants hiding their sexual orientation and/or gender identity. Confidentiality concerns include clinical settings that segregate HIV services from other health services, fear that healthcare providers would publicly disclose their status, and problems at LGBT-friendly clinics that peers would discover their intention to get tested or their HIV status. HIV-related stigma contributes to fear of testing HIV-positive and intersects with the stigma of HIV as a "gay" disease. Reports about the difficulties of starting HIV prevention program among MSM in some countries, in correlation with a strong sexual discrimination, has led to the legal invisibility of MSM serologic status. Heavy reliance on international funders and donors for HIV programs is compounded by limited in-country institutional capacities, increasing the vulnerability of high-risk populations (Dunbar et al. 2020c, 2021).

An exploration of Haitian medical students' attitudes towards MSM was conducted to understand better the extent to which stigma and other factors impair actual and future healthcare and, secondly, to explore suggestions of opportunities for making such services socially accountable. Medical students represent the next generation of clinicians responsible for HIV care efforts and often reflect attitudes held in their society and community of practice (Dunbar et al. 2020a). This research was developed with the School of Health Sciences of the Université Quisqueya and GHESKIO's training center. Quisqueya University School of Health Sciences is a medical school located in Port-au-Prince, the capital city of Haiti. As the largest private university, the School of Health Sciences comprises 800 students from all the country's administrative departments. The six-year medical program is divided into two-year basic sciences and four-year clinical sciences in partnership with associated academic hospitals in the capital city and several rural and urban regions of the country, ensuring practice through various cultures and contexts. The program also entails clinical placements in infectious diseases and HIV settings in partnership with GHESKIO centers, where students work under the supervision of clinical tutors. As part of the social accountability reform process for accreditation renewal, efforts are being made to have a substantial basic science, clinical, and epidemiological community-oriented research activity within the university and associated academic hospitals. As with any research team and participants, biases and power asymmetries were always possible. All the participants and research team members were encouraged to develop new ideas, codes, and analyses aligned with their research interests or personal lived experiences, giving them more space to contribute to the data collection and analysis process.

All students indicated that they were or would be comfortable serving MSM, although a few of them expressed some level of discomfort. They expressed their willingness to provide MSM with comprehensive HIV care based on the right for MSM to receive care, the moral responsibility of healthcare professionals, and the perceived health disparities regarding MSM in the population. The participants stated that everyone has the right to receive adequate healthcare services regardless of their sexual practices and sexual orientation. They indicated that in their capacity as soon–to–be graduated physicians, taking care of MSM is a moral duty under the Hippocratic Oath. Thus, they were compliant with providing MSM with services the same as they would for other patients and maintaining the expected confidentiality level. Stigma was also identified as a reason MSM may be reluctant to take up healthcare services (Dunbar et al. 2020a).

However, the findings revealed that the medical education curriculum does not consider MSM specificities. Students identified their limitations in relation to attending to the health of sexual minorities. Some of them explained that their professors and clinical instructors do not address MSM particularities and explained some stigmatizing attitudes they had noted from them.

*"I don't think we learn much because some professors laugh when we bring discussions about gay people. They don't like talking about them; it's a sensitive topic…."*
[Medical Student 8, male, 24 years old].

Although they all agreed that caring for MSM is an obligation, some male participants expressed discomfort by affirming that MSM could try to harass them during a medical examination. Moreover, some students think that taking care of not only MSM but also any PLHIV required specific protection equipment, like gloves and masks. Some students expressed a level of discomfort when it came to holding discussions with MSM about sexual relationships. When we probed further about the discomfort, some expressed disagreement with same-sex relationships and their disposition to convince MSM to stop such practices.

*"I would feel uncomfortable asking questions about their private life. I don't need to know their private life; it's disgusting. This is why they are sick…."*
[Student 14, male, 26 years old]

These findings suggest the need to continue questioning their ability to adequately address sexual health issues and confirm the need for a medical curriculum to address MSM-sensitive topics. Finally, these sentiments suggest a lack of medical and communication skills in the HIV and sexual health (Dunbar et al. 2020a).

## 6 Stigma Reduction Mechanisms Through Community Partnership and Societal Engagement

Through this work, we identified 6 sets of stigma reduction mechanisms:

(a) Self-acceptance—through self-esteem, awareness and pride, perception of HIV risk, and acceptance of HIV status—is a critical component in addressing the intrapersonal barriers. The MSM can be more confident by focusing on greater self-awareness of their emotions, goals, behaviors, and associated obstacles while fostering acceptance of parts of the self that cannot be changed.

*"...We can only achieve great things once we reach pride regarding our homosexuality. When I was hiding, I didn't have the mental freedom to take care of myself, even after knowing my HIV status."*

[IDIMSM0015]

(b) Comprehensive and tailored MSM HIV services. This can be achieved through sexual stigma reduction training for healthcare providers, engagement of peer support, financial assistance, and adapted services delivery through drug dispensing points and mobile technologies to improve comprehensive care.

(c) Support of research initiatives to better understand the experiences and needs of MSM living with HIV and the drivers of stigma. Collection and analysis of data on stigma-related incidents and their impact to inform evidence-based interventions and policy development. Advocacy allows for developing and implementing non-discriminatory policies and laws that protect the rights of MSM living with HIV. Engagement with policymakers raises awareness about the impact of stigma on MSM and promotes inclusive practices in healthcare, employment, and social services.

(d) Strengthening community support by addressing community stigma, societal acceptance, and tolerance, strengthening MSM organizations and community networks. Fostering partnerships with community-based organizations, networks, and support groups to empower MSM living with HIV and promote their involvement in decision-making processes. Community-led initiatives to address stigma and discrimination include peer support groups, educational workshops, and social events promoting inclusivity. Engagement with media outlets to ensure accurate and positive representation of MSM living with HIV, highlighting their achievements, stories of resilience, and contributions to society. Development and testing of media campaigns that challenge stereotypes and promote acceptance, under-

standing, and empathy towards MSM living with HIV. These mechanisms would allow MSM to help their peers with stigma reduction, engagement, and retention in care.

(e) Foster collaboration between sectors, including government agencies, healthcare providers, NGOs, and community-based organizations, to create a united front against stigma. Establish coordination mechanisms to share information, resources, and best practices among stakeholders working towards reducing stigma and discrimination.

(f) Development of comprehensive educational campaigns targeting the general public, healthcare providers, and key influencers to raise awareness about MSM, HIV transmission, and the realities of living with HIV. Promotion of accurate and up-to-date information about HIV prevention, treatment, and care to dispel misconceptions and reduce fear and stigma. Development of training and capacity-building programs for healthcare providers, social workers, and other relevant professionals on culturally competent care for MSM living with HIV. Empowerment of community-based organizations to support and advocate for the rights and needs of MSM through training and resource allocation.

Existing intervention strategies for MSM living with and at risk for HIV include self-motivation to access better quality and more integrated HIV services, confidentiality protection, peer support on accessing the steps of the continuum, understanding needs in a non-stigmatizing way, community tolerance, and meaningful opportunities for community engagement.

Several intervention strategies, such as training for healthcare providers and religious leaders, aim to drive changes in stigmatizing attitudes and behaviors against MSM. However, these strategies need to consider the intrapersonal mechanisms of stigma generation sufficiently. Stigma interventions are more effective when multiple strategies are implemented together to address complex health programs, such as the HIV prevention and care continuum. Our case study provides sufficient evidence to claim that multi-level intervention strategies are essential for stigma mitigation (Rouzier et al. 2014; UNAIDS 2017).

Political will and resources are crucial to support and scaling up stigma reduction activities throughout healthcare settings (Delany-Moretlwe et al. 2015). Public messaging, communications, and educational campaigns should be reshaped and targeted to eliminate stigma and discrimination, resulting in a more efficient, equitable, and acceptable HIV response. Creating "safe" spaces for MSM to receive education and access health information is also crucial (Dunbar et al. 2020d).

Our collaborative work provided strong evidence that HIV interventions for MSM need to be tailored according to cultural contexts and structural values. We provide a unique opportunity to build comprehensive intervention strategies from theory-based mechanisms. Yet, many challenges persist, including limited health system capacity, stigma and discrimination, violence, and discriminatory attitudes. These factors reduce MSM access to resources and result in low social status and exclusion of MSM from meaningful spaces of dialogue. There is also a lack of government support to scale up and sustain MSM services currently funded by donors.

## 7    Conclusion

HIV and sexual stigma can have profound effects on MSM's health and need to be addressed. Beyond militancy, real societal engagement, strong intersectoral partnerships, and interventions acknowledging contextual factors are urgently needed. The activities were developed under the leadership of the GHESKIO centers. However, several entities were involved in the activities, such as the Université Quisqueya, which facilitated the recruitment of participants and gave space for discussions, meetings, and conferences; several LGBT and community organizations, which accepted to sit down and discuss to formulate their issues, their views and gave directions to the overall activities. Also, we must acknowledge the financial support from the

Université libre de Bruxelles in Belgium and the Fogarty.

The path through our research was long and filled with concurrences and controversies. Parts of those concurrences and controversies may largely be over in public and global health research communities, but the work of questioning, exploring, assessing, disseminating, implementing, and evaluating has just begun. We still have a long way to go to combat stigma, discrimination, ostracism, and injustice to restore tolerance and respect. Nevertheless, every effort matters to give visibility to marginalized populations. Above all, anything that seems inalterable can change, nothing can be taken for granted, and everything is possible.

## References

Aho J, Hakim A, Vuylsteke B, Semde G, Gbais HG, Diarrassouba M, et al. Exploring risk behaviors and vulnerability for HIV among men who have sex with men in Abidjan, Cote d'Ivoire: poor knowledge, homophobia and sexual violence. PLoS One. 2014;9(6):e99591.

Albert-Hope C, Gustav R, Simon Y, Castellanos E, Irwin R. PLHIV in the Caribbean: many islands, same issues. Lack of resources, fragmented health/care systems: an under-resourced community response. J Int AIDS Soc. 2016.

Alvarez-Jimenez M, Bendall S, Lederman R, Wadley G, Chinnery G, Vargas S, et al. Stigma: notes on the management of spoiled identity. Proc SIGCHI Conf Hum Factors Comput Syst. 2011.

Castro A, Farmer P. Understanding and addressing AIDS-related stigma: from anthropological theory to clinical practice in Haiti. Am J Public Health. 2005;95(1):53–9.

Daniels JP. Haiti's complex history with HIV, and recent successes. Lancet HIV. 2019;6(3):e151–2.

Delany-Moretlwe S, Cowan FM, Busza J, Bolton-Moore C, Kelley K, Fairlie L. Providing comprehensive health services for young key populations: needs, barriers and gaps. J Int AIDS Soc. 2015;18:19833.

Dube F. Key populations in Haiti. 2012.

Dunbar W, Jean-pierre MCA, Raccurt C, Pape JW, Coppieters Y. Attitudes of medical students towards men who have sex with men living with HIV : implications for social accountability. Int J Med Educ. 2020a:233–9.

Dunbar W, Sohler N, Coppieters Y. Outcomes along the HIV continuum of care for men who have sex with men in Haiti. Eur J Pub Health. 2020b;30(Supplement_5):2020.

Dunbar W, Sohler N, Coppieters Y. Loss to follow up among men who have sex with men and heterosexual men living with HIV in Haiti. Eur J Pub Health. 2020c;30(Supplement_5):2020.

Dunbar W, Labat A, Raccurt C, Sohler N, Pape JW, Maulet N, et al. A realist systematic review of stigma reduction interventions for HIV prevention and care continuum outcomes among men who have sex with men. 2020d. Available from: https://doi.org/10.1177/0956462420924984.

Dunbar W, Pape JW, Coppieters Y. HIV among men who have sex with men in the Caribbean: reaching the left behind. 2021;1–7.

Figueroa JP. Review of HIV in the Caribbean: significant progress and outstanding challenges. Curr HIV/AIDS Rep. 2014;11:158–67.

Figueroa JP, Weir SS, Jones-Cooper C, Byfield L, Hobbs MM, McKnight I, et al. High HIV prevalence among men who have sex with men in Jamaica is associated with social vulnerability and other sexually transmitted infections. West Indian Med J. 2013;62(4):286–91.

Jones J, Sullivan PS, Curran JW. Progress in the HIV epidemic: identifying goals and measuring success. PLoS Med. 2019;16(1):e1002729.

Judgeo N, Moalusi KP. My secret: the social meaning of HIV/AIDS stigma. Sahara J. 2014;11(1):76–83.

Knight R, Shoveller JA, Oliffe JL, Gilbert M, Goldenberg S. Heteronormativity hurts everyone: experiences of young men and clinicians with sexually transmitted infection/HIV testing in British Columbia, Canada. Health (London). 2013;17(5):441–59. Available from: http://journals.sagepub.com/doi/10.1177/1363459312464071

Koenig S, Ivers L, Pace S, Destine R, Leandre F, Grandpierre R, et al. Successes and challenges of HIV treatment programs in Haiti: aftermath of the earthquake. HIV Ther [Internet]. 2010;4(2):145–60. Available from: http://www.futuremedicine.com/doi/10.2217/hiv.10.6

Lieb S, Thompson DR, Misra S, Gates GJ, Duffus WA, Fallon SJ, et al. Estimating populations of men who have sex with men in the Southern United States. J Urban Health. 2009;86(6):887–901.

Pape JW, Liautaud B, Thomas F, Mathurin JR, St Amand MM, Boncy M, et al. Risk factors associated with AIDS in Haiti. Am J Med Sci. 1986;291(1):4–7.

Pape JW, Stenger M, Fitzgerald D. HIV disease in the Caribbean. Int Antivir Soc [Internet]. 2011;19(1):e1–5. Available from: https://www.iasusa.org/sites/default/files/tam/e1_pape.pdf

Pape JW, Severe PD, Fitzgerald DW, Deschamps MM, Joseph P, Riviere C, et al. The Haiti research-based model of international public health collaboration: the GHESKIO centers. J Acquir Immune Defic Syndr. 2014;65(SUPPL.1):1–7.

Rouzier V, Farmer PE, Pape JW, Jerome J-G, Van Onacker JD, Morose W, et al. Factors impacting the provision of antiretroviral therapy to people living with HIV: the view from Haiti. Antivir Ther [Internet]. 2014;19(Suppl 3):91–104. Available from: http://www.intmedpress.com/journals/avt/abstract.cfm?id=2904&pid=88.

Sharma J. Reflections on the construction of heteronormativity. Development [Internet]. 2009;52(1):52–5. Available from: http://link.springer.com/10.1057/dev.2008.72

Surkan PJ, Mukherjee JS, Williams DR, Eustache E, Louis E, Jean-Paul T, et al. Perceived discrimination and stigma toward children affected by HIV/AIDS and their HIV-positive caregivers in Central Haiti. AIDS Care. 2010;22(7):803–15.

UNAIDS. Global AIDS monitoring 2018. J Occup Rehabil. 2017.

UNAIDS. UNAIDS Data 2018. 2018;1–376.

UNAIDS. Fact sheet—global AIDS UPDATE 2019. Unaids; 2019.

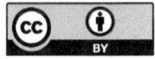

# Building Partnerships to Empower Women Through Home Self-Sampling for Sexual and Reproductive Tract Infections

Comfort R. Phiri, Namakau Chola, and Amaya L. Bustinduy

*If girls are given the chance, they can transform Africa.*

Angelique Kidjo

## Abstract

This team actively created strong bonds with stakeholders to successfully research the validity and feasibility of rolling out sexual and reproductive health (SRH) self-screening programs. The success of this effort relied on local and external support from all involved, from the field to the policy-making level. This resulted in a novel transdisciplinary approach to integrate surveillance for well-researched infections, such as HIV and human papillomavirus, with less understood and hence neglected diseases, such as female genital schistosomiasis. Active support from local institutions was also crucial. In this chapter we will elaborate on the experience of the first partnership built to integrate several SRH issues in an endemic community in Zambia, with a special emphasis on how the partnership was developed. Through the prism of a case study, we review the lessons learned that could be applied widely across different sectors as a woman-centered approach. Barriers to implementation are also discussed.

## Keywords

Self-sampling · Female genital schistosomiasis · Partnerships · Empowerment · Sexual and reproductive health

## Acronyms

| | |
|---|---|
| BILHIV | Bilharzia and HIV |
| COVID-19 | Coronavirus -2019 |
| FGS | Female Genital Schistosomiasis |
| GH | Global Health |
| HIV | Human Immune-deficiency Virus |
| HPTN 071 | HIV Prevention Trial Networks 071 |
| HPV | Human Papillomavirus |
| PI | Principal Investigator |
| PopART | Population effects of Antiretroviral Therapy |
| RAs | Research Assistants |
| SH | Schistosoma haematobium |

C. R. Phiri · N. Chola
Zambart, Lusaka, Zambia
e-mail: comfort@zambart.org.zm

A. L. Bustinduy (✉)
Clinical Research Department, London School of Hygiene & Tropical Medicine, London, UK
e-mail: Amaya.Bustinduy@lshtm.ac.uk

A. Stewart Ibarra, A. D. LaBeaud (eds.), *Transforming Global Health Partnerships*, Sustainable Development Goals Series, https://doi.org/10.1007/978-3-031-53793-6_16

SRH        Sexual and reproductive Health
SSA        Sub-Saharan Africa
STI        Sexually Transmitted Infections
UK         United Kingdom
WHO        World Health Organization

**Author Perspective**

The preparation of this chapter brought together three women from different backgrounds and cultures but with a common interest in partnering for a shared goal: improving the lives of women suffering from stigmatizing reproductive tract infections. They partnered in Zambia on a project that dared to be different in its approach by decentralizing care and bringing screening to the homes of women. They brought different views and expertise, building a common understanding of the issue at hand, and identifying the importance of everyone to successfully achieve the goals. Together with the wider team, their collaboration yielded excellent scientific results and encouraged more work with the same vision. They also learned valuable lessons of women's empowerment and partnership that are shared in this chapter.

# 1    Introduction

In this chapter, we will cover how partnership and community empowerment enabled women in a sub-Saharan country to break forth from barriers of stigma and isolation and embrace home-health interventions—self-sampling and self-testing for Sexually Transmitted Infections (STIs) and other reproductive tract infections. Partnership through transference of skills and participant empowerment allowed women to control their environment and gain the autonomy to conduct sensitive self-genital sampling at home. They were able to trust themselves to make their health decisions despite societal and, often, partner opposition. In addition, women were able to manage their own health without exposing themselves to external scrutiny. The

**Key Tenets**

1. A transdisciplinary approach involving all key players is needed from project inception.
2. Regular communication between all members of the teams to keep the work transparent and equitable allows problem-solving in real time.
3. Community engagement focusing on potentially vulnerable populations (e.g., adolescent populations) emphasizes project ownership by community members, and it empowers those directly involved.
4. Participant involvement in disseminating results facilitates timely feedback to the study participants.
5. This chapter addresses the following SDGs: #3 Good health and wellbeing, #5 Gender Equality, #10 Reduced inequalities, #17 Partnerships for the Goals

relationships built through this process provided a fertile ground for mutual learning, common understanding, and capacity strengthening amongst all parties involved (Brown et al. 2012). Further, good communication among all key players facilitated the building of good relationships, leading to a successful building of trust (Jenkins et al. 2021).

Based on our experience in Zambia working on sexual and reproductive health (SRH) community-based diagnosis and surveillance, we proposed a simple structural diagram for women-centered equitable partnerships as shown in Fig. 1. Following the basic tenets exposed in this chapter, this structure can be easily adapted to different environments and settings with a patient centered approach.

As an introduction to our work, Fig. 1 illustrates how community women were *core-partners* in the implementation of our research. Our work and partnerships were built up from their needs.

**Fig. 1** A model of women-centered equitable partnership, based on our experience in Zambia working on sexual and reproductive health via community-based diagnosis and surveillance

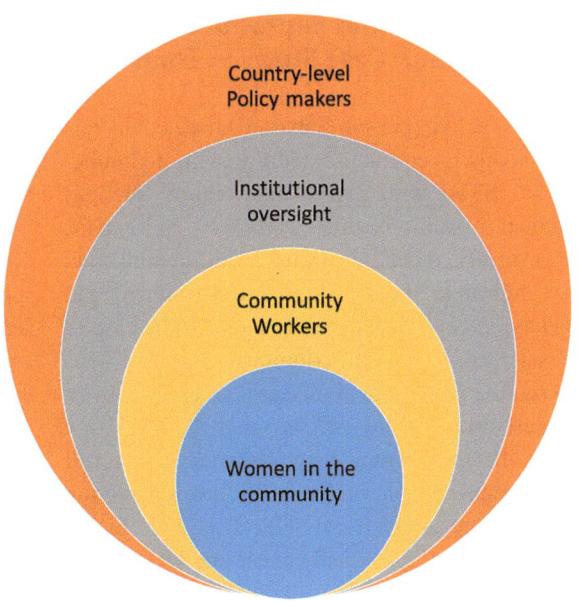

Women community workers were responsible for the delivery of the information that women in the community needed to make an informed choice. They were at the forefront of empowerment. Institutional oversight was essential for the logistical and regulatory aspects of the research. Lastly, country-level spheres followed with their distinct roles and responsibilities.

This chapter will address the following topics:

I. Sexual and reproductive health case study in Zambia—The BILHIV study is an example of a successful transdisciplinary team that managed to create strong partnerships with diverse stakeholders working as advocates for women's sexual health and rights. This study strongly promoted the role of community health workers as the front-line workforce to empower women in the community potentially living with multiple reproductive tract infections.

II. The process of building partnerships—Working with numerous players in building strong, global, and effective partnerships for the delivery of our work was a complex endeavor. We will elaborate on the different approaches we used to create a cohesive and strong group.

III. Partnering with key stakeholders—The authors worked together with a core stakeholder team and closely with large external teams working on different areas in health, policy, advocacy, and education in Zambia. These important links allowed our study team to share important research findings with ministerial bodies.

IV. Overcoming hurdles through empowerment—Strict societal structures became the study's biggest hurdles as they limited personal choices. We will elaborate on some concrete examples and how these were overcome through strong team efforts.

V. Conclusions and the way forward—We will elaborate on several key interventions that can be jointly implemented through strong transdisciplinary partnerships, which can prove useful when applied at scale across settings.

## 2    Sexual and Reproductive Health Case Study in Zambia

A woman living in sub-Saharan Africa could harbor at any given time sexually transmitted infections (STIs) with global distribution, such as human papillomavirus (HPV) and HIV. Conversely, other infections of the genital tract are linked to their particular environment and behavior, beyond sexual activity, as is the case of female genital schistosomiasis (FGS). This chronic gynecological disease is caused by a waterborne parasite, *Schistosoma haematobium (Sh)*, that is transmitted by freshwater contact. It is estimated that around 40 million women living in SSA are affected by FGS. This adds to the global burden of cervical cancer and HIV, which have the highest incidence and mortality rates in Africa, particularly in young women (Bray et al. 2018; UNAIDS 2019; WHO 2015).

FGS is associated with severe sexual and reproductive health manifestations that include infertility, pain and bleeding during and after sex, and other symptoms indistinguishable from STIs (Bustinduy et al. 2022). Awareness of disease is largely absent in endemic communities and there information is scarce (Hotez et al. 2019). This is despite growing evidence of increased prevalence of HIV, suggestion of increased incidence and transmission of HIV (male to female) in the presence of FGS, and increased cervical dysplasia in women affected with FGS (Bustinduy et al. 2022).

Conventional FGS diagnosis is challenging, as it relies on costly equipment and high-level specialized training seldom available in resource-limited countries. This severely limits accurate estimations of disease burden. To address this gap, novel screening and diagnostic strategies closer to the point-of-care were urgently needed.

The BILHIV (bilharzia and HIV) study was conducted in Zambia, and piloted genital self-sampling for community-based diagnosis of FGS. The study involved a complex network of partners who worked together from inception to conclusion. Nested within a large HIV prevention trial (PopART (Hayes et al. 2014)), the initial partnership involved institutional-level support with complex permissions, different levels of

ethical clearance, and multi-country partners and funders. This was due to the complexity and breadth of the parent trial. The work for the BILHIV study was almost entirely conducted in Zambia, despite funds coming from a UK funder through a UK institution.

Local research and health institutions in Zambia owned the study and led the team recruiting and supervising the field team, a named field supervisor, an institutional supervisor, a team of midwives and local laboratory support. For the field team, the study investigators recruited an all women team of BILHIV community workers (BCWs) who were the front-line workforce and champions in the field. There was multilevel leadership at different stages. This structure worked well, empowering different members of the team with their own tasks. For example, the BCWs had a field supervisor who is an author of this chapter (NC) who worked very closely with the institutional supervisor (CRP) and overall chief investigator (AB). The hierarchy was mostly conceptual as each member acted as specialist in their areas, which provided reassurance and empowerment to all members of the team. The success of these team dynamics was reflected in the positive results of the study, relying greatly on high rates of follow-up of the study participants (Sturt et al. 2020). Self-sampling procedures were very well accepted by participants (Phiri et al. 2020).

## 3    The Process of Building Partnerships

A single-disease approach for reproductive tract infections is inherently flawed in the wider context of global health. This is, however, how science has historically studied diseases like HPV leading to cervical cancer, HIV, or schistosomiasis. This approach has deepened the understanding of individual infections but misses the broader global picture of sexual and reproductive health in settings where a woman or man can suffer from multiple genital tract infections and diseases at any given time. The BILHIV study offered a broader approach to reproductive tract co-infections and focused not only on the best possible diagnostic possibilities at the point-of-care, but also looked at disease interactions to help risk-stratify women in their pathway to health (Bray et al. 2018). As a fairly small project, the BILHIV team worked very closely with the following key partners mentioned below:

(a) The PopART (HPTN 071) parent study team: The HPTN 071 (PopART) trial's intervention arm provided a door-to-door package of HIV prevention strategies that included HIV home testing and other supportive measures. This was the largest HIV prevention trial ever conducted. Since the PopART study had not yet finished data collection, the BILHIV team worked closely with their Research Assistants (RAs), who introduced the BILHIV study to PopART female participants who were eligible to participate. The good communication flow between RAs, BCWs and key supervision were paramount at the field stage. The BILHIV principal investigator (PI) and study manager had regular meetings with the PopART leadership team to ensure practices complied with all ethical and funder regulators. This relationship continued throughout the study and further into the analysis and publication stage. Careful oversight of study procedures and transparent communication was paramount at this stage. A particular challenge was to work nested within a clinical trial operating under stringent ethical regulations pertaining to four different countries [South Africa, Zambia, USA and UK).

(b) BILHIV community health workers (BCWs): The BCWs were purposefully selected from those that initially worked in communities under HPTN 071 (PopART) study (Hayes et al. 2014). The all-women team were chosen for their communication skills and their track record of knowledge and acceptance by the communities. Trust is crucial when interventions have a door-to-door approach, encouraging participation without coercion. They had to endure arduous field work in communities with difficult conditions, often under scorching sun or flooded during rainy season. The BCWs were trained to understand the study protocol and other study-related procedures which included: providing eligible participants with information about the study and obtaining written informed consent, providing instructions for obtaining urine, demonstrating how to self-collect a vaginal and cervical swab using a 3D model, administering electronic questionnaire, storage of samples while in the field, and FGS teaching using WHO-developed visual aids (WHO 2015). Beyond this 'formal' training, their skills as educators became their greatest asset. As they deepened their own understanding of FGS and the consequences relating to HIV acquisition and cervical cancer, they went from adequate field workers, to experts in the matter. Participants felt at ease and trusted the information given to them (Chola, N, Personal Communication).

(c) Health care providers. The clinical team for the BILHIV study comprised three medical staff: a trained medical doctor specialized in obstetrics and gynecology and two qualified nurse-midwives. With the aim to decentralize services for the diagnosis of FGS and other reproductive tract infections, all procedures in clinic were performed by the midwives, with referral to the gynecologists only for those women with suspicion of cervical cancer. Tasks, procedures, and treatment all took place at the point of care and were based on the information available from the study procedures. As samples were transported between the clinic and laboratory, rapport between the clinicians, the BCWs and the laboratory personnel were essential. Support from the clinic and hospital, widening the partnership, was also crucial.

## 4 Partnering with Key Stakeholders

Forming a multi-level equitable partnership with high-level in-country partners was crucial in the implementation of the BILHIV study. The partnership included relevant interested parties that were key in achieving the study aims. Following the ongoing research structure in Zambia, all activities and ethical requirements in-country were coordinated and led by the local institution at Zambart in Lusaka (https://www.zambart.org.zm/). There was also collaboration with Ministry of Health personnel from the department of Neglected Tropical Diseases, who guided the team to those areas that could be targeted for the study. Through different levels of involvement, all parties were notified of the progress of the study. WHO was informed on the results of the study, and investigators and key study personnel were invited to present on the topic. The overall study oversight and funding were located at a UK institution (London School of Hygiene & Tropical Medicine) where the PI (AB) kept the communications flowing regularly among partners, from the field to the ministries. This strategy aimed to minimize the risk of miscommunications that can easily hinder the progress of the work. Transparency and a collaborative approach to multiple partnerships were essential qualities required from all team members, but most importantly, from the leadership team.

## 5 Understanding Global Health Partnerships

The basic tenets of equitable partnerships hinged on mutual participation, trust and respect, mutual benefit, and the equal value placed on the contribution of each partner across the stages of the research process. In applying these principles to health agendas under the umbrella of "Health for all and equity in health," strong bonds of the partnership were established with commitments from all parties involved, from the individual (participants) level to the collective health perspective (Witteman et al. 2018; Mangold et al. 2014).

Put into the context of the BILHIV study, all parties involved in the study understood their roles and responsibilities, and this led to a concerted effort in achieving not only the research goals but also thinking beyond the strictly scientific deliverables and working towards a broader

health agenda. Research is cardinal in promoting evidence-based novel ways of understanding and delivering health. An equitable partnership was the backbone in our research, and it facilitated good practices respectful of culture, diversity, and justice for all those involved. However, in order for research to have a truly tangible impact, the vision and the equitable partnerships have to hold core values beyond the duration of the funding.

Following this principle, in the BILHIV study, we encouraged every member to give their thoughts and personal visions in different ways. The BCWs recorded a video with their own thoughts about FGS with suggestions for improvement. Some BCWs went on to become midwives because they felt compelled to become hands-on practitioners to have a more clinical role, as they had observed with their nurse colleagues from the BILHIV study. Both supporting institutions in the UK and Zambia worked together to promote the results and organize dissemination events and publications. Ministerial representatives were invited and included in the process.

These strong multi-leveled partnerships also provided a framework for unforeseen threats such as when the COVID-19 pandemic occurred. The BILHIV study had already concluded. However, a follow-up study was about to commence building on the existing networks that BILHIV had provided. The dire effects on staff, participants, implementation programs, and community members were ameliorated thanks to the strong commitment of the previously built partnerships (Chatterjee and Chakraborty 2021). As in any emergency, those most affected by the pandemic are the ones with limited forms of communication.

## 6 Overcoming Hurdles Through Women's Empowerment

Tradition and culture are symbols of identity that are accepted and even revered in most African communities. From time immemorial, women have had been viewed as being inferior to males and often regarded secondary in family matters, especially in most African cultures and settings (Agbemabiese P., unpublished)(See Chapters "Gender Equity in African Academia: An Implementation Science Evaluation of the Kenya Context", "Collective Learning: Power and Trust in Partnerships in the 3D Program for Girls and Women in Rural Pune District, India", and "Role of Social Science in Infectious Disease Research: a Case Study of Partnering with Communities in Vector Control in a Kenyan Village"). This has resulted in many women looking down on themselves, not believing in their own power, or thinking that they are not capable of making wise decisions, independent from their father and husband (Banda and Sitali 2019). In some cultures, during an initiation ceremony when a girl reaches puberty, they are taught to blindly obey their husbands and male elders as a sign of a well-behaved woman (Fumpa-Makano 2019). A woman raised in such environments is likely to feel inferior to men and to grow up believing that she is not worthy of making her own decisions about any aspect of her life. It is the husband's or elder's responsibility to choose for them (See Chapter "Role of Social Science in Infectious Disease Research: a Case Study of Partnering with Communities in Vector Control in a Kenyan Village") (UNAIDS 2019; Bustinduy et al. 2022). Aware of these differences, women raised with such limitations can also feel disadvantaged compared to fellow women that were not exposed to such traditions. There is not an easy way out for them. However, education and information can play an important role in empowering women and giving them a greater voice (Fumpa-Makano 2019; Shabaya and Konadu-Agyemang 2004). These very sensitive issues have to be well known to the community workers who navigate their daily work between the waters of cultural respect and empowerment, not always aligned and always challenging.

In the BILHIV study, some women struggled to participate despite their willingness, due to husband or elderly opposition (Chola, N. personal communication). Some women were not recruited and some could not complete all study procedures because their husbands or relatives stopped them or discouraged them after the initial household visit. However, there were also women who overcame their difficult cultural constraints and decided on their own to join the study- a bold and risky step opposing their own communities. They understood that it was their choice to keep healthy. Many of these women are now the biggest promoters of health choices and self-empowerment in their communities, gaining respect and inspiring change around them.

## 7    Lessons Learnt

Forming equitable partnerships with all key parties was essential for the implementation of the BILHIV study. In addition, the broad vision for the study allowed different partners to contribute equitably in their own disciplines and through their unique expertise. Working closely together towards a common goal gave purpose to the teams that were better suited to understand and resolved the hurdles that inevitably arose at different stages. These stages included BCWs working under the scorching sun and making door-to-door visits to participants. finding participants for follow up, processing samples in real time, communicating with overseas laboratories and partners, safeguarding confidential data, and disseminating results. Every step of the way required strong leadership and delegation to team members, who in turn were also recognized as leaders in their areas.

Including participants in the partnership was a key element in delivering on the global goals for the research. It was also essential to provide clear information via effective communication so that participants could complete subsequent study visits (see Chapter "Foundations and Future Directions of Global Health Communication"). *With them and for them* became the ultimate motto. Women who entered the study began to understand that performing the study procedures was their choice, for their health.

# 8　　Conclusions

Allowing women to decide when and where to be screened for sexual and reproductive health diseases is a way to actively empower them, but they cannot do this alone. Successful partnerships in research in global health, such as the one discussed in this chapter, are key to design, develop, implement and safeguard women on the path to health. In our case, to achieve the success of these self-strategies, cultural context needed to be understood, acknowledged and included in the team's decision-making process. This is the case for most topics in Global Health. It is important to help women step up, sometimes against their own environment, for their own health and well-being. Issues around stigma remain. Changing this paradigm will require time and the resolve of the women who have walked that path of self-determination, women who can lead the way for others.

# References

Banda M, Sitali M. Myths and practices of initiation ceremonies among the Bemba of Kasama District: implications on early marriages and quality education. J Hum Educ Dev. 2019;1(3):128–37.

Bray F, Ferlay J, Soerjomataram I, Siegel RL, Torre LA, Jemal A. Global cancer statistics 2018: GLOBOCAN estimates of incidence and mortality worldwide for 36 cancers in 185 countries. CA Cancer J Clin. 2018;68(6):394–424.

Brown CH, Kellam SG, Kaupert S, Muthén BO, Wang W, Muthén LK, et al. Partnerships for the design, conduct, and analysis of effectiveness, and implementation research: experiences of the prevention science and methodology group. Admn Policy Ment Health. 2012;39(4):301–16.

Bustinduy AL, Randriansolo B, Sturt AS, Kayuni SA, Leustcher PDC, Webster BL, Van Lieshout L, Stothard JR, Feldmeier H, Gyapong M. An update on female and male genital schistosomiasis and a call to integrate efforts to escalate diagnosis, treatment and awareness in endemic and non-endemic settings: the time is now. Adv Parasitol. 2022;115:1–44. https://doi.org/10.1016/bs.apar.2021.12.003. Epub 2022 Feb 17

Chatterjee I, Chakraborty P. Use of information communication technology by medical educators amid covid-19 pandemic and beyond. J Educ Technol Syst. 2021;49(3):310–24.

Fumpa-Makano R. Initiation ceremonies in Zambia: reflections on their role in girl child educational advancement. Int J Arts Social Sci. 2019;2(4)

Hayes R, Ayles H, Beyers N, et al. HPTN 071 (PopART): rationale and design of a cluster-randomised trial of the population impact of an HIV combination prevention intervention including universal testing and treatment – a study protocol for a cluster randomised trial. Trials. 2014;15:57.

Hotez PJ, Harrison W, Fenwick A, et al. Female genital schistosomiasis and HIV/AIDS: Reversing the neglect of girls and women. PLoS Negl Trop Dis. 2019;13(4):e0007025.

Jenkins C, Hien HT, Chi BL, Santin O. What works in global health partnerships? Reflections on a collaboration between researchers from Vietnam and Northern Ireland. BMJ Global Health. 2021;6(4):e005535.

Mangold K, Denke NJ, Gorombei D, Ostroski TL, Root L. Principles of successful partnerships. Nursing Admin Q. 2014;38(4):340–7.

Phiri CR, Sturt AS, Webb EL, Chola N, Hayes R, Shanaube K, Ayles H, Hansingo I, Bustinduy AL, BILHIV Study Team. Acceptability and feasibility of genital self-sampling for the diagnosis of female genital schistosomiasis: a cross-sectional study in Zambia. Wellcome Open Res. 2020;5:61. https://doi.org/10.12688/wellcomeopenres.15482.2.

Shabaya J, Konadu-Agyemang K. Unequal access, unequal participation: some spatial and socio-economic dimensions of the gender gap in education in Africa with special reference to Ghana, Zimbabwe and Kenya. Compare. 2004;34(4):395–424.

Sturt AS, Webb EL, Phiri CR, et al. Genital self-sampling compared with cervicovaginal lavage for the diagnosis of female genital schistosomiasis in Zambian women: the BILHIV study. PLoS Negl Trop Dis. 2020;14(7):e0008337.

UNAIDS. No more neglect: Female genital schistosomiasis and HIV. 2019. Accessed 10/01/2020.

WHO. Female genital schistosomiasis: a pocket atlas for clinical health-care professionals. In: Organisation WH, editor. Geneva, Switzerland; 2015.

Witteman HO, Chipenda Dansokho S, Colquhoun H, Fagerlin A, Giguere A, Glouberman S, Haslett L, Hoffman A, Ivers NM, Légaré F, Légaré J. Twelve lessons learned for effective research partnerships between patients, caregivers, clinicians, academic researchers, and other stakeholders. J General Internal Med. 2018;33(4):558–62.

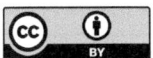

# An Autobiographical Perspective on Community-Based Participatory Research, an Approach for More Inclusive Research in Nicaragua

Harold Agusto Suazo Laguna

*To be a good [participatory researcher] means above all to have faith in people; to believe in the possibility that they can create and change things... Liberation begins to the extent that men [and women] reflect on themselves and their condition in the world -the world in which and with which they find themselves. To the extent that they are more conscientized, they insert themselves as subjects into their own history.*

(adapted from Freire, 1971, p.61) quoted in Nina Wallerstein and Bonnie Duran (2017)

## Abstract

In this chapter, I share my perspective on the role that we, researchers, play when developing a community-centered research project. Through my autobiographical narrative, I share experiences and lessons learned over two decades as a social scientist, facilitating and implementing diverse methodologies that have been oriented towards the development of the organizational skills of communities and their role as protagonists in identifying solutions for their own health problems.

## Keywords

Community-based · Participatory research · Mosquito-borne disease · Evidence-based communication · Inclusion in research · Nicaragua

H. A. Suazo Laguna (✉)
Department of Community Projects and Entomology, Sustainable Sciences Institute, Managua, Nicaragua
e-mail: hsuazo@icsnicaragua.org

## Author Perspective

The idea of writing this autobiographical chapter comes from my friend and mentor, Dr. Josefina Coloma, Executive Director of the Institute of Sustainable Sciences (SSI), a research professor with extensive experience in Scientific Research in Health, who inspired me to take this step to share my experience and knowledge in this in this book, with new researchers, program managers, students, teachers, reviewers, editors and funders who are interested in developing scientific research projects that involve communities.

## Key Tenets

1. The researcher has to be aware that community members are capable of self-reflection and have agency with feelings and thoughts. They are "sentient-thinking" beings.
2. Working with communities is a learning opportunity for all. Researchers are external agents of the community. We must recognize that, just as we share our

A. Stewart Ibarra, A. D. LaBeaud (eds.), *Transforming Global Health Partnerships*, Sustainable Development Goals Series, https://doi.org/10.1007/978-3-031-53793-6_17

knowledge and experiences, we also learn from "local wisdom."

3. The best approach to promote community action is when the researcher places the human being first—an approach that respects communities' own identities and the sense of belonging and promotes the free choice of the community, whether or not they want to participate in the research.

4. Any researcher designing a study with people or human subjects considers delivering the results to the people involved.

5. In times of crisis, local evidence and science play an essential role in reconstructing the social fiber.

6. This chapter addresses SDG #3, Good health and well-being and SDG#17 Partnerships for the goals.

# 1 Introduction

In this chapter, I share my perspective on the role that we, researchers, play when we develop a research project that involves communities. Here I relate my experiences and lessons learned from what have been almost two decades of my life as a social scientist, facilitating and implementing diverse methodologies that have been oriented towards developing the organizational skills of communities and their role as protagonists in identifying solutions for their health problems. Examples include the implementation of proven methodologies such as the strategy to socialize the evidence and discuss alternatives (SEPA by the Spanish acronym) for dengue prevention (Ledogar et al. 2017) Community-Based Participatory Research (CBPR)(Wallerstein et al. 2017), Dengue Chat: A social platform and software platform for community-based arbovirus vector control (Holston et al. 2021), The Innovative Use of the Care Group Model and Mobile Health (mHealth) to Reduce Zika Virus

Transmission (David et al. 2016), and the methodology of Communication for Social and Behavioral Change (C4D) (UNICEF 2022).

Here, I will pause because it is important for you to know where I come from and who I am. There is a phrase from the book *The Little Prince*, "All great people have been children before. (But few remember)." I identify with this phrase because today, I find myself in a position as a Social Scientist dedicated to scientific research in health. Still, to become the person I am, I had to travel a life path full of challenges and adversities. I, too, "was a child before," and the one who brought me to this world, my beloved mother, was also "a child before." That is why it is important to look at where we come from. We all have a story to tell, and in my case, my experiences from childhood to now where I am, breathing in this life, are the main points of reference that I have applied in my career as a social scientist. The challenge I always have in mind is: How to do scientific research without losing my human sensitivity.

# 2 Doña Adita

I can only tell you about myself if I tell you about my origin and the origin of my mother, Ada Laguna. She was born in 1949 in the city of La Libertad, Chontales, 175 kilometers from the capital of Nicaragua. My maternal grandmother raised her with her younger brother Ricardo Laguna. My grandmother died when my mother was only eleven years old, and she did not know her father. My mother told me, "Ricardo and I were given away like two little animals." It was then that the siblings were separated. One of my mother's aunts took her to live in town, but one day she told her, "Adita, I can't give you an education and I can't support you anymore," so they looked for my mother's father to care for her. My grandfather decided to send my mother to a farm where they raised cattle, and there she was reunited with her younger brother Ricardo. The move from the city to the countryside ended my mother's schooling, and she was obligated to learn tasks such as milking cows, making cheese, fixing fences, and performing other activities typical of the countryside.

Years went by, and my mother's life on the farm was very sad because she suffered much violence. Her only source of affection and protection was her younger brother Ricardo. Then she met my father, and they had their first children. When she was 21 years old, in 1970, they decided to leave the countryside to move to the capital city, Managua. They used money from the sale of land that my grandfather gave to my mother, but my father's mismanagement of money made him go bankrupt soon after. One day my father told me, "I'm leaving," and he never returned. He decided to create a life with another person and he abandoned us. My mother was already 33 years old; I was only six years old. My mother was left holding my newborn brother in one arm and my other one-year-old brother in the other. I have no pleasant memories of my relationship with my father; only sad memories come to mind because he gave a life of violence to my mother and her children. Maybe it was better that he left.

By 1982, my mother was left utterly alone with the responsibility of raising 13 living children (seven boys and six girls) from her 18 births. She faced a hard reality. She had not finished primary school, and without opportunities to work, she did not have a house of her own, so we were living, as my mother tells me, "In a situation like this, where the pain goes deep into your being." Many nights passed when my mother cried in silence because she did not know how she would feed us each day.

## 3    A New Home

That same year, very close to where we were living, a process of re-distribution of land was ongoing. The "Quinta," a small farm, had been abandoned by its owners, the Pacheco family, after the Sandinista Popular Revolution. On this land, there was an old house, a place where the owners of the land used to live. The community leader, Teodoro López, was coordinating the re-distribution of land. He was informed about the case of my mother and her children, who had nowhere to live, and he permitted my mother to live with her children in this large house. Soon the land began to be populated by people who came from the countryside to the capital. There were very basic services; eight public water pumps supplied around 100 families. This settlement is now called the La Quinta Pacheco neighborhood, the place where I grew up and where I have lived for 40 years.

My mother's first step to improving her family's situation was to organize with the community. She began to receive workshops for Adult Education Promoters, a program supported by the Ministry of Education to eliminate illiteracy, which affected more than 50% of the Nicaraguan population. Soon after, my mother started working as a teacher of adult education. She began to exercise this noble work in my community, La Quinta, and then she earned a distinction as Promoter of Adult Education Vanguardia of Managua. She was promoted to assist the Adult Education Program at several government companies and other neighborhoods of the capital.

Education transformed my mother's life. Now she was recognized in her community with great respect; forty years later, people in the neighborhood said to her with a smile, "You are my teacher."

In the years that followed, my mother continued to organize in the community. She was a health promoter and a promoter for the Ministry of the Family, which had a program called Hogar Sustituto, where they provided care and a safe space for children in vulnerable conditions. My mother tells me that in addition to being the mother of 13 children, she was a temporary mother of 8 more children; some came, and some went. She also managed a children's dining room where 45 children from the community came to eat. This program of the Ministry of the Family focused on supporting vulnerable families with food. The program provided basic grains, and the community prepared the food.

All of the community activities in which my mother participated were not paid. She received some support as a promoter, which was not enough to maintain us, so she dedicated herself to other jobs. In the '80 s in Nicaragua, no foreign products entered, so the country produced its own soap. My mother started buying and selling artisanal soap, then innovated and made her own artisanal soap to wash clothes. She took us to the market to buy from the ladies who sold meats. We would buy the hides with fat and transport them in sacks on the public bus. The passengers complained about the foul smell of the grease emanating from the sacks. Then we fried the hides, and from there came the raw material to prepare the soap. My mother (with much effort) obtained the other components to make the soap. I and several of my siblings would go out to sell the handmade soap my mother made. Carrying a bucket on our heads, we would walk up to 5 kilometers in each direction. From then on, we never lacked food in our house.

## 4     My Early Years

In 1984 my mother taught me to read and write. I was eight years old, and she enrolled me in a public school, and I went straight to second grade. My elementary school at that time did not have desks. We sat on the floor. I remember my mother bought me used shoes so that I would have shoes to attend school, and sometimes they were broken, and she had to fix them. Once a month, she would cut our hair because she could not afford to pay for so many haircuts.

The years passed, and I continued my studies, but I also continued selling. I went from selling soap from house to house to selling gum and candy, carrying a small basket on my arm. I did this in an ambulatory way on the buses of Managua. I would go out to sell with my younger brother Franklin in the afternoon. A woman would give me the products each day (on credit), and I would pay her at the end of the day. We always returned home with food. We were like little ants carrying our backpacks with products to sell and food to bring home.

By the time I was thirteen years old, I had become an independent salesman. I would go to the market with my younger brother, the largest market in Central America, to buy cases of gum, milk candy bars, and colored gummy candies. I began to give jobs to other children in my community. That leap from being a dependent to an independent vendor was disliked by other older vendors, who wanted to decide who would get on the buses to sell and who would not. They were upset because we did not listen to them, but they were not the owners of the buses. Several times they beat us and stole our products. The street hit me hard, and the only thing I could do was take a deep breath and find the strength to go on, even with tears in my eyes.

One day my brother Franklin and I were selling candy at a traffic light in La Subasta. When the light turned red, we ran towards the cars and offered the candies, raising our arms to show the basket. At that moment, a large truck stopped, and the driver lowered his window and took out a bill. My brother Franklin ran over to take the bill and asked the driver what candy he wanted. The driver answered, "Nothing, nothing, just leave it there." My brother started yelling, "daddy, daddy, daddy." I ran to where he was standing, and the driver raised the window and left. The driver was our father. This kind of thing hits hard in the heart of a child. That day I told myself that when I became a father, I would not be like mine.

## 5     Teachers Making a Difference

In 1989, I went from elementary to a public high school, and my first year did not go well. I failed math with 58 points and needed a minimum of 60 points to pass. I took a make-up exam and failed again. I remember the teacher telling my mother, "He is young and can repeat the year."

The following year I felt discouraged to continue studying. I told my mother that I was already earning money and supporting myself. What good would my studies do? But my mother insisted that I should study. She finally convinced me and we changed high schools. In the new public high school, I met teachers who I still remember with great affection, teachers who admired me because they knew that I was a street vendor and that I studied. That was exceptionally motivating for me. In 1992, I was in my second year of high school and became the best student at the Enrique Flores Guevara Institute. That same year I won first place in the Mathematics Olympics of Managua, and I represented Managua capital at the Mathematics Olympics at the national level, winning third place.

From that year on, my life changed. I remember that the director of the Institute called me to the Director's office and said to me, "Son, they tell me that you sell candy in the streets." I answered yes; she was amazed at how I, being a street vendor, was the champion of the Math Olympiads. That year they gave me an award to go to Costa Rica for a student exchange. It was my first trip on a plane and my first experience interacting with people from other countries. I enjoyed representing the students of my country and I felt important.

# 6    Student Organizing

The following year, I was appointed student representative to the Board of Directors of the Institute, representing 3550 students. My life as a student and community leader defending the rights of students began. This experience helped me grow as a person. I began to develop the ability to empathize and identify and feel other students' problems. I learned to organize and lead groups to solve conflicts. I coordinated 60 section presidents, who daily raised different issues, such as conflicts between students, between students and teachers, problems of public safety, domestic violence, diseases, etc. This daily hustle and bustle made me a more sensitive person, and at a young age, I had the responsibility and the burden to make decisions that affected the lives of others.

At the age of 16, I stopped selling on the streets and continued studying and working, beginning an office job as an accounting assistant. I finished high school when I was 19 years old. That same year, I married Ulda del Carmen Centeno, a beautiful girl who had just finished her high school studies. She came from a difficult childhood, with a story very similar to mine. She also grew up without a father, and as a child, with her mother and brothers, they sold different products as informal vendors in a market in Managua.

In 1996, we both applied for a scholarship to a prestigious private university (Central American University), and based on merit and grades, we each got a 100% scholarship. I studied Economics with a Major in Macroeconomics, and she studied Business Administration. After a year of college, our son Harold Steven Suazo Centeno was born; this was one of the most important moments of my life. A son is the most precious gift from God, and he became our life incentive. We had to get ahead. During the day we worked, and at night we studied. Sometimes we carried our infant son to our classes. At the beginning of our careers, it was very difficult to be parents; although we were scholarship holders, our income was limited. However, we were presented with opportunities that allowed us to grow as people and as professionals. We both managed to graduate, thus improving our family economy, and we built a little house of our own next to my mother's at Barrio La Quinta, which is still our home. Fifteen years after my first child, our beautiful daughter Fernanda Suazo Centeno was born. She brought much joy to the family; a baby girl always brings hope to us adults. Since the day she was born, I sing a song to her when I wake up, and it makes me the happiest dad in the world.

I decided to study Economics because I like numbers. The Economics major was new, therefore, the students did not have representation before the higher authorities of the university, similar to the other majors. We needed to have our voice, to be represented by our major. As a group of university students, we requested to hold elections for our representatives, and I organized a slate in the election. Each student voted, and our slate won. I became the secretary for the department of Economics. I was part of a committee to evaluate and approve new scholarship applications from applicants for the economics major nationwide. This experience reinforced my interest in youth organizations and motivated me to help the underserved.

## 7    My First Work Experiences, then Consultancies, and Research

At the beginning of my university studies, I had the opportunity to apply for my first formal job. I joined the Ministry of Labor (MITRAB) when I was 19 years old, starting in a technical position as a Socio-labor Researcher in the office of Projects and Technical Cooperation. This marked a new stage of my life. I remember my first day of work, I was assigned an old computer with the MS-DOS system, which I could not use because I had never used a computer.

It was six years of learning. I developed competencies in project design and development. I learned about resource management and administration in the areas of Labor Inspection, Alternative Dispute Resolution, Occupational Health and Safety, Employment, and Child Labor.

In 2005, the Senior Management of MITRAB made me an offer to be part of a team of AECI-UNDP-MITRAB Consultants of the Occupational Training and Labor Insertion Program (FOIL), a regional program with Spanish funding through the United Nations. I could not believe that I had come from the streets and was now a well-paid "consultant." I worked for two years as a Technical Assistant in the FOIL Program, and despite offers to continue with this office-based work, the community had a stronger pull on me, and I left.

In parallel, I started working at CIET international, an organization dedicated to scientific research in social science, public health, and epidemiology. I started as a data entry person, then as an interviewer. I became field team coordinator, then field director, coordinating fieldwork with up to 130 people under my responsibility. I developed several projects in Nicaragua and Central America. I participated in data analysis and preparation of the reports with the results of the investigations. I also held responsibilities as executive director of the country office.

At CIET, I participated as a key researcher in the Pilot Project called Camino Verde for Dengue Control. It centered its strategy on SEPA: Socializing Evidence for Participatory Action, or Socializing Evidence and Discussing Alternatives to Prevent Dengue. The project focused on implementing an evidence-based communication strategy that motivated families and communities to develop actions to control mosquito breeding sites without relying on chemical larval control and spraying. This successful pilot experience allowed us to scale up the SEPA strategy in a Cluster Randomized Controlled Trial that we implemented in communities in Nicaragua and Mexico (Andersson et al. 2015). Through this project, I met Dr. Josefina Coloma and Dr. Eva Harris from UC Berkeley and SSI. Both are prestigious Professors at the University of California Berkeley and Research Scientists of Global Health, recognized internationally for their work to in transferring scientific capacities in Latin American countries and the world.

## 8    Sustainable Sciences Institute

Once the Camino Verde concluded in 2014, Dr. Josefina Coloma invited me to be part of her research team at the Sustainable Sciences Institute (SSI Nicaragua), trusting me to coordinate the new community intervention project in Nicaragua. We teamed up with Dr. James Holston, an anthropologist from the University of California Berkeley, to develop a platform and app with mobile technology DengueChat (www.denguechat.org) to pilot an entomological surveillance system in the neighborhoods of Managua, with the participation of communities to control the *Aedes aegypti* mosquito vector of dengue, Zika, and chikungunya. This experience in Nicaragua motivated other organizations in Colombia and Paraguay to use the DengueChat app for community entomological surveillance. Once the project ended in 2017, SSI decided to open a Community Projects Division, under my direction.

One interesting aspect of this project was that my neighborhood, La Quinta Pacheco, a coastal neighborhood on the shores of Lake Managua, was selected as an intervention neighborhood.

This allowed me, for the first time, to work in my local environment, and to connect with the families of my community. Besides being a resident, I was also "The Researcher" who directed a community intervention focused on dengue prevention in my neighborhood. Before this opportunity, I always felt indebted to my community because I had been working in other neighborhoods of Managua for several years and not in La Quinta. It was extremely fulfilling to be able to contribute to the development of my community.

I remember that during one of her visits to the study sites, including my community, Josefina assessed that everything was great with DengueChat. The project was developing successfully. However, while she walked on the dirt streets, followed by children crisscrossing and jumping over streams of raw sewage, she stopped and said, "The main problem here is not mosquitoes. It's the sanitary situation." She recommended to the leaders of the community and myself that something had to be done in the La Quinta neighborhood to solve the the lack of sanitary sewage and that she would support all efforts for a solution encouraging us to prioritize the problem because it would have an impact directly on the quality of life and health of families.

## 9 Community Leader, Water and Sanitation for La Quinta

In 2016, the residents of La Quinta proposed that I be the community leader, which I accepted. My experience as a researcher and coordinator of community work was tested by this new challenge because in my community, there were many problems, and the main one was to resolve the sanitary sewer system. The first step we took was to organize ourselves by blocks. For each block, we chose a coordinator, and we carried out a community diagnosis, which included a population and housing census. We used a survey to determine the conditions of health, education, and environmental conditions, specifically sanitation. We also held meetings with the residents to present and discuss the results.

The results of the diagnosis showed that my community had a population of 800 people (53% women, 47% men), with 200 families living in 150 homes. None of the families had sanitary sewer service. 76 used latrines and 74 used toilets connected to septic holes (not tanks). 52% of the dwellings were in poor condition. In relation to health, we found that in 28% of households there was at least one person with a chronic noncommunicable disease, mainly diabetes mellitus and hypertension. The most common diseases affecting the population in the last year were influenza 58%, diarrhea 22%, other diseases 15%, and dengue 5%.

We prepared a report for the municipal authorities showing the state of vulnerability of my community. We included photographs of collapsed septic holes and latrines, because every winter the heavy rainfall caused direct damage to homes and streets. We officially requested the Mayor's Office to carry out the Sanitary Sewage Project. A Neighborhood Committee regularly followed up on our requests. That same year our Sewage Project was approved by the Municipal Council, and the Majors office installed a main pipe in 5 neighborhood streets. As for the home connections, they left it as the residents' responsibility.

Households with better economic means connected to the sewage pipe, but 76 families with latrines could not connect for lack of resources. We followed up with a second request to the Mayor's Office and the FISE (Emergency Social Investment Fund) and obtained approval for a second Improved Sanitation Project with funds from FISE, which have loan funds from the Central American Bank for Economic Integration (CABEI) for water and sanitation projects in rural areas.

Although barrio La Quinta is not located in a rural area, it is quite peripheral to Managua, and the project was approved based on the conditions of the critical state of emergency that the community was experiencing. The 76 families that still used their latrines were the protagonists of this project, which included the provision of a sanitation module (hut with a toilet, shower, sink, laundry washbasin, and installation of a drinking water system), delivered to each family.

This Improved Sanitation Project was executed under the Community Guided Projects (PGC) modality, a methodology implemented by FISE with the objective that the community participates in the physical and financial execution of the project. For this purpose, we created a project administration committee comprised of community members. Through the committee, all purchasing and contracting services of technical personnel were carried out by the community. We received approximately $100,000 in a community bank account, with co-signatories being a community member and the mayor herself. The committee executed the funds, audited by the municipality and FISE, and ultimately supervised by BESIE. Residents made their contributions through unskilled labor and transport of construction materials. We underspent, and from the savings, electrical connections and painting were completed in all the modules, which was not expected in the original design. We also built a concrete room with the installation of a sanitation module for a senior person with disabilities who had nowhere to live. This is how, after forty years, my community, Barrio La Quinta, has a sanitary sewage system that reaches 100% of the families. They now have infrastructure that has provided collective self-esteem and dignity to all. In the past few years, we have also paved most of our streets and improved trash collection and flood control.

## 10    Director of Community Projects for SSI

In 2016, the World Health Organization declared the Zika pandemic as an international public health emergency, which led our organization, SSI, in collaboration with local partners at the NGO AMOS Health and Hope and UC Berkeley, to prepare a project on Zika in Nicaragua, to support a coordinated response with the Nicaraguan Ministry of Health.

Between 2016 and 2020, I coordinated implementing the Community Prevention Project for Zika and other arboviruses on behalf of SSI, funded in part by USAID and with the collabora-

tion of UNICEF. The project focused on strengthening the capacity of communities to prevent the transmission of Zika and other arboviruses. The project applied the Family and Community Health Mode. It implemented house-to-house visits to conduct entomological and epidemiological surveillance through a network of 500 health volunteers in 34 neighborhoods in districts 3 and 6 of Managua using our SEPA strategy, CareGroups (Care Group Info 2021) and DengueChat.

## 11    Public Health and Other Crises

The sociopolitical events that occurred in 2018 in Nicaragua affected community relations. Social cohesion was broken, respect and trust were lost, and home violence increased. Concerning the Zika project, we, as an organization, took a step back because different neighborhoods that participated were in conflict zones. We suspended activities for six months. When we returned, we focused on developing relief groups, generating spaces where the brigadistas could process their traumas and resume community participation, with health at the center. Local evidence and science played an essential role in the reconstruction of the social fabric.

In 2020, the SARS-CoV-2 pandemic brought many deaths and illnesses to my community. Eighteen people died, and we were in permanent mourning for our close ones. I was in a state of very delicate health as a result of COVID. I had never felt so much pain in my life as thinking that I would die. I was not afraid of death, but it was the thought that my little daughter would grow up without a father to accompany her in life. She was only eight years old. Thank God we got ahead, beating COVID-19.

In 2021, SSI delegated a new responsibility to me as a member of the Coordination and Research team of an Arbovirus Surveillance Population Study in Managua called A2CARES (Asian-American Center for Arbovirus Research and Enhanced Surveillance) as part of the Centers of Research in Emerging Infectious Diseases (CREID) of the NIH.

I have completed my Master's Degree in Epidemiology at the Center for Research and Studies in Health (CIES) of the National Autonomous University of Nicaragua. My graduate studies are part of the Capacity Building initiative of A2CARES to promote a new generation of researchers in global health. Thus completing a personal goal.

## 12    Designing My Research Study: Community Intervention

As researchers, we make enormous efforts to design research projects that meet the scientific quality standards demanded by funders and evaluators. Examples include specifying a sample size and a sample selection method that are statistically valid or presenting a method of scientifically validated analysis of results. However, when it comes to working with the community, you may find challenges in meeting those scientific parameters in the reality of community life. I refer to this as an issue that goes beyond the availability of resources for your research.

Here, I highlight the importance of considering the community from the study's design stages. Most of the time, research topics are imposed by a global agenda rather than based on the local priorities or needs of the communities. Here, a question arises: Is the research topic a community priority? To illustrate this conflict, I share the following experience.

In August 2010, within the baseline framework for the Camino Verde cluster randomized controlled trial (evidence-based community mobilization for dengue prevention), we asked 8402 households in 60 neighborhoods of Managua: What is the main problem in this neighborhood? One-third of households answered safety, alcohol, and drugs; 20% answered drinking water, sanitary sewerage, and storm drainage; 17% mentioned streets. One in ten indicated no problem, 4% did not know, and the rest mentioned other issues. Only 38 households mentioned mosquitoes and dengue (<1%) as the primary neighborhood problem.

With these results, we realized that dengue, my research topic, was not a priority of the study communities. Here we were faced with a challenge: how to carry out more inclusive research? We designed a strategy to share and discuss the results of the baseline with the communities where the study was developed. They interpreted their own data, such as costs of care for people with dengue, spending on chemical products to avoid mosquitoes, time spent looking for and eliminating larvae and pupae, and identification of neighborhood priorities. Their perspectives guided the design of the intervention. The community appropriation of their data facilitated their involvement in the intervention.

This process that I experienced made me reflect on the importance of sharing the results of my research with families and communities. I suggest that every researcher who designs a study with people or human subjects considers delivering the results to the people involved, a principle that we must practice when researching in communities.

Another example of the importance of data return is the following. On one occasion, I was invited as an evaluator by a group of researchers doing a community health intervention project using SEPA principles in another country in South America. I shared a week with them, visiting the sites where the study was being carried out. I spoke to the families and with the researchers to get to know their perspectives on the project. The study contemplated intervention and control communities. In both groups, baseline data were collected. The results were returned only to intervention communities, and from there, the intervention was born. However, the control communities did not receive any information. They were only providers of data to meet a scientific requirement that demonstrated that the intervention had an impact compared to a group of control communities.

At the end of my visit to the project, I met with the principal investigator, who asked for my feedback. I reflected with her on the fact that she had in her hands the power to save many people's lives and prevent others from getting sick because she had information on confirmed cases of infections of people from intervention and control communities. Still, she could not share it because her protocol did not allow her to share this information with the latter. The researcher shed tears and became very frustrated as she realized the internal ethical conflict. A month later, I received an email in which she told me that the university's Ethics Committee approved an amendment to their protocol so that they could share the information with control communities. With peace of mind, knowing that she did what was morally correct, she continued and completed her investigation successfully.

## 13   Conclusions

My life trajectory and my time as a researcher have allowed me to build a perspective of self-critical thinking. It is a continuous exercise to reflect on whether I, as a researcher, am complying with my research protocol, but even more importantly, whether I am complying with the basic principles of the ethics of scientific research, respecting the integrity of the participants of the research study that I am implementing.

Here, I share some of the lessons I've learned on this journey:

Working with communities sounds nice, but it is not an easy matter. It requires much tact. The researcher has to be aware that community members are capable of self-reflection and have agency with feelings and thoughts. They are "sentient-thinking" beings. Often we researchers assume that "we are the saviors" and that we will solve their problems. We even go so far as to express that we are going to the community to "educate them," something that subtly reveals the assumption that "we have the knowledge." In this context of these expressions of language, I reflect: As a researcher, I am an external agent of the community. I must recognize that, just as I am going to share my knowledge and experiences, I also get to learn from local wisdom. Working with communities is a learning opportunity for all. My experience tells me that the best approach

to promote community action is when the researcher places the human being first and not their ego—an approach that respects communities' own identities and the sense of belonging and promotes the free choice of the community, including whether or not they want to participate in the research.

Finally, I hope to be a motivational reference for many by telling my life story, where I come from, and how far I have come. How a resilient child who came out of the streets became a sentient-thinking person and, through education opportunities, became a scientific researcher. I am an example that it is possible to get ahead in life and collaborate with prestigious researchers from the global North, with a horizontal relationship of mutual benefit. The most significant message I want to leave you with is that through education, dedication, and commitment to the community, one can contribute to the development of our nations on small and large scales.

I identify with the words of Nina Wallerstein, DrPH, a University of New Mexico Distinguished professor and the Center for Participatory Research Director, who stated "Community-based participatory research (CBPR) is not just a methodological approach but a commitment to equity, inclusivity, and social justice."

**Acknowledgments** To my mother, Ada, I express my enormous gratitude, respect and admiration; you are a powerful, courageous woman with an enormous capacity for resilience who has overcome many adversities. Thank you for supporting me and accompanying me in facing the challenges of my life. Thank you for giving me your unconditional love and because you never stopped believing in me. Because of you, I am a better person and a professional. I always carry with me your good advice and healing words. How nice it feels to have a mom that everyone admires for being a benchmark for self-improvement; you are a leader in our community, with all my love and gratitude.

I want to express to my wife Ulda, my son Harold, and my daughter Fernanda the most important things I have in my life. We have faced many challenges and moved forward, and life has had many beautiful moments of joy—a huge thank you for your support and inspiration, and are the most beautiful blessing in my life. I thank my extended family, brothers, and sisters, whom I love wholeheartedly.

I thank life for putting Dr. Josefina Coloma on my path, who has been my mentor during the last ten years of my professional life and has become a great friend. I am very grateful to her for trusting me and allowing me to work in her team. Having her as a mentor has been a true honor. She has contributed significantly to my growth as a person and as a scientific researcher. She has been present in many meaningful moments of my life, listening to me and giving me sage advice and words of motivation; she is a sentient-thinking being whom I respect and admire as an example human being and a scientist to follow. Thank you for working with me on this chapter- it has been a journey! Today I tell you with great affection, amiga Josefina, thank you very much!

I also want to express my special thanks to Drs. Eva Harris, Leah Katzelnick and James Holston, who believed in the communities and me, as we successfully developed community studies with a new paradigm of doing science with the community and for the community.

I want to highlight the contribution of my community team, María Mercedes López Quintero, Jacqueline del Carmen Mojica Díaz, Juana Rosa Ruiz Torres, Rosa Villareal Dávila, Engel Antonio Méndez García, Julia Esmeralda Mena Castillo, Jennifer Ruiz Hernández, Damaris de los Ángeles Zavala, Jorge Alberto Ruiz Salinas, who have accompanied me in my career as a scientific researcher, the success achieved has been due to the collective effort, where each one of them has given himself with great dedication and social commitment.

To Don Carlos Augusto Suazo Miranda, my father, who, after 20 years of absence, life brought us together again and has been part of my team, doing excellent work as a driver and logistical support.

My immense gratitude to the community leaders and health brigades of the community network, who became community entomologists and citizen scientists. They are the protagonists that generate and communicate evidence. Thank you for all your teachings and for sharing moments of growth together. A special memory of Isaac Mendez, who at age 8 was a stellar brigade member, a living example of enthusiasm, solidarity, and love for his neighborhood. You will always be remembered. Special thanks to the families for allowing us to enter their homes and learn together a different way of taking care of our health.

I also express special thanks to Dr. Anna Stewart-Ibarra and Dr. Desiree LaBeaud, for allowing me to tell my story and my experiences in this book, a beautiful effort to bring together the voices of many people around the world, which will serve as motivation and reference to carry out better scientific research, research with human sensitivity.

# References

Andersson N, Nava-Aguilera E, Arosteguí J, Morales-Perez A, Suazo-Laguna H, Legorreta-Soberanis J, Hernandez-Alvarez C, Fernandez-Salas I, Paredes-Solís S, Balmaseda A, Cortés-Guzmán AJ, Serrano De Los Santos R, Coloma J, Ledogar RJ, Harris E. Evidence based community mobilization for dengue prevention in Nicaragua and Mexico (Camino Verde, the Green Way): cluster randomized controlled trial. BMJ. 2015;351 https://doi.org/10.1136/bmj.h3267.

Care Group Info. About Care Group. 2021. https://caregroupinfo.fh.org/about-us.

Davis T, Suazo H, Parajon L, Coloma J. Innovative use of Care Groups, Home Inspection. In: APHA 2016 Annual Meeting & Expo (Oct. 29-Nov. 2, 2016); 2016, November. APHA.

Fondo de las Naciones Unidas para la Infancia. Comunicación para el Desarrollo (C4D). 2022. https://www.unicef.org/nicaragua/comunicacion-para-el-desarrollo#:~:text=C4D%20es%20un%20enfoque%20que,calidad%20de%20vida%20para%20todos%E2%80%9D.

Holston J, Suazo-Laguna H, Harris E, Coloma J. DengueChat: a social and software platform for community-based arbovirus vector control. Am J Trop Med Hygiene. 2021;105(6):1521–35. https://doi.org/10.4269/ajtmh.20-0808.

Ledogar RJ, Arosteguí J, Hernández-Alvarez C, Morales-Perez A, Nava-Aguilera E, Legorreta-Soberanis J, Suazo-Laguna H, Belli A, Laucirica J, Coloma J, Harris E, Andersson N. Mobilising communities for Aedes aegypti control: the SEPA approach. BMC Public Health. 2017;17(1) https://doi.org/10.1186/s12889-017-4298-4.

Wallerstein N, Duran B, Oetzel JG, Minkler M, editors. Community-based participatory research for health: advancing social and health equity. John Wiley & Sons; 2017.

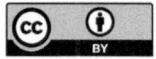

# Gender Equity in Academia Thriving as a Clinician-Scientist, Establishing Partnerships, and Driving Policy for Change in the Kenya Context

Miriam Mutebi, Jacqueline Kitulu, and Christine Ngaruiya

*Stories Matter. Many stories matter. Stories have been used to dispossess and to malign. But stories can also be used to empower, and to humanize.*

Chimamanda Ngozi Adichie

## Abstract

In global health, the mantra that men lead while women do the work is one that is not lost on us. As women in global health, who have also been part of many global health partnerships, we are keen to challenge the status quo on how we think about impact of global health—a viewpoint that must account for gender equity at every level of partnership and global health initiatives. Our stories provide a window into the experiences of what that status quo currently looks like, with personal reflections on how that has impacted us and our own potential impact—by and large negatively so. We also describe potential solutions based on these experiences supplemented by literature on this topic; these are samples of the problem, albeit not comprehensive. To be sure, the challenges go beyond our own in breadth and depth. They will need continued purposeful and intentional work at the core of addressing the educational pipeline, advancing female academics equitably to their male counterparts, promotion and sponsoring for leadership positions equitably among others. This mindset and paradigm shift needs to start at the level of developing global health experts, with the students, trainees, and learners who will soon take over in our stead—it needs to start with you.

M. Mutebi
Department of Surgery, Aga Khan University, Nairobi, Kenya

J. Kitulu
Kenya Medical Association, Hospital Holdings B.V., PATH, Nairobi, Kenya

C. Ngaruiya (✉)
Department of Emergency Medicine, Stanford School of Medicine, Stanford University, Stanford, CA, USA
e-mail: cngaruiy@stanford.edu

## Keywords

Gender equity · Gender parity · Physician · Academia · Global health · Policy

**Author Perspective**

Drs. Mutebi, Kitulu and Ngaruiya are physicians from Kenya with global experiences in training, research, leadership and clinical practice. They collectively bring more than 50 years of lived experience training and working in medicine and global health. These experiences have been

A. Stewart Ibarra, A. D. LaBeaud (eds.), *Transforming Global Health Partnerships*, Sustainable Development Goals Series, https://doi.org/10.1007/978-3-031-53793-6_18

fraught with being "the only" in many scenarios: the only woman in their classroom, the only woman to have sat in a particular role, the only woman participating in closed door meetings where key decisions are being made. These are their stories framed through a gendered lens, and their associated recommendations, for those pursuing global health initiatives through partnership in research, clinical care and policy setting.

**Key Tenets**

1. There are not enough in women in the pipeline for medicine and academia in Sub-Saharan Africa, which hampers future potential for gender-inclusive global health partnerships and decision-making opportunities.
2. Lack of mentorship and leadership training are key impediments to the advancement and spotlighting of women and their contributions in global health research.
3. The model for academia in Sub-Saharan Africa needs to be transformed to one that highlights, and supports, the importance of developing an academic career including the nuances and particular challenges faced by women in academia.
4. Diasporans play a potentially pivotal role in bridging the gap and enhancing global health partnerships between HIC and LMIC stakeholders by leveraging personal will, lived experience and cultural awareness, in addition to essential content expertise.
5. This chapter addresses the following SDGs: #3 Good health and well-being; #4 Quality Education; #5 Gender Equality; #8 Decent Work and Economic Growth; #10 Reduce Inequality; #16 Peace, Justice and Strong Institutions; #17 Partnership for the Goals.

# 1 Introduction

Acclaimed Nigerian writer, Chimamanda Ngozi Adichie best encapsulates the power of stories when she states in her famous Ted Talk "The Danger of a Single Story" that: "Stories Matter. Many stories matter. Stories have been used to dispossess and to malign. But stories can also be used to empower, and to humanize." In this chapter, we have shared our personal stories. These encompass decades of experience as bonafide global health practitioners with practice spanning Low- and Middle-Income Country settings (such as Kenya, Uganda, Tanzania, Congo and South Africa), High-Income Country settings (such as the US and the UK), and in partnership roles acting as bridges between the two–all with the aim of achieving health equity that is trans-continental (Koplan et al. 2009). Consequently, we ascribe to the definition of "global health" by Koplan et al.: "an area for study, research, and practice that places a priority on improving health and achieving health equity for all people worldwide" in presenting our views (Koplan et al. 2009).

Moreover, we use African animal prototypes to further characterize our stories, as an ode to the relevance of their role in the African tradition of storytelling. This concept was recently reclaimed by palliative care specialist, Dr. Christian Ntizimara, who originates from Rwanda (unpublished work). We close with recommendations based on our collective experiences and ultimately propose efforts to ensure advancement of women in global health. These efforts are critical to equitable global health partnerships.

There is evolving evidence to support the use of story-telling as a primary contributor, or adjunct to, more conventional research approaches. This is especially relevant in the case of marginalized populations, where nuance is key in driving new hypotheses and codifying findings. This level of vulnerability and representation of the African woman's story is underrepresented in literature (McCall et al. 2021; Rieger et al. 2020). We hope that our stories serve to triangulate, to humanize, and to empower.

## 2    The Female African Academic Clinician by Dr. Miriam Mutebi

*Genus/ species: Cheetah—Acinonyx jubatus*

*Strengths: Intelligence, flexibility, coalition building*

*Weaknesses:    Occasional    tendency    to self-isolate,*

*The cheetah is the smallest of the big cats and frequently underestimated. As a cheetah, one has to move faster to keep up with the other big cats who frequently steal their prey. The cheetah has adapted to this by hunting during the day as other cats are nocturnal. Despite their aerodynamic dominance, cheetahs have a success rate of 25–50%. Cheetahs are highly intelligent, sensitive cats with a strong sense of community, and are prone to form coalitions where all members have equal access to the hunt. They are light on their feet and extremely flexible to allow for rapid shifts and changes when hunting. Female academicians have to be similarly agile in dealing with all the different curveballs faced in academia. While making many endeavors, they may have a lower success rate, however they continue to build their communities and keep reaching forward.*

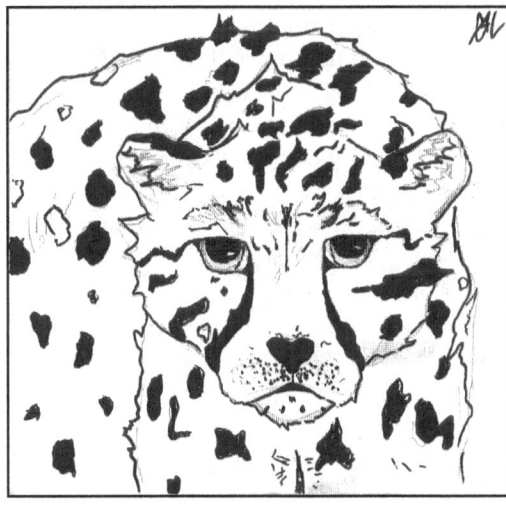

Cheetah. Art by Everest Lavery

## 2.1    The Road Less Travelled: Forging New Paths

Completing surgical residency in 2012 made me pause as the seventh woman in Kenya to complete a degree in general surgery. Surgical programs have existed in the country since the fifties, but until recently there were very few females in surgery. *Cheetah trait: constantly needing to move quickly to hunt its prey or achieve its target.* Luckily this has started to change, with an exponential increase in the number of women enrolled and graduating from surgical specialties in recent years. My gravitation towards a specialty in breast surgery was based on the fact that the women I was seeing in clinic were very different from the textbook definition of who gets breast cancer. These were young women, with multiple children who had all breastfed which were traditionally protective factors. In addition, I noticed that many of our patients were diagnosed with advanced cancers and anecdotally had very aggressive disease. I felt that someone needed to make sense of these variations in clinical presentation, identify these barriers, and do something to change this. *Cheetah trait: being led by a strong sense of community.* That is how my training in breast surgical oncology and my foray into clinical epidemiology and health systems research started.

The role of the *academic* surgeon is an old one but perhaps not as well embraced in the Africa context. *Cheetah trait: frequently overlooked, bullied or sequestered by larger animals in the wild.* As an academic scientist there is a triple expectation of delivery: f clinical service to address the needs of patients, teaching and the inherent responsibility to train the next generation of surgeons with this new knowledge, and research, meaning the opportunity to push the needle and generate new region-specific, culturally appropriate data that will help to enhance patient care. Tensions invariably set in when these three factors come into direct competition.

Sub-Saharan Africa has the greatest health workforce deficits and more than two million workers are needed to address this (Crisp and Chen 2014; World Health Organization 2016). As such, many clinicians are faced with large patient volumes and often struggle to provide optimal care to patients. *Cheetah trait: often hunting prey much bigger than itself, it must deploy tact and strategy to survive.* At the same time, one needs to produce a reasonable body of work in terms of research and this aspect is one that frequently suffers in academic practice in Africa. Fewer faculty engage in research due to a lack of protected time to conduct research, lack of skills in basic research methodology, and a failure of institutional and infrastructural support for many aspects of research such as grant applications and management, manuscript preparation, statistical support and data management .

## 2.2    Structural Barriers for the Developing African Clinician Scientist

Additional barriers may be institutional ethics boards which can sometimes be more obstructive than supportive of young researchers. *Cheetah trait: often disadvantaged as one of the smallest carnivores.* Thus, the need to do research is unfortunately frequently begrudged. Starting out in surgery, however, I had always clung to the somewhat I ideal of the 'renaissance of the African scientist' and an old video taken in my second year of surgical training had me aspiring to develop 'research for Africa, by Africa'. *Cheetah traits: agility and intelligence.*

Looking back on the journey, I realized early that I would need to be proactive to achieve my goals. As with any life decision, I turned to my mentors who pointed me in the right direction, but it took a lot of letter writing, online searches, bids and networking to ultimately arrive at some of the tools I needed, in order to acquire the skills I looked for. *Cheetah traits: tact and strategy.* Many African institutions, however, are underfunded and do not have the capacity to support young fac-

ulty along a research career track. This means that one needs to actively compete for the limited global research funding opportunities for career support in order to develop. Counterintuitively, one needs to develop a robust enough portfolio to attract any significant funding. *Cheetah traits: while smaller than most carnivores in the wild, it must still use its inherent skills to tackle the same prey and fend off competitors.*

## 2.3    On Africa-Centered Solutions for Africa-Centered Research

How then do we shift the narrative around the deficits in research in academia in Africa? What innovations could we envision to address some of these needs? I founded the Pan African Women's Association of surgeons (PAWAS) in 2014 as a means of providing peer mentorship to women interested in or considering a career in surgery. *Cheetah trait: aerodynamic.* This provided an online platform for clinicians across Africa to consult over patients and share their successes and complications as an impetus to shared learning—our so-called popular 'gory Wednesdays'. It also provided a safe space to discuss common gendered and universal challenges such as unconscious biases, remuneration and mentorship concerns. As it has grown, PAWAS has evolved more into looking at some of the gaps in surgical residency and serving to expand the needs of the clinicians in the group. For the first time last year, PAWAS, in collaboration with AuthorAid, was able to have a mentorship cohort in research methodology.

This involved pairing a mentor and mentee to work on some aspect of research methodology, with the mentor and mentee partnering to develop the m'ntee's idea or project over a couple of months. The preliminary results and feedback were promising and are an area that could potentially be amplified going forward. *Cheetah trait: ultimately one of the most determined and successful hunters in the wild.* These efforts cannot stand alone and require an intentional restructuring of research approaches in institutions in Sub-

Saharan Africa (SSA) and their compensatory mechanisms. Real investment in local research including national funding opportunities and capacity building are needed along with grant support and administration. The basics of research methodology also need to be introduced early in medical school curriculums, along with more structured support for early career researchers.

## 2.4   On Gender Equity in the African Academy, and the Pregnancy Penalty

How do we then achieve a diverse, inclusive, academic community in this setting, that is also more engaged in research? This demands that we challenge old academic models of compensation, remuneration and support for research activities. *Cheetah trait: as one of the oldest living carnivores on the planet, it has had to continually evolve to succeed and thrive.* Unless we think critically about models that support both men and women in the workplace, we are bound to continue along the same trajectory. Early introduction of research into the undergraduate curriculum may provide an opportunity to develop an interest in research. Mainstreaming the audit of clinical outcomes in surgery, medicine etc., could serve as the basis for reflective clinical practice and a springboard for research ideas and development.

During the COVID-19 pandemic, the challenges faced by women in academia became even more apparent. Women scientists became less prolific due to expanding roles at home (Shamseer et al. 2021). How can we ensure productivity in the workplace as we move forward in this context of global change, to support all faculty? How can we customize this to African institutions? Practical measures in the workplace, such as creches and areas to breastfeed or express milk for mothering staff, can go a long way towards enabling productivity among working mothers. *Cheetah trait: mothering and conscientious caregiver.* Taking this a notch higher and offering on-site daycare services at institutions helps to ensure that mothers are more engaged. Clear actionable policies around maternity and paternity leave ensure a balanced outlook and wellness for all staff. While policies around these exist in many large institutions, victimization continues to occur at an individual level. Anecdotally, cases have been reported where academic clinicians have been forced to pay their institutions as a result of going on maternity leave. Other women have been compelled to not sit for their exams etc. while pregnant, even when they personally felt capable of doing so. Sadly, these cases are not unique (Matotoka and Odeku 2020; Fathima et al. 2020) and should give us pause in the process of developing a more inclusive workforce.

## 2.5   Take Me to Your Leader

Finally, there is a clear lack of female role models in the academic workforce. There is a dearth of leadership opportunities, coupled with the socialization in many cultures in low and middle-income countries (LMIC) where females are discouraged from speaking and are expected to be deferential. This results in a lack of female voices in leadership, even in traditionally women-led specialties like nursing. We need to develop different leadership styles and encourage networks that support young faculty, of all genders, providing them with the skills they need to develop into leaders. Having more women in leadership roles would certainly encourage individuals to take up these positions.

Conclusion: A paradigm shift is needed in our approaches to research and inclusion for the equitable and sustained advancement of global health partnerships. This will require a critical look at research models and creation of new opportunities to develop the desired research culture. The mission should be focused on the needs of Africans, driven by African expertise. *The cheetah's ingenuity, perseverance, tenacity and willingness to evolve are traits that would serve the African academic environment in its mission.*

## 3 The Female African Health and Global Policy-Maker By Dr. Jacqueline Kitulu

*Genus/ species: African elephant—Loxodonta Africana*

*Strengths: wise, long-suffering, resourceful*

*Weaknesses: Tendency to perseverate and dominate*

*The elephant is a community-based animal that is invested in family and community values. Towering at a great height the elephant is able to see the '30,000 foot view' or bigger picture. Due to their large size, elephants have a huge impact on the communities around them and are considered a 'keystone species" and can use this dominance either positively or negatively. Their contribution is largely positive. They generally co-exist peacefully with other species and are keen to look after and protect their own. Due to its excellent memory and recall, the elephant can occasionally get trapped in repeating the same patterns over and over again, despite changes in circumstances and new developments. In addition, positions of power are held till death suggesting a need to intentionally prepare for and transition leadership.*

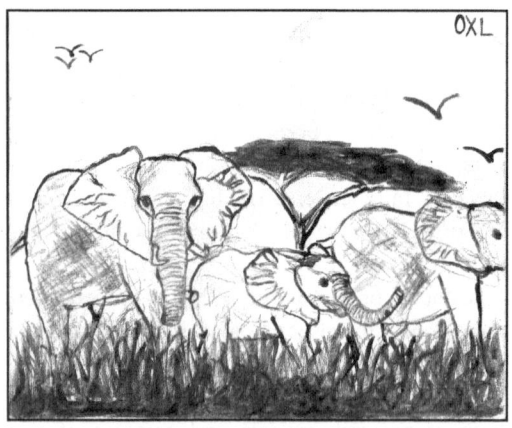

Elephant. Art by Orion Lavery

## 3.1 The Beginning of a Fortuitous End: Foundations in Leadership Development

As a trainee in medicine at one of the top medical schools in Kenya, completing my medical training at the University of Nairobi was my foremost concern at the time. *Elephant trait: wise.* Looking back now more than two decades, however, I realize that leadership, evasive as it might have seemed back then, was going to be an eminent part of my story. I was one of only ten ladies in a class of around 100 medical students. *Elephant trait: impactful.* This was a far cry from the all-girls high school that I attended, not an uncommon phenomenon in Kenya, where I led as a prefect in my senior years. But the lack of representation of women at my medical school did not stop at students. Our lecturers were majority male, and there were no female heads of departments.

After internship, the mandatory year of training one must complete after medical school in Kenya, I joined the Kenya Medical Women's Association (KMWA), an affiliate of The Medical Women's International Association (MWIA). This threw me into my first real experience in the leadership arena in the health sector. Not long after joining the organization, in 2006, I became the Assistant Treasurer for KMWA. Two years later, in an unexpected turn of events, I was elected National Chair of the Association, serving two terms from 2008 to 2012. I was privileged to receive generous mentorship from senior lady physicians in KMWA, and through leveraging partnerships, was able to reroute the association towards a successful future. *Elephant trait: community keystone.*

After this inaugural experience with national leadership, as they say, the rest was history. I was nominated to the National Economic and Social Council (NESC) from 2008 to 2014, a private sector team nominated by the country's President to spur economic and social development in Kenya towards achieving Vision 2030 (Vision 2030 Delivery Secretariat 2022). *Elephant trait: way-maker, little can stand in the way of this gentle giant.* This initiative aims to "transform Kenya into a newly industrializing, middle-income country providing a high quality of life to all its citizens by 2030 in a clean and secure environment." This gave me a novel experience in working with partners nationally and internationally, and across sectors.

In the 43-member council of the initiative, there were only three women– including myself. I soon came to be known as "Dr. Social Issues" as I consistently called out that all items on the agenda were matters on the economic pillar and seldom on the social pillar, which is where health lies. *Elephant trait: community-focused.* Consequently, it became my mission to push this important pillar to the forefront. I watched in dismay as time and again, our articulation of important matters in the health sector were overlooked. Our issues sounded like good "sob stories" that were returned with somber looks and tearful eyes but that did nothing to appeal to the policymakers. Ultimately, it became apparent that to effectively communicate across this chasm, they needed to hear the matters framed from a perspective of economic impact. I realized that if I was to impact any change in health policies through this group, I had to change how I framed health issues. *Elephant trait: versatile and deciphering.*

Around the same time, I began my pursuit of an MBA in Healthcare Management at the Strathmore Business School from 2014 to 2016. This was the most impactful training I received during my entire career because it shifted my world view from dealing with individual patients as a clinician, to striving to impact more people in the health policy space. In addition, I learned the language of the policymaker. *Elephant trait: effective communicator.* To that end, while formal training through a master's degree was the best option for me, other informal training in leadership and governance overall are still lacking, and could be harnessed to help advance more women into leadership positions in policy.

## 3.2 On Being a "One of One" and the Role of Male Mentorship in Developing Women Leaders

Concurrently, in 2012, the national umbrella professional association for doctors in Kenya—The Kenya Medical Association (KMA)—nominated me to sit on their National Executive Council as Assistant Secretary. Between 2012 and 2016 I was promoted from National Assistant Secretary to National Vice Chair, and in a ground-breaking election, to National Chair. As a result of my election to this position, I became the first ever female chair in the history of KMA In −016— after 48 years of the organization's existence! *Elephant trait: matriarchal lead tendencies.* This prestigious society led by and consisting mainly of senior male colleagues, suddenly had a female at the helm. I was relieved to find great mentors in senior male colleagues who enabled me to be my authentic self, quite different from any other leadership position that I had taken on before. In turn, they also made sure that I could step into leadership with my solid credentials backing me, but also bringing my emotional intelligence, respect, and willingness to collaborate with other like-minded societies.

My tenure saw a more collaborative approach to engaging with the Kenya Ministry of Health on matters related to the profession. This resulted in press statements signed by various medical associations. This was unprecedented, and I believe it resulted from relationships that were based around true partnership. We widened this to include societies across the health cadres so that instead of soloists, we could begin to act more like an orchestra playing a beautiful symphony in the health sector. We could begin to act more like an orchestra playing a beautiful symphony in the health sector. This was not easy as a siloed approach among the various health cadres had always prevailed in the sector, but I am proud to have been a part of the era that helped to realize this change.

I am a firm believer that women and men look at issues differently. If you don't have enough women in the room, health suffers. Kamani et al. in a recent paper highlighted the effectiveness of women in leadership during the COVID-19 pandemic. One of the core reasons was that women leaders have a "drive for equity." (Kamani et al. 2020) The Harvard Business Review highlights three contributions that women make that men are less likely to make in leadership as well: women broaden discussions representing a wide set of stakeholders, they are more dogged than men in pursuing answers to difficult quest–ons—perhaps as males feel a gender-based obligation to know everything, and women bring a collaborative approach to leadership. *Elephant trait: effective leaders.* This impact is best realized when there are at least three or more women in the proverbial room. I continue to aspire towards the day when I will no longer be the 'one of one', or the only in the room, as we seek more equitable outcomes in global health.

### 3.3 On Mentoring the Next Generation of Leaders and Policymakers

I am astutely aware that, given my own experiences, it is crucial to build a strong pipeline of female leaders to fill this space. Throughout my varied positions, I consistently encourage other lady doctors to join in the leadership space. An example of this impact, my second term as KMA president had a very cohesive and result-oriented national executive council that had four out of six members (five elected and the CEO) being female. This was unprecedented, as mentioned previously, given that the society had always been male dominated. Our tenures changed the look and feel of KMA to one that encouraged more females and youth to join via a very strong Young Doctors Network Committee. *Elephant trait: mothering, provider, caregiver.* Mentorship, in this way, has opened the doors for many others on the local and global stage in recent years. Ultimately, we need more women in the leadership space. As Sheryl Sandberg has famously been quoted to say, women need to "lean in." My own leadership journey, that began with a first courageous step, consequently led me to sit on

multiple different boards including the NHIF, The Kenya Medical Practitioners and Dentists Council, PATH Kenya Board, and Safaricom Health Advisory Committee to name a few. These opportunities have provided me with the opportunity to make an impact on the health sector and society as a whole.

### 3.4 On Encountering Leadership Among Global North and Global South Partners

In my role as president for KMA, I was also a delegate to the World Medical Association (WMA). There, I realized that I was once again underrepresented—in this case as an African delegate—and our voices seemed to be largely muted by other countries that had more sizeable delegations based on the respective size of the countries that they represented. I pushed for more collaboration with our fellow African Medical societies and served as Deputy Coordinator of the novel Coalition of African National Medical Associations (CANMA) bringing together sixteen countries that would help to push some of our agendas forward in a more concerted effort. *Elephant trait: community driven, herd mentality.* We even set up a legal entity. In sum, at The World Medical Association, I got KMA back to positively impacting the world stage. I am delighted to report that this will ensure we can "sit at the table" having become members of various committees. Furthermore, I ensured that we had representative participation during the election process for WMA. In 2023 for the first time ever, KMA will host the WMA Council session in Kenya. This experience showed me that intentionality and inclusive partnership across South-South partners is also key.

### 3.5 On Maintaining One's Roots

As a physician by training, I believe firmly that maintaining a close link between clinical practice and policy has been important in my career. I still maintain a foot in both worlds, continuing with a primary care clinic load that I love. I also see this as crucial to test the policy on the ground! Sometimes the theory is not practical. I have seen the value of being in clinical practice demonstrated in my roles in the boards over and over. Each time I go back to see my patients, I immediately see the impact of policy decisions and can take the feedback to improve on the policy table. Our spheres of impact do not have to be mutually exclusive, and in fact are very complementary in my mind.

Finally, I would be remiss not to highlight the importance of a support network from the family which for me has constituted a firm base—and one that has certainly enabled me to excel. I have brought my family into my world by involving them as much as I can in my leadership activities, and they have given me the room to go out and be the change I want to see! If it were not for them, this would not have been possible. For that reason, I also advocate for transformative change in communities that would rigorously support women in leadership.

Conclusion: More women leaders are needed across all sectors. Increased access or pathways to leadership for young girls and women, increased capacity-building and training for women leaders, mentorship, willingness to take initiative by the women themselves, and openness among communities are all key to realizing equity at these levels. The traits of the elephant: wise, herd-driven, and with effusive matriarchal strengths in leadership, also highlight key points for the way forward in gender equity for academia.

## 4 The Diaspora Perspective: The Good, the Bad and the Opportunity Quotient

*Genus/ species: Black rhinoceros—Diceros bicornis*

*Strengths: Strong, close relationship with offspring until completely weaned, strong sense of hearing*

*Weaknesses: Tendency towards solitude, nervous and untrusting, 'tunnel vision'/poor eyesight*

*Rhinos tend towards solitude in adulthood, and while caring for the next generation inti-*

*mately for a prolonged period, they otherwise fend for themselves. Given their poor vision and resultant short-sightedness, they tend to charge blindly even at the most benign obstacles; this also comes from feeling easily threatened. Once other rhinos are in their pack, if challenged or under threat, they group together and charge as one. They are have excellent hearing, are intelligent, emotional, and expressive of their feelings. By comparison, the diasporan can sever ties by approaching partnerships brashly and in a short-sighted nature. While there may be a tendency towards working alone, this is actually the quickest way to shortchange trusting relationships and effective change.*

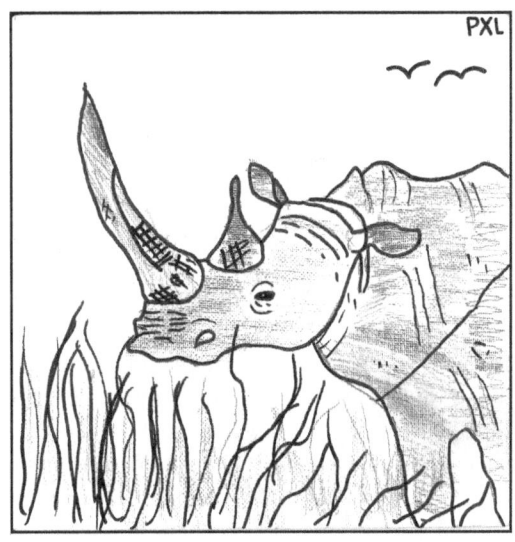

Rhinoceros. Art by Phoenix Lavery

The unique position of the African diasporan is one that lies at the intersection of cultural appreciation and lived experience in the Africa context, and experience and knowledge in navigating Western institutions. It is also one that constitutes an as-yet poorly tapped population in global health and global health partnership-building today. Meanwhile, the diasporan struggles with opportunities to contribute to their home context in Africa. For women, these issues are compounded on a gendered basis.

The term "African diasporan" has had varied definitions as far as which population it encompasses. For the sake of this section, I will use the term to refer to "Africans abroad" or those of

"African descent who live outside of their ancestral continent" (Colin Palmer 1998). I will particularly hone in on the relationships involving those diasporans living in High Income Countries (HICs) such as the US and UK, given my own personal experiences as well as the recent spotlight by the decolonization movement on best practices for engagement by those in HICs (Abimbola and Pai 2020) (see chapters "Colonialism, Decolonization, and Global Health" and "Gender Equity in African Academia: An Implementation Science Evaluation of the Kenya Context"). This movement seeks to take on power differentials that leave those in LMICs—a majority of African countries—with the short end of the stick. Decolonization should be incorporated into discussions around how African diasporans engage with partners on the continent.

## 4.1     The Good

The role for African diasporans living outside of their ancestral country positions them as ideal bridges to partnerships between the diverse cultures and regions which they inhabit and rear from, respectively. They have the unique opportunity to do so by overcoming common barriers to global health partnerships such as cultural understanding, language, and establishing trust. They are experts through lived experience, training and/or academic careers on the continent. As such, they are able to contribute to enhancing global partnerships through knowledge sharing on navigating the host and ancestral country's work environments. *Rhino trait: groups together.* This might include awareness of key organizations in each respective country for a given subject or expertise area, familiarity with cornerstone stakeholders and their roles in the given subject or expertise area, and knowledge of grant sources for both sites. They may also bring insights on ideal outlets for reporting outcomes from projects such as key conferences to attend or major academic journals from each of the respective nations. Additionally, the desire to engage in partnerships has been demonstrated to be inherently preferred by those hailing from these African nations, as is the case for many diasporans (Madhukar Pai 2022). So, why then, has the focus on Africans abroad as instrumental in establishing global health partnerships lagged, and why have interventions to ensure increased availability for such roles not been put in place?

## 4.2     The Bad: Conventional Frameworks for Global Health Partnerships Prevail as the Mainstay for Global Health Relationships

Collaborative opportunities for global health research and collaboration between partners in the global North and the global South have conventionally revolved around relationships with longstanding organizations such as the Kenya Medical Research Institute (KEMRI)-Wellcome Trust program (McCall 2014), with origins, source funding, or persistent funding in this case, from Western nations. With increased development and time, formidable institutions that have originated on the continent have grown, such as the KEMRI (KEMRI 2023) and the African Academy of Sciences (The African Academy of Sciences 2023). More African diasporans continue to seek to build bridges, or in fact wholly repatriate in Africa (Madhukar Pai 2022; Minta 2007). However, it is often difficult for these individuals to establish partnerships, jobs, or meaningful interactions with these Africa-based institutions. This is due in part to lack of social networks, know-how on navigating institution-specific infrastructure, or resources to afford travel and other networking opportunities, thus limiting connections and sustained partnerships. In sum, establishing new global health partnerships as a diasporan may be intimidating or even wholly unattainable as the predominant partnerships are dominated by a small quorum of impenetrable networks. These issues are further compounded for women in the diaspora, many of which I have experienced personally, and the reasons for this are further explored below.

## 4.3 The Bad: The One that Responded—On Personal Challenges to Engaging with Africa-Based Counterparts

As far as establishing partnerships on an individual basis, and spearheading connections on behalf of an organization/ institution, a common challenge is how to get started. My own journey started with initiative, which entailed "cold-calling" and "cold-emailing" everyone — and every institution — that I could remember from growing up in Kenya as a child in attempting to identify potential collaborators to partner with. *Rhino trait: imposing stature can easily give the wrong impression.* To be sure, I was young, bright-eyed and bushy-tailed, and didn't have much guidance on how to go about this despite well-intentioned mentors in the US. *Rhino trait: clumsy.* As a result, this process led to a series of open and shut doors that in turn led to my career today—because someone finally responded. This path was marked by organizational red tape, bureaucracy, and a significant amount of personal funds, such as for travel and project work, before I had stable partnerships or grant funding, among other roadblocks.

As intimidating as these factors seemed, the barrier that I found the most challenging and surprising was a lurking suspicion of me—as a diasporan—and the steady treatment as an outsider. *Rhino trait: anomalous, different from other species.* As a returning diasporan, having finally completed my medical school and residency and making a solid income as a fellow, I was eager to go back to what I considered "home" and to be able to contribute. But this benevolence (at least on my end) was hardly matched by the reception that I received. In fact, it was quite the contrary. This is probably best encapsulated by an early experience where one organization categorically stated that they would not work with me unless I was "mentoring a Kenyan trainee" as part of a project. It was a wakeup call. I, a Kenyan trainee myself (as a fellow, pursuing a master's degree at the time) would not suffice. But there was also the softer side of intangible discomfort with me as foreign ("when is the last time you were in Kenya?"), as representing the unknown ("are you really Kenyan? Do you still speak Swahili?"), as being perceived as a potential threat and an assumption that I thought that I was "better than" those on the ground in one way or another. Looking back, I realize that this could have easily curtailed my global health career if not for my perseverance and dogged commitment to what really mattered—a focus on improving public health and the people that my work affects. At the time, I lacked key mentorship to facilitate what I now know was better navigation of my privilege as an African abroad (Madhukar Pai 2022; Nixon 2019). *Rhino trait: charging blindly.* Many years and relationships later, thanks to my own reflection, grant support, and experience, this has led to multiple collaborations with different partners, countless academic outputs, grants, and hundreds of trainees and junior scientists taught or mentored.

All the same, it is incumbent upon diasporans to be well-equipped to approach home institution partnerships with humility. Equity should be the cornerstone of those relationships. I also trust that systems in HIC institutions and governments that have the capacity to regulate equity in relationships with LMIC sites, will do better to protect LMIC partners in the future on issues such as authorship, grants administration, and project directions. Finally, I continue to hope that the trepidation, fear, and sometimes even disapproval of the diasporan (I still see some of it today) that pervades novel partnerships with partners based in LMICs will continue to wane as protective systems, exposure, and increased mindfulness in navigating partnerships increases. Capacity building and leadership training for LMIC trainees and junior scientists can also contribute to equitable partnerships and averting missed opportunities that might occur due to misplaced assumptions.

## 4.4 Missing the Diaspora Opportunity Quotient

While diasporans have been cited to contribute upwards of $58 billion annually (Ratha 2021) to the African continent, constituting significant portions of whole country GDPs in some cases, I would argue that much more in terms of knowledge and human resource capacity strengthening could occur. The infrastructure to facilitate this simply has not taken off at the same rate as opportunities to facilitate money transfer (The World Bank 2020). The reasons likely center around the immediacy of the need for money. However, we should not lose sight of the importance of long-term investments such as those to help overturn limited human resources due to migration and brain drain (African Union 2018). In the 2011 book "Diaspora for Development in Africa", Ratha and Plaza highlight that in addition to money transfer, buildings, wells, and other such physical structures constitute the majority of contributions made to the continent (Ratha and Sonia 2011).

Meanwhile, I see a gap in opportunity to advance the human resource quotient, while tapping into an accessible population—diasporans. I propose that human resources and skills investment should be accessed in the academic or global health realm through: making visiting professorships accessible, publicizing job positions or opportunities through diaspora networks with clear routes to facilitate resettlement, and facilitating partnership-based grant applications that encourage Africa-based/ diaspora-based research partnership initiatives. This is not to say that continued capacity-building on the continent should not continue. Rather we can think of ways to strategically enhance the existing capacity through tapping into our own "resources"—human resources. *Rhino trait: resourceful and strong.* This may not be the correct approach for all sectors.

Where gaps in skillsets exist (World Economic Forum 2019), I propose prioritizing the pool of diasporans instead of off-shoring contracts to expensive consultants from Western nations who may or may not have the continent's best interest or cultural appreciation at heart. This example is best demonstrated by the brain drain of Africa's health professionals (Zimbudzi 2013). This could be tempered through the creation of channels for contributions from diasporans such as visiting clinical opportunities, establishing specialty training programs for those with advanced training that may not currently be available in the host

country, and optimizing and legitimizing tele-health channels. The pathway to return as a clinician once trained abroad is fraught with challenges, expensive re-certifications, and no promise of placement in one's specialty/ specialty expertise, or of a job position. These are missed opportunities.

The Carnegie Mellon program is a prime example of a successful program that facilitates diaspora scholar visiting opportunities at African institutions (iie 2023). The exchange can be North-South or South-South in nature. The program was founded fairly recently in 2012, but has been successful in already placing and funding more than 500 scholars to date. Limitations include that the program only supports placement in six African countries, and funding (while laudable) is limited. I propose that African countries as well as African institutions should build strategic plans that make these and other such opportunities for exchange the norm rather than the exception. Rather than being supported by external funding that may not be sustainable, the responsibility should be turned over to local universities that have the capacity to plan and incorporate this sustainably if prioritized.

At the international level, the African Union should also develop fora for discussion on this, as well as set targets or mandates for member states to develop improved policies on diaspora collaboration and resettlement.

African countries too need to see the value of the diaspora beyond solvent cash, and such programs like Carnegie Mellon could easily be replicated and augmented in terms of their scope. *Rhino impacts: an endangered species where protections have not been implemented by countries, devaluating it and causing further dwindling of its presence.* Ghana's president Nana Akufo-Addo previously stated with reference to Ghana that "we believe we have a responsibility to extend a hand of welcome back home to Africans in the diaspora," and in 2019, the country explicitly focused on tapping the diaspora through a movement dubbed the "Year of Return." This initiative not only saw a surge in new visitors to the country but also brought a $2 billion surge in the economy (BBC News 2020). The "Right of Abode" policy

(Dovi 2015) passed by the country in 2000 allows a person of African descent to apply and be granted the right to stay in Ghana indefinitely. These and other priorities have contributed to a rise in resettlement in Ghana. More should be done in other African countries.

Moreover, development agencies and funders with work on the African continent could increase opportunities for contributions by diasporans, while acknowledging the key importance of elevating Africans based on the continent. This could be done by recruiting African diasporans for key positions that are not filled by Africa-based counterparts, developing unique partnership roles in their organizations that are filled by diasporans, and providing opportunities or pathways to repatriate through positions. Additionally, funders and agencies should encourage Africa-based and African diasporans alike to be in leadership positions that drive the mission and funding priorities of their organizations. *Rhino impacts: outsiders can observe, appreciate and avoid poaching.*

Universities based in HICs can also play a role in developing strategic programs that facilitate partnerships with Africa-based institutions. They can facilitate diaspora participation or involvement in their home country which otherwise may be challenging for individuals. At Yale University, President Peter Salovey spearheaded the Yale Africa Initiative (Yale Africa Initiative 2023) "a university-wide effort to prioritize and expand Yale's commitment to Africa." This effort highlights both organizational partnerships as well as individually led activities (including those of diaspora) by faculty, staff and students at the university. The President took an inaugural trip (for a Yale president, and one of the first of any US university president) to the continent and highlighted this work, including those of Yale diaspora Africans, while visiting their respective countries. These diasporans were invited to attend the trip as delegates and to help formulate the nature of the program. This simple act of sponsorship and inclusion also contributed to advancing their existing networks and contributed in enriching the content of these trips (Fuchs 2018).

Finally, individuals in the diaspora of HICs can also play a role in advancing partnerships and spotlight key issues on the continent. This author (CN) spearheaded the "Through the Eyes of She" conference in 2021, a virtual conference that highlighted "equity in health, education, business and leadership for the African Woman in the twenty-first Century." (Yale Macmillan Center Council on African Studies 2023) Specifically, this unique conference brought together 500 registered attendees from Africa, Africa diaspora, and HIC counterparts (primarily in the US, and affiliated with Yale) to discuss these issues through didactics, discussion, and workshops. This program is now codified as a sustained program through Yale for perpetuity. Naturally, the funding and logistics of coordinating such novel programs may be challenging for individuals. HIC university infrastructure that prioritizes and facilitates such opportunities will be beneficial.

Conclusion: African diasporans sit at a unique intersection that bodes well for global health partnerships in Africa. However, navigating the challenges of privilege, trust, and intersectional disparities in funding, leadership and job opportunities short-change the potential for their success. *The rhino, while sometimes short-sighted and clumsy in approach, is resourceful, strong and unique; its value could be better appreciated and its rich resource put to better, long-term gain by outsiders and locals alike.*

## 5    Conclusions

There is a burgeoning role for women in the workplace, in global health and in academic spaces, especially in Sub-Saharan Africa. There is a need to build a diverse and inclusive global health workforce to improve global public health outcomes. These solutions will include ensuring women across the pipeline are included in global health partnerships in the Africa context, for example, through inclusion of early career women in research consortia or memoranda of understanding. Additionally, mentorship and training to match these efforts should be implemented to ensure the pipeline has the necessary skillsets to match what is needed for respective roles. The old adage "teach a man (or woman, equitably in this case) to fish…" holds true here. The promotion and advancement of women from Africa-based institutions and global health organizations is also key. Organizations must create appropriate interventions to offset challenges with maternity leave and childcare, and tackle the pervasive disparities in remuneration by increasing transparency in salaries. Furthermore, the diasporan can contribute to enhancing the number and content of partnerships based on existing commitment to one's home country/ country of origin, knowledge of diverse country cultures, and ability to connect networks from each setting. Deliberate efforts to develop institutional, in-country, regional and international collaborations and strategies are key to enabling the full participation of all genders in developing and implementing effective solutions for global health in the twenty-first century.

# References

Abimbola S, Pai M. Will global health survive its decolonisation? Lancet. 2020;396(10263):1627–8.

African Union. The revised migration policy framework for Africa and plan of action (2018–2027); 2018.

BBC News. African diaspora: did Ghana's year of return attract foreign visitors? 2020. Available from: https://www.bbc.com/news/world-africa-51191409

Colin Palmer. Defining and studying the modern African Diaspora. 1998 [January 2023]. Available from: https://www.historians.org/research-and-publications/perspectives-on-history/september-1998/defining-and-studying-the-modern-african-diaspora

Crisp N, Chen L. Global supply of health professionals. N Engl J Med. 2014;370(10):950–7.

Dovi E. African-Americans resettle in Africa. 2015. Available from: https://www.un.org/africarenewal/magazine/april-2015/african-americans-resettle-africa

Fathima FN, Awor P, Yen YC, Gnanaselvam NA, Zakham F. Challenges and coping strategies faced by female scientists-a multicentric cross sectional study. PLoS One. 2020;15(9):e0238635.

Fuchs H. Salovey visits Ghana, Kenya. 2018 [March 2018]. Available from: https://yaledailynews.com/blog/2018/03./28/salovey-visits-ghana-kenya/

iie. Carnegie African Diaspora Fellowship Program. 2023 [February 2023]. Available from: https://www.iie.org/programs/carnegie-african-diaspora-fellowship-program

Kamani L, et al. Redesigning the landscape for women and leadership: insights gained from the Covid-19 pandemic. On Behalf of Women in Gastroenterology Network Asia Pacific (WIGNAP) and Women in Endoscopy (WIE). Clin Endosc. 2020;53(5):620–2.

KEMRI. 2023 [February 2023]. Available from: https://www.kemri.go.ke/background/

Koplan JP, Bond TC, Merson MH, Reddy KS, Rodriguez MH, Sewankambo NK, et al. Towards a common definition of global health. Lancet. 2009;373:1993–5.

Madhukar Pai. Double Agents in Global Health. 2022 [February 2023]. Available from: https://www.forbes.com/sites/madhukarpai/2022/02/06/double-agents-in-global-health/?sh=4a7c200c1a2e

Matotoka MD, Odeku KO. Discrimination on the grounds of pregnancy, denial of maternity leave and lack of conducive environment for nursing mother in the workplace in South Africa. Obiter. 2020;41(3):593–607.

McCall B. Profile: KEMRI-Wellcome Trust Programme celebrates 25 years. Lancet. 2014;383(9931):1796.

McCall B, et al. Storytelling as a research tool used to explore insights and as an intervention in public health: a systematic narrative review. Int J Public Health. 2021;66

Minta K. The Reverse Diaspora: African Immigrants and the Return Home. Undergraduate Humanities Forum 2006–7: Travel. 2007;10. https://repository.upenn.edu/uhf_2007/10

Nixon SA. The coin model of privilege and critical allyship: implications for health. BMC Public Health. 2019;19(1):1637.

Ratha D. Keep remittances flowing to Africa. 2021 February 2023. Available from: https://www.brookings.edu/blog/africa-in-focus/2021/03/15/keep-remittances-flowing-to-africa/

Ratha D, Sonia P. Diaspora for development in Africa. World Bank. © World Bank. 2011. https://openknowledge.worldbank.org/handle/10986/2295.License: CC BY 3.0 IGO

Rieger KL, et al. Elevating the uses of storytelling approaches within Indigenous health research: a critical and participatory scoping review protocol involving Indigenous people and settlers. Syst Rev. 2020;9(1):257.

Shamseer L, Bourgeault I, Grunfeld E, Moore A, Peer N, Straus SE, Tricco AC. Will COVID-19 result in a giant step backwards for women in academic science? J Clin Epidemiol. 2021;134:160–6. https://doi.org/10.1016/j.jclinepi.2021.03.004. Epub 2021 Mar 8. PMID: 33705957.

The African Academy of Sciences. 2023. Available from: https://www.aasciences.africa/about

The World Bank. COVID-19: Remittance Flows to Shrink 14% by 2021. [2020 February 2023]. Available from: https://www.worldbank.org/en/news/press-release/2020/10/29/covid-19-remittance-flows-to-shrink-14-by-2021?utm_source=Triggermail&utm_medium=email&utm_campaign=Post%20Blast%20bii-payments-and-commerce:%20Legacy%20remittance%20firms%20could%20emerge%20strong

Vision 2030 Delivery Secretariat. Kenya Vision 2030. 2022 [January 2023]. Available from: https://vision2030.go.ke/

World Economic Forum. Why the skills gap remains wider in Africa. 2019 [February 2023]. Available from: https://www.weforum.org/agenda/2019/09/why-the-skills-gap-remains-wider-in-africa/

World Health Organization. Global strategy on human resources for health: workforce 2030. Geneva: WHO; 2016.

Yale Africa Initiative. 2023 [January 2023]. Available from: https://world.yale.edu/yale-africa-initiative

Yale Macmillan Center Council on African Studies: Through the eyes of she. Our Mission. 2023 [February 2023]. Available from: https://african.macmillan.yale.edu/through-eyes-she/our-mission

Zimbudzi E. Stemming the impact of health professional brain drain from Africa: a systemic review of policy options. J Public Health Afr. 2013;4(1):e4.

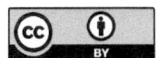

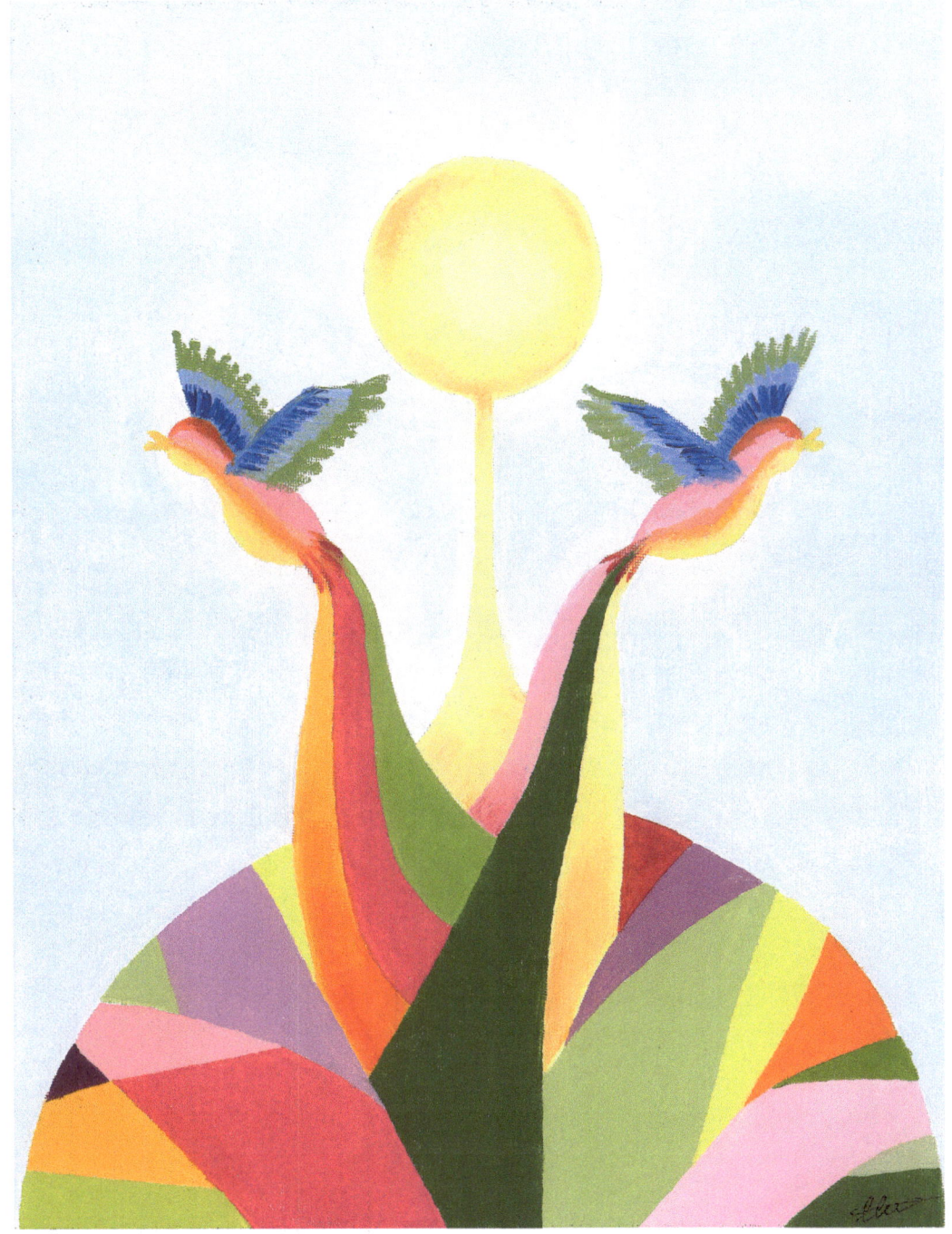

"What is yet to be" by Mira Cheng

# Transforming the Planetary Health Crisis Through an Indigenous Land-Based Meta-Narrative

Nicole Redvers and Kelly Menzel

*"Let's do our work in a world not full of resources but full of relatives"*

~Dan Wildcat

## Abstract

Our current biodiversity, pollution, climate change, and pandemic crises are deep and complex yet have similar underpinnings and a clear road map out. Indigenous Peoples have long asserted the importance of their enduring and dynamic relationship to ancestral lands, seas, waterways, and wildlife as a protective road map for people and the planet. As we are all dynamic beings with the potential for direct kinship relationships to all planetary elements ranging from the micro to the macro level, it leaves open the possibility of large-scale and emergent positive change. This means that as action-based planetary relatives, we can all enact great change around us by precipitating these emergent processes within our own bodies and in the environment around us. Therefore, we provide an interconnected narrative that centers Land and Country, our Ancestors, and story as we consider the path we need to walk going forward. We premise that the story we need to co-walk is an ecologically derived one with the complexity of the world expressed through the simplicity of being of Nature.

## Keywords

Indigenous Peoples · Traditional knowledge · Planetary health · LAND-based · Climate change

N. Redvers (✉)
Schulich School of Medicine & Dentistry, University of Western Ontario, London, ON, Canada

Arctic Indigenous Wellness Foundation, Yellowknife, NT, Canada
e-mail: nredvers@uwo.ca

K. Menzel
Gnibi College of Indigenous Australian Peoples, Southern Cross University, Lismore, Australia
e-mail: kelly.menzel@scu.edu.au

## Author Perspective

We are Indigenous Scholars seeking to amplify Indigenous voices and to uplift strengths-based dialogues from within Indigenous Nations to improve relations between individual, community, and planetary health. We are committed to challenging race-based violence in institutions; decolonizing systems; understanding and exploring Indigenous Knowledge Systems; and challenging and decolonizing Western, anthropocentric approaches to planetary health. From Australia to the sub-Arctic Canada, we root our work in relationship to Land and Country.

A. Stewart Ibarra, A. D. LaBeaud (eds.), *Transforming Global Health Partnerships*, Sustainable Development Goals Series, https://doi.org/10.1007/978-3-031-53793-6_19

### Key Concepts and Tenants for Indigenous Global Health Partnerships

1. **Relational obligation:** Relationality means that one experiences the self as a part of others, and that others are part of the self (Walters et al. 2020; Tynan 2021). Relationality is learned from stories—listening and watching Elders and community members 'story' or 'yarn' while sitting with Land or Country. Relationality is an informed practice bound with responsibilities to planetary kin and Land or Country (Tynan 2021). Therefore, to enact relational obligation in practice is to feel the world as kin and to enact a relational ethos with the responsibilities and accountabilities that accompany it (Tynan 2020).

2. **Autonomous regard:** A specific form of conduct and ethical disposition that evokes the lawful relationship of the self with the world by the process of actively considering, weighing, and scaling one's relations with others and the world (Briggs and Graham 2021). Autonomous regard enables such diverse relations (i.e., relational obligation) and "necessarily promotes ways of being that resonate with classical virtues in diverse traditions — qualities such as temperance, humility, self-management, and prudence" (Briggs and Graham 2021).

3. **Indigenous self-determination:** Article 3 of the United Nations Declaration on the Rights of Indigenous Peoples (UNDRIP) states, "Indigenous Peoples have the right of self-determination. By virtue of that right they freely determine their political status and freely pursue their economic, social and cultural development" (United Nations 2007). Understanding UNDRIP and Free, Prior, and Informed Consent (FPIC) concerning Indigenous Peoples under UNDRIP are fundamental to any potential partnerships with individuals, communities, and/or Indigenous Nations (Food and Agriculture Organization of the United Nations 2021).

4. You can never be an expert in Indigenous Nations or on Indigenous Peoples. Honor the collective expertise and local knowledge within Indigenous communities by 'listening' and 'relating' to support their planetary health solutions.

5. We are no more important than the tiniest ant with our gifts and roles in a collective community. Remain humble in what is known and not clearly apparent. Remember in the struggle that you are in and of Nature—a part of her.

6. Indigenous knowledges are not owned but stewarded carefully by Indigenous Peoples through strict protocols of living and relating to the world. The knowledge does not exist without Indigenous Peoples and their sovereign rights in any circumstance.

7. This chapter addresses the following SDGs: #3 Good health and well-being, #12 Responsible consumption and production, #13 Take urgent action to combat climate change and its impacts, #5: Achieve gender equality and empower all women and girls, #17 Partnership for the Goals.

## 1    Introduction

Indigenous Peoples have long asserted the importance of their enduring relationship to ancestral lands, seas, waterways, and wildlife. We know that if a person or community is disconnected from Land or Country (see *Glossary*), or the Land or Country itself is ill, this can lead to illness in the person and the community (Albrecht 2005). This illness can be referred to as "crying for country" (Westerman 2004). More specifically, Westerman (Westerman 2004) realized a condition termed "longing for, crying for, or being sick for country (Westerman 2004)." The cause of this condition is the dislocation of the person from Land or Country, or from their "dreaming place" for extended periods of time or as a result of distress caused by damage to and destruction of Land or Country (including from that of climactic change). Additionally, solastalgia is a form of psychic or existential distress caused by environmental change, such as loss of or removal from Land or Country (Albrecht 2005). The condition of "Crying for Country" and the concept of solastaglia are fundamental foundations to understanding our response to and the lasting effects of the multiple interrelated crises occurring on the planet.

We, as Indigenous Peoples, do intimately feel the constant stress currently placed upon the ecosystem (solastaglia) and the resulting ill health of Mother Earth ("crying for country") because we are of her—existentially, physically, spiritually, socially, and emotionally. We position ourselves explicitly here in this narrative as descendants of our ancestors, the Ngadjuri Peoples of the mid-north of South Australia and the Bundjalung Peoples of far northern New South Wales (K.M), where sovereignty was never ceded, and the Dene Peoples of Denendeh, located in Treaty 8 territory in sub-Arctic Canada (N.R). Despite our variant geographies and traditional protocols, we are deeply interconnected in worldview and purpose.

As Indigenous Peoples, we have learned, adapted, and have been forced to "walk in two worlds" (Styres et al. 2010) while navigating complex and colonized systems. In general, "walking in two worlds" (Styres et al. 2010) or more specifically our "Two-Eyed Seeing" perspective (i.e., "the gift of multiple perspectives" (Bartlett et al. 2012)) enables our Indigenous Nations to be leaders in supporting Mother Earth while also acting as an important conduit for solutions to complex health and eco-systems management, climate change, and sustainability processes. Indigenous leadership is firmly predicated, however, on acknowledging our Land and rights on the road to reconciliation of people, communities, and the planet.

Our current biodiversity, pollution, climate change, and pandemic crises are deep and complex yet have similar underpinnings and a clear road map out from our perspective. *We need to remember where we come from.* For the Dene Peoples of Denendeh, the word *De* means flows, and *ne* means land. The Dene Peoples flow from the Land ("we come from the land") (Redvers 2016), and are therefore directly interconnected with it. This means that to understand any crisis as it pertains to people, communities, and the planet, we need to deeply understand our interconnection with Land and Country through the concept of *relationality*.

Relationality is a fundamental tenet of Indigenous Peoples' way of valuing, knowing, being, and doing. Relationality requires us to understand and embody our connections with all things "… and consider what it means to live as part of the world, rather than distinct from it" (Country et al. 2016). For Bawaka et al. (2016), "everyone and everything is in a bounded relationship to each other […] so this relationality is both bounded and constituted through flows and relationships" (Country et al. 2016, p. 460). Relationality also refers to the web of interconnectedness, the intersectionality between all things. Dudgeon and Bray (Dudgeon and Bray 2019, p. 4) contend that "Indigenous relationality is recognized as the life force, and that which supports and nourishes life." Greenwood (2005) further encapsulates the relational nature of Indigenous ways of valuing, knowing, being, and doing:

> The foundations of Indigeneity, then, are comprised, in part, of values that privilege interrelationships among the spiritual, the natural, and the self; reflect a sacred orientation to place and space; encompass a fluidity of knowledge exchanged between past, present, and future, thereby allowing for constant and dynamic knowledge growth and change…
>
> (Greenwood 2005, p. 554)

We firmly agree that our multiple crises, including the COVID-19 pandemic and the climate crisis itself, are "a relationship problem" (O'Brien 2020). Yet, despite our communities' essential knowledges, and being at the frontline of witnessing climate change, Indigenous voices generally have not been adequately privileged or acknowledged in mainstream scientific, institutional, global health, or planetary health dialogues—irrespective of the plethora of Indigenous scholars, community, and cultural expertise (Ratima 2019; Ratima et al. 2019; Redvers 2018; Redvers et al. 2020a; Whyte 2017; Jones 2019). An Australian glossary on Health and Climate Change was recently launched by 'leading' climate-change scholars at the University of Sydney in Australia (Zhang et al. 2021). This document failed to include Indigenous voices or Indigenous scholars, did not include any definitions or details about the complex nature of Indigenous knowledge systems, nor were the concepts of a holistic relationship to Land or Country discussed. These glaring and significant omissions perpetuate the silencing of Indigenous voices and uplift colonial ideology in the mainstream climate and health debate—which ultimately harms us all.

Colonialism is grounded in the tenets of othering and marginalizing and the perpetuation of systemic race-based violence. These underpinning tenets are evident in the disconnected and dislocated manner in which Western capitalist society often engages with diverse groups, the planet, and all beings that inhabit it. This has wrought havoc on all beings and eco-systems. Thus, it makes it even more crucial that global and planetary health endeavors are hinged upon a decolonial framework and practice that place Indigenous Peoples, communities, and voices at the forefront of expertise in their own right (Gram et al. 2021). This may be our last hope for a healthy and sustainable future for our grandchildren.

## 2  Proper Story, Rights Story, and Wrong Story

Our Indigenous colleague, Dr. Tyson Yunkaporta, a member of the Apalech Clan in the far north of Queensland, Australia, recently penned an essay explaining why "[a]ll our landscapes are broken (Yunkaporta 2021)." Dr. Yunkaporta discusses the Indigenous knowledge system concepts of "proper story, rights story, and wrong story" (Yunkaporta 2021). *Proper story* (the way we are supposed to be living in dynamic balance), *rights story* (our Indigenous Natural Laws that underpin how we live), and *wrong story* (how society currently operates) are framing concepts that can help us understand planetary boundaries and our place within them. Dr. Yunkaporta states more specifically that "… [p]roper story is a living landscape model that allows you to make accurate predictions, shows you the limits and obligations of your relationship with the Land, and teaches you how to move with it as it transforms over time" (Yunkaporta 2021). *Proper story*, therefore, can be seen as a culmination of collective and dynamic story knowledge that embodies proper knowledge transmission mechanisms within communities and songline knowledges (i.e., ancestral knowledges) from countless community knowledge holders who have stewarded and spoken for different areas and diverse ecosystems over millennia. *Proper story* decentralizes and distributes capital, power, and governance structures,

> …throughout social systems in patterns that align with the complex ecosystems … [and i]n this way, story speaks the law that is in the Land. [The law of the Land is the foundation of] … rights story, which regenerates every entity of the landscape in perpetuity, including our own species, the custodial species of the Earth.
>
> (Yunkaporta 2021)

*Rights story* is a necessary underpinning of sustainable and equitable planetary health endeavors, including both adaptation and transformations in addressing ecosystems' collapse and planetary ill health. *Rights story* is a strengths-based perspective that can pave the way forward. We can conceptualize *rights story* through Natural or First Law (i.e., the law of the Land). "Indigenous Peoples associate their own laws with the laws of the natural world, which are formally known as or translated as Natural or First Law" (Redvers et al. 2020b). Natural Law or First Law clearly characterizes our reciprocal responsibility to Mother Earth as it has been passed on for generations. Following Natural, or First Law, avoids being in a state of *wrong story.*

*Wrong story* is grounded in the disconnection from ecosystems, unequal power differentials that prioritize inequitable expansion, and emphasize profit growth as the underlying incentive.

When *wrong story* is the foundation of systems development, the wrong model emerges, and "it can only result in self-terminati[ng] algorithms in every landscape, even digital ones (Yunkaporta 2021)." Consequently, Mother Earth and all her beings endure deeply and profoundly the ongoing catastrophic effects of this *wrong story* modeling. Currently, this *wrong story* continues to facilitate ongoing colonialism and ecocide, which needs to be nullified and redirected to a new *proper story* and *rights story*. This is urgent and emergent and can pave the way for a strengths-based approach to healing Land and Country, complex ecosystems, and ourselves.

> The culture's vitality is literally dependent on individuals, in community with the natural world. Indigenous cultures are an extension of the story of the natural community of a place and evolve according to ecological dynamics and natural relationships.
>
> (Cajete 2018)

## 3     The Path We Walk

In some traditional medicine systems, the lungs are intimately connected with feelings of grief. It could be said that the COVID-19 pandemic was Mother Earth grieving through our lungs. Through our Indigenous knowledges, there is purpose and meaning in everything as long as we keep our eyes and other senses open to receiving this purpose and meaning. What is key is that we not only listen with all senses, but embody the messages the Land gives us and take it forward with us on our journeys and in our decisions.

Our Haudenosaunee brothers and sisters have a core value that represents this embodiment called the "Seventh Generation Principle." The "Seventh Generation Principle" ensures that any decision we make must consider those who are not born yet, as they will inherit the world (Haudenosaunee Confederacy n.d.; Miller et al. 2008). As we are borrowing the world from future generations, we must treat Mother Earth with great respect and keep our teachings alive through our cultures so this respect can be actioned in a good way. The "Seventh Generation Principle" is intergenerational equity in action.

Our Elders are clear with us that to be able to steward our knowledges and contribute to our communities in "a good way," we must first ensure we ourselves are in dynamic balance. It is sometimes hard to imagine how just one person can make a difference in this complex world; however, it is the complexity itself that allows for this to happen. When we spend focused time and sit in relationship with Land and Country, we start to remember who we really are. This is why Indigenous Peoples' sacred ceremonies are always interconnected with Land and Country—the two are indivisible. When you remember through Land relationship who you really are, you are better able to give away your special gifts to others. We become true planetary relatives when we give our gifts away instead of hoarding them.

As we are dynamic beings with a direct kinship relationship to all planetary elements ranging from the micro to the macro level, it allows for the possibility of emergence, even if from one instance in one place in time. This means that as action-based planetary relatives, we all have the ability to enact great change around us as we can precipitate emergent processes within our own bodies and in the environment around us. Our ancestors went into sacred ceremony as conduits of interconnected systems; however, if ego ever came into being, the conduit would be closed, and the process of positive emergence stopped. Our Natural and First Laws describe the importance of being humble for this reason, as bringing ego into being will only create disconnection and thereby stop the development of relationship.

So how do you turn the understandings of interconnection and relationship to all entities into a methodology for research and practice? Well, there is already a methodology. There has been a scientific, evidenced-informed method in existence for thousands of years in how to live and know the world around us. Traditional Indigenous knowledge systems are based within sacred Natural Laws (i.e., *rights story*), which then define traditional protocols and give a framework for both old-world and modern-world ways of knowing and healing (i.e., *proper story*). Yet in the spirit of scientific hegemony that has pervaded most branches of Western inquiry, research, and clinical practice, knowledge democracy has not prevailed (*wrong story*).

Epistemological pluralism is a complex term that recognizes and appreciates that there may be several valuable ways of knowing in any clinical or practice context, and accommodating this plurality can lead to more successful integrated study and practice (Haudenosaunee Confederacy n.d.; Miller et al. 2008). We are stronger and better able to solve complex problems with respect for the great diversity of knowledges that exist on the planet. However, epistemological pluralism has not been prioritized in our healing systems or within applications to real world complex problems. So, before we can truly address issues of planetary ill health and health inequity more broadly, we must understand how ways of knowing, being in the world, and carrying out inquiry are steeped in considerations of social justice and the mere democracy of our knowledges.

The lens of the world we take (i.e., our worldview) affects how we view planetary hierarchy or lack thereof (see Fig. 1), how we create research questions, and how we operationalize projects. We are in dire need of epistemological pluralism to disrupt notions of what constitutes progress and for whom. "We cannot solve complex problems from the same worldview that created them in the first place, as it will continue to perpetuate a disconnect between us and the planet as 'relatives' (Redvers 2021)." There is continued and urgent need within this space as well as many other spaces to prioritize epistemological pluralism that elevates and grounds greater planetary health discourse and movements with the stewardship practices, the relation-building, and the innate sense of reciprocity embodied in traditional Indigenous knowledges around the globe. But this is first and foremost with Indigenous Peoples themselves.

We have in fact seen increasing appreciation and calls for the inclusion of Indigenous traditional knowledges in climate change and biodiversity spaces; however, this has not been consistent or uniform in action. However, it is critical to understand that Indigenous knowledges do not come without the peoples themselves. There has been an increasing pattern of attempting to draw and appropriate from Indigenous traditional knowledges without the consequent elevation of Indigenous Peoples themselves. This pattern perpetuates colonial ideals. Article 31 of the UN Declaration on the Rights of Indigenous Peoples clearly states the rights of Indigenous Peoples themselves to maintain, protect, and control their culture and traditional ecological knowledge (TEK); however, these rights have consistently been violated.

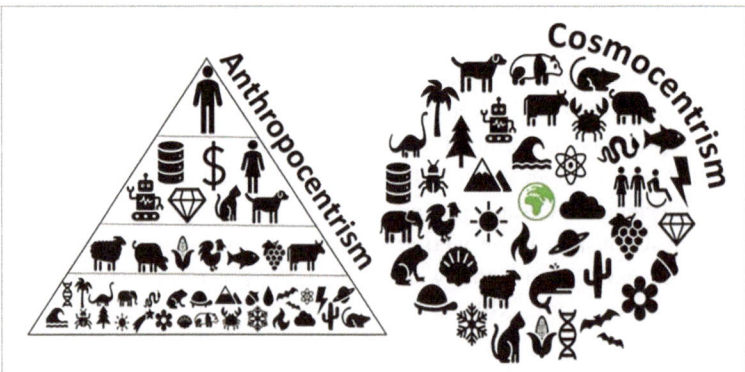

**Fig. 1** Humancentric (i.e., anthropocentrism) on the left versus the Maya cosmocentric worldview (CWV) on the right. CWV is a cosmology of conservation, or merged existence, where people, animals, plants, rivers, stones, clouds, etc., each played a role in maintaining the world. (From Lucero and Cruz 2020)

We are concerned that the current momentum of large global climate and health goals and movements will continue to promote Traditional knowledge extraction that further perpetuates inequities and discrimination of Indigenous Peoples. If the world wishes to partner and work with Indigenous communities leading traditional ecological knowledge efforts, it needs to understand and respect established international agreements and Indigenous-defined ethics. Potential partners must be proactive in protecting Indigenous Peoples' intellectual property and the data-sovereignty rights of local communities, first and foremost. There needs to be increasing focus on amplifying Indigenous Peoples and their voices, as opposed to their knowledges alone. **The knowledges do not exist without the Peoples themselves.** We are in a time that demands system transformation; however, we need to ensure that transformation is led and governed by the stewards of the systems we are trying to affect.

We are reminded of our own Indigenous methodologies that help pave the way for system transformation through reconnection with who we are and where we come from. These Indigenous methodologies stem from a rooted decolonized state of being that can be premised on six *Rs*, so aptly described by Karina Walters and colleagues (2009): Reflection, Respect, Relevance, Reciprocity, Responsibility, Retraditionalization, and Revolution, all of which are interconnected through the conceptualizations of relationality (Walters et al. 2009).

Here we specifically highlight Revolution, which we define as the purposeful transformation from the micro- through to the meta-levels of being and living in the world. The idea of self-revolution goes beyond transformation. Self-revolution is the act of going inwards to our very being so that we can better see outwards the world around us. This is depicted well by the yogic state of Samadhi, which is seeing and realizing just "what is." Indigenous Peoples have also known "what is," as they have known "*proper story*," and "*rights story*" from being interconnected within Nature.

This is the key lesson in our moment of multiple crises. The complexity of the world is expressed through the simplicity of being of Nature. "In the vision for a healthy future, it is important to create the conditions that enable the overcoming of the dissonance between 'being in nature' (i.e., nature that surrounds us) and 'being of nature' (i.e., nature that embodies us)" (Redvers et al. 2020a).

*You cannot understand true medicine power (in whatever capacity that may be) unless you have an understanding of the nature of things. To understand the nature of things, you need to be [with] nature, and you need to connect to the animals, the rocks, the plants, the stars, and the winds.*

(Redvers 2018)

## 4    The Journey Forward

As we contemplate what comes next, we urge you to consider the following questions along your journey. How is your interconnected narrative fulfilled? How will you move forward as a steward and relative of the planet and all other living entities? How will you take notice of the importance of epistemological pluralism in research and practice? Where are you Land-rooted? Whose traditional territory do you reside on? How will you elevate the Indigenous knowledge holders and voices in your respective regions or institutions? We also refer you here to Table 1, an adaptation of prior work, that gives concrete steps you can take within your institutions to further the elevation of Indigenous voices and therefore epistemological pluralism.

## 5    Conclusion

Ensuring safe decolonizing spaces for Indigenous voices creates the possibility for emergent and transformative dialogue and action within varied spaces. Ensuring safe decolonizing space for Indigenous Peoples means stepping back, listening, and engaging in action as a planetary relative. Our Elders and knowledge holders are our

**Table 1** Recommendations for the Indigenization of global and planetary health

| | |
|---|---|
| 1 | A truth-telling process is a necessary requirement to acknowledge and privilege Indigenous voices. With this, value the inherent and often uncomfortable tensions that can be felt while walking through difficult historical truths, as by acknowledging these truths, such as the continued marginalization of Indigenous Peoples, the path to health equity for all on the planet is more likely to be attainable (Warne 2018) |
| 2 | Colonization is a fundamental determinant of Indigenous health (Czyzewski 2011). Health organizations and institutions must acknowledge their historical and contemporary role in the colonial project and engage in an organizational and institutional decolonization process |
| 3 | Understand and better acknowledge the 'patterns of privilege' in current health professions education and planetary health/global health landscapes (Wikaire et al. 2016), including the recognition that colonization is a fundamental determinant of both Indigenous (Jones et al. 2019) and planetary health. To do this requires cultural humility and the understanding and embodiment of 'right relations' (Gram et al. 2021, p. 1). Embodying 'right relations' requires deep listening, self-reflexivity, creating space, and being in action. It is a continuous process of becoming and co-becoming. One must be open and willing to be in relational and reciprocal collaborative relationships to imagine decolonial ways of valuing, knowing, being, and doing, and in so doing, generating sustainable and equitable planetary health endeavors and transformations |
| 4 | Prioritize and increase the intake of Indigenous students at health professions institutions through active support of institutional pathway programs and admittance support starting in grade schools (Indian Health Service (IHS) n.d.) |
| 5 | Prioritize and increase the appointment and retention—including leadership and decision-making positions—of Indigenous faculty in health profession institutions globally, including the mobilization of sufficient funds to do so (Glauser 2019) |
| 6 | Ensure and actively support *direct* Indigenous involvement at local, national, and global scales in global health and planetary health work (Ratima 2019) as well as in research, research opportunities, and grants in this area |
| 7 | Recognize and include Indigenous-led *Land-* and *Country*-based understandings of health and wellbeing into health professions' education and professional development through supporting and expanding institutional Indigenous leadership (Lewis and Prunuske 2017) |
| 8 | Cultural safety training integration in all health profession education and medical systems (Curtis et al. 2019), including active and ongoing reconciliation work with Indigenous healing and pluralistic medical systems (Redvers et al. 2019) |
| 9 | Expand global and planetary health frameworks to include a broader culturally sensitive planetary- and ecosystems-based lens into the operationalization of health profession practices in diverse settings (Ratima et al. 2019) through a direct community engagement process |

Adapted from Redvers et al. (2020c)

brilliant scientists whom we have been honored to learn from in various capacities. As Indigenous Peoples, this has required great sacrifice to operationalize their teachings as we walk in a modern world that is not our own. It is part of our responsibility to sustain our Elders' teachings. It is your time now to embody "*proper story*" and "*rights story.*"

The story we need to co-walk is an ecologically derived one, and as interconnected beings your path is intimately connected to our path. This path is not easy. We need to remember along the way that often it is the suffering in life that helps us come to terms with our place in the world. Our multiple crisis will continue to challenge us; however, do not forget that your humble intentions and the dedicated emergence to understandings of where you come from—the Land—does have the capacity to make an impact on the world around you.

With this, we would like to thank you (mahsi cho) for taking this complex journey with us. Mother Earth and the next seven generations that will come after us are very much worth our time and effort.

*Land-based is one of those words, it's a beautiful, wonderful term. It is bringing people back to the land and helping them become alive and remembering their humanity and their connection to all living things. We are the land. So, if we remember who we are, then the same miracle that we see all around us, will be us.*

(Redvers 2020)

# Glossary

**Epistemological pluralism:** Recognizes that, in any given research or practice context, there may be several valuable ways of knowing, and that accommodating this plurality can lead to more successful integrated study [and practice] (Miller et al. 2008).

**Intergenerational Equity:** The principle that every generation holds the Earth in common with members of the present generation and with other generations, past and future. Their knowledge and practices are guided by the principle of how one's action will affect the wellbeing of generations to come (United Nations: Climate Change 2019).

**Country:** When Australian Aboriginal Peoples use the term Country it is has a unique and specific meaning. For Aboriginal Peoples culture, nature, and land, and all that surrounds these are interconnected and interdependent. Aboriginal communities have a cultural connection to Country, and it is based on each community's distinct culture, traditions and laws. Country includes the entirety of the landscape—landforms, waterways, the air, flora, fauna, minerals, materials, medicines, food sources, stories, artefacts and sacred places (Menzel 2020).

**Land or Land-based:** Relationship with the land as a central feature or concept rooted in Indigenous epistemology and pedagogy. Land-based implies a deep connection with and non-separation between human beings and the natural world. A reference to land includes all aspects of the natural world: plants, animals, ancestors, spirits, natural features, and environment (air, water, earth, minerals) (Redvers 2020).

**Planetary Health (Indigenous):** Planetary health as a 'field' is primarily a Western construct as Indigenous Traditional Knowledge systems have no clear separation between the health of the planet and the health of self or that of the community and ecosystem at large (Convention on Biological Diversity 2014). This means that the meaning and applications of planetary health are directly rooted in community values based on protocols for living in harmony with all that have existed for thousands of years (Redvers et al. 2020b).

**Planetary Health (Western):** A field focused on characterizing the linkages between human-caused disruptions of Earth's natural systems and the resulting impacts on public health (Working Party on the Environment (WONCA) et al. 2019).

**Relationality:** Indigenous relationality is recognized as the life force, and that which supports and nourishes life (Dudgeon and Bray 2019). Relationality is reciprocal as well as spatial, given it does not move forward and backward in time, but rather encompasses all directions simultaneously (Walters et al. 2020).

**Solastalgia:** Is the distress that is produced by environmental change impacting on people while they are directly connected to their home environment (Albrecht 2005).

**Strengths-based approach:** Strengths-based approaches support the generation of research findings that are focused on strengths in order to reward and reinforce positive change (Thurber et al. 2020). It is a relational practice, which reconfigures the usual relationship of client and service provider, to fellow community member while centering people, rather than projects, policies, programs, or careers (Askew et al. 2020).

**Traditional Knowledges:** Are systems of knowledge, know-how, skills and practices that are developed, sustained and passed on from generation to generation within a community, often forming part of its cultural or spiritual identity (World Intellectual Property Organization (WIPO) n.d.).

**Traditional protocols:** The term protocol includes many things, but overall, it refers to ways of interacting with Indigenous Peoples in a manner that respects traditional ways of being. Protocols are not just "manners" or "rules"—they are a representation of a culture's deeply held ethical system (BCcampus n.d.).

**Two-Eyed Seeing:** To see from one eye with the strengths of Indigenous ways of knowing, and to see from the other eye with the strengths of Western ways of knowing, and to use both of these eyes together (i.e., "the gift of multiple perspectives") (Bartlett et al. 2012).

# References

Albrecht G. 'Solastalgia': a new concept in health and identity. PAN, 2005;3 [cited 2021 Sept 14]. Available from: https://doi.org/10.4225/03/584f410704696

Askew DA, Brady K, Mukandi B, Singh D, Sinha T, Brough M. Closing the gap between rhetoric and practice in strengths-based approaches to Indigenous public health: a qualitative study. Aust NZ J Pub Health. 2020;44(2):102–5. [cited 2021 Sept 14]. Available from: https://onlinelibrary.wiley.com/doi/full/10.1111/1753-6405.12953

Bartlett C, Marshall M, Marshall A. Two-Eyed Seeing and other lessons learned within a co-learning journey of bringing together indigenous and mainstream knowledges and ways of knowing. J Environ Stud Sci. 2012;2:331–40. [cited 2021 Sept 14]. Available from: https://ceaa-acee.gc.ca/050/documents/p80156/132968E.pdf

BCcampus. Engaging with Indigenous communities: respecting protocols. n.d. [cited 2021 Sept 14]. Available from: https://opentextbc.ca/indigenizationcurriculumdevelopers/chapter/respecting-protocols/

Briggs M, Graham M. The relevance of Aboriginal political concepts (7): Autonomous regard. ABC Religion & Ethics; 2021. [cited 2021 Nov 10]. Available at: https://www.abc.net.au/religion/aboriginal-political-concepts-autonomous-regard/13472098

Cajete G. Native science: natural laws of interdependence. In: Nelson MK, Shilling D, editors. Traditional ecological knowledge. Cambridge: Cambridge University Press; 2018. p. 15–26.

Convention on Biological Diversity. Nagoya protocol on access and benefit-sharing. 2014 [cited 2021 Sept 14]. Available from: https://www.cbd.int/abs/

Country B, Wright S, Suchet-Pearson S, Lloyd K, Burarrwanga L, Ganambarr R, Ganambarr-Stubbs M, Ganambarr B, Maymuru D, Sweeney J. Co-becoming Bawaka: Towards a relational understanding of place/space. Progress in Human Geography. 2016;40:455–75. [cited 2021 Sept 14]. Available from: https://doi.org/10.1177/0309132515589437

Curtis E, Jones R, Tipene-Leach D, Walker C, Loring B, Paine SJ, et al. Why cultural safety rather than cultural competency is required to achieve health equity: a literature review and recommended definition. Int J Equity Health. 2019;(1):18, 174. [cited 2021 Sept 14]. Available from https://equityhealthj.biomedcentral.com/articles/10.1186/s12939-019-1082-3

Czyzewski K. Colonialism as a broader social determinant of health. Int Indigenous Policy J. 2011;2(1) [cited 2021 Sept 14]. Available from: https://ojs.lib.uwo.ca/index.php/iipj/article/view/7337#:~:text=A%20proposed%20broader%20or%20Indigenized,along%20with%20other%20global%20processes.&text=Colonialism%20can%20also%20be%20enacted,influencing%20scholarly%20and%20popular%20perceptions.

Dudgeon P, Bray A. Indigenous relationality: women, kinship and the law. Genealogy. 2019;3(23) [cited 2021 Sept 14]. Available from: https://doi.org/10.3390/genealogy3020023

Food and Agriculture Organization of the United Nations. Indigenous peoples- free, prior and informed consent. 2021 [cited 2021 Nov 10]. Available from: https://www.fao.org/indigenous-peoples/our-pillars/fpic/en/

Glauser W. The many challenges of increasing Indigenous faculty at medical schools. CMAJ. 2019;191(37):E1036–7. [cited 2021 Sept 14]. Available from https://www.cmaj.ca/content/191/37/E1036

Gram-Hanssen I, Schafenacker N, Bentz J. Decolonizing transformations through 'right relations.' (Originally The "how" of transformation: integrative approaches to sustainability.). Sustain Sci. 2021;17:673–85. [cited 2021 Sept 14]. Available from: https://doi.org/10.1007/s11625-021-00960-9.

Greenwood M. Children as citizens of First Nations: linking Indigenous health to early childhood development. Pediatr Child. Health. 2005;10(9):553–5. [cited 2021 Sept 14]. Available from: https://www.ncbi.nlm.nih.gov/pmc/articles/PMC2722642/

Haudenosaunee Confederacy. Development consultation on Haudenosaunee lands. n.d. [cited 2021 Sept 14]. Available from: https://www.haudenosauneeconfederacy.com/values/

Indian Health Service (IHS). Indians into medicine program. n.d. [cited 2021 Sept 14]. Available from https://www.ihs.gov/dhps/dhpsgrants/indiansmedicineprogram/

Jones R. Climate change and Indigenous health promotion. Glob Health Promot. 2019;26(3_suppl):73–81. [cited 2021 Sept 14]. Available from: https://journals.sagepub.com/doi/full/10.1177/1757975919829713.

Jones R, Crowshoe L, Reid P, Calam B, Curtis E, Green M, et al. Educating for Indigenous health equity: an international consensus statement. Acad Med. 2019;94(4):512–9. [cited 2021 Sept 14]. Available from https://journals.lww.com/academicmedicine/fulltext/2019/04000/educating_for_indigenous_health_equity__an.28.aspx

Lewis M, Prunuske A. 2017. The development of an Indigenous health curriculum for medical students. Acad Med 2017:92(5):641–648 [cited 2021. Sept 14]. Available from https://journals.lww.com/academicmedicine/Fulltext/2017/05000/The_Development_of_an_Indigenous_Health_Curriculum.35.aspx.

Lucero LJ, Cruz JG. Reconceptualizing urbanism: insights from maya cosmology. Front Sustain Cities. 2020;2:1. [cited 2021 Sept 14]. Available from https://doi.org/10.3389/frsc.2020.00001

Menzel K. Indigenous pedagogy is good pedagogy: applying indigenous pedagogical approaches in the United Kingdom. In: Lock D, Caputo A, Hack-Polay D, Igwe P, editors. Borderlands: the internationalization of higher education teaching practices. Lincoln: Academy of Management; 2020.

Miller T, Baird T, Littlefield C, Kofinas G, Chapin F, Redman, C. Epistemological pluralism: reorganizing interdisciplinary research. Ecol Soc 2008:13(2) [cited 2021 Sept 14]. Available from http://www.jstor.org/stable/26268006

O'Brien K. You matter more than you think: quantum social change in response to a world in crisis. Unpublished manuscript. Ed. Adaptation CONNECTS, University of Oslo, 2020 [cited 2021 Sept 14].

Ratima M. Leadership for planetary health and sustainable development: health promotion community capacities for working with Indigenous peoples in the application of Indigenous knowledge. Glob Health Promot. 2019;26(4):3–5. [cited 2021 Sept 14]. https://doi.org/10.1177/1757975919889250.

Ratima M, Martin D, Castleden H, Delormier T. Indigenous voices and knowledge systems—promoting planetary health, health equity, and sustainable development now and for future generations. Glob Health Promot. 2019;26(3_suppl):3–5. [cited 2021 Sept 14]. https://doi.org/10.1177/1757975919838487.

Redvers JM. Land-based Practice for Indigenous Health and Wellness in Yukon, Nunavut, and the Northwest Territories. Master of Environmental Design thesis, University of Calgary, 2016.

Redvers N. The value of global Indigenous knowledge in planetary health. Challenges. 2018;9(2):30. [cited 2021 Sept 14]. Available from: https://doi.org/10.3390/challe9020030.

Redvers J. "The land is a healer": perspectives on land-based healing from Indigenous practitioners in northern Canada. Int J Indigenous Health. 2020;15(1) [cited 2021 Sept 14]. Available from: https://jps.library.utoronto.ca/index.php/ijih/article/view/34046.

Redvers N. The determinants of planetary health. Lancet. 2021;5(3):E111–2. [cited 2021 Sept 14]. Available from: https://www.thelancet.com/journals/lanplh/article/PIIS2542-5196(21)00008-5/fulltext

Redvers N, Marianayagam J, Blondin B. Improving access to Indigenous medicine for patients in hospital-based settings: a challenge for health systems in northern Canada. Int J Circumpolar Health 2019:78(2):1589208. [cited 2021 Sept 14]. Available from https://www.tandfonline.com/doi/10.1080/22423982.2019.1589208

Redvers N, Yellow Bird M, Quinn D, Yunkaporta T, Arabena K. Molecular decolonization: an Indigenous microcosm perspective of planetary health. Int J Enviro Res Public Health. 2020a;17:4586. [cited 2021 Sept 14]. Available from: https://doi.org/10.3390/ijerph17124586

Redvers N, Poelina A, Schultz C, Kobei DM, Githaiga C, Perdrisat M, et al. Indigenous natural and First Law in planetary health. MDPI Challenges. 2020b;11(2):29. [cited 2021 Sept 14]. Available from: https://doi.org/10.3390/challe11020029

Redvers N, Schultz C, Prince MV, Cunningham M, Jones R, Blondin B. Indigenous perspectives on education for sustainable healthcare. Med Teacher. 2020c;42(10) [cited 2021 Sept 14]. Available from: https://www.tandfonline.com/doi/full/10.1080/0142159X.2020.1791320.

Styres S, Zinga D, Bennett S, Bomberry M. Walking in two worlds: engaging the space between Indigenous community and academia. Can J Educ. 2010;33(3):617–48. [cited 2021 Sept 14]. Available from: https://www.researchgate.net/publication/264038226_Walking_in_Two_Worlds_Engaging_the_Space_Between_Indigenous_Community_and_Academia

Thurber KA, Thandrayen J, Banks E, Doery K, Sedgwixk M, Lovett R. Strenths-based approaches for quantitative data analysis: a case study using the Australian Longitudinal Study of Indigenous Children. SSM – Popul Health. 2020;12:100637. [cited 2021 Sept 14]. Available from: https://www.sciencedirect.com/science/article/pii/S2352827320302743.

Tynan L. Thesis as kin: living relationality with research. AlterNative Int J Indigenous Peoples. 2020;16(3):163–70. [cited 2021 Nov 10]. Available from: https://journals.sagepub.com/doi/abs/10.1177/1177180120948270

Tynan L. What is relationality? Indigenous knowledges, practices and responsibilities with kin. Cult Geogr. 2021;28(4):597–610. [cited 2021 Nov 10]. Available from: https://journals.sagepub.com/doi/abs/10.1177/14744740211029287?journalCode=cgjb#:~:text=Knowledges%2C%20practices%20and%20responsibilities%20with%20kin,-I%20can%20almost&text=For%20human%20geography%2C%20relationality%20actually,kin%20and%20research)%20with%20respect.

United Nations. United Nations declaration on the rights of indigenous peoples. United Nations; 2007. [cited 2021 Nov 10]. Available from: https://www.un.org/development/desa/indigenouspeoples/declaration-on-the-rights-of-indigenous-peoples.html

United Nations: Climate Change. Values of Indigenous peoples can be a key component of climate resilience. News, 2019 [cited 2021 Sept 14]. Available from: https://unfccc.int/news/values-of-indigenous-peoples-can-be-a-key-component-of-climate-resilience

Walters KL, Stately A, Evans-Campbell T, Simoni JM, Duran B, Schultz K, et al. "Indigenist"collaborative research efforts in Native American communities. In: Stiffman A, editor. The field research survival guide. Oxford: Oxford University Press; 2009. p. 146–73. https://doi.org/10.1093/acprof:oso/9780195325522.003.0008.

Walters KL, Johnson-Jennings M, Stroud S, Rasmus S, Charles B, John S, et al. Growing from our roots: strategies for developing culturally grounded health promotion interventions in American Indian, Alaska Native, and Native Hawaiian Communities. Prev Sci. 2020;21(Suppl 1):54–64. [cited 2021 Nov 10]. Available from: https://link.springer.com/article/10.1007%2Fs11121-018-0952-z.

Warne D. UND's approach to American Indian health issues stands out, says Dr. Donald Warne during Indigenous Peoples' Day talk. North Dakota University System; 2018. [cited 2021 Sept 14]. Available from https://ndus.edu/2019/10/21/unds-approach-to-american-indian-health-issues-stands-out-says-dr-donald-warne-during-indigenous-peoples-day-talk/.

Westerman T. Guest editorial: Engagement of Aboriginal clients in mental health services: what role do cultural differences play? Aust e-J Adv Ment Health. 2004;3(3):88–93. [cited 2021 Sept 14]

Whyte K. Is It Colonial Déjà vu? Indigenous Peoples and Climate Injustice. In: Adamson J, Davis M, editors. Humanities for the Environment. London: Routledge; 2017. p. 88–105. https://www.academia.edu/24999116/Is_it_Colonial_D%C3%A9j%C3%A0_Vu_Indigenous_Peoples_and_Climate_Injustice.

Wikaire E, Curtis E, Cormack D, Jiang Y, McMillan L, Loto R, Reid P. Patterns of privilege: a total cohort analysis of admission and academic outcomes for Māori, Pacific and non-Māori non-Pacific health professional students. BMC Med Educ. 2016;16(1):262. [cited 2021 Sept 14]. Available from https://doi.org/10.1186/s12909-016-0782-2

Working Party on the Environment (WONCA), Planetary Health Alliance, Clinicians for Planetary Health Working Group. Declaration calling for family doctors of the world to act on planetary health. 2019 [cited 2021 Sept 14]. Available from: https://www.wonca.net/site/DefaultSite/filesystem/documents/Groups/Environment/2019%20Planetary%20health.pd.

World Intellectual Property Organization (WIPO). Traditional knowledge n.d. [cited 2021 Sept 14]. Available from: https://www.wipo.int/tk/en/tk/

Yunkaporta T. All our landscapes are broken: right story and the law of the land. Griffith Rev. 2021;74:1. [cited 2021 Sept 14]. Available from: https://www.griffithreview.com/articles/all-our-landscapes-are-broken/.

Zhang Y, Barratt A, Rychetnik L, Breth-Petersen M. An Australian glossary on health and climate change. 2021 [cited 2021 Sept 14]. Prepared for: The Human Health and Social Impacts (HHSI) Node, The NSW Adaptation Hub.

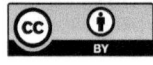

# Social Movement and Empowerment in Shaping Global Health Priorities: Past, Present, and Future Perspectives from India

Anil S. Bilimale [ID], P. Arathi Rao [ID],
Kesavan Rajsekharan Nayar [ID], Meena Som [ID],
Anjana Penugondla [ID],
and Ashok Gladston Xavier [ID]

*Social movements are at once the symptoms and the instruments of progress. Ignore them and statesmanship is irrelevant; fail to use them, and it is weak.*

Walter Lippmann

## Abstract

Social movements can play an important role in shaping the policies and local implementation of sustainable development goals and global health priorities. A major challenge is to understand the interconnectedness of the origins of social movements and their processes required to empower them. It is important to understand the pivotal role of people, partnerships, products, and policy to ensure solidarity, social security, system strengthening, and social justice. In addition to flagging existing challenges in the system, social movements can be instrumental in bringing substantive changes to systems and policies that are then reflected on the ground. A few prominent social movement examples from India are used to illustrate successful approaches that have led to lasting policy changes and positive health outcomes in local communities. Successful initiatives have focused on ensuring comprehensive coverage, community participation, collaboration with stakeholders, empowerment of women, and approach focused on equity to attain equality for healthcare access among women, underprivileged and hard to reach population. These efforts can inform future visions of global health partnerships with social movements.

A. S. Bilimale (✉)
School of Public Health, JSS Academy of Higher Education and Research, Mysuru, Karnataka, India
e-mail: anilbilimale@jssuni.edu.in

P. Arathi Rao
Prasanna School of Public Health, Manipal, India
e-mail: arathi.anil@manipal.edu

K. R. Nayar
Global Institute of Public Health, Trivandrum, India

M. Som · A. Penugondla
Independent Public Health Professional, Bhubaneshwar, India

A. G. Xavier
Loyola College, Chennai, Tamil Nadu, India

## Keywords

Social capital · Grassroots movement · Global health · Equity · Community participation · Digital era

## Abbreviations

| | |
|---|---|
| ASHA | Accredited Social Health Activist |
| ANC | AnteNatal Checkup |
| ART | Antiretroviral Therapy |
| CSO | Central Statistics Office |
| CEPI | Coalition for Epidemic Preparedness Innovation |
| CHV | Community Health Visitor/Worker |
| COVID | CoronaVirus Disease |
| DOTS | Directly Observed Treatment Short course |
| GAVI | Global Alliance for Vaccine and Immunization |
| HIV | Human Immuno Virus |
| IMR | Infant Mortality Rate |
| IEC | Information Education Communication |
| ICDS | Integrated Child Development Services |
| JSA | Jan Swastya Abhiyan |
| JSY | Janani Suraksha Yojana |
| KROSS | Karnataka Regional Organization for Social Service |
| KSSP | Kerala Sastra Sahitya Parishad |
| MAS | Mahila Arogya Samiti |
| MMR | Maternal Mortality Rate |
| MFC | Medical Friend Cycle |
| MIC | Middle Income Country |
| NHM | National Health Mission |
| NRHM | National Rural Health Mission |
| NUHM | National Urban Health Mission |
| NHG | Neighborhood Groups of Women |
| NGO | Non-Governmental Organization |
| ORS | Oral Rehydration Salts |
| PLHIV | People Living with HIV |
| PHM | People's Health Movement |
| PNC | Postnatal Checkup |
| PHC | Primary Health Centre |
| SDG | Sustainable Development Goals |
| SVYM | Swami Vivekananda Youth Movement |
| UN | United Nations |
| UNICEF | United Nations Children's Fund |
| USD | United States Dollar |
| USA | United States of America |
| UHC | Urban Health Centre |
| WHO | World Health Organization |
| WTO | World Trade Organization |

## Author Perspective

The authors have experience in the public health and development sector belonging to various international NGOs and academic institutions. Three of them have worked together in maternal and child health programs, especially in health system strengthening projects. They have worked in the eradication and elimination of vaccine-preventable diseases involving large-scale immunization programs. Four authors from the team have academic experience and have been working in the social sector field for more than 10–20 years. One of them has worked in refugee programs in various south-east asian countries. Together, they have amalgamated their experiences with grass root movements in this article.

### Key Tenets: People's Health in People's Hands

1. The solution for a societal problem exists in the society itself. We need to be open to listen to all perspectives and work together to achieve health goals.
2. Empower the people even before a social movement originates and support them in sustaining the movement later on.
3. *Vasudhaiva Kutumbakam*—India's philosophy of 'World is one family,' emphasizing oneness and the spirit of co-existence, is facilitated by digital media platforms that create communication beyond horizons.
4. Successful approaches to partnering with social movements in the Indian context include: (OECD 2021) Initiatives to ensure comprehensive coverage of different sections of population for awareness and access to health services; (The 2018 Astana Declaration on Primary Health Care 2021) Bridging the communication and cultural gaps by community participation with leadership roles; (Kraef and Kallestrup 2019) Working with actors from health services and NGOs to ensure healthcare coverage; (World Social Capital Monitor 2021) Empowering women and target-

ing approaches to eliminate the gender-based differences for health care access, and (Adams 2008) Ensuring equity and equality with interventions to reach the unreached

5. This chapter addresses the following SDGs: #3 Good health and wellbeing, #10 Reducing inequities, #11 Sustainable cities and communities, #16 Peace, justice, and strong institutions, and #17 Partnership for the Goals.

# 1    Context Setting

Human beings develop networks and connections in a society over a considerable period based on norms, values, and understandings. Social networks include families, urban localities, rural villages, organizations, and ethnic groups, depending on where they reside, work, or share. These networks gather under a common purpose and work towards achieving common goals–but few will lead to movements. Many sociologists have coined such phenomena as "Social movements" or "Grassroot movements." A few researchers have gone a step further and conceptualized them as "social capital"as they may benefit society or nation.

Ultimately, social movements are primed to shape global health priorities by exposing them to perspectives beyond any particular nation's knowledge, domain, or norm (OECD 2021).

In the nineteenth century, India went through many social movements against caste, gender inequity and colonization. Following the colonial era, India developed as one of the strongest nations in the world over six decades through many of these social movements, which reformed and brought values to the existing democratic constitution.

*Social capital provides the glue which facilitates cooperation, exchange, and innovation.*
—The New Economy: Beyond the Hype

**At the end of this chapter, the reader will be able to understand the following concepts:-**

What is a Social Movement?

Why do we have to empower Social Movements?

How are social movements connected to the Public Health/Development sector?

How can a Public Health/Development Professional empower and collaborate with this capital?

The development sector's critical driving force is the development agenda set by the United Nations, World Bank, non-governmental organizations, and national governments. Health is a vital development sector whose importance has gained more attention in recent decades. The UN General Assembly and World Health Assembly have ensured that countries work towards the goals set for the development sectors.

Healthcare is a major part of the development sector. From the declaration of Alma-Ata in 1978 to the declaration of Asthana in 2018, organizations have realized and ratified the importance of Primary Health Care (PHC) for delivering healthcare. One of the approaches of PHC is community participation- "empowering individuals, families, and communities to take charge of their health." (The 2018 Astana Declaration on Primary Health Care 2021) Multiple participatory approaches have been designed to improve community participation. However, governments, NGOs, and Civil Society Organizations (CSO) mobilize the vast majority of community involvement in working toward sustainability (Kraef and Kallestrup 2019).

Grassroots movements depend on community processes and purposes for their genesis. Empowering such movements is an ongoing phenomenon. If there is a higher level of awareness and diverse understanding of developmental issues, these movements can move toward constructive goals. Development and public health professionals often work to promote the enrollment and mobilization of community members through existing health systems to adopt the solutions and services that are designed globally and nationally. However, community involvement is more likely to be sustainable and accepted if it evolves from within the community (World Social Capital Monitor 2021). Professionals need to identify and tap into the existing resources available in the community.

Building on Millennium Development Goals, countries came together to define and formulate a broader development agenda, namely the Sustainable Development Goals (SDGs) to be achieved by 2030. The development of SDGs is informed by multiple data sources including people of different age groups, women, people with disabilities, civil society leaders, and activists (Organization WH, Fund (UNICEF) UNC 2014). SDG Agenda 2030 has three closely linked dimensions—Economic, Environmental and Social. Any change in one dimension impacts the outcomes of the other, which is measured by the 17 goals and 169 targets defined in the agenda (Social Development for Sustainable Development 2021). Sustainable change has to occur locally through community-led movements to realize these goals. Designing strategies and evaluating their benefits in the target population requires community participation and guidance from subject matter experts, technocrats, and bureaucrats. This bottom-up approach, interwoven with technical support, ideas, and innovations from supporting organizations would promise better outcomes.

Without social cohesion, it will be challenging to achieve SDGs, and individuals could potentially be left behind (The forgotten dimension of the SDG indicators 2021). Specific core values like trust, solidarity, helpfulness, and hospitality play a vital role in influencing community involvement and will enable stronger social ties to achieve SDGs. For any action plan to materialize effectively, communities must be examined at a granular level to understand particular people's persistent and emerging needs. To understand and establish community-specific priorities, it will be especially important to understand the interplay and interdependence of factors that have implications on health. Ultimately, the success of any social movement or development agenda lies in inclusion and diversity.

That said, the success of any social movement also needs a sensitive and sensible political mobilization that can advance reforms in population health, rearrange priorities based on a bottom-up approach, and hold government bodies responsible for people's "right to health." A healthy and developed society is not only one that is free of pathogens– but it is also an environment that allows people to grow to their fullest potential.

In the current chapter, readers will learn about factors that influence grassroots movements and opportunities to empower social movements through various examples of health-related issues from a developing country's perspective drawing on the authors' deep expertise in India.

## 2 Framework

*Give a man a fish, you feed him for a day. Teach a man to fish, and you feed him for a lifetime.*
—Old Chinese Proverb

Robert Adam writes, "Empowerment is the capacity of individuals, groups, and communities to take control of their circumstances, exercise power, and achieve their own goals, and the process by which, individually and collectively, they can help themselves and others to maximize the quality of their lives." (Adams 2008) Thus, social empowerment is the key to building an inclusive environment for making informed choices. Such social empowerment visualizes a world in which every person can contribute to the collective good and progress of the community. In other words, social empowerment enables grass-root organizations to lead movements addressing local problems. When these movements gather support beyond local or regional boundaries, they can shape national and international movements advocating for changes at respective levels (Alexandra Bettencourt n.d.). In this section, we will present a framework focused on People, Partnership, Product, and Policy to ensure Solidarity, Social Security, System Strengthening, and Social Justice (Fig. 1). Physical, social, cultural, and environmental determinants also must be considered in the context of empowering communities to achieve health for all. Once empow-

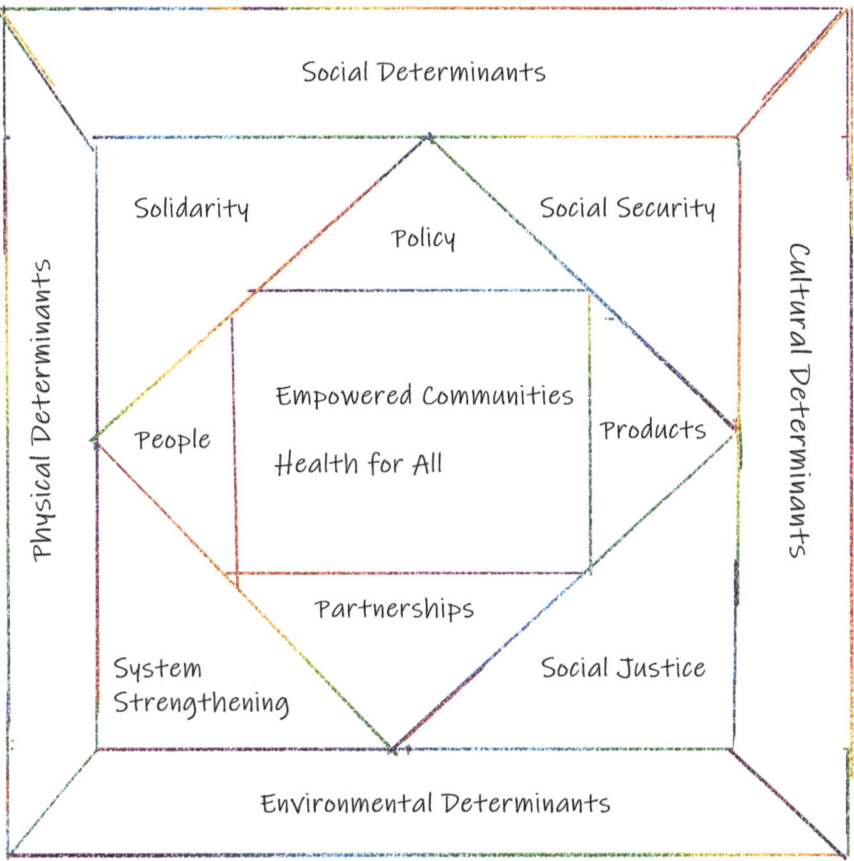

**Fig. 1** Illustration of Conceptual model for community solutions to promote health equity (National Academies of Sciences Engineering, Medicine 2017)

ered, the communities will in turn impact the determinants of health.

Solidarity means "the emotional cohesion between the members of the social movements and the mutual support they give each other in their battle for common goals" (Bayertz 1999).

Social security is a human right and all people, regardless of where they live, should be guaranteed at least a floor of basic social protection which should consist of at least four basic social security guarantees: essential health care and basic income security during childhood, adulthood and old age for all residents and all children.

System strengthening happens by social participation as a part of social movement.

The recognition of collective injustice is proposed to motivate participation in social movements, collective protests and political rebellions to achieve Social Justice.

Social determinants of health such as poverty, unequal access to health care, lack of education, stigma, and racism are underlying, contributing factors of health inequities. To impact social determinants of health, we have to work towards reducing inequities.

**People.** Community engagement through grassroots initiatives is vital for alleviating health inequities. A community-based participatory approach led by informed individuals at the local level paves the way for community members to express their ideas and solve the problem. The incorporation of local solutions based on the felt needs of the community leads to effective policymaking. All communities operate within a frame of social norms and customs that influence the behavior of their community members, impacting health and wellness, including health-seeking behavior amongst communities. Hence empowering communities with appropriate knowledge helps bring us closer to a world where everyone enjoys the right to attain the highest form of health and healthcare. Social capital, as defined by the Organization for Economic Cooperation and Development (OECD), refers to the "networks together with shared norms, values, and understandings that facilitate cooperation within or among groups." (Human Capital 2021) Strengthening and enriching social capital at the grassroots level is essential for shaping strategies to help make people-centric decisions for sustainable development and progress.

**Partnership.** Collaboration and cooperation between public and private entities, civil society organizations, faith-based organizations, and non-governmental organizations coupled with collective efforts lead to accumulative effects which pursue health for all, paving the way towards a community's overall development. With the onset of globalization, information & communication technologies, including the internet and social media, have connected the world. Marshall McLuhan aptly mentions that the "world is a global village." In the era of social media, in particular, real-time information is now accessible concerning several areas of interest like personal, professional, health, development, etc. (Marshall 1995) As a result, some communities have become closer, prioritizing health issues, searching for possible solutions, recognizing and mobilizing human capital, providing leadership, fostering innovations, and transforming existing systems to positively impact people's lives. "Vasudhaiva kutumbakam" is an ancient Indian saying, which means the world is one family. The speed with which the COVID pandemic has spread aptly demonstrates global interconnectedness. At the same time, the response to this pandemic by individuals and societies guided by experts from various domains is a living example of the strengths of these interconnectedness and

collaboration. The interconnectedness among different groups of society during the digital era empowers direction and enhances the partnership and collaboration.

**Product.** With the COVID pandemic, the world has witnessed the rapid spread of information and misinformation through social media channels. Therefore, harnessing the potential of digital technology in the right way for social mobilization is an essential task, and is one example of a product.

Digital technology helps us understand and solve complex problems that need a multisectoral approach involving government and individual engagement. Such technology has enormous potential for helping us better understand issues. Particularly, analytics can help identify the root causes of such issues, which would allow policymakers to make evidence-based decisions. With the access and availability of digital literacy, digital solutions can achieve desired outcomes. Increased access to large parts of the world gives rise to democratic movements which foster integral values like accountability and transparency, giving everyone a fair opportunity to share their voice and emotions. Such access can ultimately shape and amend opinions to encourage new ways of overcoming challenges through people's participation.

Challenges regarding access to digital tools include poor access in remote regions, rural-urban divide, and lack of digital literacy. Most of the time, those communities with limited digital access also encounter difficulty with primary health care needs. As such, having digital infrastructure empowers nations and communities as it enables faster responses to problems by faster delivery of solutions.

**Policy.** The people, partnership and products can effectively work when there are robust policies in place. The governments and other stakeholders must invest in primary health based on social justice and equity principles, community participation, and solidarity. Restructuring health systems around people's needs and expectations by integrating comprehensive health services will empower them to actively engage in health matters. Robust financing structures, community insurance mechanisms, compulsory funding sources (for example, tax revenues), and higher investments into the public health systems can act as a safety net to mitigate catastrophic expenditure for various illnesses, which can push families "below the poverty line." Designing multi-sectoral policies, leveraging public and private partnerships, using reliable, accurate health information systems, harnessing the power of data intelligence for decision-making, and establishing effective governance structures can help achieve the goal of Health for All (Universal health coverage (UHC) 2021).

Access to quality and affordable health care, in turn, allows people to earn and sustain their livelihoods while ensuring that children can grow up healthy and ultimately contribute to nation-building. For optimum utilization, we need to design services to suit the needs of the local communities. Empowering people and encouraging community participation strengthens community ownership and meaningful involvement in "Health for all." Responsive primary health care systems can help manage most health needs and provide care close to the community. This would reduce the burden on health facilities that provide specialized and secondary or tertiary care services. One example of social capital's influence on health is a community fund pooling mechanism run locally by a small group of individuals in the community. The community fund pooling strengthens the economic development of women in rural areas and helps them build self-reliance and access to their resources and support them in income generating activities. Unless communities actively participate in the change process, sustaining such goals is difficult.

Evidence-based decision-making, problem-based interventions, people-centric policies, and a focused programmatic approach with community engagements rooted in social equity are vital to closing health disparity gaps. The world can enjoy the fruits of sustainable development only when collective efforts emphasize the need for caring and sharing with others across the globe,

guiding local leaders, organizations, and nations to act consciously.

The interconnectedness of various aspects of the framework has been described in Fig. 2. Ultimately, social media, education, and research will influence the empowerment of social movements, thereby bringing people's felt needs to shape global health priorities. Social movements can support health system reforms, transparency and equity, governance and accountability, thereby attaining the SDGs (Fig. 2).

## 3    Success Stories

In Table 1, eleven success stories from the Indian context have been compiled based upon two major factors: -

- State-led initiatives on empowerment of the marginalized
- Decentralization of power and health

*People's health in people's hands.* People realize their role in decision-making and governance through the decentralization of power. National efforts in Asia have implemented several decentralization initiatives to address de-concentration, delegation, and privatization (Rondinelli 1983). Decentralization involves local people and communities in the essential functions of health systems, such as service provision, resource generation, financing, and stewardship (Alliance for Health Policy and Systems Research 2004). Bossert's decision space approach considers power transfer from the center (principal) to the periphery (agent), considering how local agents evolve innovative programs to maximize health programs' impact (Bossert 1998).

The Bhore Committee (1946) report emphasized that we could achieve sustainable improvement of public health only with the active participation of people in local health programs (Bhore committee 1946). In the light of the Alma Ata Declaration, this document highlights the role of grass root level workers and direct health-care workers who formed the first contact with the community for the public healthcare delivery

**Fig. 2** Schematic illustration of the interconnectedness of the framework

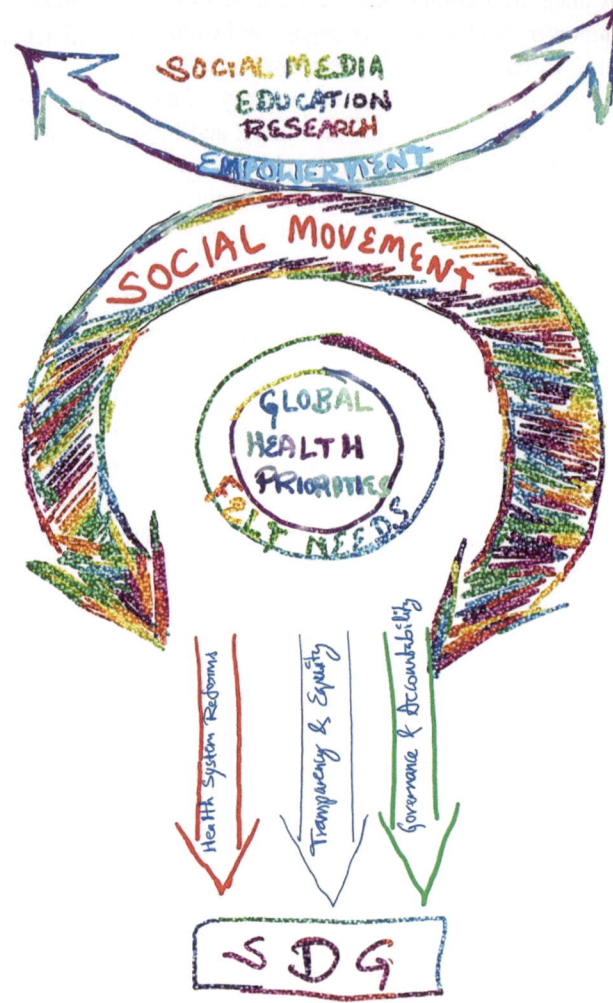

system. Many initiatives have been implemented, of which the Community Health Workers/Volunteers (CHVs) and the Accredited Social Health Activists (ASHA) require primary mention due to their voluntary status. The strategy that emphasized participation, democratization, and community ownership of public health programs was necessary and considered a fundamental right (Kumar et al. 2016).

The various successful approaches to partnering with social movements in the Indian context include:

1. Initiatives to ensure comprehensive coverage of different sections of the population for awareness and access to health services as mentioned in examples 3, 4, 5, 6, 7, and 8 in Table 1. The diverse social and economic parts of society in India present a challenge to create awareness and provide access to healthcare services.

2. Bridging the communication and cultural gaps by community participation in leadership as mentioned in examples 1, 2, and 10 in Table 1. Identifying and empowering community members to take leadership in health matters ensures ease of communication and is culturally acceptable.

3. Working with actors from health services and NGOs to ensure healthcare coverage as mentioned in examples 1, 2, 3, 4, 5, 6, 7, 8, and 9 in Table 1. To ensure Healthcare coverage,

**Table 1** Success stories of grass root movements in India and their positive impact on health care service delivery

| S1 No | Name of the initiative | Location | Partners involved | Best practices | Key outcomes |
|---|---|---|---|---|---|
| 1 | Community Health Volunteer Scheme (CHV Scheme) | Rural India | Community-Primary health care centers | Mainly centralized and clinically oriented health services (Maru 1983) | Strengthened the linkage between people and health services (Critical reflections on health services development in India: the teleology of disorder–NLM Catalog–NCBI 2021) Succeeded in emphasizing primary care (Maru 1983) |
| 2 | Accredited Social Health Activist (ASHA) | Pan India | National Health Mission (NHM) | Filled the gap of workforce unavailability, bridging cultural and communication gaps Steered the rural population toward a formal health care system Coordinated with other community health workers, village health and sanitation committees, and women's self-help groups Door-to-door visits to rural households Imparted health information customized to the family members Promoted health awareness on various schemes and programs of the public health sector Encouraged family participation (Scott et al. 2019) Ensured access to antenatal care and institutional delivery among women (Agarwal et al. 2019) Immunization in children played a vital role in the elimination of polio in India Extensively used for COVID-19 control activities (Kumar et al. 2020) DOTS (Directly Observed Treatment Short Course) for ensuring adherence during the treatment of Tuberculosis cases in the community. | Linking community and health system in accessing and utilizing the services. (nrhm-framework-latest.pdf 2021; About Accredited Social Health Activist (ASHA) 2021) Significant communication efforts were undertaken in India, primarily focusing on women's health It is one of the most successful community health programs in India. |

(continued)

**Table 1** (continued)

| S1 No | Name of the initiative | Location | Partners involved | Best practices | Key outcomes |
|---|---|---|---|---|---|
| 3 | People's Health Movement (PHM) | LMICs | | A global network of grassroots health activists, civil society organizations, and academic institutions Universal access to quality health care is according to people's needs and not their affordability (Critical reflections on health services development in India: the teleology of disorder–NLM Catalog–NCBI 2021) | One of them is Jan Swasthya Abhiyan (JSA). JSA at present is the major national platform that co-ordinates activities and action on health and health care across the country on a non-State platform (http://phmindia.org) |
| 4 | Jan Swasthya Abhiyan (JSA) | India | Feminist organizations, people's science organizations | Formed in 2001 with 18 national networks across the country in 2000 The primary national platform that coordinates activities and action on health and health care | Represented in the first Global People's Health Assembly, in Dhaka, in December 2000 Philosophy of "people's health in people's hands." Demonstrates the disturbing evidence of rising disparities in health status between people in India and worldwide Increasing commercialization in health worldwide, including settings like Kerala, where health service availability and health indicators have been favorable. |

(continued)

**Table 1** (continued)

| S1 No | Name of the initiative | Location | Partners involved | Best practices | Key outcomes |
|---|---|---|---|---|---|
| 5 | Kerala Sastra Sahitya Parishad (KSSP) | Kerala, India | People's Science movement | Popular movements and people's action in health have been largely initiated by smaller groups and localized. The Kerala Sastra Sahitya Parishad (KSSP) has been the most prominent in Kerala which focused on campaigns for awareness and policy change and initiatives for alternatives and focus on health issues. But importantly KSSP has also been involved in surveys, research and advocacy. The organization has been actively involved in publishing and disseminating materials which have highlighted the limitations and strengths of health care in Kerala. The notion of Kerala model of health care which focused on cost-effective, accessible and available health services to majority of the population has been popularized by KSSP studies. The better health indicators in Kerala had been attributed to this model apart from social and economic factors. | Researching, advocating and popularizing model Healthcare system |
| 6 | Swami Vivekananda Youth Movement | Karnataka, India | NGO | Health sectors focus on remote and tribal communities. The organization was established with the intent to serve the tribal and remote villages. In the process, they learnt that health is a part of larger development process and started working on development issues pertaining to livelihood, women empowerment, education, skill building, etc (https://svym.org) | Education and empowerment of the tribal population |

(continued)

**Table 1** (continued)

| Sl No | Name of the initiative | Location | Partners involved | Best practices | Key outcomes |
|---|---|---|---|---|---|
| 7 | Karuna Trust | Karnataka, India | NGO | Adopted more than sixty primary health centers to support the workforce, and improve infrastructure Information Education and Communication (IEC) activities for the health and family welfare of the rural population in nearly six states in India, including Karnataka (www.karunatrust.org) | Ensuring skilled health care delivery to remote areas |
| 8 | Medico Friend Circle (MFC) | New Delhi, India | Health activists | Health activists from varied backgrounds and interests Forum for debate and sharing ideas relevant to the health movement (Shukla 2021) Functions without any institutional funding and has considerable ideological diversity Emphasis on understanding, discussing, and debating issues within a broad, people-oriented, but pluralistic and humanist framework | Fostered a wave of broader democratization, and conscientization in the society at large, including among the intelligentsia (thinkers and policy makers) |
| 9 | People Living with HIV (PLHIV) | Global initiative | PLHIV | The successful fight for getting generic drugs for antiretroviral treatment by research and analysis and getting involved in country wide movements | Bill in the parliament for safeguarding the patent law amendments Rejecting a patent against Boehringer Ingelheim, which manufactured the pediatric antiretroviral drug, Nevirapine India filed patent opposition against more than eight international drug manufacturing companies. (People Living With HIV in India n.d.) |

(continued)

**Table 1** (continued)

| S1 No | Name of the initiative | Location | Partners involved | Best practices | Key outcomes |
|---|---|---|---|---|---|
| 10 | Mahila Arogya Samiti (MAS) | India | National Health Mission (NHM) | Community participation in health at all levels. Planning, Implementing, and Monitoring health programs Collective action on Health, Nutrition, Water, Sanitation, and social determinants at the community level Chaired by the ASHA, MAS - is one of the mechanisms to improve Universal Health Coverage for urban poor and slum dwellers through active community engagement and mobilization | Decentralized health planning as 'Local Collective Action' Intended to improve monitoring and accountability of services, and community mobilization, ultimately leading to community empowerment and realization of rights Re-emphasize the need for people's involvement and role in prioritizing health issues, voicing concerns, and bridging the gap between health service providers and beneficiaries. (Mahila_ Arogya_Samiti.pdf 2021) |
| 11 | Kudumbashree | Kerala | Government of Kerala | Neighborhood Groups of Women (NHG), empowers in financing and realizing their fundamental rights Working areas are - Health, Nutrition, Agriculture, Education platform for income generation, microcredit organization for individual enterprises | Covers every woman in rural and urban households. Broad research and community interface for all activities related to local government It ensures awareness, accountability, ownership, and participation of the community in various public sector initiatives Better education and health of the family by empowered women. (Kudumbashree 2021) |

partnerships must be built with various NGOs and actors within health services.

4. Empowering women and targeting approaches to eliminate the gender-based differences for health care access, as mentioned in examples 5, 10, and 11 in Table 1. Women were empowered in their diverse roles as healthcare workers, village leaders, decision makers, and as members of the social and health systems.

5. Ensuring equity and equality with interventions to reach the unreached, as mentioned in examples 5, 6, 7, and 10 in Table 1. The geographical isolation and exclusion from the current advancement of health care and society has been addressed by these interventions by focusing on equity and equality principles.

## 4   Conclusion

*Major social movements eventually fade into the landscape not because they have diminished but because they have become a permanent part of our perceptions and experience.*

—Freda Adler

The chapter provides you insights from our experiences in India on social movements and empowerment in shaping Global health priorities.

The social movement's origin is based upon the perceptions of an issue and the community's concerns toward a larger goal. The empowerment of these social groups toward emerging issues and goals warrants new deliberation. Social media and the digital era have propelled these perspectives, and deliberations torrent sparked new social movements. In some cases, the philanthropic nature of humans emerged during the recent COVID-19 crisis. Many formed local groups and mobilized funds and resources to help their communities. However, these groups often dissolved once the purpose was attained. Documentation of these movements, education, and inspiration of the communities using these examples can spark a willingness to work toward a more just society. Platforms for communication, digital technology, and training in digital literacy and reaching out to people in the system will help these movements work efficiently. As a development/public health professional, recognizing this potential resource in the community and developing sustainable solution models will support countries in improving health for all.

These success stories from India exemplify community empowerment and grassroots movements that continue to influence policy responses to health issues. These examples illustrate the interplay between determinants of health, geographical variations, sociocultural norms, state planning, implementation, and the community at large. They bring in examples of sustainable primary health care solutions and the roles of government, civil society organizations, and community members. Finally they emphasizes the increasing realization during the COVID pandemic that the world is becoming a "Global Village".

Digital media platforms can be used to empower communities. However, community participation, democratization, ownership, and decentralization of power are key principles to be adopted. Effective utilization of people, products, policy, and partnership is the key to empowered social movements in society. Policies need to be set up to encourage these movements by providing platforms, training, resources, and sustainability.

# References

About Accredited Social Health Activist (ASHA) :: National Health Mission [cited 2021 Sept 15]. Available from: https://nhm.gov.in/index1.php?lang=1&level=1&sublinkid=150&lid=226

Adams R. Empowerment, participation and social work. New York: Palgrave Macmillan; 2008. p. xvi.

Agarwal S, Curtis SL, Angeles G, Speizer IS, Singh K, Thomas JC. The impact of India's accredited social health activist (ASHA) program on the utilization of maternity services: a nationally representative longitudinal modelling study. Hum Resour Health. 2019;17(1):68. [cited 2020 Jan 21]. Available from: https://human-resources-health.biomedcentral.com/articles/10.1186/s12960-019-0402-4

Alexandra Bettencourt, Associate Governance and Public Administration Officer—Further reading Grass roots; n.d.

Alliance for Health Policy and Systems Research. Strengthening health systems: the role and promise of policy and systems research. Geneva: Alliance for Health Policy and Systems Research; 2004.

Bayertz, K. (1999). Four uses of "Solidarity". In: Bayertz K, editor. Solidarity. Philosophical Studies in Contemporary Culture, vol 5. Springer, Dordrecht. https://doi.org/10.1007/978-94-015-9245-1_1

Bhore committee. | National Health Portal of India 1946 [cited 2021 Sept 15]. Available from: https://www.nhp.gov.in/bhore-committee-1946_pg

Bossert T. Analyzing the decentralization of health systems in developing countries: decision space, innovation and performance. Soc Sci Med 1982. 1998;47(10):1513–27.

Critical reflections on health services development in India: the teleology of disorder–NLM Catalog–NCBI [cited 2021 Sept 15]. Available from: https://www.ncbi.nlm.nih.gov/nlmcatalog/101629030

Human Capital. The value of people, OECD [cited 2021 Sept 15]. Available from: https://www.oecd.org/insights/humancapital-thevalueofpeople.htm

Kraef C, Kallestrup P. After the Astana declaration: is comprehensive primary health care set for success this time? BMJ Glob Health. 2019;4(6):e001871. [cited 2021 Sept 14]. Available from: https://gh.bmj.com/content/4/6/e001871.

Kudumbashree [cited 2021 Sept 15]. Available from: https://www.kudumbashree.org/

Kumar A, Nayar KR, Bhat L. Where is 'public' in the public health discourse? Rochester: Social Science Research Network; 2016. [cited 2021 Sept 15]. Report No.: ID 2761737. Available from: https://papers.ssrn.com/abstract=2761737

Kumar A, Rajasekharan Nayar K, Koya SF. COVID-19: challenges and its consequences for rural health care in India. Public Health Pract. 2020;1:100009. [cited 2021 Sept 15]. Available from: https://www.ncbi.nlm.nih.gov/pmc/articles/PMC7199699/.

Mahila_Arogya_Samiti.pdf [cited 2021 Sept 15]. Available from: https://nhm.gov.in/images/pdf/NUHM/Training-Module/Mahila_Arogya_Samiti.pdf

Georgiadou E. Marshall McLuhan's 'global village' and the Internet 1995. [cited 2021 Sept 15]; Available from: http://rgdoi.net/10.13140/RG.2.1.1490.1282

Maru RM. The community health volunteer scheme in India: an evaluation. Soc Sci Med. 1983;17(19):1477–83. [cited 2021 Sept 15]. Available from: https://www.sciencedirect.com/science/article/pii/0277953683900461

National Academies of Sciences Engineering, Medicine. In: Weinstein JN, Geller A, Negussie Y, Baciu A, editors. Communities in action: pathways to health equity. Washington, DC: The National Academies Press; 2017. Available from: https://www.nap.edu/catalog/24624/communities-in-action-pathways-to-health-equity.

nrhm-framework-latest.pdf [cited 2021 Sept 15]. Available from: https://nhm.gov.in/WriteReadData/l892s/nrhm-framework-latest.pdf

Human and social capital are keys to well-being and economic growth. OECD [cited 2021 Sept 14]. Available from: https://www.oecd.org/social/humanandsocialcapitalarekeystowell-beingandeconomicgrowth.htm

Organization WH, Fund (UNICEF) UNC. Social mobilization: key messages for social mobilization and community engagement in intense transmissions areas. World Health Organization; 2014. p. 6.

People Living With HIV in India: The struggle for access; n.d.. Available from: https://phmovement.org/wp-content/uploads/2018/07/E3.pdf

Rondinelli DA. Secondary cities in developing countries: policies for diffusing urbanization. SAGE Publications; 1983. 296 p.

Scott K, George AS, Ved RR. Taking stock of 10 years of published research on the ASHA programme: examining India's national community health worker programme from a health systems perspective. Health Res Policy Syst. 2019;17(1):29. [cited 2021 Sept 15]. Available from: https://doi.org/10.1186/s12961-019-0427-0.

Shukla P. Role of civil society in achieving health for all [cited 2021 Sept 15]. Available from: https://phmovement.org/wp-content/uploads/2018/06/19_IndiaReportFinal.pdf

Social Development for Sustainable Development | DISD [cited 2021 Sept 15]. Available from: https://www.un.org/development/desa/dspd/2030agenda-sdgs.html

The 2018 Astana Declaration on Primary Health Care, is it useful? [cited 2021 Sept 14]. Available from: https://www.ncbi.nlm.nih.gov/pmc/articles/PMC6445497/

The forgotten dimension of the SDG indicators – Social Capital [cited 2021 Sept 15]. Available from: https://blogs.worldbank.org/voices/forgotten-dimension-sdg-indicators-social-capital

Universal health coverage (UHC) [cited 2021 Sept 15]. Available from: https://www.who.int/news-room/fact-sheets/detail/universal-health-coverage-(uhc).

World Social Capital Monitor – United Nations Partnerships for SDGs platform [cited 2021 Sept 14]. Available from: https://sustainabledevelopment.un.org/partnership/?p=11706

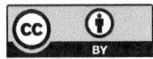

# When Women Lead in Global Health: Alternative Mobilizations

Cristina Alonso, Irene Torres, and Barbara Profeta

*People ... in a single day, reproduce, resist, are complicit in, rage against, celebrate, throw up hands/fists/towels, and withdraw and participate in uneven social structures— that is, everybody.*

Tuck (2009)

## Abstract

Ongoing discussions on what is "wrong" with global health or how to decolonialize global health tend to focus exclusively on structural shortcomings, such as effectiveness of global platforms and institutions or lack of truly participatory consultation strategies (downstream perspective). Thereby they fail to capture alternative approaches to global health leadership (upstream perspective) and to recognize the sovereignty of non-Western knowledge and the intrinsic value of community regeneration in all its forms as a key ingredient for effective global health practice.

Women's perspectives have been largely relegated to the gender agenda (balance, parity, equity) or proposed as models on "how to lead better" based on preconceived, male-based notions of what constitutes "effective" leadership, including setting and prioritizing goals. Instead of creating hierarchies of priorities, we must understand the complexity of human experience and the power and inequality patterns it is embedded in, and remain open to or embrace apparent contradictions when designing support mechanisms. This chapter centers on the disproportionate impact of COVID-19 in the lives of Latin American immigrants in Chelsea, Massachusetts, United States, during the 2020 pandemic. The chapter explores how public health prioritization of basic needs neither captured the relationship between impact and social response nor acknowledged the interplay between the different needs of people. Employing an insider's look, we describe how the women leaders of the local organization La Colaborativa called upon culturally accepted codes to reverse power roles, questioned scientific definitions of needs and led their community out of potentially irreversible consequences of the crisis in a holistic and sustainable way. Their leadership serves as an example of how self-governed, women-

This chapter is based on Cristina Alonso's DrPH thesis.

C. Alonso (✉)
La Colaborativa, Chelsea, MA, USA

Harvard T.H. Chan School of Public Health, Boston, MA, USA

I. Torres
Inter-American Institute for Global Change Research, Montevideo, Uruguay

Uruguay and Fundación Octaedro, Quito, Ecuador

B. Profeta
Independent consultant, Bern, Switzerland

© The Author(s) 2024
A. Stewart Ibarra, A. D. LaBeaud (eds.), *Transforming Global Health Partnerships*, Sustainable Development Goals Series, https://doi.org/10.1007/978-3-031-53793-6_21

led organizations that are rooted in the community may address the real needs of its members during a global catastrophic event.

### Keywords

Infectious disease · Health emergency · Community · Women leadership · Equity

## Author Perspective

Sharing a cultural understanding of solidarity although coming from different backgrounds and countries, the authors have worked in health-related research and interventions, for or with funding from international organizations, but also self-funded and independently. They are interested in social justice, scientific sovereignty, recognition of practical experience and other forms of knowledge and what is relevant and desired by communities, in other words, they value participation, equity, as well as alternative and critical ways of thinking.

**Key Tenets for Global Health Partnerships**

1. Research and interventions in health require awareness and recognition of alternative forms of knowledge.
2. Openness and attention to possibilities help pave the way to alternative ways of thinking.
3. Partnerships must be based on mutual trust and respect, not on the need to fill quotas.
4. Partnerships require fair (in accordance to each parties' real possibilities) contributions (responsibilities) from all partners, granting equitable access (right) to spaces and opportunities for visibility and recognition.
5. Serving a community holistically requires designing programs and interventions that are built from the ways it is

already functioning. Communities already have systems to solve problems, create support networks, and ensure the wellbeing of its members. Working with these make programs more sustainable and engender trust.

6. Equity in health involves ensuring diversity at the policy and implementation levels; while each cohort may prioritize their needs, together they ensure the regeneration and wellbeing of the most vulnerable.
7. This chapter addresses the following SDGs:

Goal 3: Ensure healthy lives and promote well-being for all at all ages

Goal 5: Achieve gender equality and empower all women and girls

Goal 10: Reduce inequality within and among countries

## 1 Situating Women's Leadership in Action

Powerful journals based in high income countries have gained attention lately by proposing that researchers discuss what is "wrong" with global health (The Lancet Global Health 2021) or calling for "action" to decolonize global health (Khan et al. 2021). Although we have been tempted to engage in the debate, we find that doing so would not help to subvert the existing power imbalances that actively prevent change from happening. On the one hand, the debate's set up suggests that these leading journals and their academic acolytes declare themselves ready to "open their space" for "others" to "have a voice" or become "visible", with the "others" representing less dominant perspectives from researchers in low and middle income countries, as if the latter were silent or dormant unless "graciously" prompted. The leading narrative diverts the attention away from a purposely entertained power imbalance, fed by self-preservation interests, to the benefit of a "feel good" pseudo-participatory approach. On the other hand, and quite similarly to this "decolonization" scenario, the conversation on women's leadership is rooted in dry land, one where women are lumped into the "bodies with a vagina" category in a *Lancet* cover (The Lancet Global Health 2021). This effectively pushes the right to discuss anything women-related to the corner that we continuously struggle to break away from. On the same dry land, women's perspectives have been largely relegated to the gender agenda (e.g., balance, parity, equity) in global health. Successful leadership models are automatically associated with pre-conceived (male-driven or male-typologized) notions of what "effective" leadership consists of in the first place, including the goals such a leadership must set.

This chapter seeks to respond to the question of what is wrong with "global health" and associated forms of leadership in the terms imposed against a background of predominantly linear mindsets all too often referring to "universal standards" meant to bring to reason non-existing average countries. Typically a response would legitimize a damage-centered approach that consciously ignores the option of really engaging with alternative ways of thinking and doing. These nevertheless resemble the natural variety of real life, than the dominant scientific and narrative perspective is keen to show and embrace.

Rather than take a damage-based or -centered approach to evaluate what is "wrong" with global health, we propose to look at alternative understandings and actions that are working well at local levels. We move beyond a focus on morbidity and mortality caused by the COVID-19 pandemic and examine aspects of regeneration, community strengthening and program sustainability.

In this chapter, we reflect on women leadership and its ability to effectively subvert power relationships. It does so by challenging linear approaches to needs assessments and response designs, and addressing inequities through a much theoretically promoted, but seldom truly embraced or implemented, whole-health/well-being or whole-life approach. Public health tends to divide the implementation of social protections and interventions into categories and specific cohorts (women, people of color, immigrants, etc.). However, a group of postcolonial feminists argue that this perspective necessarily sustains colonial categories of domination and submission. Viveros Vigoya argues that, in the US, intersectionality[1] ignores the issue of class by focusing on race, and gender (Viveros 2016).

While the COVID-19 pandemic disproportionately impacted people of color in the United States (US), negative effects were more acute on populations living under multiple layers of inequities. Specifically, this chapter describes the impact of the pandemic on poor, essential workers, belonging to Latino families frequently led by women. These families live near the city of Boston and have immigrated from poor, rural areas of Central America where access to education and rights is virtually non-existent, and Indigenous identity is denied through post-settler policies. These layers exceed a description of "ethnicity" and "gender", and co-exist in individuals' bodies and experience and at the community level. Tuck and Yang (2012) remind us that Indigenous People are rendered "visible as 'at risk' and as asterisk people", a compromise that "erases and then conceals the erasure of Indigenous Peoples... to the margins of public discourse" (Tuck and Yang 2012).

---

[1] Intersectionality was defined by Kimberle Crenshaw in 1989 the interconnected nature of the social categorizations such as race, class, and gender as they apply to a given individual or group, regarded as creating overlapping and interpedent systems of discrimination or disadvantage (Oxford Languages 2023).

In this same way, "Hispanics" become a catch-all category for anyone who was born, or whose parents (or even grandparents) were born in Latin America. This category negates the deep structural inequities within Latin America that necessarily include gender, geographic location, political participation, sexuality, and degree of Indigenous-ness. Recognizing the sovereignty of Latinx bodies (in all their intersectional identities) requires creating social protection programs that acknowledge what is distinct about levels of access to social protections, how community members relate internally, and how much agency that community has.

The reason this rests within feminist theory is because ensuring families have what they need to survive (in this case during a pandemic) is the burden of women in Latinx societies. Hence, it is not surprising that it is women who lead organizations that design the most relevant responses, because they act informed by needs but also represent access to safety and wellbeing as matriarchs. We question whether this form of leadership is actually empowerment, or just another burden for women to carry, or what Cornwall (2018) has termed "empowerment lite".

As a form of reflection, we document the actions of women leaders of La Colaborativa in Chelsea, Massachusetts, as they interplay with the impact of COVID, Latinx cultures, and social inequities. Our focus is on what is strong, regenerative, and worthy in a health-oriented intervention. We acknowledge the values that guide our own work as researchers, trying to capture the complexity of human experience while remaining open to apparent contradictions.

The mission of La Colaborativa is to empower Latinx immigrants to enhance the social and economic health of the community and its people; and to hold institutional decision-makers accountable to the community.

Currently La Colaborativa focuses on food and housing security, economic advancement, cultural celebration, and immigrant leadership to drive policy and systems change. During the pandemic La Colaborativa established a Health Equity department in response to the health and economic crisis brought on by COVID-19.

To learn more about La Colaborativa visit: https://la-colaborativa.org/

The city of Chelsea occupies about two square miles just north of Boston. It has an estimated formal population of 40,000 residents, but informal estimates claim there may be up to 75,000 residents (Editorial Board, Boston Globe 2020). A city of mostly low-wage Latinx immigrants, it is known for having overcrowded and substandard housing, high levels of poverty, and food insecurity. The underlying social and economic realities of this community might have predicted a major catastrophe with the arrival of COVID. In April 2020, an exploratory study found antibodies to COVID among 30% of Chelsea residents (Saltzman 2020), almost six times higher than the state average. Also, testing rates were low, i.e., positivity rates were high (Barry 2020).

**La Colaborativa, a community based organization in Chelsea, MA**

Founded in 1988 in Chelsea, MA, La Colaborativa is a Latina-led organization that has worked to design and deliver an array of programs, initiatives and community organizing campaigns that serve, protect, celebrate and uplift Latinx immigrants in the Greater Boston area.

## 2 Situating the Conversation on Health Equity

Systemic failures including social marginalization, economic poverty, high rates of low-wage essential jobs, and low access to healthcare services (Velasco-Mondragon et al. 2016), have impacted Latinx communities in the US. Even before the pandemic, Latinx suffered disproportionately from low quality social and

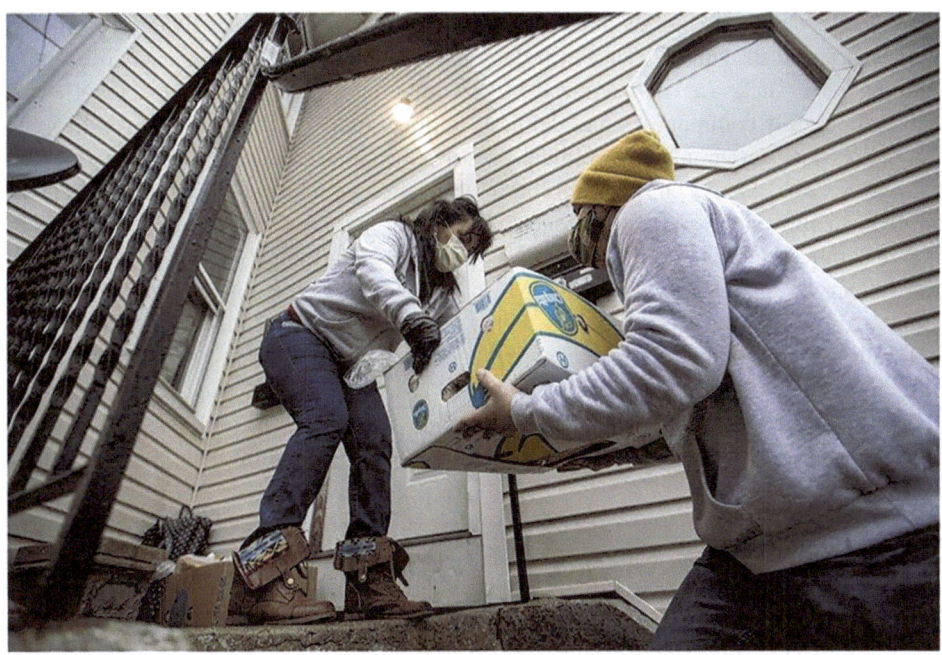

La Colaborativa staff distribute a box of food to Chelsea residents during the pandemic. Home deliveries wereenabled for people who were positive for COVID, the elderly and people with disabilities

physical environments in the US that impacted their health outcomes (Velasco-Mondragon et al. 2016). Many of them have fled violence in their countries of origin,. The experience of collective and personal trauma on Latinx immigrants impacts their decision to leave their homes and their physical and mental health in adverse ways throughout their lives and in future generations (Shonkoff and Garner 2012; van Steenwyk et al. 2018). Immigration policies and fear of deportation among those lacking permanent residency or citizenship deter access to healthcare services, increase stress, and exacerbate prior trauma lived in the home country or during migration (Torres et al. 2018).

By October 2020, half of all Latinx workers in the US had lost their jobs or taken a pay cut due to the COVID pandemic, exceeding the rates of any other ethnic group in the country (Shiro and Klein 2020). Many were uninsured and essential workers that could not switch to remote work. Similar to their countries of origin, the uprooted Latinx population in the US is lacking the health and economic equity (OECD 2020; Pan American Health, Organization 2020; Von Haldenwang

2005) that serve as the water and light that a tree needs to thrive.. Unsurprisingly, rates of hospitalization for COVID among Latinxs were 4.1 times higher and mortality among Latinx was 2.8 times higher than among whites (CDC 2020).

## 2.1 From Damaged to Self-Fulfilled

It is well established that wider social determinants have an impact on health outcomes. Marginalized communities are at higher risk of infections, even when they do not have underlying health conditions (Keyes and Galea 2021). Unsurprisingly, researchers focus on documenting the loss of individuals, families, and communities, commonly defining them as broken (Tuck 2009). The social sciences, argues Tuck, have presented an inevitable dichotomy: communities are bound either to reproduce social inequities or to resist unequal social conditions. However, communities and individuals operate in malleable and dynamic ways. In a single day, communities and individuals "reproduce, resist, are complicit in, rage against, celebrate, throw

up hands/fists/towels and withdraw and participate in uneven social structures" (Tuck 2009).

According to Tuck, a damage-centered
approach pathologizes communities and defines
them by oppression, commonly for political or
material gains. The focus on vulnerabilities
inhibits the identification and knowledge of
strengths. It implicates a colonialist perspective,
which is intent on finding "what is wrong."
Correspondingly, asking what is wrong with
global health reiterates the damage-centered
approach. It implies a need to be critical, but
again fails to recognize existing approaches that
transcend the intention of saving lives and move
towards rebuilding communities.

In contrast, a desire-based framework
accounts for the hope, vision, and wisdom of
lived experience and allows for multiplicity,
complexity, and contradiction. It accounts for
sovereignty, as well as for the survival and regeneration strategies that are inherent and ever-
evolving in a community. As a woman, Tuck
proposes that communities are more than their
collective illnesses and trauma. We must understand them through the lens of regeneration,
which involves "turning our back" to narratives

of fear, oppression and depletion (Tuck 2009).
Indeed, Chelsea serves as a vivid example of a
community that is much more than its vulnerabilities. In a city that suffers from deep disparities, women leaders from La Colaborativa
activated an unusual and effective response that
was unique in Massachusetts, going far beyond
the more traditional public health-oriented testing and contact tracing coupled with social protection measures. Under the leadership of Latinx
women, Chelsea harnessed its collective strength
to establish a supportive, mycorrhizal network
addressing the needs for physical survival, meaning, and self-fulfillment, which made the
response sustainable.

## 3    Collective Survival as a Path Towards Self/Fulfillment

Prioritization of needs is a common tenet of public health responses, and pandemic management
was no exception. Physical distancing, for example, was viewed from the pragmatic standpoint of
prevention measures with limited consideration
for its non-physiological aspects or consequences

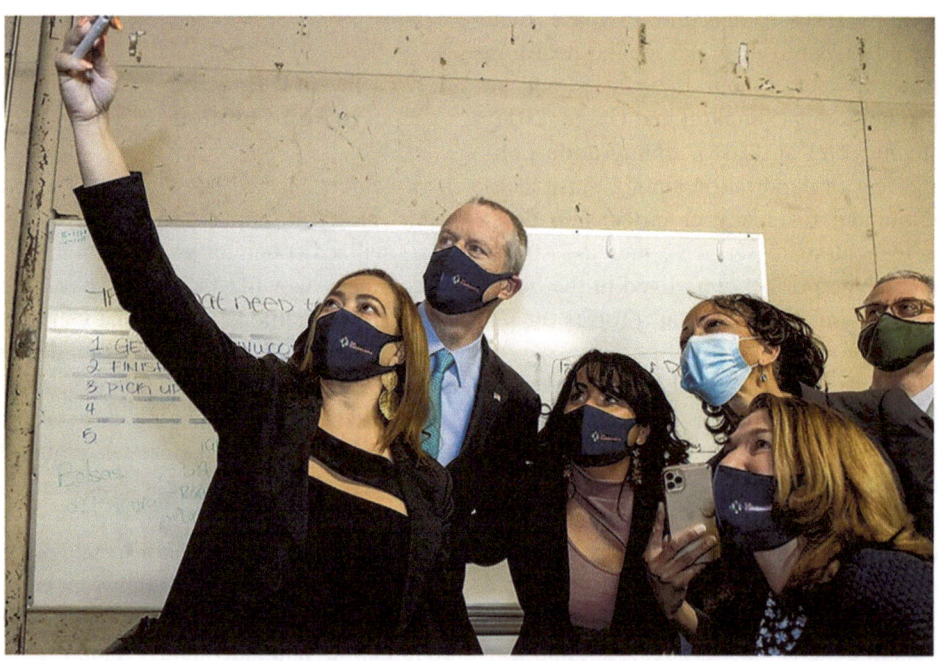

Food pantry

(Ryan et al. 2020). According to such a "hierarchy of needs", Maslow (1943) argued that humans evolve on a progressive scale. First, they are concerned with their basic needs, which include food, water, warmth, rest, security, and safety. Once these are met, people move on to concern themselves with psychological needs, which include belonging, love, and prestige, or a sense of accomplishment. Finally, when these needs are met, people can finally concern themselves with self-fulfillment, which includes being creative and achieving one's full potential. Maslow (1943) argued that when basic needs are unmet, "the organism is then dominated by the physiological needs, all other needs may become simply non-existent or be pushed into the background (p. 5)."

## 3.1 Basic Needs

Without downplaying the stress of the dire economic and health impacts of the pandemic, La Colaborativa organized rapidly and with agility at the onset of the pandemic to meet the basic needs of Chelsea's residents, while maintaining existing programs. As an organization that supported community development, La Colaborativa hired local mothers who desperately needed income to establish the largest food pantry in Chelsea. The pantry operated almost every day of the week from March 2020 onward, and still operates today (June 2023). The organization also organized a system to support residents to process rental assistance applications, prevent evictions, and find emergency housing for evicted families, all while maintaining previously existing immigration support, English language classes, and youth training programs.

Unconditional support for basic needs, including rent, food, diapers, sanitary pads, and transitional housing, created a deep sense of gratitude from the community to La Colaborativa, as an organization that responded quickly to alleviate residents' hardships. According to surveys, people recognized that they would not have been able to afford these costs on their own, apply for rental assistance through the Residential Assistance for Families in Transition (RAFT) program, or obtain useful information on COVID prevention from a trustworthy source. La Colaborativa was identified as the main source of social support, often in comparison to their countries of origin—for example, Honduras, El Salvador, and Guatemala—where governments have mostly failed to provide protection.

Key to this work was the immediacy of assistance. The organization bypassed complex bureaucratic processes to provide assistance immediately, based on residents' requests. At the same time, the organization's leadership acknowledged the complexities of time management and began offering services in conjunction. For example, once COVID vaccines were made available, they were offered together with knowledge on and means to prevent the disease during food and diaper distribution to make things easier and more efficient for families. Integrating services to overcome bureaucratic silos when serving families was a key element to this women-led response. This built on women's lived experience as heads of the household.

Perhaps it was through the leadership of La Colaborativa that people came to realize a sense of pride and belonging to their community. It could also be argued that this sense of belonging and loyalty to family and loved ones existed before the pandemic and served as the impetus to provide quick solutions to the catastrophe that rolled into Chelsea in the shape of the coronavirus pandemic.

## 3.2 Psychological Needs

The mental health impacts of the pandemic have been and will continue to be devastating for this community. During 2020 and 2021, according to the ethnographic research used for reflection in this chapter, families were deeply stressed about meeting basic needs and emotionally exhausted by the never-ending nature of the pandemic. In interviews, residents reflected that many were already suffering from deep life-long trauma and the insecurities exacerbated by COVID. Persistent trauma was exacerbated by lockdown and social distancing contradicted values that are deeply sowed in Latinx culture. Getting together for Sunday lunch at the matriarch's house, having coffee with friends, and celebrating life transitions in community are just a few of the many cultural rituals that are non-negotiable to members of a Latinx household. But common practices, such as families convening to support each other through joy and hardship, were largely eliminated during the pandemic.

Despite increased isolation and distancing, in-depth interviews conducted with female heads of households in Chelsea revealed that the pandemic brought families closer together. They pooled their resources and looked out for each other's mental and physical health. During the darkest months of uncertainty, families expressed their joy in spending more time with their children and watching them grow in ways they had not been able to before. Women expressed the perception that their marriages were strengthened through problem-solving and emotional support. Friendships and church groups became spaces for regeneration, joy, and strength.

Planning and execution did not depend on women's leadership only at the organizational level, but also at the family level, which La Colaborativa also depended on and trusted. It was assumed that Chelsea residents self-identify in relation to their families and the support networks they are part of. Food and resources are distributed among these networks, and parents rely on extended childcare through social networks. During the pandemic, family members were brought into homes if they were unable to pay rent. Families prayed together. They strategized on how to join forces to survive the pandemic, sometimes extending to other countries where remittances were expected to arrive or where the power of prayer was magnified in the case of an ailing family member. Food pantry boxes were often shared with other families in the building or those they considered more vulnerable and in need of assistance.

The food pantries at La Colaborativa would fill up with women who were there not just to lend a hand. They would show up early to huddle and share time together. Leaving the pantry open so that women could answer the ancient call to huddle, gossip, and problem solve within a collective, even during restrictions to physical proximity, became an important space and tool to a whole-wellbeing approach to tackling the COVID-19 pandemic.

## 3.3 Self-Fulfillment Needs

Despite the constant stress of having to meet basic needs for their families, Chelsea residents still grappled with issues of meaning and purpose in life. They felt that the extreme hardship of the pandemic required a deeper search for fulfillment. A combination of a sense of belonging to a family and a more extensive social network, faith in God, and trusting that things would work out were key to getting through the pandemic's challenges.

Although residents struggled with unemployment and poverty, they felt there was always a relative or another person who was worse off than them. Regardless of undergoing dire hardship, women felt obligated to give the little they had to support others' wellbeing. Not only did they understand this as a community obligation, but also as a spiritual mandate to be a better person. Chelsea residents understand that their personal self-fulfillment is intimately linked to their family and community. They perceived fulfillment as resulting from members of a community sharing with and helping others.

How residents found meaning and in doing so achieved self-fulfillment through community service and response helps to explain why La Colaborativa was able to pivot so quickly to address the multiple needs of Chelsea residents during the pandemic. For staff and volunteers, there was no question that fulfilling the mission of La Colaborativa was through providing full scope, wrap-around services for anyone who needed them. Volunteers were not difficult to find since Latinx are always volunteering to support their family and loved ones through cooking, childcare, housing, and taking care of others. While such values could be described as having the burden of care placed on the women, Chelsea volunteers of La Colaborativa signaled that they considered this network their family. Their loyalty and obligation made it natural for them to help out.

## 4    A View into Women's Leadership in a Health Response

La Colaborativa did not prioritize needs following mainstream public health guidelines in the US. Instead they integrated all levels of need in their actions. While the organization supported testing, monitoring and, eventually, vaccine distribution, it also attended to the yearning for meaning and belonging, and even inspiration, through collective action. Parents would look for open food pantries, many experiencing the sadness and humiliation of having lost a job that they

were proud of and needed, while hanging on to their families and faith for strength. It was important that residents learned to take care of themselves as they also kept their bonds with the community.

The approach and impact of women's leadership in Chelsea's response to COVID-19 can be described in the figure below, which integrates the self-described social response from the Chelsea community by adapting Maslow's categorization of needs from a hierarchy into a circle that informs and shapes community capacity. A circular format acknowledges that needs build on each other. This shifts away from the prioritization of needs and highlights how successful leadership in health may help navigate a continuing crisis and adapt to abrupt changes by focusing on all three levels of needs at the same time. Outside of the circle are listed some of the factors that impact local communities (Fig. 1).

**Fig. 1** Theory of change for Chelsea, MA

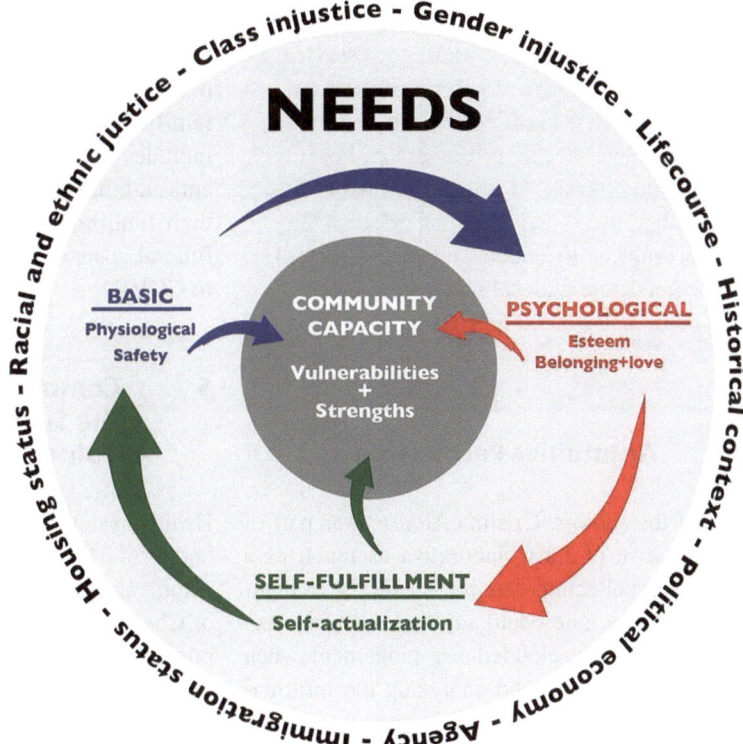

**Cristina Alonso, on getting involved with Chelsea during the pandemic.**

At the start of the pandemic (March 2020), I became involved in leading a statewide initiative that placed public health students and professionals with local departments of public health in Massachusetts. I was surprised that the Chelsea Department of Health and Human Services rejected any level of support and referred us to the Department of Strategy.

After the murder of George Floyd, I witnessed that surge in activism and street protests across the United States. As a longtime resident of Latin America, I was curious where and how Latinos were mobilizing. The Hispanic community was severely hit by COVID-19 and at a time of racial reconning across the country, I knew there had to be a movement, but it was not being covered by the media. I asked around my contacts in Boston, and was told connect with Gladys Vega, in Chelsea. I took the bus to Chelsea in mid-June 2020 and found a line 6 blocks long that was waiting for services at La Colaborativa. I offered myself as a volunteer, first in the food pantry and then as a public health professional. For my doctoral thesis I worked with La Colaborativa and the Chelsea City Government to understand the impact of the pandemic on local residents and design a community-based response.

## 4.1 An Intuitive Partnership

One of the authors, Cristina Alonso, was part of the initiative of La Colaborativa as much as a researcher collecting data for her thesis. In regular conditions, one could say that such involvement could have clouded her judgement when designing her study and analyzing the information. However, the widespread uncertainty of the COVID pandemic required a close collaboration between research and practice (Leach et al. 2021)

for decision making. As the leadership of La Colaborativa expressed, it was natural that they and Cristina (a researcher) would tend to "the needs of our people" (Gladys Vega, CEO of La Colaborativa).

Key to this was the "on the ground" formal and informal iterative process of listening and adapting of La Colaborativa, as it expanded its original programs to meet in flexible manners the complex layering of needs that emerged in Chelsea. Each life story was taken seriously, perhaps because staff and volunteers of La Colaborativa were beneficiaries themselves, or were immersed in and a part of community life. The food pantry was not just a place to fill an empty stomach. The leadership spent time there asking people how they were doing and what had happened since the last time they spoke. In addition, the food distribution line served as triage for additional services from rental assistance to domestic violence referrals. Connections were made through consecutive links shared across family and social networks.

Finally, unlike in city and state programs, beneficiaries were not turned away because they lacked paperwork or proof of certain status. There was an acknowledgement that Latinx family composition is flexible and often includes more than the nuclear family of parents and their children. La Colaborativa adapted their funding to meet unexpected needs such as funeral costs of families who had lost members to COVID.

## 5 Communities Are More Than the Sum of Their Vulnerabilities

Health systems are composed of more than a body of formal institutions, pre-established actors, and standardized norms. The community of Chelsea has demonstrated it is a crucial component of the health system of the state of Massachusetts in the US, even though it is not formally recognized as such and does not act according to expectations within an infectious disease response (Brower 2018). Therefore, when emphasizing the importance of working with local communities, global health researchers should consider self-governed local initiatives in equal terms as other institutions.

The partnership between the researcher, La Colaborativa and Chelsea City Govennrment was aimed at creating a greater understanding of the expressions and strengths of local systems. This work has taught us important lessons from La Colaborativa's leadership that may have otherwise been missed. Being as much a participant as an observer, the researcher moved under the surface of La Colaborativa, acquiring the understanding of an insider while providing the organization the alternative outlook of a different discipline (the social sciences). Consequently, alternative points of view from different terrains were planted together and grew in constant cycle of renewal and regeneration.

While the ethos of public health is to address population health and not focus on the individual, centralized government COVID task forces concentrated in hierarchical tiers of service delivery. This left populations scrambling for information and support practically on their own, or by piecemeal. In contrast, a desire-based framework is rooted in a collective effort towards decolonization to understand the design of resource sharing and social problem solving. This allows us to challenge traditional delivery design, which focuses on interventions that enable access to essential goods and services only by those deemed "at-risk."

The leadership values and skills of the women of La Colaborativa allowed the community to make the best of their capacities, relying less on government-mandated solutions, which were scarce or ineffective in the US prior to vaccination. There wasn't a need to rely on external assistance, which is the capacity building mantra of global health.. Ultimately, women leaders in this case were showing people the best they had within. They knew strengths were latent and needed some tending to sprout and grow strong.

Every crisis, instead of constituting pure tragedy (without forgetting the negative side of the experience) is an opportunity for any system to adapt and improve. In this case, the women lead-

ers of La Colaborativa were able to seize the opportunity, consciously or perhaps unconsciously as a product of their intentional monitoring of "what works". Concurrently, this entailed that the researcher did not need to pollinate the ground with her ideas, securing some form of "consensus" on her research agenda and plans. Like the Chelsea community, the researcher became driven by the community's desire-based framework. The study took place in an organic manner similar to the work of the organization. As practitioners, the actors involved did not expect to predict or control the results of their actions (contrary to what enthusiasts of "log-frames," "theories of change," and planned responses would prefer).

The experiences in Chelsea highlight that when a catastrophe hits and significantly alters our ways of living, communities naturally deploy their adaptive skills to survive. They manage to somehow mitigate the devastating collateral damages of the crisis. Lack of community participation in high-level decision making and practice was been a constant during the pandemic (Torres and López-Cevallos 2021). Perhaps public health should focus on helping families thrive. For that to happen, public health should be led by specialized departments in cities and regions in alliance with civic organizations. This alliance should serve to link patients to health care institutions and providers for care with the understanding that needs go beyond the damage caused by a disease and extend into many other aspects of daily life.

Interviews and participant observation with staff and volunteers revealed that it was through the women's leadership of La Colaborativa in meeting basic needs that the community came to realize a sense of pride and belonging to their community. Therefore, public health professionals can learn the broader lesson from Chelsea about how vulnerabilities can activate grassroots responses that go beyond the basic needs of residents to establish systems for strength and resilience.

Understanding Chelsea's vulnerabilities and strengths can give public health practitioners and policymakers insight into approaching the response to COVID-19 and other health challenges in similar communities. It is becoming more widely accepted that responses must include a strategy for addressing health inequities (Bleser et al. 2022). These insights are relevant to other Latinx immigrant communities in the US and even in Latin America, where response and social protections have been significantly weaker than in the US. While some of the specifics may vary, the synchronous approach to needs adopted in Chelsea may be relevant for all communities.

This insider's analysis of a researcher's collaboration with a community has helped us tot understand the nature and form of a potentially successful partnership in (global) health research. While there are no magic seeds for unpredictable yet irreplaceable nutrients such as opportunities (political momentum) and human factors (leadership skills), the COVID-19 response capacity of La Colaborativa points at four key tenets that are crucial to research alongside practice:

1. Global health is inevitably embedded in concrete realities, with their history, societal dynamics, knowledge and intrinsic capacities. Attempts to standardize partnerships in the interest of over-simplistic intervention policies and approaches are bound to fail their targeted ambition.

2. The ability to manage the unknown (and unknowable) and adaptability to embrace alternative (at times unorthodox) forms of practice and knowledge are crucial features of a regenerating health system. Avoiding disruption of such natural regeneration should be the minimum standard expected from any partnership (including in research) in global health

3. Semantically, partnerships suggest equal participation, rights, and conditions, as well as symmetrical benefits, regardless of the platform (channels) and rules set up to facilitate the collaboration. In sum, mutual trust and respect are the primary roots of any partnership that can face incoming challenges in an agile manner, where solutions germinate while continuously becoming renewed.

4. In designing solutions that garner trust and respect, participants in global health leadership and practice must consider that all communities already have existing systems designed to solve their own problems. Holistic programming must learn, understand and embed within said structures, since they may very well enable the sustainability of new initiatives because they engender trust in local capacity.

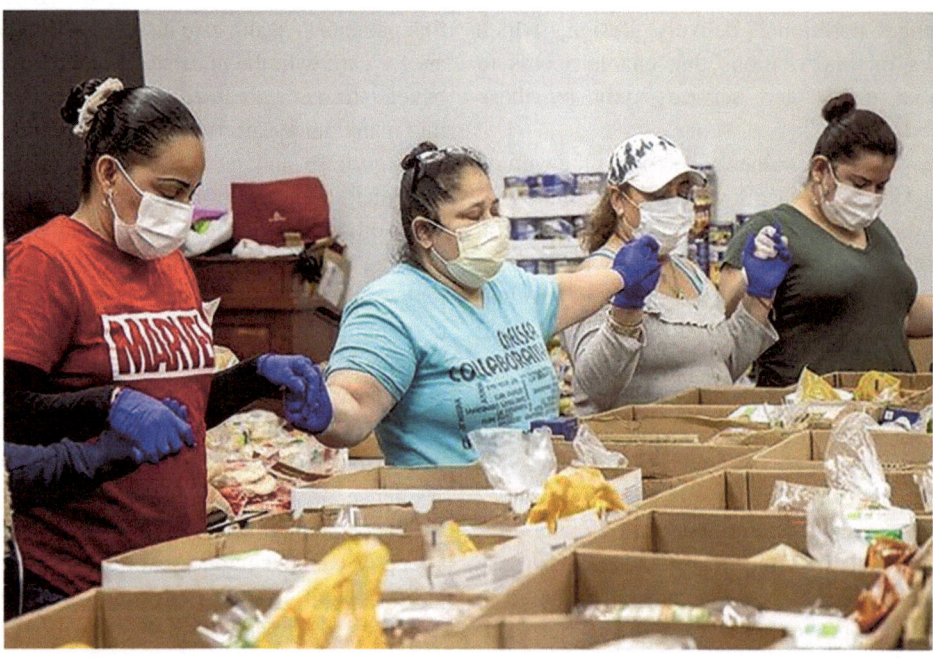

Governor Baker Visits

## 6    Conclusions

Chelsea's experience highlights that when catastrophe hits and significantly alters our ways of living, communities quickly build networks and systems to survive. These systems go beyond resolving the basic needs of food and shelter. They include love, protection, ritual, reflection, negotiation, finding meaning, bonding, and collective problem solving that embrace the complexities of human survival. By developing a collective vision, strategy, and sharing the burden for public health action, Chelsea is a model of recovery and resilience.

Our chapter provides critical insight into a recurrent flaw of the "aid" industry paradigm that, despite claims to the contrary, continues to reach communities with imported solutions, presuming that before and after the arrival of external "saviors" there is sheer emptiness and that communities that function differently from the expected standard lack fundamental creativity.

This persistent paternalism may act as a "disruptor," undermining the organic manifestation of coping strategies by communities, whose energy and resources are all too often mobilized in mimicry exercises aimed at the assimilation and reproduction of "international good practices." Also, to receive external aid, people must change their ways.

What the Chelsea case shows is that the best help is to avoid "disruption" as much as possible, so the community may quickly recover its capacity to react after the initial shock caused by a crisis and organize itself according to guidelines held by its members. Expending time and energy to align to other people's standards should not be the priority of affected communities, instead, resources including time should focus on learning to manage and managing a crisis. The reproduction of unequal social structures depends on how we condition aid and external technical assistance. Perhaps, instead, the key to resilience lies in resistance to external forces of change.

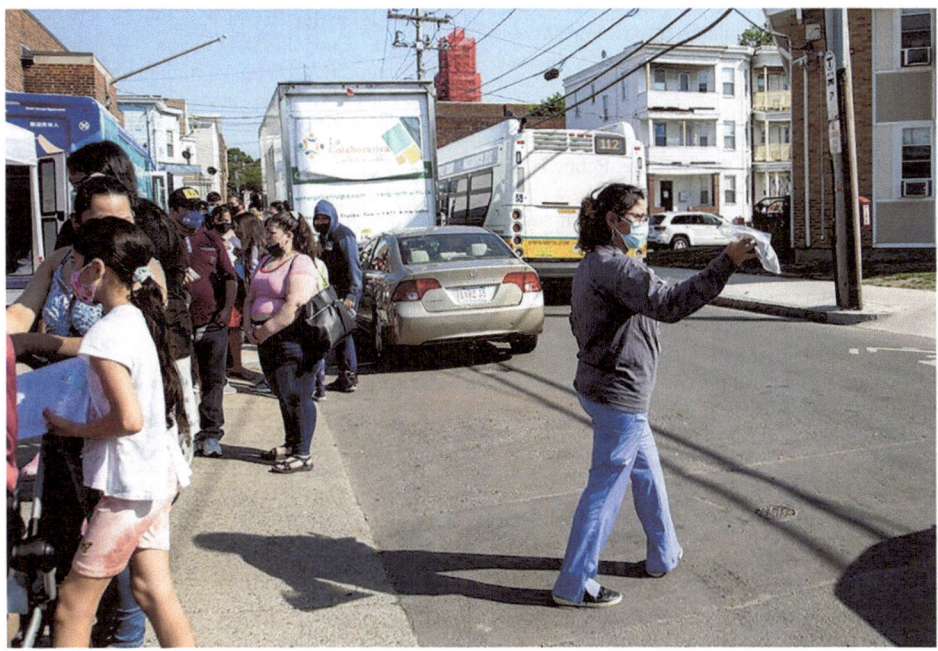

Youth vaccines

# References

The Lancet Global Health. Global health 2021: who tells the story? Lancet Glob Health. 2021;9(2):e99.

Khan M, Abimbola S, Aloudat T, Capobianco E, Hawkes S, Rahman-Shepherd A. Decolonising global health in 2021: a roadmap to move from rhetoric to reform. BMJ Glob Health. 2021;6(3):e005604.

Viveros VM. Interseccionality: a situated approach to dominance. Debate Fem. 2016;52:1–17.

Tuck E, Yang KW. Decolonization is not a metaphor. Decolonization Indig Educ Soc. 2012;1(1):40.

Cornwall A. Além do "Empoderamento Light": empoderamento feminino, desenvolvimento neoliberal e justiça global. Cad Pagu. 2018 [cited 2022 May 12]; Available from: http://www.scielo.br/j/cpa/a/9zJqwjXHP4KbgfsLRCY7WpC/?lang=pt

Editorial Board, Boston Globe. Low-balling the Chelsea population threatens the state's coronavirus epicenter. The Boston Globe; 2020. [cited 2020 Jun 17]; Available from: https://www.bostonglobe.com/2020/06/14/opinion/an-undercounted-population-threatens-chelsea-states-coronavirus-epicenter/

Saltzman J. Nearly a third of 200 blood samples taken in Chelsea show exposure to coronavirus – The Boston Globe. Boston Globe; 2020. [cited 2021 Jan 29]; Available from: https://www.bostonglobe.com/2020/04/17/business/nearly-third-200-blood-samples-taken-chelsea-show-exposure-coronavirus/

Barry E. In a Crowded City, leaders struggle to separate the sick from the well. The New York Times. 2020 [cited 2020 Jul 6]; Available from: https://www.nytimes.com/2020/04/25/us/coronavirus-chelsea-massachusetts.html

Velasco-Mondragon E, Jimenez A, Palladino-Davis AG, Davis D, Escamilla-Cejudo JA. Hispanic health in the USA: a scoping review of the literature. Public Health Rev. 2016;37(1):31.

Shonkoff JP, Garner AS. The commitee on psychological aspects of child and family health, Commitee on early chidhood, adoption and dependent care, and section on developmental, and behavioral pediatrics, Siegel BS, Dobbins MI, Earls MF, et al. The Lifelong Effects of Early Childhood Adversity and Toxic Stress. Pediatrics. 2012;129(1):e232–46.

van Steenwyk G, Roszkowski M, Manuella F, Franklin TB, Mansuy IM. Transgenerational inheritance of behavioral and metabolic effects of paternal exposure to traumatic stress in early postnatal life: evidence in the 4th generation. Environ Epigenetics. 2018;4:dvy023. [cited 2021 Feb 9]. Available from: https://doi.org/10.1093/eep/dvy023.

Torres SA, Santiago CD, Walts KK, Richards MH. Immigration policy, practices, and procedures: the impact on the mental health of Mexican and Central American youth and families. Am Psychol. 2018;73(7):843–54.

Shiro AG and Klein A. The COVID-19 recession hit Latino workers hard. Here's what we need to do. Brookings. 2020 [cited 2021 Jan 29]. Available from: https://www.brookings.edu/blog/how-we-rise/2020/10/01/the-covid-19-recession-hit-latino-workers-hard-heres-what-we-need-to-do/

OECD. Panorama de la Salud: Latinoamérica y el Caribe 2020. OECD Publishing; 2020. [cited 2021 Feb 8]. Available from: https://www.oecd.org/health/panorama-de-la-salud-latinoamerica-y-el-caribe-2020-740f9640-es.htm

Pan American Health, Organization. Equity in Health policy assessment: region of the Americas. Washington DC: 3; 2020. Report No.: License: CC BY-NC-SA 3.0 IGO

Von Haldenwang C. Systemic governance and development in Latin America. RevCEPAL. 2005;85:35–52.

CDC. Coronavirus Disease 2019 (COVID-19) in the U.S. Centers for Disease Control and Prevention. 2020 [cited 2020 Jun 16]. Available from: https://www.cdc.gov/coronavirus/2019-ncov/cases-updates/cases-in-us.html

Keyes KM, Galea S. Population Health science. Population Health science. Oxford University Press; [cited 2021 Nov 9]. Available from: https://oxfordmedicine.com/view/10.1093/med/9780190459376.001.0001/med-9780190459376

Tuck E. Suspending damage: a letter to communities. Harv Educ Rev. 2009;79(3):409–29, 539–540

Ryan BJ, Coppola D, Canyon DV, Brickhouse M, Swienton R. COVID-19 community stabilization and sustainability framework: an integration of the Maslow hierarchy of needs and social determinants of Health. Disaster Med Public Health Prep. 2020;14(5):623–9.

Maslow AH. A theory of human motivation. Psychol Rev. 1943;50(4):370–96.

Leach M, MacGregor H, Scoones I, Wilkinson A. Post-pandemic transformations: how and why COVID-19 requires us to rethink development. World Dev. 2021;138(105233):105233.

Brower J. The threat and response to infectious diseases (revised). Microb Ecol. 2018 Jul;76(1):19–36.

Torres I, López-Cevallos D. In the name of COVID-19: legitimizing the exclusion of community participation in Ecuador's health policy. Health Promot Int. 2021;36:1324–33.

Bleser W, Shen H, Crook H, Thoumi A, Cholera R, Pearson J, et al. Pandemic-driven Health policies to address social needs and Health equity | Health affairs. Health Aff Health Policy Brief; 2022. [cited 2022 May 26]; Available from: https://www.healthaffairs.org/do/10.1377/hpb20220210.360906/

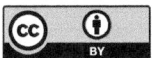

# Funding for Equitable Infectious Disease Research and Development

Meggie Mwoka ⓘ

*The essence of global health equity is the idea that something so precious as health might be viewed as a right.*

—Dr. Paul Famer

## Abstract

Research and development (R&D) are critical to develop effective solutions to address the prevention, control, elimination, and even eradication of infectious diseases globally. Financing global health and infectious diseases research is complex. It involves diverse and overlapping sources of funding; multiple recipients and mechanisms of funding; limited coordination, and lack of comprehensive data and impact assessment. Public funding for neglected diseases mainly comes from high income governments and multilateral organizations. Domestic contribution by most LMICs governments to R&D remains low and reliant on external funding from HICs. As a result, funding priorities may not always be aligned to country priorities.

Funding for research and development of infectious diseases has largely focused on HIV, TB and malaria, however with the pandemic, there is increasing focus on pandemic preparedness and response, and platform technologies for vaccine delivery and general diagnostics. Several initiatives have been developed over the years to address gaps in the research funding landscape such as establishment of public private partnerships including product development partnerships.

Shifting disease burdens and demographic changes, re-emergence and emergence of epidemic prone diseases in the face of climate change and a high globalized world, is impacting current and future approaches to infectious disease research and thus the funding priorities. Advancements have been made in establishing research institutions especially in LMICs in collaboration with HICs partners. However systemic challenges persist at institutional, political and global level limiting the growth of research and development especially in LMICs. Addressing these challenges at domestic level will require governments to take on greater responsibility towards investments in research, while leveraging external partnerships to strengthen and sustain relevant research and development that meets country and global needs.

M. Mwoka (✉)
Rockefeller Foundation-Boston University 3D
Commission, Nairobi, Kenya

© The Author(s) 2024
A. Stewart Ibarra, A. D. LaBeaud (eds.), *Transforming Global Health Partnerships*, Sustainable
Development Goals Series, https://doi.org/10.1007/978-3-031-53793-6_22

**Keywords**

Funding · Infectious diseases · Research and development

**Author Perspective**

The author is a dynamic global health specialist with a medical background, who has been practicing in Africa for the last 8 years with a focus on health systems strengthening, infectious diseases, health financing, public private partnerships in health, sexual and reproductive health, and diagnostics. She has expertise in research, knowledge translation, project implementation, and policy engagement. She has worked with different stakeholders ranging from regional bodies, national governments, and civil society to develop strategies, policies and programs towards advancing health and well-being in the region. She is passionate about amplifying the African voice in the global health space, transdisciplinary collaboration, and equitable action-oriented partnerships in global health.

**Key Tenets**

1. The current funding system for infectious disease research is not sustainable for long-term impact on research and development globally, especially in low- and middle-income countries.
2. Collaboration between public and private sectors, provides an opportunity for the advancement of research and development (R&D) related to infectious diseases.
3. Equitable, sustainable, and inclusive funding for infectious diseases R&D, requires a context specific, multi-stakeholder, and multi-sectoral approach.
4. This chapter addresses the following SDGs: #3: Good Health and Wellbeing, #10: Reducing Inequities, and #17: Partnerships for the Goals.

# 1 Background

Research and development (R&D) are critical to develop effective solutions to address the prevention, control, elimination, and even eradication of infectious diseases globally. Funding for R&D however remains precarious in low- and middle-income countries (LMICs) which bears the greatest burden of infectious disease and remains reliant on external funding. Countries such as Mozambique, Burkina Faso and Uganda receive more than 50% of their R&D funding from foreign sources such as philanthropic foundations, and multilateral organizations (Arvanitis and Mouton 2019). Less than 10% of global health research spending is dedicated to diseases that primarily afflict the poorest 90% of the world's population, the majority of whom are found in LMICs (Vidyasagar 2000). This reveals the misalignment of funding to disease prioritization and raises questions regarding the level of ownership and responsibility of national government funding for endemic diseases and epidemics that are likely to extend beyond borders.

**Funding Cuts**

In 2021, international research and development funding cuts by the UK government led to an outcry from researchers not just in the UK but across the globe. These budget cuts were deemed unlawful and a threat to human rights, health, and well-being across the globe (Foreign aid 2021; Kanja et al. 2021; GCRF African Science for Weather Information and Forecasting Techniques (SWIFT) 2021; Worley 2021). The budget cuts impacted projects focused on infectious disease research and interventions, including a withdrawal of over £150 million of funding toward interventions to control neglected tropical diseases (NTDs), a group of diseases that are intimately linked to poverty (Uniting to combat neglected tropical diseases 2021; Engels and Zhou 2020). This announcement revealed the unstable nature of infectious disease research funding especially in low- and middle-income countries (LMICs) which remain reliant on external funding for research and development (R&D) from few key investors.

As the COVID-19 pandemic ravaged the social, economic and health systems of the world, the global community was shocked into recognizing the urgency of setting up infectious disease surveillance, preparedness and response systems and increasing research and development targeting emerging infectious diseases. These are diseases that are newly recognized in a population or have existed but are rapidly increasing in incidence or geographic range such as zoonotic, food-borne, air-borne and vector-borne diseases (Hotez et al. 2008).

The COVID-19 pandemic has magnified the characteristic shortcomings of financing for infectious diseases R&D. That is, financing for R&D is disproportionately insufficient, uncoordinated, and tied to an unjust system of intellectual property (IP) rights. While 70.3% of the world population had received at least one dose of a COVID-19 vaccine (as of June 2023), only 32.2% of people in low-income countries have received at least one dose (Our World in Data 2021). The lack of equitable distribution of available COVID-19 vaccines has spurred conversations and initiatives towards improving local capacity to conduct infectious diseases research and to manufacture vaccines and improve diagnostics (Zhan 2020; Unitaid 2021). Amidst these conversations, are appeals to the World Trade Organization (WTO) to waive IP protection for

products and technologies related to COVID-19 prevention, treatment, and containment, which currently restrict LMICs such as India and South Africa from contributing to the manufacturing of COVID-19 related products and technologies (Rubin and Saidel 2021).

The current funding system for infectious diseases research is not sustainable for long-term impact on R&D globally, especially in LMICs. Disparities in funding infectious disease research exists between regions, within regions, across and within countries. A look at research output, in comparison to disease burden and the main actors in research, reveals these disparities. In Africa, for example, despite the gradual increase in research productivity, major capacity limitations exist as evidenced by university rankings, numbers of researchers, numbers of publications, clinical trials networks, and pharmaceutical manufacturing capacity (Arvanitis and Mouton 2019). Only 3% of scientific production is contributed by Africa, which is home to 15% of the world's population (Arvanitis and Mouton 2019). This comes as no surprise considering that it receives 1.3% of global investment in R&D and has 98 researchers per million inhabitants in comparison to regions such as East Asia and Pacific with 1623 researchers per million inhabitants, Latin America and Caribbean with 580 researchers per million inhabitants, and North America with 4404 researchers per million inhabitants (UNESCO Science report 2021; UNESCO Institute for Statistics (UIS) Science 2021; World Bank 2021).

In Africa, for example, scientific contributions are unevenly distributed across the continent. Countries in the North, East and Southern parts of Africa are in a much more favorable situation than countries in West and Central Africa, especially Francophone countries (Arvanitis and Mouton 2019). Only 13 countries in the region (out of 54) account for 89% of all research output (Arvanitis and Mouton 2019). Studies on the scientific contribution of African Researchers of infectious disease research showed under-representation of Africans in first and last author-ships positions in papers published from research done in Africa (Adetokunboh et al. 2021; Mbaye et al. 2019). Where both first and last authors have an African Institutional Affiliation, the researchers were predominantly from either South Africa or Kenya (Mbaye et al. 2019). Human Immunodeficiency Virus/Acquired immunodeficiency syndrome (HIV/AIDs), malaria, tuberculosis (TB), and Ebola virus disease are the most researched infectious diseases in the region currently (Adetokunboh et al. 2021).

## 2    Where We Are Now?

**Current Funding Landscape** Financing global health and infectious diseases research is complex. It involves multiple, diverse, and overlapping sources of funding; multiple recipients for funding; multiple mechanisms of funding, a multiplicity of roles, limited coordination, and lack of comprehensive data and impact assessment (McCoy et al. 2009; G-FINDER 2022). The three main sources of funds for R&D for neglected diseases are: (i) the public sector (e.g., governments and/or aid agencies); (ii) the private sector (e.g., multinational/small pharmaceutical companies or biotechnology companies); and (iii) philanthropic foundations and individuals such as The Bill & Melinda Gates Foundation and the Wellcome Trust (G-FINDER 2022).

> **Definition**
> Neglected diseases are defined as diseases disproportionately affecting people in developing countries, with need for new products (i.e., no existing products or improved or additional products are needed) and where there is market failure. For example: Chagas disease, schistosomiasis, dengue fever, and snake bites (World Health Organization (WHO) 2012).

The main funders for neglected diseases are public funders accounting for two-thirds of global funding (G-FINDER 2022). High income countries (HICs) governments provided most of the public funding (95%), followed by multilateral organizations (2.9%) and LMIC governments (1.7%) (G-FINDER 2022). Private sector funding for neglected diseases from multinational pharmaceutical companies (MNCs) and small pharmaceutical and biotechnology firms has grown over the years from USD 118 m in 2017 to USD 694 m in 2018 (G-FINDER 2022). The Bill and Melinda Gates Foundation and the Wellcome Trust accounted for 93% ($9792 m) of philanthropic sector funding for neglected disease research (G-FINDER 2022).

As signaled above, domestic contribution by most LMICs governments to R&D remains low. In 2007 African Member States committed to investing at least 1% of GDP in R&D, acknowledging the importance of R&D in sustainable development. However, this goal remains unrealized (World Health Organization n.d.). In Latin America, only Brazil allocates more than 1% of its GDP to R&D (World Health Organization n.d.). This is followed by Argentina and Chile at 0.65% and 0.36% respectively (STISA-2024 2014). This creates a ripple effect in terms of research output in the countries, with Brazil, Argentina, and Chile having the highest number of publications and researchers in the region (UNESCO Institute for Statistics (UIS) 2021). A study done in Serbia, showed a correlation between GDP growth and increased investment in R&D at the national level (SCImago 2007), demonstrating the important role of domestic funding by governments to the growth of research and development in a country.

Differing ideologies of the value of R&D for social and economic advancement may play a role as well in investment in infectious disease R&D. Low contribution by governments, especially LMICs, could be due to the low value and importance attached to science and technology as drivers of national development (World Health Organization n.d.; STISA-2024 2014; UNESCO

Institute for Statistics (UIS) 2021; SCImago 2007; Kutlača et al. 2020). In comparison, many HICs prioritize science and technology as core to social and economic development (Kutlača et al. 2020; Assessing the needs of the research system in Kenya 2019; World Health Organization Regional Office for Africa 2016; Estenssoro et al. 2016; Ciocca and Delgado 2017). In LMICs research is sometimes seen as a vehicle to leverage external funding versus a core contributor to national development (Kutlača et al. 2020). Additionally, it could signal the risk-averse nature of governments in LMICs to commission research where clear benefits to society are not guaranteed. The weak research culture and lack of ownership of research agendas in most LMICs thus, leads to reliance on funding from external donors (Kutlača et al. 2020; Assessing the needs of the research system in Kenya 2019; Estenssoro et al. 2016). Additionally, political and economic priorities and/or instability contribute to limited domestic funding towards research and development including for global health and infectious diseases in LMICs (World Health Organization Regional Office for Africa 2016; Estenssoro et al. 2016; Ciocca and Delgado 2017).

## 2.1    What Is Funded?

Funding priorities are influenced by multiple factors such as the prevalence of infectious diseases, burden of diseases (mortality and morbidity), research capacity, infrastructure, the potential to commercialize a product, and other social and political factors. For example, bacterial and parasitic diseases receive less research priority compared to viral diseases, according to a study done by Furuse Yuki (Daszak et al. 2020). Moreover, diseases transmitted from the environment compared with those with other transmission modes, and vaccinable-diseases versus those without a vaccine are likely to have higher research attention (Daszak et al. 2020).

Current research investments in selected infectious diseases are not commensurate with their burden of disease (Engels and Zhou 2020; Adetokunboh et al. 2021; G-FINDER 2022; Kutlača et al. 2020; Estenssoro et al. 2016; Abutu 2017; Head et al. 2016; Head et al. 2020; Ault 2007; Institute for Health Metrics and Evaluation (IHME) 2020). For example, HIV/AIDs-related research received more than double the research investment compared to TB, malaria, and pneumonia combined (Head et al. 2020; Ault 2007), despite, those diseases having a higher global burden in terms of disability-adjusted life years (DALYS), years lived with disability (YLDs) and deaths (Ault 2007). Other under-funded infectious diseases include some sexually transmitted infections (syphilis and gonorrhoea), neglected skin infections (e.g., scabies), diarrhoeal diseases, and helminth infections (World Bank 2021; Head et al. 2016). Of note is decreased funding for product development partnerships by 40% between 2008 and 2022 contributed by cuts from the UK Foreign, Commonwealth and Development Office (FCDO), USAID and Gates Foundation. However, funding seems to have been reallocated towards emerging infectious diseases. Increased investment in platform technologies with potential application across a wide range of disease groups has also been noted in the last few years. These include vaccine delivery technologies and devices, general diagnostic platforms, drug-delivery technologies and devices and adjuvants and immunomodulators.

Looking at previous pandemics (e.g. Ebola), investments in R&D in disease surveillance, preparedness and response are often reactive, following a major outbreak and dwindle thereafter (Head et al. 2016). For example, in response to the 2014, West Africa Ebola pandemic, funding for Ebola and Marburg virus more than tripled between 2014 and 2015 (McArthur 2019). As the Ebola pandemic waned, so did funding, by around USD125 million in both 2016 and 2017 (McArthur 2019). The drop was also due to the emergence of Zika virus, which began in Brazil in 2015 and was declared a Public Health Emergency of International Concern in February 2016 (McArthur 2019).In many cases, the priorities of funding bodies, largely situated in the Global North, dictate who is funded, what diseases are funded, and even type of research conducted (Arvanitis and Mouton 2019). Infectious disease funding to LMICS is often channeled through HIC institutions. As a result, the research agenda is driven by external researchers and research institutions. There are steps being taken to increase the role of LMICs in setting the research and funding agenda, as mentioned in the section below on Setting Research Priorities.

**Funding Design** Funding design can either promote or weaken institutional growth in research. An analysis done by Arvanitis R. & Mouton J (Arvanitis and Mouton 2019) found research funding in LMICs tends to have an individualistic design of funding (consultancy-based) versus institutional funding often seen in HICs. That is funding tends to flow directly to individuals in the form of consultancies, versus, towards institutions with a focus on building institutional capacity. This individualist funding approach likely leads to fragmentation of skills and competencies versus synergizing and building strong institutions that nurture collaboration, promote growth of strong research cultures and infrastructure to support research and development (Arvanitis and Mouton 2019).

Additionally, limited and competitive funding, weak infrastructure, and limited growth opportunities have contributed to the brain drain of researchers from LMICs to HICs (Arvanitis and Mouton 2019). About 30% of African researchers leave for HIC institutions, such that there are more African researchers in the USA than the whole of Africa (Arvanitis and Mouton 2019). In Argentina, a leader in science in South America, with half of the people with doctoral education are absorbed into the national scientific systems, and one in five leaving the country (Mbaye et al. 2019). Argentina provides fully funded research career tracks for Argentinian scientists paid by the national science funding agency. Moreover they have highly trained PhD scientists who support national university systems. However, the current financial crisis in Argentina has led to severe research budget cuts and low salaries for researchers, contributing to brain drain..

## 2.2 Type of Research and Development Activity

Funded infectious diseases research activities range from basic research, applied research, translational research, and public health-oriented research and interventions, including implementation research (Abutu 2017; Head et al. 2016).

**Types of Research Activities**
**Basic research** refers to experimental or theoretical work primarily to obtain new knowledge of the underlying foundation of phenomena and noticeable facts, without having any specific application or use in view (Chapman et al. 2020).

**Applied research** is original work aimed at attaining new knowledge while focusing on a precise, actual aim or objective (Hotez et al. 2008).

**Translational research** fosters the multidirectional integration of basic research, patient-oriented research, and population-based research, with the long-term aim of improving the health of the public.

**Implementation research** describes the scientific study of the processes used in the implementation of initiatives as well as the contextual factors that affect these processes.

According to the OECD Frascati Manual (2015), R&D includes three kinds of research activities: basic research, applied research, and experimental development (Hotez et al. 2008; Dujardin et al. 2010). All these activities are essential to addressing infectious diseases challenges. In most instances, publicly funded research, usually focuses on basic research, which is the case in most developing countries (Head et al. 2016; Frascati Manual 2015). Basic research can generate fundamental knowledge to develop new techniques, methodologies, and instruments that can later be applied in the process of developing and commercializing novel therapeutics, diagnostic tools and vaccines. This is an essential source of knowledge to drive innovation (Martin 1996). In HICs, there has been considerable investment in basic research. This has generated significant amounts of knowledge to support increased investment in applied research and experimental development (Martin 1996) that leads to improved or novel biomedical interventions to reduce the burden of disease. This suggests the potential benefit of increasing investment in basic research in LMICs.

Finding a balance between these research funding categories at national and global level is critical to ensuring efficient allocation of funding towards the prevention, control, management, elimination, and eradicate of neglected infectious diseases. Hotez PJ et al. (Institute for Health Metrics and Evaluation (IHME) 2020) argued that despite the high burden of many neglected diseases in Latin America and Caribbean many could be significantly reduced with existing tools. In this case, funding should be allocated to applied research focused on implementation science (see Chapter "Gender Equity in African Academia: An Implementation Science Evaluation of the Kenya Context") to improve public health service delivery (Institute for Health Metrics and Evaluation (IHME) 2020).

Integrating social sciences and related disciplines in infectious diseases research is increasingly recognized as highly valuable to understand patterns of exposure, health-seeking behaviour, infection outcomes, the likelihood of diagnosis and reporting of cases, and the uptake of pharmaceutical and non-pharmaceutical interventions (see Chapter "Role of Social Science in Infectious Disease Research: A Case Study of Partnering with Communities in Vector Control in a Kenyan Village") (Castillejos-Petalcorin and Kim 2020). For example, social science research funding is critical for the management of stigmatized neglected tropical diseases such as scabies, where effective treatments are readily available (see also Chapters "Addressing Sexual and HIV-Related Stigma in Haiti: Need for Societal Engagement" and "Building Partnerships to Empower Women Through Home Self-Sampling for Sexual and Reproductive Tract Infections" on stigma) (Head et al. 2016).

The importance of social sciences was also demonstrated during pandemics such as the Ebola and COVID-19 response (see Chapters "Building Partnerships and Confronting Challenges: Implementation of an Ebola Virus Vaccine clinical Study During an Outbreak in the Democratic Republic of the Congo" and "When Women Lead in Global Health: Alternative Mobilizations") (Buckee et al. 2021). The politicization of public health decisions in the USA during the COVID-19 pandemic led to public confusion over the value of non-pharmaceutical interventions and eroded public confidence in government decisions around COVID-19. This contributed to high mortality and morbidity and vaccine resistance (Jones et al. 2008; Daszak et al. 2020; Furuse 2019; Yong 2020). Research on the political economy of disease outbreaks is key in preparing to respond to the next pandemic. Despite this recognition, research investment related to Ebola Virus between 2000–2017 largely focused on preclinical research, with minimal funding toward public health or social sciences (Head et al. 2016).

## 3　Where Are We Headed?

### 3.1　New Global Health Approaches

Several approaches have emerged over the last 10 years that have influenced the trajectory of funding and partnerships in the field of infectious diseases research. The era of the millennium development goals (MDGs) saw a rise in funding for research on HIV/AIDs, TB, and malaria. The current era of the sustainable development goals (SDGs) has seen growth in the type and number of actors in the global health space (especially private sector participation). The areas of focus have also expanded e.g., environmental health and climate action.

Global health frameworks such as One Health and Planetary Health (see Chapter "A Holistic Systems Approach To Global Health Research, Practice, And Partnerships") provides new lenses for funding infectious diseases R&D. These frameworks recognize that the patterns of occurrence and distribution of emerging and persistent diseases are influenced multiple social-ecological drivers, such as urbanisation, climate change, increasing travel and trade, human population growth, human behaviour and the emergence of antimicrobial resistance (Castillejos-Petalcorin and Kim 2020; Buckee et al. 2021). One Health promotes a multisectoral strategy, to address emerging threats such as zoonotic diseases, vector-borne diseases, and antimicrobial resistance by promoting integration and utilization of human, animal and environmental data systems and interventions (Mackenzie and Jeggo 2019; Jones et al. 2008). Planetary health focuses on how the degradation of our planet by humans has led to climate change, loss of biodiversity, pollution, and shortage of fresh water, land, and ocean resources and in turn how this impacts human health (Myers and Frumkin 2020). This has highlighted the need for transdisciplinary and integrated systems approaches to global health and infectious disease research and practice (see Chapter A Holistic Systems Approach To Global Health Research, Practice, And Partnerships).

The growth in the number and interactions between global health actors and variations of funding mechanisms, both complicates the funding architecture but also provides opportunities to explore innovative funding structures for the advancement of infectious diseases R&D. In this section we will look at some of the key priority areas, partnerships, and funding models with potential to shape the funding landscape in infectious disease R&D.

## 3.2    Emerging Global Priorities

**Preparing for the Next Pandemic is Now a Global Priority** Increased investment in operational emerging infectious diseases research and surveillance is needed now more than ever. In Africa forty-one countries (87%) had at least one epidemic between 2016 and 2018. Twenty-one countries (45%) had at least one epidemic annually (Smiley Evans et al. 2020). There is limited funding available for research to strengthen operational infectious disease surveillance and preparedness, particularly to improve data systems, case identification, and reporting.

Increased investment in disease surveillance has proven to be highly successful in rapid response to an outbreak, thus minimizing the health, social and economic impacts of an outbreak on a population. For example, establishing a more sensitive surveillance system by the Nigerian CDC was instrumental in the detection of the index case of Monkey Pox in 2017, 39 years after the last recorded case (Talisuna et al. 2020; Nigeria Centers for Disease Control (NCDC) 2018). In addition, investment in the Nigeria CDC allowed the team to conduct genetic sequencing to identify potential sources of introduction of monkeypox virus into the human population (Nigeria Centers for Disease Control (NCDC) 2018; Yinka-Ogunleye et al. 2018; Fagbemi 2021).

Another example is Singapore's response to the SARS outbreak. SARs revealed weaknesses in its epidemiological surveillance and health care system (Government of Singapore n.d.). In response the country established the Disease Outbreak Response System Condition—a colour-coded framework for national response to any outbreak. They also replaced the 39 isolation-bed Communicable Disease Centre with the National Centre for Infectious Diseases (NCID), a 330-bed purpose-built infectious disease management facility with integrated clinical, laboratory and epidemiological functions to be the centerpiece of pandemic management in Singapore (Government of Singapore n.d.; Lin et al. 2020).

The COVID-19 pandemic saw the global community establishing or readapting funding initiatives to address the pandemic. For example Global Fund established the COVID-19 Response mechanism (C19RM) to mitigate the impact of the COVID-19 pandemic on programs to fight AIDS, TB and malaria and to strengthen health systems. As countries transition from emergency response, the C19RM funding has been extended to support resilient and sustainable health systems for health and pandemic response until 2025. The World Bank approved the establishment of the Pandemic Fund in June 2022, with the aim of providing a dedicated stream of additional, long-term financing to strengthen critical pandemic prevention, preparedness and response (PPR) capabilities in LMICs. In its first round of funding the Pandemic Fund Governing Board has approved an envelope of about USD 300 million in funding.

**Antimicrobial resistance is a global public health threat** to effective prevention and treatment of an ever-increasing range of infections caused by bacteria, parasites, viruses and fungi. To address the glaring AMR threat, there is a need for product development and strategies to addressing contextual factors appropriate antimicrobial use. Currently, 52% of AMR funding, goes towards therapeutics, 12% to transmission, 12% to diagnostics, 11% to intervention, 6% to surveillance, and 7% to environmental factors (Joint Programming Initiative on Antimicrobial Resistance, JPIAMR 2017). In addition, most funding goes towards antibiotic resistance (76.2%) followed by 20.6% in anti-parasitic and 3.2% in anti-fungal resistance research (Joint Programming Initiative on Antimicrobial Resistance, JPIAMR 2017).

Acknowledging the urgency of addressing AMR globally, led to the establishment of the Joint Programming Initiative on Antimicrobial Resistance Mapping (JPIAMR) to monitor the scale and scope of research investment in AMR research to guide decision making in funding, policy, and practice. Increased investment is needed to establish responsive AMR surveillance systems. There is a lack of data on AMR in more than 40% of countries in Africa (Joint Programming Initiative on Antimicrobial Resistance, JPIAMR 2017), and sporadic and selective surveillance in most South East Asian countries (Tadesse et al. 2017).

AMR surveillance systems should be integrated to health/hospital information management systems to monitor susceptibility patterns of micro-organisms and antimicrobial agents, improve diagnostic standardization, optimizing treatment guidelines, and thus improve infection prevention control (Joint Programming Initiative on Antimicrobial Resistance, JPIAMR 2017;

Tadesse et al. 2017; Vong et al. 2017; Prestinaci et al. 2015). AMR surveillance systems should ensure quality data arer collected, synthesized, and utilized to identify AMR research priorities, and respond early and appropriately to emerging drug resistance (Joint Programming Initiative on Antimicrobial Resistance, JPIAMR 2017; Tadesse et al. 2017; Vong et al. 2017; Prestinaci et al. 2015).

## 3.3 Setting National and Regional Research Agendas

**Identifying national and regional research priorities** to fund is a context-specific process that requires an analysis of the epidemiological context, research and public health capacities, national policy priorities, local needs, and available resources. Priority-setting should be driven by the nations and communities where the research will be conducted; the places and people that serve as the study participants and purported beneficiaries of the research.

Organizations such as African Academy of Sciences (Chapman et al. 2020) have been set up to drive the research agenda of Africa with expertise from the region. For example, the organization developed a COVID-19 research agenda that identified key research priorities for the region. The Academy also supports the management of funding and programs and growth of research infrastructure. By building capacity and providing growth opportunities, the Academy also aims t retain African researchers on the continent.

In Latin America and Caribbean, a group of researchers from the region, mapped out research priorities for neglected diseases in the region that included five groups of diseases: vector-borne diseases, soil and tissue transmitted helminths, non-arthropod emerging viral diseases, endemic mycosis and sexually transmitted diseases (African Academy of Sciences (AAS) n.d.). The exercise enabled the team to determine, which diseases required R&D for new or additional or improved drugs, diagnostics, and vaccines versus those that could be addressed via public health interventions with existing tools (Joint

Programming Initiative on Antimicrobial Resistance, JPIAMR 2017). These kinds of analyses should guide future investments in the region.

## 3.4    Creating an Equitable and Enabling Environment for R&D

Governments can catalyze investments towards infectious diseases R&D through i) increasing national financial allocation towards R&D to improve research capacities and ii) developing policies that offer a favorable environment for external investors to invest in R&D for the long-term. Funding should be context specific and guided by the country's infectious diseases research agenda. Funding should be geared to build or strengthen existing research institutions, development of national research funds and policy making bodies, create favorable learning and work environments for researchers to grow and apply their expertise, and developing centers of excellence (Arvanitis and Mouton 2019). To catalyze, private sector investment, governments need to create an enabling R&D investment environment through policies that strengthen health sector infrastructure, increased domestic capability to conduct translation research and development, and regulatory frameworks like the Food and Drugs Authority in Ghana (Fauci and Morens 2012). The importance of domestic funding cannot be over-emphasized. To address LMICs unmet health needs and ambitious social and economic targets, increased investment in R&D will play a critical role.

As LMIC governments continue to increase engagement with external funders, investors, and researchers, all need to be cognizant of power imbalances that contribute to unfair partnerships favoring career progression and priorities of external researchers over national priorities. These imbalances can be addressed by increasing domestic funding towards R&D to reduce over-reliance on external funding, establishing context-specific research agendas driven by local expertise and principles to guide research part-nerships. This requires that LMICs adopt strong ownership and responsibility to build and strengthen their infectious diseases R & D as a pillar of national development and security.

**Improving Research Infrastructure** The backbone of infectious diseases R&D is a country's research infrastructure. This includes physical infrastructure (such as laboratory capacity), technology, quality of training, and regulatory bodies, and Institutional review boards/ethics dimensions, which are detailed more in Chapter "Ethical Challenges in Global Health Research" on ethics in this volume. Responding to the challenges posed by infectious diseases requires enhancing national laboratory capacities, beyond the physical aspects of the lab (World Health Organization (WHO) 2014). This should include a long-term commitment to building local human resource capacity and skills, quality control, and biosafety systems (World Health Organization (WHO) 2014).

There is also a need to invest in robust data systems, electronic medical records, and interoperable data sharing platforms that facilitate the use of big data. One example is the Surveillance Outbreak Response Management and Analysis System (SORMAS), an open-source mobile and web application software developed to enable health workers to notify health departments about new cases of epidemic-prone diseases, detect outbreaks, and simultaneously manage outbreak response (Wertheim et al. 2010).

**Improving Data Systems for Research and Development** Data is paramount to understanding and designing interventions to address the burden of infectious disease on population health and well-being. The emergence of big data and new data sources (such as social media), coupled with artificial intelligence (AI) and increased computing power, provides an unparalleled opportunity to detect and respond to infectious disease patterns and associations. Traditional surveillance data often have time lags and lack spatial resolution. Big data have the potential to improve timeliness, spatial and temporal resolution, and reveal "hidden" populations and human behavior in response to public health interventions (Tom-Aba et al. 2020). However, most LMICs, continue to struggle in setting up robust data and surveillance systems, which are needed to generate the quality datasets that can inform AI systems. Setting up quality, robust, and responsive data systems is further complicated by diverse data types (e.g., epidemiological, genetic, clinical, laboratory, social and behavioural data), the multiple purposes of data sharing, the multiplicity of actors involved in its generation, management, analysis and use, and ethical sensitivities associated with data sharing (Tom-Aba et al. 2020; Bansal et al. 2016). Understanding specific country gaps and needs is important. For example, research funding is more often available for modelling rather than data collection, despite models being reliant on high-quality data to parametrize them (GLOPID-R 2019). COVID-19 models in LMICs were noted to be less accurate partly due to the lack of local data to contextualize the models (GLOPID-R 2019).

**Enabling innovation and access to health technologies** remains a key strategy in developing new interventions, such as diagnostics, vaccines, and drugs, to combat infectious diseases in LMICs (Deepti et al. 2020). Limited funding for translational research and product development in LMICs remains a major barrier. Other challenges include limited human resource capacity, lack of market incentives, weak regulatory and IP management mechanisms, and infrastructure (Abutu 2017). These challenges de-incentivise private sector engagement in research and development especially in low-income countries (G-FINDER 2022). As a result, the health innovation systems in LMICs remain basic and fragmented. They remain reliant on products developed outside their countries that may not be culturally appropriate, affordable, accessible, and acceptable especially in resource limited setting e.g., with un-reliable electricity, and under-resourced health systems. Product development partnerships involving public and private sectors have been established to address these challenges. In the following section, we will discuss various models of public and private sector partnerships.

## 3.5 Public and Private Funding Initiatives and Partnerships

Public and private sector funding for R&D are needed to catalyze and sustain R&D and innovation, and should be complementary, not substitutive. Evidence suggests that higher levels of public R&D expenditure induce more private R&D investment (Al-Bader et al. 2010). Over the last decade several initiatives have cropped up, with the aim of incentivizing win-win funding and partnership opportunities to advance public-private collaborations. These include:

1. **Product Development Partnerships (PDPs)** are non-profit organizations established to address the dearth of infectious diseases R&D that disproportionately affect LMICs (see examples in inset box) (Al-Bader et al. 2010). These partnerships aim to spur development and manufacturing of new products focused on global health priorities such as neglected diseases rather than economic incentives. They do this by pooling resources and leveraging expertise across public, private, academic, and philanthropic sectors for the development of drugs, vaccines, and diagnostics as public goods. PDPs differ in focus area, stakeholders, and the extent of funding contributions. For example the development of the RTS,S malaria vaccine (Mosquirix TM) which took over 30 years has been a result of collaboration between GlaxoSmithKline (GSK), a network of African research centres, PATH, MVI and BMGF which funded the late stage development (Castillejos-Petalcorin and Kim 2020). Other examples include the International AIDS Vaccine Initiative (IAVI), International Partnership for Microbicides (IPM), The Global Alliance for TB Drug Development (TB Alliance), Aeras Global TB Vaccine Foundation, Human Hookworm Vaccine Initiative (HHVI), Foundation for Innovative New Diagnostics (FIND), Drugs for Neglected Diseases initiative (DNDi), OneWorld Health, and CARB -X Combating Antibiotic-Resistant Bacteria Biopharmaceutical Accelerator.

## Examples of Product Development Partnerships (PDPs) for Advancing Infectious Diseases Research and Development

Global health Innovative Technology Fund (GHIT Fund) is an international non-profit funded by the Japanese government, Japanese pharmaceutical companies, Bill & Melinda Gates Foundation, Wellcome Trust and United Nations Development Program. GHIT has invested about USD 291,000,000 towards malaria, TB and NTD research and development (Grace 2010).

CARB -X Combating Antibiotic-Resistant Bacteria Biopharmaceutical Accelerator (Medicines for Malaria Venture 2021) is a global non-profit partnership whose mission is to support early-stage antibacterial product development via non-dilutive funding, expert support, and cross project initiatives. CARB X demonstrates the diversity of types of partnerships in infectious disease research and development. It is led by the Boston University and funded by the Biomedical Advanced Research and Development Authority (BARDA), part of the Office of the Assistant Secretary for Preparedness and Response (ASPR) in the United States Department of Health and Human Services, the Wellcome Trust in the United Kingdom, Germany's Federal Ministry of Education and Research (BMBF), the UK Government's Department of Health and Social Care (DHSC), the Bill & Melinda Gates Foundation, and the National Institute of Allergy and Infectious Diseases (NIAID). Up to US$480 million is expected to be invested into CARB-X from 2016–2022 to accelerate the development of antibiotics and other therapeutics, vaccines, and rapid diagnostics to address drug-resistant bacteria. CARB-X has an active portfolio of 92 projects (as of September 2021) comprising of early development pipeline of antibacterial projects that include 47 active therapeutics and vaccine projects and active 11 rapid diagnostics projects.

Drugs for Neglected Diseases Initiative (DNDi)is an international not-for-profit research and development organization that draws together over 200 partners from around the world to develop urgently needed treatments for neglected patients ensuring they are affordable, available, and adapted to the communities who need them. Currently the initiative is working on over 40 projects, including more than 20 new chemical entities. In addition to running over 20 clinical trials. A major success thus far has been the revolutionary development of a simple oral cure for sleeping sickness. Partners include public, private, academic, non-profit, and philanthropic sectors (Slingsby 2015).

2. **Incentive mechanisms** are geared towards encouraging greater private-sector investment and engagement in R&D for infectious diseases where limited commercial market exists. Examples of incentive mechanisms include prizes, priority review vouchers, advance market commitments.

3. **Advanced market commitment** incentivizes private-sector investment in R&D by providing an upfront financial commitment, through a legally binding contract, to guarantee the future purchase, at an agreed-upon price, of a vaccine or health product not yet developed and available (CARB 2021). A recent example is the Global Alliance for Vaccines and Immunization (GAVI) COVAX Advance Market Commitment (AMC) (CARB 2021). COVAX AMC led by the Coalition for Epidemic Preparedness Innovations (CEPI), Gavi, World Health Organization (WHO), and UNICEF was designed to leverage scale of high- and low-income economies to ensure

that people in all countries get rapid, fair, and equitable access to COVID-19 vaccines. It is the investment mechanism for the COVID-19 Global Vaccine Access Facility (COVAX Facility). COVAX Facility is purposed to pool resources, share vaccine development risk, create demand guarantees for vaccine manufacturers to promote access to substantial volumes of vaccines; better allocate capital; and support the manufacturing and procurement of sufficient volumes of vaccines to support equitable access globally. COVAX AMC funding is largely through Official Development Assistance (ODA), as well as contributions from the private sector, philanthropy and in some instances the ODA-eligible countries accessing vaccines through the COVAX AMC. Donor funding to the COVAX AMC aims to ensure people at most risk and vulnerable obtain urgent access to COVID-19 vaccines. COVAX is an unprecedented creation and has provided a great learning opportunity of the challenges and opportunities provided for AMCs in an outbreak response (Drugs for Neglected Diseases initiaitve (DNDi) n.d.; Global Health R&D Dictionary 2021)

4. **Other incentive mechanisms** include Milestone prizes that allows product developers to receive predetermined monetary rewards as they complete milestones in the R&D process for a target product (GAVI 2021). Priority Review Vouchers are intended to incentivize R&D for neglected or rare diseases by rewarding developers of a health product for these diseases with a voucher for accelerated regulatory review, which they can apply to another health product or sell to another entity (Mueller and Robbins 2021). Priority review vouchers are expected to impact the availability of products, however there is no guarantee that this translates to availability in developing countries.

**Public-public partnerships** are another model of collaboration that refer to collaboration between two or more public authorities or organi-zations, aimed at improving the capacity and effectiveness of one partner. The European & Developing Countries Clinical Trials Partnership (EDCTP) (European and Developing Countries Clinical Trials Partnership (EDCTP) 2021) is such a partnership. It's composed of between 14 European and 16 African countries with the support of the European Union. The aim of the EDCTP is to reduce the individual, social and economic burden of poverty-related infectious diseases affecting sub-Saharan Africa by accelerating the development of new or improved products for the identification, treatment, and prevention of infectious diseases, including emerging and re-emerging diseases. The partnership is focused on pre- and post-registration clinical studies, with emphasis on phase II and III clinical trials. In addition, it seeks to improve the capacity and expertise of African researchers in infectious diseases R&D.

## 3.6 Is There Value for Money?

Increased allocation towards infectious diseases R&D should be commensurate with funding being inclusive, efficient, equitable and sustainable. This means, setting up or improving systems to measure R&D activity and funding. Most countries do not have a robust research evaluation system geared towards improving research quality and its impact in addressing issues relevant to the country/region. Limited tracking or detailed analysis of investments into infectious diseases R&D makes it difficult to identify the best funding decisions. This challenge is further expounded by limited systematic coordination between stakeholders involved in funding research and development in infectious diseases (Head et al. 2016). A shift in how research is measured will be required. Funding policies can be set up to promote research quality, public health impact, and data sharing. This will be guided by the creation of national research quality evaluation institutions to monitor research quality and impact on population health in-country.

## 4    Conclusion

Funding shapes what gets done. Equitable, sustainable, and inclusive funding for infectious diseases R&D, requires a context specific, multi-stakeholder, and multi-sectoral approach. Research investment should address both the immediate needs being faced, e.g., building physical facilities where needed, but should also aim to achieve long-term goals such as building the capacity of local researchers and research institutions. Each country should establish research agendas that address their short- and long-term research priorities to guide investment allocation. Collaboration between public and private sectors, provides a great opportunity for advancement of infectious diseases R&D especially in the field of translational research and product development. Strengthening such engagements for infectious diseases research is highly dependent on the level of investment made towards R&D by national governments- an area that is lagging in LMICs. Threats to public health, such as antimicrobial resistance and emerging infectious diseases, are expected to continue being at the fore front of infectious diseases research. In line with this, advancements in data systems and technology such as AI offer exciting opportunities to enhance existing surveillances systems. As the world continues to grapple with the aftermath of COVID-19, it is paramount that each country and the world at large move quickly in addressing the shortcomings of current research and health systems that the pandemic magnified and exposed. It will be a shame to be in the same place when the next pandemic hits.

## References

Abutu A. Why African governments commit less to R&D funding. SciDevNet: Why African governments commit less to R&D funding. 2017 December 22 [cited 2021 Sept 16]. https://www.scidev.net/sub-saharan-africa/news/african-governments-commit-research-funding/

Adetokunboh OO, Mthombothi ZE, Dominic EM, Djomba-Njankou S, Pulliam JRC. African based researchers' output on models for the transmission dynamics of infectious diseases and public health interventions: a scoping review. PLoS One.

2021;16(5):e0250086. https://doi.org/10.1371/journal.pone.0250086.

African Academy of Sciences (AAS). n.d.. https://www.aasciences.africa/covid-19-updates

Al-Bader S, Daar AS, Singer PA. Science-based health innovation in Ghana: health entrepreneurs point the way to a new development path. BMC Int Health Hum Rights. 2010;10(Suppl 1) https://doi.org/10.1186/1472-698X-10-S1-S2.

Arvanitis R, Mouton J. Observing and Funding African Research, Working Paper du Ceped, n°43. Ceped, UMR 196 Université Paris Descartes IRD. Paris; 2019. https://doi.org/10.5281/zenodo.3403895.

Assessing the needs of the research system in Kenya. Report for the SRIA programme. October 2019. Available from: https://assets.publishing.service.gov.uk/media/5ef4acb5d3bf7f7145b21a22/NA_report_Kenya__Dec_2019_Heart_.pdf

Ault SK. Pan American Health Organization's regional strategic framework for addressing neglected diseases in neglected populations in Latin America and the Caribbean. Mem Inst Oswaldo Cruz. 2007;102(Suppl):199–07.

Bansal S, Chowell G, Simonsen L, Vespignani A, Viboud C. Big data for infectious disease surveillance and modeling. J Infect Dis. 2016;214(4):375–9. https://doi.org/10.1093/infdis/jiw400.

Buckee C, Noor A, Sattenspiel L. Thinking clearly about social aspects of infectious disease transmission. Nature. 2021;595:205–13. https://doi.org/10.1038/s41586-021-03694-x.

CARB -X Combating Antibiotic-Resistant Bacteria Biopharmaceutical Accelerator. [cited 21 Sept 2021]. https://carb-x.org/portfolio/portfolio-pipeline/

Castillejos-Petalcorin C, Kim J. The role of government research and development in fostering innovation in Asia. Asia Development Bank; 2020. https://www.adb.org/sites/default/files/institutional-document/575671/ado2020bp-government-rd-innovation-asia.pdf

Chapman N, Doubell A, Tuttle A, Barnsley P, Oversteegen L, Goldstein M, Borri J,Chowdhary V, Rugarabamu G, Hynen A, Kearney M, Ong M, Tjoeng I. Landscape of emerging infectious disease research and development: Preventing the next pandemic. G-FINDER 2020; 2020. Available from: https://s3-ap-southeast-2.amazonaws.com/policy-cures-website-assets/app/uploads/2020/10/30095357/EID_Report.pdf

Ciocca DR, Delgado G. The reality of scientific research in Latin America; an insider's perspective. Cell Stress Chaperones. 2017;22(6):847–52. https://doi.org/10.1007/s12192-017-0815-8.

Daszak P, Keusch GT, Phelan AL, Johnson CK, Osterholm MT. Infectious disease threats: a rebound to resilience. Health Aff. 2020; https://doi.org/10.1377/hlthaff.2020.01544#B14. https://www.healthaffairs.org

Deepti M, Baker P, Buckley E, Maida J, Chalkidou K. We must stop flying blind: building on existing systems in low- and middle-income countries to improve the COVID-19 response. Center for Global Development.

2020. https://www.cgdev.org/blog/we-must-stop-flying-blind-building-existing-systems-low-and-middle-income-countries-improve

Drugs for Neglected Diseases initiaitve (DNDi). n.d.. https://dndi.org/about/how-we-work/

Dujardin JC, do Rosario HS, et al. Research priorities for neglected infectious diseases in Latin America and the Caribbean Region. PLoS Negl Trop Dis. 2010;4(10):e780. https://doi.org/10.1371/journal.pntd.0000780.

Engels D, Zhou XN. Neglected tropical diseases: an effective global response to local poverty-related disease priorities. Infect Dis Poverty. 2020;9(10) https://doi.org/10.1186/s40249-020-0630-9.

Estenssoro E, Friedman G, Hernández G. Research in Latin America: opportunities and challenges. Intensive Care Med. 2016;42:1045–7. https://doi.org/10.1007/s00134-016-4342-3.

European & Developing Countries Clinical Trials Partnership (EDCTP). [cited 2021 Sept 21]. Available from: https://www.edctp.org

Fagbemi SE. WHO confirms three cases of Monkey pox in Nigeria. [cited 2021 Sept 15]. https://www.tribuneonlineng.com/115703/

Fauci AS, Morens DM. The perpetual challenge of infectious diseases. N Engl J Med. 2012;366:454–61. https://doi.org/10.1056/NEJMra1108296pmid. http://www.ncbi.nlm.nih.gov/pubmed/22296079

Foreign aid: Government decision to cut budget 'unlawful', says peer. BBC News 2021 March [cited 2021 Sept 22]. Available from: https://www.bbc.com/news/uk-politics-56473067

Frascati Manual 2015 Guidelines for Collecting and Reporting Data on Research and Experimental Development. Available from: https://www.oecd-ilibrary.org/docserver/9789264239012-4-en.pdf?expires=1632145799&id=id&accname=guest&checksum=E7F67843AAF5E20D1F0E5DF109C8E9EF

Furuse Y. Analysis of research intensity on infectious disease by disease burden reveals which infectious diseases are neglected by researchers. Proc Natl Acad Sci USA. 2019;116(2):478–83. https://doi.org/10.1073/pnas.1814484116. https://www.pnas.org/content/116/2/478

GAVI. GAVI COVAX AMC Explained. [cited 2021 Sept 21]. https://www.gavi.org/vaccineswork/gavi-covax-amc-explained.

GCRF African Science for Weather Information and Forecasting Techniques (SWIFT). Statement on UKRI funding cuts. 2021 April [cited 2021 Sept 22]. Available from:https://africanswift.org/2021/04/07/statement-on-ukri-funding-cuts/

G-FINDER. Neglected Disease Research and Development: The status quo won't get us there. 2022. https://policy-cures-website-assets.s3.ap-southeast-2.amazonaws.com/wp-content/uploads/2023/01/31200737/2022-G-FINDER-Neglected-Disease-Report-Executive-Summary.pdf

Global Health R&D Dictionary. [cited 2021 Sept 20] https://www.ghtcoalition.org/global-health-research-and-development-dictionary#a

GLOPID-R. Data sharing in public health emergencies. Learning from past outbreaks. 2019 March [cited 2021 Sept 21]. Available from: https://www.glopid-r.org/wp-content/uploads/2017/02/data-sharing-in-public-health-emergencies-case-studies-workshop-reportv2.pdf

Government of Singapore. National Centre for infectious diseases. n.d.. https://www.ncid.sg/About-NCID/Pages/default.aspx

Grace C. Product Development Partnerships (PDPs): Lessons from PDPs established to develop new health technologies for neglected diseases. UK Government. 2010 [cited 2023 June 18].

Head MG, Brown RJ, Newell ML, Scott JAG, Batchelor J, Atun R. The allocation of US$105 billion in global funding from G20 countries for infectious disease research between 2000 and 2017: a content analysis of investments. Lancet Glob Health. 2020;8:e1295–304. https://doi.org/10.1016/S2214-109X(20)30357-0.

Head MG, Fitchett JR, Nageshwaran V, Kumari N, Hayward AC, Atun R. Research investments in global health: a systematic analysis of UK infectious disease research funding and global health metrics, 1997–2013. EBioMedicine. 2016;3:–190.

Hotez PJ, Bottazzi ME, Franco-Paredes C, Ault SK, Roses PM. The neglected tropical diseases of Latin America and the Caribbean: a review of disease burden and distribution and a roadmap for control and elimination. PLoS Negl Trop Dis. 2008;2:e300.

Institute for Health Metrics and Evaluation (IHME). GBD Compare. [updated 2020 October 15; [cited 2021 Sept 17]. Available from: http://www.healthdata.org/data-visualization/gbd-compare

Joint Programming Initiative on Antimicrobial Resistance, JPIAMR. Mapping of AMR research funding. 2017 [cited 2021 Sept 21]. https://www.jpiamr.eu/wp-content/uploads/2019/02/Mapping-of-AMR-research-funding-2017-report.pdf

Jones K, Patel N, Levy M, et al. Global trends in emerging infectious diseases. Nature. 2008;451:990–3. https://doi.org/10.1038/nature06536.

Kanja W, Flowe HD, Cheeseman N. Cuts to UK research funding threaten critical human rights projects across the world. The Conservation 2021 April [2021 Sept 22]. https://theconversation.com/cuts-to-uk-research-funding-threaten-critical-human-rights-projects-across-the-world-158333

Kutlača Đ, Stefanović-Šestić S, Jelic S, Popovic-Pantic S. The impact of investment in research and development on the economic growth in Serbia. Industrija. 2020;48:23–46. https://doi.org/10.5937/industrija48-25209.

Lin RJ, Lee TH, Lye DC. From SARS to COVID-19: the Singapore journey. Med J Aust. 2020;212(11):497–502.e1. https://doi.org/10.5694/mja2.50623.

Mackenzie JS, Jeggo M. The One Health Approach-Why Is It So Important? Trop Med Infect Dis. 2019;4(2):88. https://doi.org/10.3390/tropicalmed4020088.

Martin BR. The use of multiple indicators in the assessment of basic research. Scientometrics. 1996;36:343–62. https://doi.org/10.1007/BF02129599.

Mbaye R, Gebeyehu R, Hossmann S, et al. Who is telling the story? A systematic review of authorship for infectious disease research conducted in Africa, 1980–2016. BMJ Glob Health. 2019;4:e001855.

McArthur DB. Emerging Infectious Diseases. Nurs Clin North Am. 2019;54(2):297–311. https://doi.org/10.1016/j.cnur.2019.02.006.

McCoy D, Chand S, Sridhar D. Global health funding: how much, where it comes from and where it goes. Health Policy Plan. 2009;24(6):407–17. https://doi.org/10.1093/heapol/czp026.

Medicines for Malaria Venture. First-ever malaria vaccine to get WHO recommendation for roll-out. https://www.mmv.org/newsroom/news-resources-search/first-ever-malaria-vaccine-get-who-recommendation-roll-out. October 2021 [cited 2023 Jun 18].

Mueller B, Robbins R. Where COVAX the vast Global Vaccine Program, went wrong. New York Times. 2021 September 8. https://www.nytimes.com/2021/08/02/world/europe/covax-covid-vaccine-problems-africa.html

Myers S, Frumkin H. Planetary health: protecting nature to protect ourselves. Washington, DC: Island Press; 2020.

Nigeria Centers for Disease Control (NCDC). Nigeria monkey pox outbreak report. Nigeria Centre for disease control. Abuja, Nigeria. 2018 November 13 [cited 2021 Sept 15]. https://ncdc.gov.ng/themes/common/files/sitreps/30abb20fe681f2c54122a307e305fb51.pdf

Our World in Data. Coronavirus (COVID-19) vaccinations. 2021 [cited 2023 Jun 18]. Available from: https://ourworldindata.org/covid-vaccinations

Prestinaci F, Pezzotti P, Pantosti A. Antimicrobial resistance: a global multifaceted phenomenon. Pathog Glob Health. 2015;109(7):309–18. https://doi.org/10.1179/2047773215Y.0000000030. Epub 2015 Sep 7. PMID: 26343252; PMCID: PMC4768623

Rubin H, Saidel N. Innovation beyond patent waivers: Achieving global vaccination goals through public-private partnerships. Brookings 2021 August [cited 2021 Sept 22]. https://www.brookings.edu/blog/up-front/2021/08/31/innovation-beyond-patent-waivers-achieving-global-vaccination-goals-through-public-private-partnerships/

Science, Technology and Innovation Strategy for Africa 2024; STISA-2024, 2014. African Union [cited 2021 September 22]. Available from: http://www.hsrc.ac.za/uploads/pageContent/5481/Science,%20Technology%20and%20Innovation%20Strategy%20for%20Africa%20-%20Document.pdf

SCImago. SJR—SCImago Journal & Country Rank. 2007. Available from: http://www.scimagojr.com.

Slingsby BT. How innovative financing and partnership are transforming the infectious disease product pipeline. Devex. 2015 [cited 2021 Sept 22] https://www.devex.com/news/how-innovative-financing-and-partnerships-are-transforming-the-infectious-disease-product-pipeline-87246

Smiley Evans T, Shi Z, Boots M, et al. Synergistic China-US ecological research is essential for global emerging infectious disease preparedness. EcoHealth. 2020;17:160–73. https://doi.org/10.1007/s10393-020-01471-2pmid. http://www.ncbi.nlm.nih.gov/pubmed/32016718

Tadesse BT, Ashley EA, Ongarello S, et al. Antimicrobial resistance in Africa: a systematic review. BMC Infect Dis. 2017;7:616. https://doi.org/10.1186/s12879-017-2713-1.

Talisuna AO, Okiro EA, Yahaya AA, et al. Spatial and temporal distribution of infectious disease epidemics, disasters and other potential public health emergencies in the World Health Organisation Africa region, 2016–2018. Glob Health. 2020;16(9) https://doi.org/10.1186/s12992-019-0540-4.

Tom-Aba D, Silenou BC, Doerrbecker J, Fourie C, Leitner C, Wahnschaffe M, Strysewske M, Arinze CC, Krause G. The surveillance outbreak response management and analysis system (SORMAS): digital health global goods maturity assessment. JMIR Public Health Surveill. 2020;6(2):e15860. https://doi.org/10.2196/15860.

UNESCO Institute for Statistics (UIS) Science, technology and innovation Human resources in research and development (R&D). [cited 2021 Sept 22]. Available from: http://data.uis.unesco.org/

UNESCO Institute for Statistics (UIS) Science, technology and Expenditure on Research and Development (R&D). 2021 [cited 2021 Sept 21]. Available from: http://data.uis.unesco.org/

UNESCO Science report. Towards 2030: Focus on Sub-Saharan Africa. 2021. https://en.unesco.org/sites/default/files/usr15_focus_sub-saharan_africa.pdf

FIND and Unitaid invest to support technology transfer and boost local production of COVID-19 rapid tests in low- and middle-income countries. Unitaid 2021 July [cited 2021 Sept 22]. https://unitaid.org/news-blog/find-unitaid-technology-transfer-covid-19/#en

Uniting to combat neglected tropical diseases. Our open letter on the UK cuts: A tragic blow for 'global Britain' and the world's most vulnerable people. 2021 April [cited 2021 Sept 22]. https://unitingtocombatntds.org/news/our-response-to-the-uks-cuts-to-foreign-aid/

Vidyasagar D. Global notes: the 10/90 gap disparities in global health research. J Perinatol. 2000;26:55–6. https://doi.org/10.1038/sj.jp.7211402.

Vong S, Anciaux A, Hulth A, Stelling J, Thamlikitkul V, Gupta S, Fuks JM, Walia K, Rattanumpawan P, Eremin S, Tisocki K, Sedai TR, Sharma A. Using information technology to improve surveillance of antimicrobial resistance in South East Asia. BMJ (Clin Res Ed). 2017;358:j3781. https://doi.org/10.1136/bmj.j3781.

Wertheim HFL, Puthavathana P, Nghiem NM, van Doorn HR, Nguyen TV, et al. Laboratory Capacity Building in Asia for Infectious Disease Research: Experiences from the South East Asia Infectious Disease Clinical Research Network (SEAICRN). PLoS Med. 2010;7(4):e1000231. https://doi.org/10.1371/journal.pmed.1000231.

World Bank. Researchers in R&D (per million people). 2021 [cited 2021 Sept 19]. Available from: https://data.worldbank.org/indicator/SP.POP.SCIE.RD.P6?name_desc=false

World Health Organization. Neglected tropical diseases. n.d.. https://www.who.int/health-topics/neglected-tropical-diseases#tab=tab_1

World Health Organization (WHO). Global Report for Research on Infectious Diseases of Poverty. 2012 [cited 2021 Sept 22]. Available from http://apps.who.int/iris/bitstream/handle/10665/44850/9789241564489_eng.pdf;jsessionid=BBB477DB6FEC0754D47E2108475F28F3?sequence=1

World Health Organization (WHO). Antimicrobial resistance: global report on surveillance. 2014 [cited 2021 Sept 21]. https://apps.who.int/iris/bitstream/handle/10665/112642/9789241564748_eng.pdf

World Health Organization Regional Office for Africa, 2016. Research for health: a strategy for the African region, 2016–2025. [cited 2021 Sept 21]. Available from: http://apps.who.int/iris/handle/10665/204490

Worley W. Tracking the UK's controversial aid cuts. Devex. 2021 August [cited 2021 Sept 22]. Available from: https://www.devex.com/news/tracking-the-u-k-s-controversial-aid-cuts-99883

Yinka-Ogunleye A, Aruna O, Ogoina D, et al. Re-emergence of human monkey pox in Nigeria, 2017. Emerg Infect Dis. 2018;24:1149–51.

Yong E. How the Pandemic defeated America. The Atlantic. 2020 [cited 2021 Sept 21]. Available from: https://www.theatlantic.com/magazine/archive/2020/09/coronavirus-american-failure/614191/

Zhan J. Ten actions to boost low and middle-income countries' productive capacity for medicines. UNCTAD. United Nations Conference on Trade and Development (UNCTAD). 2020 May [cited 2021 Sept 22]. https://unctad.org/news/ten-actions-boost-low-and-middle-income-countries-productive-capacity-medicines

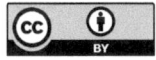

# Educational Perspectives from the Field: Pathways to the Future

Rosemary Rochford, Angela Nalwoga, Ibrahim Daud, and Gabriela Samayoa-Reyes

*Think global, act local.*

René Dubos

## Abstract

The late René Dubos, a microbiologist and an ecological philosopher, famously coined the phrase, *"Think global, act local."* This phrase presents a framework for how we might envision a new direction in education on pathogens across the globe. Infectious diseases can be considered at a global scale, as demonstrated by the recent COVID-19 pandemic, and also at the community scale, as is the case for endemic liver fluke disease in Southeast Asia. While the 30,000 foot view can help us to understand some aspects of a given pathogen and disease, it is critical that we shift our framework, such that local factors affecting disease burden are considered and relevant education is provided to the affected communities. Traditional training in microbiology has focused on knowing the pathogen. To again quote Dubos, "the etiology of disease cannot be entirely explained by the etiology of infection." If we accept this thesis, then future training in infectious diseases must also encompass knowledge of the environmental and social determinants of health. In this chapter, we will provide a brief historical framework regarding education and research in the field of Tropical Medicine. We will then offer perspectives from the field for contextualizing the current state of training. Finally, we will conclude with ideas on how to create more holistic educational pathways that build interdisciplinary teams able to tackle both infectious disease research and improved wellbeing of affected communities.

R. Rochford (✉) · A. Nalwoga · G. Samayoa-Reyes
Department of Immunology and Microbiology,
University of Colorado Anschutz Medical Campus,
Aurora, CO, USA
e-mail: rosemary.rochford@cuanschutz.edu;
angela.nalwoga@cuanschutz.edu;
gabriela.samayoareyes@cuanschutz.edu

I. Daud
CRC Laboratory at United States Army Medical
Research Directorate-Africa (MRD-A/K)| Kenya
Medical Research Institute, Kericho, Kenya
e-mail: ibrahim.daud@usamru-k.org

## Keywords

Mentorship · Partnership · Multidisciplinary · Education · Global health equity

## Author Perspective

The ideas in this chapter were shaped by our experiences as mentors and mentees. We are biomedical researchers who have worked together in different capacities in scientifically resource-limited and well-resourced settings. Our experiences researching human pathogens and

A. Stewart Ibarra, A. D. LaBeaud (eds.), *Transforming Global Health Partnerships*, Sustainable Development Goals Series, https://doi.org/10.1007/978-3-031-53793-6_23

One could consider this a "golden age" of tropical medicine research that would continue through the mid-twentieth century, and which includes the identification of many pathogens and corresponding vectors, significant advances in medical treatments, the development and implementation of infection control measures. It would be remiss to overlook the importance of this research period and the contributions made by many exceptional scientists. However, it is as important to acknowledge that during this colonial period, there were minimal, if any, efforts to build the capacity of the local populations through education in biomedical research to tackle health challenges that they suffered (see Chapter "Colonialism, Decolonization, and Global Health"). It should be noted that this failure was not unique to the public health sector, but present across all disciplines. In fact, not until the latter half of the twentieth and the early twenty-first century has there finally been a modest push to address the needs of the Indigenous Peoples, local communities and other groups excluded from scientific endeavors and resultant benefits.

Many former colonial regions, themselves sites of important scientific discoveries, found that little support remained post-independence. The effects are still felt today and have had a lasting impact on scientific education, where often an authoritarian and paternalistic approach remains the pedagogical norm (see Chapter "Learning from the Past to Inform the Future: Perspectives on Future Directions in International Health and Research"). The professor as the all-knowing source of knowledge is one of many unfortunate legacies of this period and discourages independent and critical thinking skills in trainees, which is essential to tackle the health problems of today. Good scientific research needs a robust and engaged community of researchers to exchange of ideas and methodologies. The residual imbalance from colonial times, resulting in a limited number of researchers operating in areas with high burdens of disease, results in a diminished research community (Kasprowicz et al. 2020; Sam-Agudu et al. 2016).

While there exist no shortage of global health programs—which have widely emerged in the

providing educational opportunities in varied communities provided the perspectives shared in this chapter. These experiences generated ideas for creating a world where building health equity will require us to build educational equity.

# 1 Historical Training in Infectious Disease Research

Two important scientific discoveries from the late nineteenth and early twentieth century—the identification of malarial protozoa as the cause of disease in the blood of infected patients and the mosquito vector responsible for transmission—provide a window into the impetus of tropical medicine research in this period. These findings were made by Alphonese Laveran, a French military doctor, and Sir Ronald Ross, an English physician, both who conducted research in European colonies (Algeria and India, respectively) with the primary motive to protect the colonizer and not the colonized.

early twenty-first century primarily in the US and Europe -- issues remain evident. As noted in Chapter "Learning from the Past to Inform the Future: Perspectives on Future Directions in International Health and Research", professionals from low middle income countries have to travel to high income countries to receive global health training and most global health training programs are concentrated in the global north and are very expensive making them inaccessible to the people who are most affected by the infectious diseases. Solutions continue to be predominantly defined and directed by high-income countries, with little input from local communities. Global health programs offer few ethics courses which are needed to address the unique cultural challenges of field research and the important consideration required of the needs and wants of Indigenous Peoples in these regions. Additionally, there exists the unfortunate occurrence of medical tourists and "safari" scientists, who bag their samples and go home without providing capacity building or ongoing support at the local research sites. Another notable issue is the limited allocation of the funds and resources of wealthy countries towards capacity building or infectious disease training and research that occur beyond their own borders.

A further challenge as we look to the future of education on pathogens is the categorization of the world in terms of a bimodal framework. Emerging during the Cold War were terms used to label countries as either First World or Third World. That framework shifted to the Global North versus Global South, Developed Countries versus Developing Countries or Resource Rich versus Resource Limited. More recently this has been reframed as High Income Country (HIC) to Low Middle Income Country (LMIC). Unfortunately, as long as we retain this dichotomous power structure, we will fail to see the strengths of individual countries and fail to incorporate a truly global approach to the local challenges of disease (see Chapter "When Women Lead in Global Health: Alternative Mobilizations" that discusses the need to avoid damage-centered framework that make the others a victim rather than identifying their strengths and resilience).

## 2    Perspectives from the Field

What does it take to become a scientist? It takes curiosity, aptitude, and motivation, all individual level characteristics. It also takes knowledge, including an understanding of the basic principles, technical, critical thinking, social, and communication skills, acquired through didactic or experiential knowledge transfer. It takes mentorship that coalesces and shapes both the individual with their unique aptitudes and the knowledge gained by working together. The individual characteristics are not unique to any one group of people, but the transfer of knowledge and provision of mentorship that bring that nascent scientist into being is where there are many challenges.

Scientists from research resource limited countries face a number of daunting challenges during and after their training (see Boxes). These include limited mentorship in their home country, limited access to current literature and state of the art laboratory equipment, delays in procuring laboratory supplies, restricted global engagement with peers due to paucity of funds to participate in international conferences, few peers on site, and insufficient local research funding (Ahmed et al. 2020). With these daunting challenges, it is not surprising that there is a brain drain from countries with limited scientific resources, resulting in many young scientists deciding not to stay in their home country or to seek alternative career paths that are more economically viable.

---

**Perspectives on Barriers to Training and Research from Three Trainees from Research Resource Limited Countries**

**Trainee 1 from Research Resource Limited Countries and trained in US:**

- Limited minority representation in scientific leadership roles. The few minorities you find along the way have the mentality of "if it was hard for me, I will make it hard for them."

(continued)

Instead of lending a hand they are a bump on the way.

- Tokenism—By only symbolically making an effort to include underrepresented populations, trainees are not truly valued for their contributions or as a best fit but because they bring the 'benefit" to the PI's lab of diversity.
- Discrimination based on personal identifiers (e.g., gender, ethnicity) can have direct negative impacts on trainees. While it is commonplace to have established systems to deal with discrimination as it arises, affected individuals may still have difficulty speaking out because of their vulnerable status.
- Lack of funding for non-U.S. citizens: Fellowships from the U.S. National Institutes of Health (NIH) are not available for non-U.S. citizens, making international trainees unable to get grants to support independent research, and contributing to a perceived feeling of being a financial burden to their supervisor's grant budget.
- Limited opportunities to return to their country of origin since there are few positions for individuals with advanced degrees, even if there is a need. This feeds back into the problem that there are few professors in home countries to help with capacity building and hence the same professor has to fulfill several roles (teacher, program director, PI, mentor) limiting their time for research if even they have the skills.

**Trainee 2 from a Research Resource Limited Country and trained in a Research Resource Limited Country:**

- Long delays in obtaining essential clinical and laboratory supplies needed for research, impacting progress and innovation.
- Prohibitive costs associated with research supplies and equipment, with limited vendors available to arrange affordable purchasing in LMIC.
- Limited expertise of mentors in infectious diseases beyond tuberculosis, HIV/AIDs, and malaria. This shortage results in a diminished ability to perform important research on other infectious diseases, hence those diseases remain neglected.
- Shortage of access to state-of-the-art laboratory instruments, which creates an impediment to the analysis of clinical samples and constrains research to field-based studies.
- Limited access to peer-reviewed scientific literature. Access to published scientific articles is often restricted by a paywall with few free open access articles.

**Trainee 3 from a Research Resource Limited Country and trained in the US and in a Research Resource Limited Country:**

- Lack of awareness of the importance of research among policy makers in the resource limited country, resulting in little attention and investment.
- Limited availability of motivated mentors.
- Minimal funding and training infrastructure resulting in a lack of interest or motivation to conduct research among the researchers and students
- Research priorities are often set by funding organizations from foreign countries. This, limits innovation the ability to solve local problems

(continued)

through research, and the interest or motivation to continue research.

- Minimal success in publishing in reputable journals, because editors of international journals and editorial board members exhibit limited knowledge about the region and are typically from US or European countries.

An additional challenge for the global health students from research resource limited countries who are trained outside of their home country is that very little is taught on parasitic or other infectious disease burdens found in equatorial regions of the world. For example, if a student from Peru trains in the U.S., they will likely not learn about Chagas disease, one of the most debilitating infectious diseases found in many parts of South America. This limits the trainees' capacity upon returning to their home country to tackle locally relevant diseases. In addition, there is a strong focus in biomedical research on a reductionist view of disease processes so that only if you "knock-out" the gene of interest in a mouse model, will there be importance given to the research. The current paradigm then is that students are trained in techniques and approaches that focus only on the basic science part of the scientific path, which while important, is only one part of the scientific puzzle. Research to understand "disease systems", where "mechanisms" are hard to define and correlation is more common, becomes a funding challenge for the student who takes this path. And yet this path is just as critical, if not more, to the solving of complex infectious disease challenges that face the globe. In addition, funding priorities from US or Europe dictate research areas for trainees that might not necessarily reflect research needs of the trainees' home countries (see Chapter "Funding for Equitable Infectious Disease Research and Development").

There are many programs funded through US and European agencies that focus on capacity building, e.g. increasing human capacity in the countries with the greatest burden of infectious diseases. Unfortunately, these programs often last only as long as the grants received by the US or European principal investigator (PI). After the end of these grants, the PIs can go in new directions because of other funding opportunities. This instability in funding for the PI also becomes a challenge for trainees that remain in their home country following the departure of the PI. These isolated programs supported by individual PIs from the US or Europe do train junior researchers in resource limited countries, but without an existing infrastructure to support and sustain research endeavors, the newly minted scientists are left in countries where there are no stable career trajectories (Development CoHRf 2008). Many researchers move on from these training programs to become leaders in the public health agencies, non-governmental organizations or ministries of health, but we lose their scientific training to tackle important research questions. If these researchers are able to secure an academic appointment at a local university, they are often required to devote an enormous effort to teaching and often no administrative support, leaving little time for research and mentorship of the next generation of scientists.

## 3 Pathways to the Future

Infectious disease research encompasses not just a study of the pathogen but also the burden of the pathogen or disease within the population, the clinical disease, how the host responds to the pathogen, how the pathogen is transmitted (e.g. all the phases of discovery), followed by the development of tools for intervention, and finally tools of deployment. No one person or unit can tackle all aspects of the research process for any given disease. As we saw with the COVID-19 pandemic, we need all hands-on deck to tackle the challenge of infectious diseases. As we continue to reflect on the COVID-19 pandemic and prepare the world for the next pandemic, we should learn from global health experiences in Africa. A recent article summarized, *"Too many projects on health and disease in Africa are pur-*

*sued in silos and funded only for as long as the principal investigator spearheading the project can persuade investors* (Happi and Nkengasong 2022)."

Looking to the future of education, several needs emerge based on our knowledge of where we have been. We need culturally relevant training; a forum for sharing lessons learned; new pedagogical strategies to create thought leaders; movement away from a hierarchical model of knowledge to a horizontal model, using all the minds in a team; and incorporating team culture into research programs. Identifying these needs allows us to reframe them as questions to be answered to create an educational system that is responsive to these needs. Thus, we can ask:

How do we build partnerships through educational initiatives?

How do we train for a systems approach to global health?

How do we build a culture of team-work and team problem solving?

How do we make training open and globally accessible?

While it is not feasible to have a thorough evaluation of existing capacity building programs in this chapter, we will look at two programs that tackled these questions and performed an evaluation to get a sense of possibilities. The two programs are: the Next Generation Scientists sponsored by the University of Basel and Novartis and the African Health Initiative (AHI) which funded the Population Health Implementation and Training (PHIT) partnership.

The Next Generation Scientists program was initiated as a collaboration between the University of Basel, Switzerland, and Novartis with the goal to support early-career scientists in LMIC countries (Pillai et al. 2018). This program for seven years with 143 scientists and clinicians from 25 countries participating. Researchers were brought together for a three-month intensive program based at the University of Basel. Participants selected research projects based on the research needs of their community and developed the research proposal prior to the in-person intern-

ship. Mentors were selected for each trainee. During the three months, in addition to a research project, trainees participated in face-to-face leadership workshops and seminar-style learning. Three key positive takeaways from the program assessment were: the development of peer networks, success of bi-directional mentoring, and tailoring the research to the needs of the trainees. A critical challenge was the need to increase the involvement of the home country supervisor/ mentor of the trainee to promote successful reintegration into the community. Because the program focused on the development of an individualized research training experience, an additional challenge was how to scale up the program.

A second example is the Population Health Implementation and Training (PHIT) partnership supported through the Doris Duke Charitable Foundation. This initiative focused on implementation research in five countries in Africa. Research capacity building was part of the program. An evaluation of this program identified six key lessons for creating a vision of future educational needs (Hedt-Gauthier et al. 2017). First, that funding needs to be sustained and support training that reflects local needs and contexts. Second, programs should include a continuum of activities for training that reflect the local context. Third, funds should support existing research infrastructure when possible. Fourth, research should be integrated with the implementation of health programs. The fifth lesson is the critical role of mentors. Finally, research capacity building efforts should be evaluated and monitored over both the short- and long-term.

A new vision of what is possible comes from the activities of Partners in Health and the newly established University of Global Health Equity (UGHE) based in Rwanda (https://ughe.org). The programs at UGHE have created a vision "where the field is the classroom" and "pulling people up by creating a knowledge economy while delivering care." It will be exciting to see how this new university enacts this vision.

Lessons learned from these and other programs and reflecting on the educational needs to create a global health community committed to global solidarity, we see a future for education that is based on the following key tenets for global health partnerships:

- Building and strengthening networks.
- Understanding local needs and cultural settings.
- Expanding areas of training to address the disconnect between what is taught in scientifically well-resourced countries versus what is needed in low resource settings.
- Breaking down barriers between disciplines by moving away from siloed research and creating transdisciplinary teams.
- Moving toward a non-binary view of the global health world, e.g., truly engaging the view of "global" health where all partners are treated equitably and there is mutual learning.
- Creating a forum to share lessons learned.
- Creating opportunities for mentorship.

## 4    A Path Forward

We have identified five critical issues that need to be addressed to change global health education: (1) culturally relevant training, (2) a forum for sharing lessons learned, (3) new pedagogical strategies to create thought leaders, (4) movement away from a hierarchical model of knowledge to a horizontal model, using all the minds in a team, and (5) incorporating team culture into research programs. In the following paragraphs, we incorporate these examples into a vision for the future of global health education.

A critical first step is to create a network of global health educational partners that are interested in changing the paradigm of global health research. Following the COVID-19 pandemic, we have learned that we can be connected around the world through platforms such as Zoom, Whatsapp and social media. This has created a new dynamic that allows for greater interconnectedness, regardless of location. The goal of this new network would be to create a forum that focuses on sharing lessons learned and best practices in global health education. We envision that working groups would be created from partners

to identify gaps in knowledge in particular regions. The groups would then work together to fill those gaps by creating educational content that is relevant to the particular groups based on shared discussions. The result of these educational working groups would be a peer-to-peer network that could also identify culturally relevant research priorities. The Consortium of Universities for Global Health is an education and advocacy network of academic institutions which can serve as a model. However, we need to move academia and reach out to other institutions where biomedical and public health research occurs, such as national research institutes. Understanding the determinants of health requires more than just the study of a pathogen. Any educational program will need to encompass the social and environmental determinants of health.

Beyond the nuts and bolts of training on the didactics of science that is culturally relevant, there is a more fundamental challenge in changing the culture of how we do science. We would like to propose that we borrow from the "Partners in Health" approach to form "Partners In Education and Research (PIER)" to encompass the idea of our interconnectedness. With PIER, we would create teams around themes. These teams would be across regions and scientific fields, with each member learning how different disciplines tackle scientific questions. This would help to break down silos between scientific groups. Mentorship would be a fundamental underpinning of PIER. PIER networks would be created from the start with an agreement on the fundamental principles that all members of the team have a voice in how to do the research.

## 5    Conclusion

As we look to the future, we need to acknowledge that building health equity requires us to build educational equity. The path forward that we have outlined in this chapter outlines both the challenges and a potential solution through creating PIER networks. By creating holistic educational pathways we can ensure that the next generation of scientists can tackle the infectious disease challenges that remain and improve the wellbeing of affected communities.

# References

Ahmed A, Daily JP, Lescano AG, Golightly LM, Fasina A. Challenges and strategies for biomedical researchers returning to low- and middle-income countries after training. Am J Trop Med Hyg. 2020;102(3):494–6.

Development CoHRf. Changing mindsets Research capacity strengthening in low-and middle-income countries, Geneva, COHRED, Global forum for health research and UNICEF/UNDP/World Bank/WHO special programme for research and training in tropical diseases (TDR). 2008.

Happi CT, Nkengasong JN. Tow years of COVID-19 in Africa: lessons for the world. Nature. 2022;601:22–5.

Hedt-Gauthier BL, Chilengi R, Jackson E, et al. Research capacity building integrated into PHIT projects: leveraging research and research funding to build national capacity. BMC Health Serv Res. 2017;17(Suppl 3):825.

Kasprowicz VO, Chopera D, Waddilove KD, et al. African-led health research and capacity building- is it working? BMC Public Health. 2020;20(1):1104.

Pillai G, Chibale K, Constable EC, et al. The Next Generation Scientist program: capacity-building for future scientific leaders in low- and middle-income countries. BMC Med Educ. 2018;18(1):233.

Sam-Agudu NA, Paintsil E, Aliyu MH, et al. Building sustainable local capacity for global health research in West Africa. Ann Glob Health. 2016;82(6):1010–25.

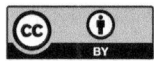

# Learning from the Past to Inform the Future: Perspectives on Future Directions in International Health and Research

## Denisse Vega Ocasio, Aude Bouagnon, and Anita Hargrave

*Education is the most powerful weapon which you can use to change the world.*

Nelson Mandela

*Of all forms of inequality, injustice in healthcare is the most shocking and inhumane.*

Martin Luther King Jr.

## Abstract

The field of global health has increasingly captured international attention in recent years. The spread of infectious diseases across international borders has sparked significant public attention as well as interest among healthcare workers, researchers, and educators. While the field provides a wide range of exciting opportunities, its historical roots in colonialism and saviorism remain in our current approaches to training and implementation. This chapter presents an overview of the challenges faced in global health training from the perspective of current and recently graduated trainees. Key issues include the gender disparity in leadership positions and insufficient efforts to improve the diversity, inclusion, and retention of minoritized trainees. We also address the growing calls to decolonize global health training and curriculum, examine the role that medicine plays in perpetuating these practices, and discuss how training costs hinder people from low- to middle-income countries and diverse socio-cultural backgrounds from advancing in the field of global health. We highlight our collective experiences in global health research and clinical training to emphasize the need for a new vision and approach to training future global health leaders. Furthermore, we aim to offer constructive criticism of the existing institutional system frameworks, and most importantly, we aim to align ourselves with the voices of those who have fiercely advocated for a more inclusive field.

D. Vega Ocasio (✉)
Rollins School of Public Health, Emory University,
Atlanta, GA, USA

A. Bouagnon
School of Medicine, University of California San
Francisco, San Francisco, CA, USA

A. Hargrave
Department of Internal Medicine, University of
California, San Francisco, San Francisco, CA, USA
e-mail: anita.hargrave@ucsf.edu

## Keywords

Global health · Training · Decolonization · Leadership

A. Stewart Ibarra, A. D. LaBeaud (eds.), *Transforming Global Health Partnerships*, Sustainable
Development Goals Series, https://doi.org/10.1007/978-3-031-53793-6_24

## Author Perspective

This chapter perspective is written based on the experiences of current and recent trainees in the public health sciences and health science professions. This authorship team is composed of researchers and clinicians who have worked internationally conducting investigations, studying in local institutions and/or providing medical care primarily in North America, Latin America, Africa, and Europe. This chapter represents their own experiences and perspectives and they do not reflect the opinions or beliefs of their affiliated institutions. We hope that by sharing our collective experiences surrounding global health training we can provide an argument for critical reflection, and subsequently, an inclusive and transformative learning approach.

**Key Tenets for Global Health Partnerships**

1. Power imbalances are prevalent among global health institutions, with systemic inequities shaping interactions and decision-making processes.
2. There are significant systemic inequities within global health training reflecting power dynamics and disparities.
3. Global health training must critically examine the field's colonial roots, behaviors, and ethical issues.
4. Students and trainees are essential agents of change in global health activism, driving efforts toward equity and justice.
5. Unequal representation in health and global health research sectors perpetuates a cycle of power dynamics that favors historically dominant groups in power and decision-making roles.
6. This chapter addresses the following Sustainable Development Goals (SDGs): #4. Ensure inclusive and equitable quality education and promote lifelong learning opportunities for all, #5: Achieve gender equality and empower all women and girls, #17: Strengthen the means of implementation and revitalize the Global Partnership for Sustainable Development: Multi-Stakeholder Partnerships and Voluntary Commitments.

## 1 Introduction

*The man or woman who proclaims devotion to the cause of liberation yet is unable to enter into communion with the people, whom he or she continues to regard as totally ignorant, is grievously self-deceived. The convert who approaches the people but feels alarm at each step they take, each doubt they express, and each suggestion they offer, and attempts to impose his "status," remains nostalgic towards his origins.*

Paulo Freire, Pedagogy of the Oppressed

Paulo Freire was a Brazilian philosopher and educator renowned for his revolutionary philosophy that education is not merely a method for mastering academic standards but rather an organic process of developing political consciousness. In his book, *the Pedagogy of the Oppressed*, Freire argues that successful education involves equal dialogue, mutual respect, and cooperative engagement. Freire's philosophy argues that educational systems play a role in maintaining systems of oppression and, therefore, should be revolutionized to transform society. He places respect and honor in the voices and experiences of those who are marginalized, "the oppressed" as he referred to them. He asserts that their contributions and knowledge are as valuable as of those considered the "experts". Freire's vision is founded on the idea that education is about equal dialogue between the educator and the trainee, rejecting the traditional teacher-student dichotomy (Freire 1970). Freire's vision of education has profoundly influenced many scholars and activists alike—many of them involved in building a more equitable and sustainable health sciences training.

In recent decades, the intersection of science, global health, and international partnerships has gained significant international visibility. The spread of infectious diseases across borders, such as SARS-CoV-2, rightfully attracted significant public attention and increased interest among current trainees in high-income countries (HIC) in the field of global health. The field attracts professionals from diverse backgrounds, and each year the number of training and job opportunities increases with more research programs, public health initiatives, and funding sources (Adams et al. 2016). However, at the same time, many of us are questioning whether the field provides adequate training. Training that builds a generation of professionals willing to challenge and disrupt the entrenched colonial roots of global health (see Chapter "Colonialism, Decolonization, and Global Health"). A new vision for global health, inspired by critical consciousness education, such as that proposed by Freire, is needed. This chapter recognizes the necessity for a revised approach to infectious disease and global health research training. Recognizing that to move forward we must first address the current systemic and institutional challenges present in today's educational systems.

## 2    Learning from the Past

*Imperialism leaves behind germs of rot which we must clinically detect and remove from our land but from our minds as well.*
— Frantz Fanon, *The Wretched of the Earth*

In 2019, Koplan and colleagues defined global health as "an area for study, research, and practice that places a priority on improving health and achieving health equity for all people worldwide (Koplan et al. 2009)." Despite the field's ongoing efforts to foster equitable relationships among partners, it continues to be influenced by unequal power dynamics stemming from a long history of colonial and neocolonial power structures.

The concept of global health can be traced back to the sixteenth and the seventeenth centuries, when European countries began to travel and occupy many countries in the Southern Hemisphere. Tropical medicine—as we know it today—emerged due to colonial settlements when European explorers frequently carried foreign pathogens that rapidly ravaged native populations (Anderson 2006; Worboys 1996). Consequently, when "tropical diseases" threatened imperial economies, medicine and medical missionaries played significant roles in establishing and reinforcing power dynamics. Colonial medical systems grew, linked to state power, and served as a mechanism through which religious and cultural norms were transmitted and imposed on Indigenous populations (de Barros and Stilwell 2003).

Colonial logics remain deeply embedded within the modern medical and academic research systems. Knowledge production, including many university discourses, curricula, and journals, often center Eurocentric and monocultural epistemologies while interiorizing or omitting Indigenous and other non-Western ways of knowing and being (Fregoso Bailón and De Lissovoy 2019). Neocolonial dynamics within academic medical systems can generate epistemic "illusions" by systematically excluding the knowledge, perspectives, norms, and priorities of historically or socially marginalized communities (Richardson 2020). This exclusion distorts understandings of the underlying determinants of health disparities, fueling mistrust in medical and academic research institutions, and biases public health strategies in favor of existing power structures.

Recent racial reckonings within academic medical centers have amplified calls to "decolonize" medicine and for institutions to address past harms through the frameworks of truth, reconciliation, and reparations (i.e., Repair Project, Lancet Commission of Reparations and Redistributive Justice) (Medical Reparations: A Resolution Paper 2022; Bassett et al. 2020). In 2020 alone, the topic of "decolonizing global health" was subject to more than 50 academic articles, discussed at numerous conferences, and was featured in public statements by leaders of global health institutions (Khan et al. 2021). This emerging movement has been fueled by student-led efforts and advocacy from other professionals, seeking more in-depth conversations and public health curricula that centers on recognizing the field's colonial roots, power dynamics and imbalances, and issues of racism, xenophobia, homophobia, and bias (Boston 677 Huntington Avenue 2019; Duke Decolonizing Global Health Working Group 2022).

The recognition stems from the understanding that neither the organization of academic research systems nor the construction of medical knowledge is scientifically or politically neutral. The COVID-19 pandemic has further exposed and amplified long-standing inequities in healthcare outcomes, and highlighted the interwoven nature of healthcare and sociopolitical dynamics. The "legacies" of global health roots continue to perpetuate power imbalances and structural inequities in different shapes and forms: ongoing silencing, discrimination and barriers faced by students of colors and other marginalized communities; HICs controlling the majority of funding programs (see Chapter "Funding for Equitable Infectious Disease Research and Development"); a scarcity of diverse mentors; English being the standard language in international science and medicine; and the maintenance of neocolonialism roots by global health efforts, including short-term projects undertaken by medical and other health students (Abimbola et al. 2021; Langer et al. 2004) (cite) By engaging in advocacy efforts, students can develop a critical consciousness of the power dynamics embedded within medical systems and accelerate the development of anti-oppressive curricula, research directives, and institutional policies.

---

**Box 1: Medical Student and Youth Action at Standing Rock, North Dakota**

In 2015, the Standing Rock Sioux Tribe passed a resolution regarding the proposed construction of the Dakota Access Pipeline (DAPL) because it threatened their access to clean water and would destroy ancient burial grounds and cultural sites (Standing Rock Sioux Tribe 2022; Smithsonian National Museum for the American Indian 2018). The Standing Rock Sioux Tribe, particularly Native youth and their mentors, began to organize events to raise awareness of the oil pipeline (Elbein 2017). In 2016, they worked with surrounding Native Nations to form the Sacred Stones Camp on the Standing Rock Reservation to stand in opposition to DAPL. As their movement grew, Indigenous People and non-Native allies from around the world began to demonstrate their solidarity with the DAPL opposition. Many supporters gathered in and around the camp, including a reported 180 tribes. During medical school, I was involved in creating a coalition of students, healthcare workers, and activists dedicated to accompanying communities in a collective movement to protect health and wellbeing (Do No Harm Coalition 2016). As a member of this coalition, I was invited by the Sioux Tribe to go to Standing Rock to collaborate with local health workers and emergency medics in coordinating clinical options and supplies for the Standing Rock Lakota Dakota and their supporters. When I returned, I worked with the Native American Health Alliance (NAHA), my mentors and the coalition to organize an event to raise support for and awareness of the First Nations People at Standing Rock and in the local Bay Area. This included a panel discussion with Native Rumsen Ohlone community members and a report back from the coalition members who had gone to Standing Rock. Over 200 people attended the event, and I was able to leverage my position as a medical student to speak about health concerns related to the Dakota Access Pipeline to reach a larger medical community.

Although this experience occurred in the United States, my identity as a white, cisgender North American woman gave me unearned privilege, as it often does in international spaces. The Native People at Standing Rock thoughtfully reminded me of my ancestral and ongoing ties to colonialism. They taught me that cultural competence means understanding your own culture and how it affects the people you seek to work with, as much as understanding the cultures of others. Importantly, Standing Rock showed me the power of youth, trainees, and students in organizing social movements and challenging oppressive systems. It also illustrated the vital role that mentors have in protecting students and youth in their advocacy work, particularly those from historically minoritized groups, as these younger generations often do not have the security afforded by longitudinal positions in traditional power structures. By supporting the leadership, activism, and insight of students and youth, we will make important advancements in health equity and scientific discovery in the U.S. and internationally.

(continued)

## 3    Learning From the Past to Understand the Present

*Even if HIC universities made their degrees more accessible, we should still ask why an African trainee must go to London or Boston to learn about control of sleeping sickness or malaria (and pay top dollars for such training)?*
— Anita Svadzian et al. 2020

Global health opportunities are increasing at every stage of training and professional careers, especially in HICs. These opportunities can take form of internships, fellowships, short-term teaching, or practice for faculty and medical students. While these opportunities can open doors to graduate programs and jobs for early-career scientists, and are crucial for the development of students' practice, institutions and training programs are still perpetuating longstanding power imbalances between countries in the Global North and the Global South. Though these imbalances manifest in many forms, we will focus on the following issues experienced during our training: (1) power and gender imbalances, (2) cost of education, and (3) systematic barriers in the study of sciences.

Power imbalances are experienced first-hand from the beginning of training. Most institutions and organizations focused on global health are primarily located in HICs, and most of their leaders are men from these regions. Experts from the Global South remain significantly underrepresented in both academic research and leadership positions across sectors (Downs et al. 2014; Dhatt et al. 2017; World Health Organization 2019). The gap in underrepresentation widens with gender. For instance, in 2015 women represented less than 27% of Ministers of Health globally, and in the United States, less than a fourth of global health institutions at the top 50 U.S. medical schools were directed by women (World Health Organization 2019; Gender and global health – Global Health 50/50 2022). For women of color, this gap is much wider, as they face intersectional challenges—understood as the relationships and interactions between social identities and stratifiers across multiple levels of society—including race, gender and classism in the workplace, resulting in unequal pay, tokenism, limited retention, and underrepresentation (Armstrong et al. 2020; Ong et al. 2018).

Another way in which institutions uphold colonial roots is the prohibitive cost of higher education. Since most global health institutions are located in HICs, the high cost of tuition is a major barrier to accessing training, especially for those with non-privileged socio-economic backgrounds. At study conducted by Svadzian and et. al, reported that the mean tuition fee across 41 international degree programs, was USD $41,790 for international students, compared to USD $33,603 for domestic students (Svadzian et al. 2020). These financial barriers perpetuate a cycle where mostly financially privileged students access training and become the 'experts' who train the next generation, reinforcing elite global health leadership, power asymmetries, and hindering efforts toward diversity, inclusion, and retention (Gender and global health – Global Health 50/50 2022; Svadzian et al. 2020). Education, and global health education more specifically, should reconsider their current economic model to generate revenue, to reduce the barriers to both low- and middle-income countries (LMICs) and low-income groups in accessing their programs. At the same time, the notion that only institutions in HICs provide quality education reflects an ethnocentrism present in many research articles, practices, and academic curriculum.

Researchers from HICs continue to benefit from the local scientific expertise contributed by researchers from LMICs. Yet, researchers from LMICs remain underrepresented in academic scientific literature and conferences (Busse and August 2020). A systematic review conducted from 2014 to 2016, described that among research papers analyzed from sub-Saharan Africa, 14% had no local authors, and only half of the first authors were local. Several studies have found that local authorship representation decreases when its collaborators are from Canada, the U.S., and Europe (Hedt-Gauthier et al. 2019; Kelaher et al. 2016). Systemic inequities in academic journals take various forms, such as: English serving as the primary language for research and publications, high fees associated with publishing in high-impact journals, and a lack of diversity on journal editorial boards and among peer reviewers (Nafade et al. 2019; Bhaumik and Jagnoor 2019). Similarly, scientific collaboration and participation in conferences for LMICs scientists are hindered by visa restrictions, political and financial barriers (i.e., high conference registration rates, travel expenses and visa fees), racism, discrimination, language barriers, and limited representation among presenters and speakers (Velin et al. 2021). If authors from LMICs are deterred from participating in scientific activities such as publications and grant development due to HICs policies, then HICs are restricting LMICs scientists potential to become independent researchers and advocate for research priorities for their own region; thereby perpetuating the dominance of scientists from HICs (Busse and August 2020; Beran et al. 2017).

Global health conferences should center the voices of those who are directly affected by the health issues being addressed. These spaces should play a key role in identifying solutions rooted in people's lived experiences by fostering equitable co-production processes. The work presented at these conferences should reflect direct and equal exchange between partners with the goal of achieving effective, thoughtful, and locally relevant strategies to tackle global health challenges. A practice that should begin during our training years. It is imperative that scientists and institutions from HICs recognize the importance of intersectionality and inclusion in global health beyond the classroom.

Ultimately, global health conferences and academic papers are meant for sharing knowledge, networking, building collaborations, and supporting professional development. When we exclude partners from the Global South and other marginalized communities in HICs, we are only serving and benefiting those who comfort themselves with neocolonialism. We stifle creativity, innovation, and the potential search for impactful and sustainable solutions in global health. When we continue stigmatizing those who do not speak English as their primary language and limit their ability to share their in-country data in their native language, or we don't include our research partners on our publications, we continue reinforcing colonial behaviors in our work and sustaining a system of privilege that oppresses those who are already marginalized.

Conversely, by increasing the diversity of presenters, speakers, and authors, we expand the body of critical scientific knowledge and open ourselves to new ideas and frameworks that are desperately needed to address the global health challenges today (for example, the Indigenous land-based meta-narrative in Chapter "Transforming the Planetary Health Crisis Through an Indigenous Land-Based Meta-Narrative"). We also increase a sense of belonging to the field for other historically minoritized and underrepresented groups.

## 4    Learning from the Past to Shape the Future

*As researchers, we need to reject the idea of fixing the lives and conditions of marginalized people. Our role is to become allies in the process and use our voice and privileged position to redistribute and challenge power structures in ways that would prioritize communities' voices as the experts of their own lives and experiences.*

– Seye Abimbola

As we look toward the future of global health, we must rethink and restructure the current power dynamics that prioritize HICs institutional needs over those of local research institutions in the Global South and other marginalized communities within HIC institutions. For this, each of us needs to deliberately reflect and deconstruct our colonial mindset that was conditioned through our education. To do so, we must make a conscious and collective effort to learn the history of colonization in science and health and its past and current impact. We must think critically about how it shapes our education and the common perception that research systems in HICs are the primary means of effecting change, rather than valuing and centering local and Indigenous knowledge systems (Abimbola et al. 2021). It is essential to acknowledge the impact of the language we use, how we work in partnership with people from diverse backgrounds, and how we react when given criticism about local culture and socio-political influences. While this chapter does not aim to provide a comprehensive analysis of the global health education situation, we have identified several critical needs based on our experience as recent trainees. We will focus on three key areas: intersectional training, partnership, and underrepresentation.

## 4.1  Intersectional Training

We propose that current global health training should challenge trainees and create a curriculum that questions the field's colonial roots and behaviors, the ethical issues that can arise from such work (see Chapter "Ethical Challenges in Global Health Research"), and the power imbalances presented when interacting with the communities the trainees work with (see Chapter "Collective Learning: Power and Trust in Partnerships in the 3D Program for Girls and Women in Rural Pune District, India"). Today, many HICs continue to enforce both domestic and international policies that endanger the livelihoods of people within their own countries as well as those in other regions. Global health trainees must be aware of their positioning within systems of oppression, both domestically and internationally, to effectively recognize and transform their colonial mentality. Addressing colonialism in global health is deeply connected to Critical Race Theory, which sheds light on how race, as a social construct, contributes to global health disparities. As the Global North increasingly acknowledges the pervasive nature of structural racism, it is crucial for global health programs and institutions to confront their own ties to white supremacy and Euro-American cultural dominance with a firm commitment to antiracism in their work and training. This commitment should include teaching students to conduct research and/or provide health care that prioritizes the voices of historically marginalized groups and is grounded in race consciousness. It should also involve critical self-reflection on the power or privilege associated with each person's uniquely intersecting identities (Ford and Airhihenbuwa 2010; Yam et al. 2021). Moreover, we must promote curricula that fosters multilingualism and multiculturalism, enhancing intercultural competence and understanding. By integrating these elements into global health training, we can better prepare future professionals to engage with and address the complex dynamics of global health disparities.

The current movement for "decolonization of global health" aims to implement an anti-colonial environment and curricula for research and practice that reflects on the power asymmetry and highlights the intersectional nature of science and global health. However, "decolonization" should not be reduced to a trendy metaphor for needed societal changes without a critical introspective analysis of power and sociopolitics. Critical analysis of colonialism in science and medicine should aim to dismantle the structures of oppression that have perpetuated colonial dynamics for generations. It tackles imperialism and colonialism at every level, and it demands centering Black and Indigenous sovereignty. While the movement for "decolonizing global health" is well intentioned, global health training needs to be wary about how it is centering and shaping the narrative with conceit and hubris in the Global North and whether the conversations are being made more palatable to the Euro-American vision.

Finally, as current trainees and/or recent graduates we should continually question our roles and privileges that may perpetuate the status quo. For those of us in HICs who come from marginalized, underrepresented communities in science, we must be cautious about complicity in preserving power imbalances inherent to global health. This is whether it is done consciously or unconsciously or enforced by societal power structures and its institutions. For that it is imperative to acknowledge transparently and with gentleness to oneself the intersection of privileges that exist within our experiences. That is, whether that privilege was obtained when receiving higher education, our immigration status, job positions, gender identity, socio-economic means, or physical location. Acknowledging privileges within ourselves does not mean that we do not also experience discrimination or increased systematic barriers to achieving success. It means that we should use our privilege to continue dismantling systems of oppressions, and to continue uplifting and opening a more equitable path for others in our own communities. Similarly, for global health trainees who come from privileged or overrepresented communities in science we have a responsibility to understand our histories and how they tie to systems of oppression. Acknowledging our own privilege and not becoming defensive when faced with this truth are essential aspects of working in global health. Leveraging the unearned social capital, when used at the request of and in collaboration with communities who do not hold the same privilege, can be a tool to address inequities.

## 4.2    Fostering Equitable Partnerships

Global health partnerships involve two or more organizations working together to reach a common goal. When implemented effectively, these partnerships amplify the voices and agendas of LMIC institutions and other organizations serving marginalized communities, to focus on local needs, visions, and priorities essential for cross-sectoral community-based solutions. These partnerships require an active and continuous process of review and consultation necessary to refine equitable practices and processes. As we look to the future of global health partnerships, we present key ways in which students and trainees can contribute to fostering equitable partnerships.

In Freire's vision of critical pedagogy, learning experiences hold transformative potential when students actively challenge established norms and perspectives, giving rise to ways of thinking and being in the world (Melling and Pilkington 2018). Indeed, student-led efforts at a number of health professional schools around the globe have catalyzed important conversations about the colonial vestiges inherent within global health work and have led to the development of

more ethical frameworks for global health partnerships (Brocher Declaration – ICMDA 2022). By integrating their lived sociopolitical experiences and technological prowess to learning environments, trainees have a heightened ability to create or adapt innovative approaches to the field of global health.

Participatory action or community-engaged research paradigms are emerging as a method through which equitable and meaningful partnerships can be formed between trainees and researchers, and communities that have historically been excluded from dominant forms of academic knowledge production (Lenette 2022). The foundational aim of participatory research is to co-create knowledge with impacted communities such to develop insights and solutions that lead to transformational social change (Page-Reeves 2019). By centering the narratives and experiences of historically marginalized groups, participatory action research seeks to democratize research processes, bring visibility to knowledge and understandings that have been erased or marginalized through colonial processes, and identify structural changes necessary for equitable health care systems. While not perfect, participàtory action models aims to challenge the implicit norm within global health that communities and countries facing inequities are incapable of addressing their own problems (Kwete et al. 2022). Instead, this engagement paradigm emphasizes that through collaborative partnerships and shared prosperity, affected communities can determine their own priorities and achieve the transformative changes necessary for global health equity. By shifting the narrative, partners from LMICs are not left as passive victims to be saved by the external researcher, but rather they are active agents of change, innovation, resources, and resilience.

Successful and equitable partnerships require a profound understanding of inherent inequalities, historical legacies, and power differentials between groups members. Transforming global research partnerships necessitates a reflective approach to ensuring transparency, equity, and shared decision-making in every step of the collaboration process. Mentors and trainees should practice open-hearted, empathy, active listening, kindness, effective communication, and cultural consciousness to foster meaningful relationships. By working in partnership, scientists can help design and advocate for research and educational programs that are responsive to local needs. They can ensure that methods and data collection align with local practices and advocate for the results to serve both the community and research goals. Moreover, empowered and supported students can improve transparency in daily communications, distribution of resources or responsibilities, decision-making, and dissemination of research findings to communities and partners. Both students and their mentors should ensure that all partners receive appropriate credit for their contributions, including recognition for grants, authorship, presentations, and benefits.

While it is not feasible to offer a comprehensive review of best practices within global health partnerships in this chapter, we want to emphasize that students play vital and active roles in reimagining institutions, identifying and disturbing entrenched power dynamics and fostering relationships built on mutual trust, respect, and equity.

intersectionality of health, sciences, and the environment. Applying this during and after my training has allowed me to understand how different populations perceive diseases, local priorities, experiences, and conditions, and sustainable solutions focused on their specific needs. This approach has opened the door for trust, communication, collaboration, and equal partnerships at every step of the research. While I received support from mentors, the "emic" perspectives on my research were not always welcomed by other peers. Often techniques such as qualitative research were placed in opposition to quantitative research and dismissed as a "lesser" science. As a student, I often found myself being forced to follow the more "traditional" routes in science and research and overexplaining how this would improve the quality of our data and project overall. Despite pushback, I was able to incorporate "emic" techniques into my research, which resulted in a broader study that amplified the voices of local partners and the communities I worked with and allowed my audience to understand social determinants of health on a more personal and local level.

---

**Box 2: Changing the "I" to "We" in Global Health**

During my PhD training, my mentors emphasized early on that, *"the communities you work with know best their community concerns and the solutions to tackle such problems. All you need to do is to listen."* With these words, my mentors wanted to emphasize the value and importance of understanding and applying "emic" perspectives in research and global health. That is understanding practices, behaviors, and norms that are specific within a group or culture "from people's experience" (Mostowlansky and Rota 2020). In practice, it meant placing myself as a "spectator" rather than an "expert" to understand the

(continued)

## 4.3  Creating Equal and Inclusive Representation

In the global health field, unequal representation across all sectors of health, research, and practice perpetuates power structures that favor those who have traditionally held decision-making roles; that is predominantly white, cis-gendered, heterosexual, male and European/American. This inequality creates a system that silences historically marginalized communities by underrepresenting them in the spaces where decisions are made about what kind of research or intervention is "needed" in their communities. Constructing a new vision for global health will require both individual and collective introspection. Students and trainees can play a crucial role in challenging themselves and their institutions to recognize that global health solutions cannot be 'one size fits all.' These solutions should be intersectional, sustainable and co-created with those directly impacted by the issues.

At an educational level, students have increasingly called for a leadership shift, one that reflects the diversity of populations that privileged academic institutions, agencies and organizations intend to serve. Women, and especially women of color, need to be centered and lead policy decision making, programmatic formulation, and the global health agenda setting. Students have also advocated for more equitable representation in academic journals, greater linguistic diversity in publications, training platforms and other research networks, and increased diversity among faculty and students at academic institutions. Trainees can contribute by creating new platforms and spaces for equitable and safe engagement in global health, where partners can come together to share their successes and challenges, lessons learned, and recommendations.

Efforts to foment an equal, inclusive, and safe environment must include classroom discussions that ensures flow of knowledge is factual, compassionate, reciprocal, anti-racist, and anti-colonialist. Students need to be taught about the racist and colonial histories that gave rise to inequitable global diseases burdens. The scientific curriculum should also be expanded to include a stronger presence of sociology, anthropology, history, and political science and emphasize sociocultural and structural determinants of health and illness (Montenegro et al. 2020). In turn, educators and institutions should recognize that students, especially those from racially minorized groups, are more vulnerable to distress due to the cumulative emotional and psychological impact of systemic inequities and racism in higher education and that pervade many aspects of their lives. Therefore, efforts should include providing the necessary tools needed for restoration and healing such as, but not limited to, equitable access to educational resources, opportunities to learn in an inclusive environment, and comprehensive support services (see

Chapter "Courageous Authenticity: Bringing Our Inner Wisdom to Our Work, Partnerships, and Communities").

As for trainees motivated to pursue global health work outside of their own communities, it is imperative to commit to ethical principles in conducting global health and to actively challenge the status quo to advance health equity and inclusion. Trainees should also reflect on the ways that they might unintentionally cause harm and recognize the intersectionality of their own social and political identities compared to those of the communities they serve or partner with. This self-awareness will enhance their understanding of the complex factors that influence health, how these factors interact across multiple levels of society, and ways to reckon them (Kapilashrami and Hankivsky 2018). Only by doing so, will we be able to reach our transformative potential, develop thoughtful global health curricula, and rebuild a field that prioritizes the voices of those who are more socially and/or politically vulnerable.

## 5    Conclusion

As we end this chapter, we hope our experiences prompt readers to reflect on their own lived experiences and spark deeper conversations about advancing equitable global health training. We recognize that this chapter covers only a small fraction of the broader discussion around steps needed to dismantle the current system of training. While some institutions in the Global North have committed to making global health a more equitable and diverse field, we still have a long way to go to achieve a field that truly practices equity, addresses colonial roots, and recognizes intersectionality. Student and trainee voices have been a constant powerful, and necessary force for change within global health. We hope this chapter empowers you to continue critically analyzing the global health training you are receiving, have previously received, or are teaching, to catalyze the transformative changes necessary for just and equitable international work.

# References

Abimbola S, Asthana S, Montenegro C, et al. Addressing power asymmetries in global health: Imperatives in the wake of the COVID-19 pandemic. PLoS Med. 2021;18(4):e1003604. https://doi.org/10.1371/journal.pmed.1003604.

Adams LV, Wagner CM, Nutt CT, Binagwaho A. The future of global health education: training for equity in global health. BMC Medical Education. 2016;16(1):296.

Armstrong A, Lomax J, Traylor-Knowles N, Samba-Louaka A, Towers C. On being black in the ivory tower. Cell. 2020;183(3):559–560.

Anderson W. Colonial pathologies: American tropical medicine, race, and hygiene in the Philippines. Duke University Press; 2006. https://doi.org/10.1215/9780822388081.

Bassett MT, Galea S, et al. N Engl J Med. 2020;383(22):2101–3. https://doi.org/10.1056/NEJMp2026170.

Beran D, Byass P, Gbakima A, et al. Research capacity building—obligations for global health partners. Lancet Global Health. 2017;5(6):e567–8. https://doi.org/10.1016/S2214-109X(17)30180-8.

Bhaumik S, Jagnoor J. Diversity in the editorial boards of global health journals. BMJ Glob Health. 2019;4(5):e001909. https://doi.org/10.1136/bmjgh-2019-001909.

Boston 677 Huntington Avenue, Ma 02115 +1495-1000. Challenging the status quo in global health. News. Published February 19, 2019. https://www.hsph.harvard.edu/news/features/decolonizing-global-health/. Accessed 19 Nov2022.

Brocher Declaration – ICMDA. 2022. https://icmda.net/about/partners/brocher/. Accessed 19 Nov 2022.

Busse C, August E. Addressing power imbalances in global health: Pre-Publication Support Services (PREPSS) for authors in low-income and middle-income countries. BMJ Glob Health. 2020;5(2):e002323. https://doi.org/10.1136/bmjgh-2020-002323.

de Barros J, Stilwell S. Introduction: public health and the imperial project. Caribbean Q. 2003;49(4):1–11.

Dhatt R, Theobald S, Buzuzi S, et al. The role of women's leadership and gender equity in leadership and health system strengthening. Glob Health Epidemiol. 2017;2:e8. https://doi.org/10.1017/gheg.2016.22.

Do No Harm Coalition. Do No Harm Coalition. Published 2016. https://www.donoharmcoalition.org/. Accessed 26 Sept 2022.

Downs JA, Reif LK, Hokororo A, Fitzgerald DW. Increasing women in leadership in global health. Acad Med. 2014;89(8):1103–7. https://doi.org/10.1097/ACM.0000000000000369.

Duke Decolonizing Global Health Working Group. 2022. https://sites.duke.edu/dukedgh/. Accessed 15 Nov 2022.

Elbein S. The youth that launched a movement at standing rock. The New York Times Magazine. Published online January 31, 2017:24.

Ford CL, Airhihenbuwa CO. Critical race theory, race equity, and public health: toward antiracism praxis. Am J Public Health. 2010;100(S1):S30–5. https://doi.org/10.2105/AJPH.2009.171058.

Fregoso Bailón RO, De Lissovoy N. Against coloniality: toward an epistemically insurgent curriculum. Policy Futures Educ. 2019;17(3):355–69. https://doi.org/10.1177/1478210318819206.

Freire P. Pedagogy of the Oppressed, 30th Anniversary Edition. 1970.

Gender and global health – Global Health 50/50. 2022. https://globalhealth5050.org/gender-and-global-health/. Accessed 19 Nov 2022.

Hedt-Gauthier BL, Jeufack HM, Neufeld NH, et al. Stuck in the middle: a systematic review of authorship in collaborative health research in Africa, 2014–2016. BMJ Glob Health. 2019;4(5):e001853. https://doi.org/10.1136/bmjgh-2019-001853.

Kapilashrami A, Hankivsky O. Intersectionality and why it matters to global health. Lancet. 2018;391(10140):2589–91. https://doi.org/10.1016/S0140-6736(18)31431-4.

Kelaher M, Ng L, Knight K, Rahadi A. Equity in global health research in the new millennium: trends in first-authorship for randomized controlled trials among low- and middle-income country researchers 1990–2013. Int J Epidemiol. 2016;45(6):2174–83. https://doi.org/10.1093/ije/dyw313.

Khan M, Abimbola S, Aloudat T, Capobianco E, Hawkes S, Rahman-Shepherd A. Decolonising global health in 2021: a roadmap to move from rhetoric to reform. BMJ Glob Health. 2021;6(3):e005604. https://doi.org/10.1136/bmjgh-2021-005604.

Koplan JP, Bond TC, Merson MH, et al. Towards a common definition of global health. Lancet. 2009;373(9679):1993–5. https://doi.org/10.1016/S0140-6736(09)60332-9.

Kwete X, Tang K, Chen L, et al. Decolonizing global health: what should be the target of this movement and where does it lead us? Glob Health Res Policy. 2022;7(1):3 https://doi.org/10.1186/s41256-022-00237-3.

Langer A, Díaz-Olavarrieta C, Berdichevsky K, Villar J. Why is research from developing countries underrepresented in international health literature, and what can be done about it? Bull World Health Organ. 2004;82(10):802–3.

Lenette C. Participatory action research: ethics and decolonization. 1st ed. Oxford University Press; 2022. https://doi.org/10.1093/oso/9780197512456.001.0001.

Medical Reparations: A Resolution Paper. The REPAIR Project. 2022. https://repair.ucsf.edu/medical-reparations-resolution-paper. Accessed 19 Nov 2022.

Melling A, Pilkington R, editors. Paulo Freire and transformative education. Palgrave Macmillan; 2018. https://doi.org/10.1057/978-1-137-54250-2.

Montenegro CR, Bernales M, Gonzalez-Aguero M. Teaching global health from the south: challenges and proposals. Critical Public Health. 2020;30(2):127–9. https://doi.org/10.1080/09581596.2020.1730570.

Mostowlansky T, Rota A. Emic and Etic. Robbins J, Stasch R, Candea M, et al., eds. *CEA*. Published online December 1, 2020. https://doi.org/10.29164/20emicetic.

Nafade V, Sen P, Pai M. Global health journals need to address equity, diversity and inclusion. BMJ Glob Health. 2019;4(5):e002018. https://doi.org/10.1136/bmjgh-2019-002018.

Ong M, Smith JM, Ko LT. Counterspaces for women of color in STEM higher education: Marginal and central spaces for persistence and success. Journal of Research in Science Teaching. 2018;55(2):206–245.

Page-Reeves J. Community-based participatory research for health. Health Promotion Practice. 2019;20(1):15–7. https://doi.org/10.1177/1524839918809007.

Richardson ET. Epidemic illusions: on the coloniality of global public health. The MIT Press; 2020.

Smithsonian National Museum for the American Indian. Treaties Still Matter - The Dakota Access Pipeline. Native Knowledge 360. Published 2018. https://americanindian.si.edu/nk360/plains-treaties/dapl. Accessed 26 Sept 2022

Standing Rock Sioux Tribe. 2022. https://www.standingrock.org/. Accessed 26 Sept 2022.

Svadzian A, Vasquez NA, Abimbola S, Pai M. Global health degrees: at what cost? BMJ Glob Health. 2020;5(8):e003310. https://doi.org/10.1136/bmjgh-2020-003310.PMID: 32759185; PMCID: PMC7410003.

Velin L, Lartigue JW, Johnson SA, et al. Conference equity in global health: a systematic review of factors impacting LMIC representation at global health conferences. BMJ Glob Health. 2021;6(1):e003455. https://doi.org/10.1136/bmjgh-2020-003455.

Worboys M. Colonialism, tropical disease and imperial medicine: Rockefeller philanthropy in Sri Lanka. Med Hist. 1996;40(4):524–5.

World Health Organization. Delivered by women, led by men: a gender and equity analysis of the global health and social workforce. World Health Organization; 2019. https://apps.who.int/iris/handle/10665/311322. Accessed 19 Nov 2022.

Yam EA, Silva M, Ranganathan M, White J, Hope TM, Ford CL. Time to take critical race theory seriously: moving beyond a colour-blind gender lens in global health. Lancet Global Health. 2021;9(4):e389–90. https://doi.org/10.1016/S2214-109X(20)30536-2.

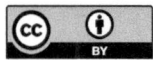

# Engaging with Heart in Global Health Partnerships

Valerie A. Luzadis ⓘ

*The best and most beautiful things in the world cannot be seen or even touched–they must be felt with the heart.*

— Helen Keller

## Abstract

What does it mean to build a more peaceful, equitable and loving world, to solve problems together? Global health partnerships are a perfect place to explore ways to do this because they rely on relationships. However, we are coming out of a dominant paradigm of Western science and colonialism that is often an invisible driver of our thoughts and actions. This frequently invisible yet insidious history still frames much of our understanding and our actions in every facet of life, including in science and global health. Continuing business-as-usual, without deep introspection and intention, leads us to replicate inequities and instabilities within our relationships with each other and between people and nature. These are experienced as traumas by all of us, some more easily seen than others. Many appear as individual and widespread human health concerns, as well as social and environmental disruption and degradation. This chapter explores ways in which we can create opportunities for healing these traumas while working together on solutions to immediate and long-term global health issues.

V. A. Luzadis (✉)
State University of New York College of
Environmental Science and Forestry and Heart
Forward Science, Syracuse, NY, USA
e-mail: vluzadis@esf.edu; http://www.
heartforwardscience.org/

## Keywords

Integrating knowledge systems · Intuition · Mind-body · Other ways of knowing · Global health

## Author Perspective

I am a woman scientist and policy practitioner working with a variety of social-ecological systems, ecological economics, and the science-policy interface locally, regionally, nationally, and internationally. My background is in forest science, adult communication and education, and ecological economics and policy. I have worked with NGOs throughout my career, serving in organizational and leadership positions at local, state, national, and international levels. I have served at all levels of academic leadership from Department Chair to Interim Provost and Executive Vice President. My research, academic, and organizational work is informed by systems thinking to enhance effectiveness and efficiency of institutions through inclusive, compassionate, and matrixed systems of shared effort, power, and respect for all. I founded Heart Forward Science to support the development of holistic knowledge through a balance of intellect, imagination, and intuition to advance equitable, sustainable scientific outcomes.

A. Stewart Ibarra, A. D. LaBeaud (eds.), *Transforming Global Health Partnerships*, Sustainable Development Goals Series, https://doi.org/10.1007/978-3-031-53793-6_25

**Key Tenets**

1. Engaging with heart means bringing our whole selves to all that we do.
2. Recognizing the extent to which one is embedded within the dominant paradigm that stems from a colonizer/settler framing is crucial to building a more peaceful, equitable, loving world.
3. Engaging diverse knowledge systems respectfully requires self-confidence with humility and humanity.
4. Intellect, imagination, and intuition all provide paths to envision and bring a more equitable, sustainable world to life.
5. This chapter addresses the following SDGs: #3 Good health and wellbeing, #10 Reducing inequities, and #16 Peace, justice, and strong institutions.

## 1    Introduction

Recognition of the power and impact of partnerships within global health initiatives brings forward the possibility of healing much more than the diseases or health concerns at their base. By expanding the scope of understanding of the "problem" to include systemic violence and inequity resulting from a colonizing-settler mentality, we can achieve much greater positive outcomes through global health partnerships.

In this chapter, I suggest that we have an opportunity to have a much greater and sustained impact by recognizing the power and influence that partnerships can have to demonstrate the respectful engagement of diverse knowledge systems within ourselves and with others. To do this, I briefly explore how we replicate the dominant paradigm of a science mentality in our current approaches to partnership and collaboration, acknowledging the trauma that this can and does cause. I then offer a few ideas to consider for bringing our whole selves to all we do as we

move toward respectful engagement of multiple knowledge systems.

## 2    Engaging with Heart

Recent worldwide attention to the Me Too and Black Lives Matter movements which emerged from northern contexts have stimulated many to begin or further our efforts on a path toward an equitable world. These movements and other influential incidents created opportunities and support for people everywhere to do their own individual work, to see and to unlearn the longstanding oppressive structures and systems of our colonizing history.

Unlearning is crucial to this process. How do we do this? It begins with acknowledgment of the traumas caused by dualistic, elitist, hierarchical power structures, including within Western science, medicine, and the public health activities stemming from them. (See Chapter(s) "Colonialism, Decolonization, and Global Health" and "Transforming the Planetary Health Crisis Through an Indigenous Land-Based Meta-Narrative" for a deeper treatment of these concepts.) Once we open to seeing this, we can go beyond acknowledgment to intending and discovering pathways that no longer replicate the harms of power-over mentalities.

The power dynamics that we see institutionally also tend to be replicated at the individual level among the "haves" and "have nots", and with gender, race, and orientation identities. This means that each of us can address this by finding ways to move in the world with love, blameless discernment, and acceptance while resisting violence and inequities. Following a path of individual awareness, empathetic listening, acknowledgment, healing, unlearning, learning, and co-creating a transformed future helps not only at the individual level but creates a ripple effect that carries much further. Just as we experience the joy of someone who enters the room with exciting and happy news such that it uplifts us, too, our work of self-healing and self-care with community awareness transforms and encourages those around us (see Chapter

"Courageous Authenticity: Bringing Our Inner Wisdom to Our Work, Partnerships, and Communities"). Recognizing this impact and adjusting one's own self-care and behavior to reflect this requires introspection, self-compassion, and emotional healing. Supporting each other in these efforts is one way in which we help to extend positive impacts.

Engaging diverse knowledge systems respectfully requires self-confidence with humility and humanity as we consider who is involved, who owns the outcomes, and how we can collaborate in truly equitable ways. It also requires self-knowledge. It is no longer enough to bring only our analytical, intellectual selves to this work. We must bring our whole selves to all that we do. I call this engaging with heart: learning and embracing the many ways we know, extending beyond the analytical and intellectual. Learning to intertwine it all to inform our actions can be described in a deliciously paradoxical way: "thinking with the heart and feeling with the mind." The results are impactful, compassionate, humble, and respectful.

## 3 Practice Seeing Embedded Oppression

Recognizing that we are steeped in oppressive structures and systems is an initial step. Practice seeing embedded oppression, supporting each other in doing so, and seeking out and listening to under-represented people helps to build within each of us the ability to better see and hear the traumas that need to be aired, acknowledged, healed, and not repeated. Being willing to let go of these structures and find new ways is vastly different from simply recognizing them. It's a natural question to ask how to let something go when (1) we can barely see it given its ubiquitous nature—like a fish seeing water; and (2) without clear ideas of what will replace it.

One way to begin to do this is to engage the use of imagination. Imagine a world where…fill in the blank here with your wildest, most loving ideas. *A world without disease? Everyone is fed and healthy? Living in harmony with nature? No violence or war; living with love? No greed?* Using imagination to envision what we want is a powerful tool. The process of imagining and envisioning helps move us toward developing intentionality—deliberate articulation of desired outcomes for our world, each program, each relationship, each day. Combining intentionality with these visions will move us collectively toward a more sustainable, equitable world. While this may seem impossible when considering it with only the analytical mind, opening to intuition and engaging with heart brings the knowledge that making these changes within each of us, one at a time, actually leads to much greater change in the world. By healing ourselves, we heal the world as it flows through us into the families, companions, and communities around us.

In addition to using imagination to individually envision the futures we want, it is also useful collectively. Science is already making use of imagination. For example, future scenario development involves going beyond data trends to imagine futures much further than data allow. I engaged this process with a national professional association to identify possible futures, the role of the organization within each, and the adjustments we needed to be relevant and useful no matter which future emerged. The outcomes were the foundation of the organization's strategic plan that was widely supported while reflecting important future possibilities. This process can be used in many different settings and in transdisciplinary approaches involving science and public health experts along with interested citizens. Interestingly, in one experience working on Great Lakes futures, I observed that science-related participants had the most difficult time letting go of data trends enough to actually engage imagination regarding possible futures. These efforts followed specific guidelines and did engage the imagination. However, they would be greatly improved by explicitly drawing together participants' individual visions and intentions for the futures they want along with the focus of the exercise, be it the management of lakes and ecosystems, planning public health programs and interventions, or the strategic plans for an organization.

## 4    Challenges of Seeing—A Personal Story

For many of us, it is difficult to reconcile the analytical power of the mind and Western knowledge with intuition, spirituality, and other ways of knowing, such as traditional Indigenous knowledge. My path to this reconciliation was a long and winding one, reminiscent of the Buddhist symbol unalome. Soon after becoming an Assistant Professor, I had two experiences so profound that they changed my entire perspective on knowledge. They shook me to the core, challenging everything I thought I understood about the world around me, including, and possibly especially, what I understood about science.

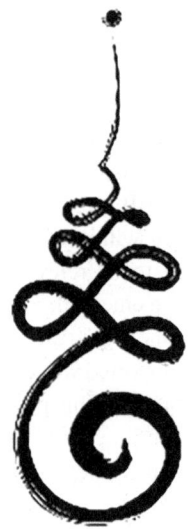

Buddhist symbol unalome

The first of these experiences involved having someone close to me, who I knew well and trusted fully, ask me a simple question: "Did you and Lorraine ever get out of that boat?" It sounds like a simple question, doesn't it? The question might seem silly since I was standing in her living room… except the night before, Lorraine and I were in a boat *in my dream*. I stood there, about to answer her question, when the realization came: *she was asking me about something I had dreamed.* How on earth would she know what I dreamed? She wasn't even in the dream! And that was it. Everything I thought I knew about the world, what we know, what we can know—science—was shattered.

The second experience took place later that year in the canopy of an old-growth forest in the Pacific Northwest. As a forestry academic colleague, I was invited to go up more than 200 feet in a gondola to the canopy where groundbreaking research was taking place. At the time, I was extremely afraid of heights, but given my interests and this extraordinary opportunity, I had to accept. I situated myself in a corner of the gondola and asked not to be disturbed because it was going to take all I had in me and much self-talk to be able to do this. Up we went, me terrified, deep breathing and self-talking, all the way to the top. The crane stopped, and we silently observed the forest from within its uppermost branches. It was astonishingly beautiful, and I found myself at complete peace. I no longer noticed the gondola nor even perceived the ground so far below us. I was enthralled by the trees and the atmosphere they created. I felt that I was a part of it. There was no separation between us. Before I knew it, the crane began to lower the gondola back to ground level.

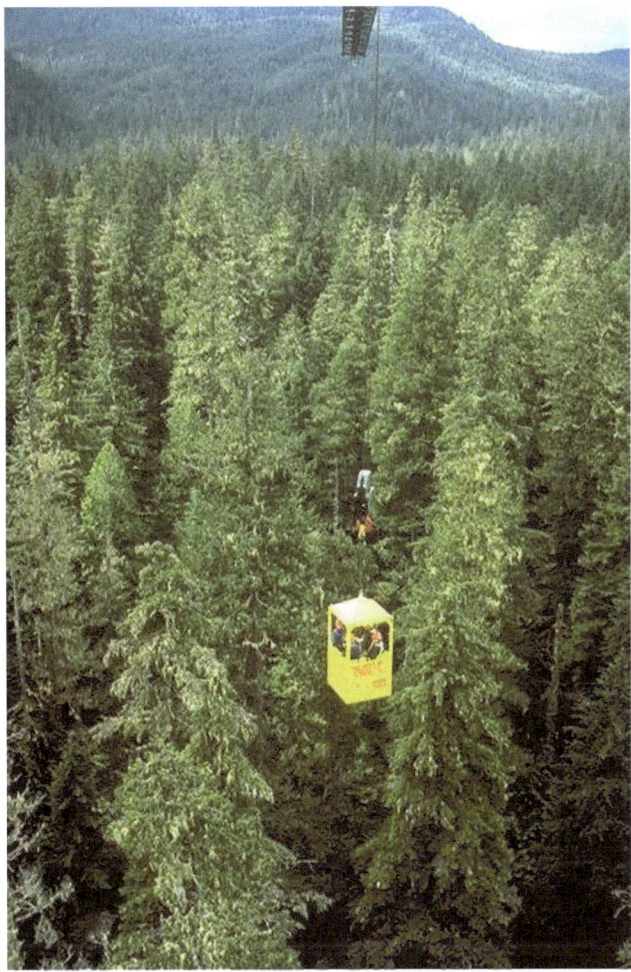

andrewsforest.oregonstate.edu

On the way down, I marveled at all that I learned while in the canopy. I now fully understood how vital energy flowed among and between trees, through intermediaries and directly, even understanding how losing trees within the forest shifted that energy and impacted the others, with clear implications for forest management. As we reached the forest floor, it hit me…there was no lecture in this gondola up in the old-growth forest canopy. How did I now know this? Where did it come from? My expertise was in forest policy and ecological economics, not biogeochemistry, the focus of this new knowledge. My Western science trained intellectual mind kicked into gear, and I asked my biophysical science colleagues about it, assuming that I must be remembering something from a forest ecology class. When the answer came back that no one had studied this energy flow, I realized that somehow this information had come to me from the trees and the forest itself. I had no idea how that could have happened, but there it was—a full understanding of something yet to be studied by Western science, and not something in my own field of expertise. The recognition of this unusual (to me) way of learning combined with the fact that I was not yet tenured resulted in me setting aside the whole experience for nearly 20 years for fear of losing credibility or even my job if I told this story. That's when I heard a radio show about scientific findings of the energetic connectedness of trees in a forest. The scientific study of what I learned nearly two decades before from the forest itself had now been done.

That radio show delivered a jolt that brought me face-to-face with the reality of something beyond science and I was no longer a professionally vulnerable Assistant Professor. It was time to explore the acquisition of this knowledge that did not fit within the definitions of science – this knowledge encountered before Western science had addressed it, what I referred to as pre-science. Read that last word without the dash. I knew it was time to share these stories. As I have done so, it validated others who, often sheepishly, offered examples of serendipity, fortunate coincidences, and unexpected sudden realizations that helped their work and everyday lives in beneficial ways. I also learned that Indigenous Peoples have known such things for millennia.

Sharing stories and validating others is an important step. We must also build the scaffolding that allows for respectful intertwining of multiple ways of knowing both within ourselves and with others. Bringing together knowledge systems allows for more complete and complementary paths toward a non-violent, equitable, sustainable world that we can pursue with confidence.

## 5      Linking Ways of Knowing Within

Engaging with heart means bringing our whole selves to all that we do. Compassion, gratitude, appropriate detachment, understanding sovereignty—individual and collective, and humility are all a part of this path. Essential to this effort is linking intellect with the other ways we know. Imagination provides a path to do this. Meditation provides a path to do this. Being still and communing with nature can do this. Recognizing and articulating what comes to us in these ways, often in deep stillness, helps to bring it into the analytical, intellectual mind. We tend to keep these parts of ourselves separate and hidden from others. By intentionally and actively connecting the non-analytical and the analytical parts of ourselves we build internal bridges that allow us to begin to intertwine these knowledges, thereby bringing more of ourselves to all that we do. By sharing

this through talking about it with others, we not only support each other in these endeavors, we build bridges between and among us, strengthening collective abilities to engage with heart. At the same time, we actively connect the specific goals of collaborations and partnerships with the broader goals of systemic change reflected by the visions of the futures we want, which for me is a peaceful, equitable, sustainable world.

Developing intuition skills is also part of engaging with heart. Unless it is the subject of a scientific study, though, many in science are uncomfortable with the notion of intuition. We have not been free as scientists to articulate our experiences with intuition without fear of damaging our credibility as scientists. It is as if having more to our life experiences, other dimensions than those expressed through the analytical mind and scientific experiences, is somehow odd and not rigorous. The usual and familiar argument goes like this: "intuition is not externally verifiable; therefore, it is not acceptable in relation to science." This stems from our understanding of intuition and intuitive knowledge being direct knowledge, not derived analytically. Therefore scientific external validation does not work to verify it. Logically, it makes no sense to use scientific external validation methods applied to a different knowledge system, yet this appears to be overlooked. It also implies that we do or would not know the difference between analytically based knowledge and intuitive knowledge. If that's so, then the answer is clear – we need skills-based training to learn how to do so.

This is an example of how science maintains and contributes to existing inequities. Rejecting knowledge from sources other than the analytical smacks of elitism and denies the experience of many cultural traditions and indeed, all individuals who have been nurtured to be and to bring more than just their analytical minds to all that they do. For example, in rural Bolivia Aymara Indigenous communities do rituals and rely on physical and biophysical indicators to predict climatic events, crop productivity, and more. This practice in Bolivia remains alive and part of the annual agricultural cycle (thanks in part to their social revolution to empower and elevate Indigenous Peoples). However, in many parts of the world, Indigenous peoples, their languages, and their practices continue to be brutally exterminated.[1]

I am keenly aware that the knowledge shared with me by the trees and forest must surely have been shared with many, many others. And yet, no one I found within the forest science community knew of these relationships—or they didn't speak of them. How could this be? We have clearly turned away, forgotten, shamed, or rejected this kind of knowledge. At what cost, I wonder, and who is paying the price? Looking at the status of environmental and social conditions, my assessment is that this forgetting or rejection has come at tremendous cost which is not borne equally within and among us. We have opportunity with every partnership to remember and to accept.

Many, if not most of us educated in the sciences were trained to limit ourselves to our analytical minds, leaving aside other parts of us. Science celebrates the analytical over all else. Understanding "mind" as more than only the analytical will help. Historically and across cultures, mind has been more widely interpreted to include conscience. In fact, definitions of mind include consciousness, yet in the practice of science in the twenty-first century, we tend toward limiting our practical engagement of mind to the analytical. Looking at the word "conscience" itself reveals broader understandings that stood at one time. Con science, from Latin, essentially meaning "with science" or "with knowledge". That's perfect! Science and conscience together reflect a breadth that would serve us well as we co-create a more equitable, sustainable world though mindful (science and conscience) global health partnerships.

## 6    Challenges to and with Western Science

Following the dominant paradigms of science, though, our tendency in practice is to take the stance that we, as experts, know something that other people need to know without giving much, if any, consideration of what they already know

or know in ways that we may not have considered. While the number of research partnerships has increased in recent years, many, maybe even most of them are based on developing relationships only deep enough for people to accept what we already know we have to offer as disciplinary experts, instead of being truly collaborative, participatory, and flexible from the start. We have learned to "be experts": to tell, to profess, to compare, to direct, and to persuade, all amounting to primarily unidirectional communication aimed at our "partners". We listen enough to make our own points better, instead of empathetic listening to deeply understand and co-create the best ways forward. Engaging communities as subjects of study is not true partnership.

Most science and public health education programs do not address the roles of imagination, consciousness, and intuition in science or ways of knowing beyond the analytical and intellectual. Nor do they teach the skills necessary to engage intuition as well as the intellect and to effectively interweave them. This combination not only results in solutions that reflect diversity in all ways, but it also welcomes all people to contribute, no matter their level of scientific education. Imagine a partnership that is designed to allow for the emergence of new ideas from anyone within the group. We may believe we are offering this simply by calling an association a partnership, but it is not so without explicitly designing and operating in ways that support every participant to bring their full selves and ways of knowing to the endeavor. To be not only allowed, but encouraged and supported by purposeful design to fully contribute. Inviting others into our world on the condition that they accept and abide by our rules does not adequately address the issues. In recent years, Western science has done just that, making an arguably weak effort to recognize Indigenous and local knowledges. In my humble opinion, this is no way to learn about and engage other knowledge systems.

Reframing partnerships with respect for all that each participant brings, balancing this with what we in Western science/medicine know— engaging differing knowledge systems with respect—will bring more people into global

---

[1] Example provided by Susana del Granado.

health partnerships, expanding and impacting them in new ways. Understandably, this raises the question of how to do so at a time when we are grappling more than ever with widespread misinformation. Discerning distinctions between knowledge systems versus misinformation is challenging, especially with social media artificial intelligence algorithms designed to misinform or to direct behavior repetition within groups with common beliefs. The primary business model of many of the largest social media companies results in increased profits by maintaining or even exacerbating separations among groups of people, limiting true dialogue and cross-pollination of ideas through these potentially powerful communication channels.

The challenges of misinformation are exacerbated by a mistrust of science. This is an important time for discernment. Continuing to reject out-of-hand anything other than the main line, dominant paradigm of Western science is likely to result in greater difficulties in managing public health issues, as trust continues to erode. We are at a difficult time in terms of managing misinformation, and we are only just beginning to develop an awareness of and respect for knowledge systems other than Western science and to tear down the colonizer/settler mentality embedded within it. This makes it more important than ever to engage with heart. Resistance to and mistrust in science may stem from values important to those resisting. Exploring these values can be a fruitful way to address this mistrust. Vaccine resistance during the COVID-19 pandemic provides many examples of public health professionals doing just this. Opportunities to do so, to engage with heart, abound. For instance, in Bolivia, chlorine dioxide, a chemical banned by the FDA, became a popular treatment against COVID-19, even approved by the National Government.[2]

In valuing ways of knowing beyond an analytical Western science approach, we can also acknowledge the value of Western science. It has brought a great deal of knowledge forward for the benefit of humanity and it continues to do so. By linking with multiple knowledge systems, we have the opportunity to incorporate many knowledges to sustain all life—human and more-than-human—and enhance its quality. Many non-dominant cultural traditions model intertwining multiple knowledges to sustain all life. We must learn how to learn without appropriating cultural and spiritual traditions of others (see Chapter "Transforming the Planetary Health Crisis Through an Indigenous Land-Based Meta-Narrative"). This is not a simple task when we are just now beginning to recognize the depth of the colonizer/settler mentality in our social structures and systems, despite many in Indigenous communities and in the global South having long called this out.

## 7    Concluding Thoughts

Engaging with communities in true participatory fashion, not simply as subjects or data providers, is an important initial step (see the case studies in this volume). Creating opportunities for solutions to emerge in more ways than only analytically with the partners—aligning with ancestral knowledge, intuitive knowledge, and imaginative and anticipatory possibilities—will transform the outcomes and our world. Stemming from our study of systems, evolution, and complexity science we have learned the limitations of prediction and the reality and value of the emergence of novelty. Discourse in policy has grown to include adaptive management, or learning from doing and making the necessary adjustments along the way as we learn. More recently, the need for an anticipatory approach to policy has been recognized if we are to adequately protect people and planet. It is not enough to adapt as we go, we need to be open to other ways of knowing. With rapidly changing conditions, anticipating the possibilities will provide a stronger means of engaging—if we do so with right relationships and intellectual humility—the recognition that what we believe in this moment might be wrong. These approaches to global health partnerships are evident in the case studies found in this volume.

---

[2]Example provided by Susana del Granado.

Systems thinking helps us to better understand both possibilities and limits (see Chapter "A Holistic Systems Approach to Global Health Research, Practice, and Partnerships") by bringing together the many threads that intertwine to create the complex situations we face in global health. One critical example is how funding sources often limit the possibilities by focusing on limited timeframes, immediate outcomes, set frameworks, and the requirement to state these outcomes *prior to* the start of the endeavor (see Chapter "Funding for Equitable Infectious Disease Research and Development"). This restricts or even precludes the possibility of new ideas, approaches, and knowledge to emerge from partnerships. As we move toward more heart-centered approaches, working with funders to adjust will also be necessary. We quickly see the systemic nature of making change and the challenges of stepping forward with change in one area without supporting adjustments in the rest of the system. None-the-less, we must carry on. As a wise friend shared with me, "it is difficult to live a post-revolutionary life in a pre-revolutionary world…and still we must."

Participating in global health partnerships provides us with the clear opportunity to have much greater and sustained impact by respectfully engaging diverse knowledge systems within ourselves and with others. Recognizing the power and influence that these partnerships have to shift us individually and collectively provides even more reason to consider exploring how we replicate trauma through the dominant paradigm of science. Finding a path to wholeness in all that we do—engaging with heart with openness and intellectual humility—is a courageous way to heal ourselves and our world.

**Acknowledgments** Gratitude to Dr. Susana del Granado, Environmental, Social and Governance Officer, Strategy and Development Department, Inter-American Development Bank, for substantive review and comments to improve this chapter prior to submission and to the reviewers following submission.

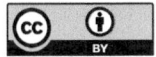

# Courageous Authenticity: Bringing Our Inner Wisdom to Our Work, Partnerships, and Communities

Amie Tyler and A. Desiree LaBeaud ⓘ

*The gift you carry for others is not an attempt to save the world but to fully belong to it. It's not possible to save the world by trying to save it. You need to find what is genuinely yours to offer the world before you can make it a better place. Discovering your unique gift to bring to your community is your greatest opportunity and challenge. The offering of that gift—your true self—is the most you can do to love and serve the world. And it is all the world needs.*

—Bill Plotkin

**Abstract**

To create the innovative solutions global health demands, we rely heavily on scientific knowledge, the scientific method to test hypotheses, and observable measurable data. However, we can also incorporate additional ways of knowing into our process, to fully honor and receive wisdom from all aspects of our humanity and to foster meaningful and impactful outcomes. We can learn to value our imagination and intuition as useful tools for innovative problem-solving. We can learn to honor ancestral viewpoints and incorporate learnings from the community, their experiences, and their land. We can learn to partner as people first, to manifest infinite possibilities of common ground and open ourselves to more connection points than scientific purpose alone. As we do this, we can become extremely fulfilled as we find deeper purpose in our work, our calling. Here, we offer ideas for global health practitioners and researchers to explore introspection to aid in deeper partnerships and engagement. First, we delve into deliberate introspection to foster greater awareness of our inner and outer landscapes. Second, we invite other ways of knowing to broaden our perspective and bring greater creativity to our global health research process. Third, we pause to consider the calling of a global health career. Finally, we approach ways to engage with others to heal collective trauma and to see ourselves as activists and healers in our capacity to build a more just, equitable and healthy world. Although it takes time to build relationships this way with oneself, our global health partners, and the work itself, this expansive way of working can be transformative. We invite you to acknowledge and honor all aspects of yourself and weave them into your global health work, partnerships, and vision.

A. Tyler (✉)
Higher Love Healing, Burlingame, CA, USA

A. D. LaBeaud
Department of Pediatrics, Division of Infectious Diseases, Stanford University, Stanford, CA, USA
e-mail: dlabeaud@stanford.edu

A. Stewart Ibarra, A. D. LaBeaud (eds.), *Transforming Global Health Partnerships*, Sustainable Development Goals Series, https://doi.org/10.1007/978-3-031-53793-6_26

**Keywords**

Authenticity · Intuition · Imagination · Other ways of knowing · Introspection · Partnerships · Self-inquiry · Science and spirituality · Collective trauma · Alignment

## Author Perspective

We are healers, trained in either medicine or psychology, who have worked with a variety of partners within our local teams and in greater social systems locally, regionally, nationally, and internationally. Our backgrounds span biology, medicine, transpersonal psychology, holistic process-oriented psychology, trauma-informed creative expression for healing, international business, pediatrics, and infectious diseases. We are American-born, working mothers who deeply value the humanitarian aspects of our work. We have both changed career paths to gain deeper alignment between ourselves and our work. On this journey, we have experienced added depth and momentum when we incorporate courageous authenticity—the commitment to remain curious, open, and vulnerable—into our work. We hope that our experiences shared in this chapter can light a path for others.

## Key Tenets

1. Through intentional probing and introspection, we can incorporate additional ways of knowing into our global health work to fully honor and receive wisdom from all aspects of our humanity and to foster meaningful and impactful outcomes.
2. A potentially helpful tool to intentionally grow our partnerships can be the incorporation of a short, introspective cycle into the research process.
3. Although the global health practitioner has many roles, and our primary role may not be to treat collective trauma, we can use our research and partnerships to ignite momentum toward systemic change and wellbeing.

4. When we allow ourselves to sink deeply into the truth of who we are—to know ourselves fully (courageous authenticity)—we bring our soul to our work, potentially allowing for more transformation and meaning in our global health practice, not only for ourselves but also for those we serve.
5. This chapter addresses the following SDGs: #3: Good Health and Wellbeing and #17: Partnerships for the Goals

## 1 Introduction

As scientists we are taught to reassess our preconceptions about the world and open ourselves to possibilities as we collect data and let it inform our thinking. We can also incorporate other ways of knowing, such as intuition and imagination, into our work to bring more of our authentic selves to our global health work, partnerships, and calling to produce insight, increase understanding, and gain new knowledge (see Chapter "Engaging with Heart in Global Health Partnerships"). In addition, if the global health work is focused on a certain community, knowing that community deeply and understanding gaps in healing for that community are essential for working together (see Chapters "Colonialism, Decolonization, and Global Health" and "When Women Lead in Global Health: Alternative Mobilizations").

We embody our best selves when we are authentic, but how do we bring forward courageous authenticity—even more curiosity, openness, and vulnerability—to better serve our communities? In this chapter we give examples and exercises to bring out our authentic selves and integrate other ways of knowing into our work to be in better service to global health and its many partnerships.

Each of us embodies our personal and unique inner and outer landscapes. Some aspects of our inner landscape include our life experiences and stories, our beliefs, our conscious and unconscious biases, our egos and personalities, our psyche—soul and spirit, and our hopes and visions for the future. We are also shaped by our outer landscape: our cultural norms and traditions, conscious and unconscious structural biases, mysteries and myths, collective experiences and stories, systems, and infrastructure.

Facing our inner and outer landscapes and integrating new ways of knowing into our work takes courage, hence the term "courageous authenticity." Owning one's truth is sure to conflict with what society expects, at least some of the time. Partnerships can go wrong because of broken trust and disharmony rooted in unspoken, deeply felt, and held value disagreements (see Chapter "Team Science and Infectious Disease Work: Exploring Challenges and Opportunities"). Knowing ourselves and others deeply can help to build trust and rapport so that when conflict arises, solutions can be co-created that center the shared vision of the work and respect and value all perspectives.

In many cases presented in this volume, authors have shared firsthand how strong partnerships impact innovation, the community, and the journey of the work. In this chapter, we explore two key tenants of courageous authenticity to help build strong global health partnerships: ways of knowing and introspection. Ways of knowing seeks to broaden access to innate wisdom that exists within each of us—trusting our instincts and our intuition (see Chapter "Engaging with Heart in Global Health Partnerships"). Introspection can be thought of as an ongoing process by which we acknowledge what has meaning for us personally and in relation to our work, as well as that of our partners and projects themselves. In our experience, these tools are not formally taught in research spaces and take practice to execute. Here, we share stories and exercises to guide the reader in exploring these inner landscapes to build better outer landscapes, particularly global health partnerships.

## 2 Using Other Ways of Knowing for Problem Solving, Creativity, and Innovation

Global health research demands immense creativity to identify solutions to complex global challenges. In this exercise, we share tools to help access other sources of knowledge to foster creative global health work. One tool to guide the explorations of other ways of knowing is the Psychological Functions diagram (Assagioli 1974) (See Exercise 1, Fig. 1). First, define what your focus will be for this exercise: it can be a question about your project, a problem you are trying to solve, or even a conflict between partners that needs resolution. Next, guide yourself around the star in a self-guided meditation, asking yourself: What do my sensations say about [my question/problem/conflict]? What do my emotions say? What do my desires say? What does my imagination say? What does my thinking mind say?" And so on. Write down your answers and revisit them as often as needed. When we trust these deeper aspects of ourselves beyond the thinking mind as valuable information, new insights and creative solutions can often be revealed.

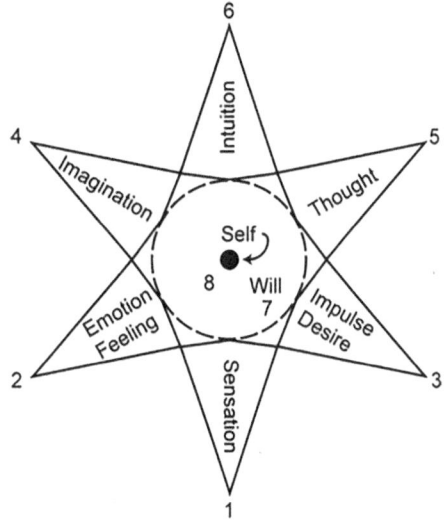

**Fig. 1** Psychological functions and their relationship to one another. (Psychosynthesis Star Diagram formulated by Roberto Assagioli)

**Exercise 1. Self-Inquiry: Ways of Knowing for Problem Solving and Innovating**

1. Complete the Star Meditation (See Fig. 1)
2. Reflect on how deeper ways of knowing can be incorporated into your projects, research process, and partnerships.
   (a) What are ways that you *know* beyond your analytical mind?
   (b) How do you involve your intuition and imagination, or a gut sense in your research and partnerships?
   (c) What does your imagination say about a solution to a problem you have been working to solve?
   (d) What would need to be adjusted in your research process to include a cycle on what your imagination is telling you about your work?

**Ways of Knowing for Problem Solving: My problem was that I didn't feel fully aligned in my global health work.**

A Reflection by A. Desiree LaBeaud

As a global public health researcher, I have led efforts to stop the world's most deadly animals: mosquitoes. My team's research has described mosquito-borne infectious disease burden in communities, linked mosquito breeding and disease risk to plastic trash, and we have conducted school and community-based interventions to prevent disease. All of this research has been done working alongside Kenyan scientists, team members, and community members and has led to increased local knowledge and community interventions, but I had a problem. I felt I was not fully fulfilled as a researcher because there was much more to do to better serve our communities, including leading grassroots efforts to effect change where it was most needed. This could not be accomplished by research alone.

Guiding myself around the star (see Fig. 1) in my identity as a researcher, I accessed these ways of knowing: (1) Sensation: Research alone felt cold, restricted/constricted, numb, and tight; (2) Feeling/emotion: As a researcher, when faced with issues of inequity, poverty, and disease that were not included in the realm of my research abilities, I felt hopeless and was left wanting to do more; (3) Impulse/Desire: My impulse was to be brave and change my foundational work to include something different; (4) Imagination: I imagined that this might be possible and I shared my dream with my long-term research collaborators in Kenya. We then brainstormed together and shared wild dreams with one another about what could be and decided on January 15, 2019, to co-found a nonprofit. (5) Thought: I had seen successful examples of nonprofits in Laos, Kenya, and elsewhere and therefore had models and teachers to turn to; (6) Intuition: If I trusted my whole self, my heart and my gut sensed that the new adventure would be both an opportunity for personal growth and for improved values alignment; (7) Will—I used my energy, time, and resources to push through the non-profit launch process by reading books, talking to other nonprofit leaders, co-designing the mission and vision with my co-founders, building an advisory board, filing paperwork, identifying a fiscal sponsor, and fundraising to support the planned work.

For years I had felt unaligned and sensed that there was a way for me to use my talents for greater good, and that research alone was not the right path for me. Something felt missing. I believe this process was an inner Call of Self. It took time to develop the confidence, faith, trust, and support that I needed to launch our nonprofit.

So, after nearly 20 years of conducting infectious disease research in Kenya, I,

(continued)

along with my two long-term Kenyan research collaborators, began this new journey: the creation of a new nonprofit, The Health and Environmental Research Institute (HERI)—Kenya. HERI-Kenya (www.heri-kenya.org) is an organization dedicated to alleviating global health inequities by focusing on the interface between health and the environment. Through education, awareness, and active engagement, HERI empowers communities to change cultural norms, destigmatize trash collection, safely clean up local environments, create recycling programs, create jobs, and improve health. Our goal is to translate the power of scientific knowledge into actionable messages in the community and to change the trajectories of health for our communities and our planet.

Initially, I felt like I was trying to do the impossible. I had no training in business or nonprofit leadership. However, as I continued to work and persist despite my uncertainty (will), I realized that everything I had learned in medicine, community-based research, and life had prepared me for this new path. Our nonprofit work is rooted in the deep inherent worth and dignity of every person and respect for the interdependent web of all existence of which we are a part. When we care for our planet, we care for all of us.

My favorite African proverb says "If you want to go fast, go alone. If you want to go far, go together." Our nonprofit work embodies this proverb and supports lasting change in our little corner of the world. The journey to launch the nonprofit is over and now the true work begins- and this work feels warm, open, exciting and true. I am in better alignment with who I am and am grateful for the opportunity to grow, learn, and transform with and through HERI.

## 3    Introspection as a Tool for Deepening Partnerships

Effective global health work requires long-standing and sustainable connections between partners (see the Case Studies section of this volume). A potentially helpful tool to intentionally grow these important relationships can be the incorporation of a short, introspective cycle into the research process (see Exercise 2). This exercise can foster deep connections with those with whom we work, revealing our inner and outer landscapes, and helping us understand what each individual brings to the partnership.

### Exercise 2: Sphere of Influence

The Sphere of Influence exercise is both a strategic and creative way to gain insight and can be done as a personal or team exercise.

Throughout a project, document what you feel each person, community, or location/land bring to the work/partnership.

To begin, first, make a mind map. A mind map is a tool to that can be used to draw out the many elements of a project so they can be visually documented and explored. This can be done on a piece of paper, whiteboard, or with sticky paper on a wall. A mind map may remain up on a wall for a long period of time, moving the notes, categorizing them, and adding to them.

1. Place the name project or central idea in the middle. From there, around your central idea, note all the contributors and players that are a part of your project. Remember to include not only the people, organizations, and partnerships, but the physical location and the community, if the project is taking place in a certain geographical area.

(continued)

2. As you review each contributor, contemplate each one and take notes about what you feel each person, community, or element bring to the partnership:
   (a) How and what am I contributing? How might they contribute to me?
   (b) What wants to be seen?
   (c) What stories want to be heard?
   (d) What injustices/injuries do I wish to highlight, if any?
   (e) Is there a hidden truth waiting to emerge?
   (f) What more wants to be revealed?

It is helpful to view this exercise not just with our physical eyes, but with our felt sense, intuition, imagination, and desires, as several aspects of our Sphere of Influence are visible and "seen," yet some are less obvious or "unseen," such as collective traumas or systematic injustices that have deepened over time.

The initial exercise can be approached as an exploration, as not all of the information will be known yet. Tracking this throughout the project can reveal deep insights over time, and the validation that each aspect of your work is part of a sphere that is there to influence and provide input, which otherwise could remain hidden or assumed without the intention to draw out deeper truths.

3. Write a post-project reflection, to capture learnings and wisdom to carry forward.

**Ways of Knowing for Launching a Project to Create a Vehicle for Collective Healing. My challenge was there had been a collective trauma that had been experienced yet largely unseen/not spoken about.**

A Reflection by Amie Tyler

Empowering communities through expressive arts can be a powerful way to foster connection and enable collective healing in a way that is accessible to everyone.

Inspired by Candy Chang's "Before I Die" wall (Chang 2011), I created the Pandemic Healing Art Wall, an interactive, public installation in central San Mateo, California, to reflect and find refuge and connection (Fig. 2). Four days after project launch, on May 17, 2022, Johns Hopkins reported, "The United States officially surpassed one million reported COVID-19 deaths today," (Donovan 2022). The project—a large, chalkboard "box" had stenciled prompts related to the COVID pandemic and an unending supply of chalk. The journey around the four walls began with the prompts, "I lost____, I am grieving_____, I am hopeful for_____, and I am grateful for_____," where participants used chalk to write their personal notes. Over a 30-day period, the wall and I became stewards to over ~10,000 handwritten notes.

When I began this project, I felt the world was returning "to normal" without a moment to contemplate the impact of the SARS- CoV2 pandemic on our lives. Many of my clients were carrying unexpressed grief and felt they had limited avenues to express it. They also felt external pressure to "keep going." I knew from my research that deep neurological wiring patterns and emotional and spiritual healing could occur for individuals when grief or trauma can be expressed in a safe environment. Yet, as I contemplated what was needed for healing, I could not readily sense the heartbeat of my city to understand what would be helpful and a catalyst for healing. The energy felt disparate and hard to articulate or grasp, and the energy my clients had described felt true: everyone had "moved on," or felt it was expected of them to move on.

As I searched for potential locations, the Sphere of Influence exercise organically

(continued)

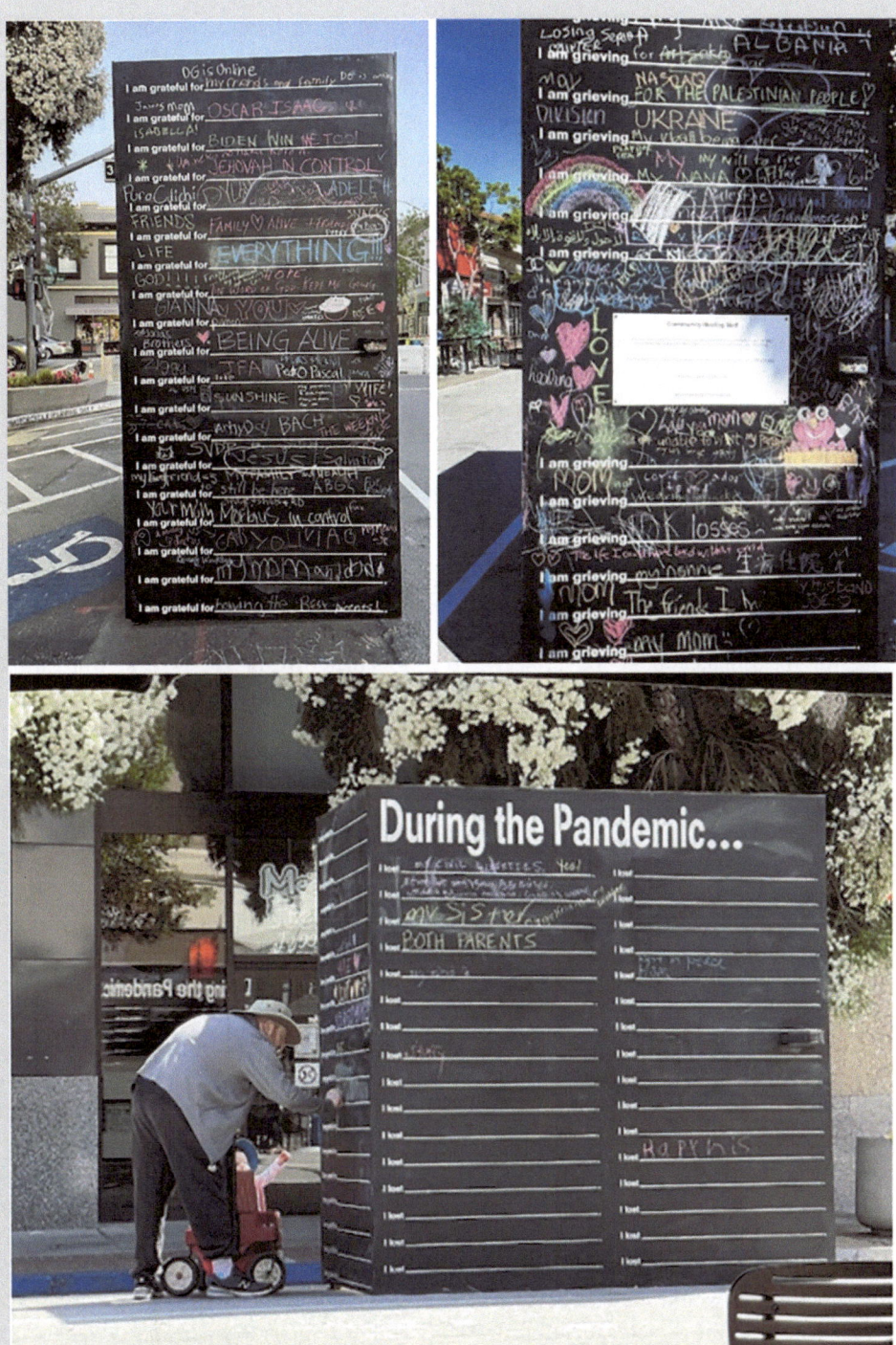

**Fig. 2** Project Images from Pandemic Healing Art Wall, an interactive, public installation in central San Mateo, California, to reflect and find refuge and connection, launched in May 2022.

emerged as a way peer into this new creation that wanted to come forward. I made a mind map of the project contributors and what I noticed they brought to the partnership.

1. The city itself: I researched the City's demographics and found them quite interesting. The city of San Mateo, California, USA, is nestled between America's third richest town and neighborhoods where 44% of the residents fall below 200% of the federal poverty level. This provided deeper meaning to my project as I wanted it to be accessible to everyone.
2. The director of the public arts commission: She was a seasoned professional with decades of experience in public art installations and working with artists. She was passionate about the project because I would be the first non-commercial artist to bring art to the city, and we could forage the groundwork for future artists to do the same—including insurance, legal contracts, and city approval.
3. The potential location: I had originally envisioned the project on the side of a wall at an old pump station building by the San Francisco Bay where there is little foot traffic. The intent was this would be a destination spot of sorts, in quiet, for families or individuals to experience peace and contemplation about their losses in a peaceful and somewhat private place. Note, while this was my original vision, I did not know at the time the key contributor to offer a location in the center of downtown with high foot-traffic would come from my partnership with the director mentioned above, who recommended a pedestrian area to reach more people.
4. The nearby business owners: At the start of this project, I did not know many of them personally. I placed the surrounding business on my mind map with the sense I would need to open the line of communication and request feedback.
5. The participants: Each day I would sit by the future installation site and observe the passersby.
6. The participant's grief: I created a placeholder for this as an important participant.

Here, I reflect on the many learnings from this project.

**Post-Project Reflection**

I was surprised by the depth of the collective experience. Visitors of all ages came to the wall to cry, celebrate, and express their emotions. On several occasions, I witnessed strangers connecting and crying together. Business owners who owned shops nearby would often make a point to come out when they saw me there, offering stories about being a witness to the wall day after day, sharing their conversations and experience. At the start of the project, I hadn't realized the role of the business owner as "witness" and the impact it would have on them to watch the wall, day after day.

Themes individuals expressed were around primary losses, such as loss of togetherness, loss of loved ones, loss of control over one's life or future, and loss of resources, but there were also secondary losses: loss of holding someone's hand, loss of inspiration gained from travel, or the pain of witnessing someone pass just before they could experience their retirement—a sense of holding others' unrealized dreams.

I was moved when one wrote he lost both parents during the pandemic and when a daughter shared that she lost her father to COVID-19 just three days after he was able to get his first COVID shot as vaccines first

(continued)

became available. I was also moved to watch a mini-phenomenon day after day, where for example, a family with a new-born baby wrote they were grateful for their grandparent and then face-timed them in Japan to show them their name on the wall during a time when it was not safe to visit. Even in unspoken ways, when one person expressed loss, others would write thoughtful notes back to that person some-times hours later. I was surprised by the immense feeling of interconnectedness that seemed to build over time. I loved watching teenagers make their visit an after-school ritual, coming by almost every day to leave notes for one another, opening a new way of sharing and connection—an outlet for communication after so much isolation. I was in awe watching people use their cour-age to speak about their truth.

The space to express oneself became a mode to allow for collectively grieving, as well as to express hope for the future. Perhaps the most surprising aspect of heal-ing is that it often takes place in the space beyond words. More than ever, this rein-forced that art allows us to feel, acting as a mirror and matching what wants to arise to the forefront within us. When at first, I thought I had to curate something more systematic, what I learned was simply holding an intentional space drew out what wanted to arise from each individual and the collective. While I could surmise "what wanted to be seen," (Exercise 2), only the participants could show me that.

Most importantly, one consistent real-ization emerged over and over: It does not matter if you are the artist, the participant, or the compassionate witness—offering a space for healing and being willing to step into that space are the two critical actions that open the door healing. The "how" it unfolded was not up to me, it was up to each soul in each moment to be present in their own way—to take their newfound

deeper sense of knowing and embody it into their own life experience. This was a beautiful reminder that our contributions—our research, our creations, our discover-ies—are our offerings. What happens thereafter cannot be controlled or pre-dicted, only experienced by the receiver: the ultimate lesson in letting go.

## 4 Understanding the Impacts of Trauma and the Opportunity for the Global Health Practitioner

The field of trauma research is vast, growing and sometimes controversial. Nevertheless, it is important to understand that trauma is universal. In a World Mental Health Study conducted by the World Health Organization across 26 countries and 6 continents, it was discovered approxi-mately 70% of those surveyed have experienced trauma and almost a third had experienced four or more traumatic events (Benjet et al. 2015).

This section explores the impacts of trauma and innovative ways to partner with local organi-zations to support your work.

Although the global health practitioner has many roles and our primary role may not be to treat collective trauma, we can use our research and partnerships to ignite momentum toward sys-temic change and wellbeing. There is an opportu-nity for global health scientists to imagine and then collectively and collaboratively build a more expansive vision of health for the people all over the world.

As activists, we can use our research to pro-mote social justice, access to basic needs and healthcare, gender equality, and quality educa-tion. As healers, we can seek opportunities to acknowledge community wounds and help restore, re-story, and re-imagine a community's vision for their future so they can regain their power.

For example, how powerful might it be, as part of your work, to fund and partner with professionals in the healing world when working with communities that have experienced trauma? As a parallel path to your research, consider partnering with a social justice & wellbeing organization to do special projects in the community. For example, an activist working for restorative justice, an artist who focuses on therapeutic expression for healing, a process work psychologist who can help groups access and establish a new identity with a collective trauma, or someone to teach or hold space for storytelling, expressive writing, music, or visual arts.

Consider partnering with a local wellness organization to establish an ongoing ritual during projects or consider partnering with a social justice activist who is working with politicians and organizations to create systemic change in your area of work. The feedback and involvement from the community is not only a welcomed offering, but this type of connection point can also fuel your work, opening doorways to depth and richness beyond research alone.

## 5    Science and Spirituality: Where Faith Meets Knowledge

The word science comes from the Latin verb "scire" to know. The root of the word is significant. Even in ancient times, science was associated with knowledge and understanding. Certainly, spiritual practice is another means of acquiring understanding. Science, based in empirical evidence and observation, informs us of the many laws which dictate the natural world. Spirituality on the other hand, illuminates the natural world in other ways and extends to the supernatural. To partake in holistic and authentic work, scientists must face the fact that we are indeed humans and with that humanity comes a departure from the objective observation that science demands of us. Our biases and our beliefs effect our science, and the interweaving of our humanity with our science potentially allows for even greater discovery.

In everyday vernacular, faith means to trust in something yet to be seen or proven. As a formal concept, faith is often confined to the realms of religion and dogma, and as such, is largely dismissed by academia and science. Yet both faith and science strive to attain an understanding of something that is limitless in its truth. Why would anyone conduct research without faith that there is something more to be discovered, something currently unknown? It is for this reason that spirituality can intersect with the scientific sphere. Science pursues a better understanding of the world to answer questions that have remained unsolved. Just as a spiritual individual meditates or prays to obtain a clearer sense of their place in the universe, a scientist conducts experiments to uncover fundamental truths. While the methods differ, the purposes are similar: to gain insight and understanding, to serve and improve humanity, and often, deeper meaning.

## 6    Approaching Your Global Health Work as a Sacred Dance

The sheer nature of life is to persist, grow, and transform. A flower can grow through a crack in the sidewalk without any tending. This is the beautiful thing about life—it will always find *some* way to participate in forward motion. However, creating a rose garden requires embedding our life force energy intentionally into the planting and tending process. We are forever pruning and curating throughout life. Life is always calling to us, providing inspiration and lighting the fire of creativity and inspiration within. Likewise, global health work can be a calling.

Bill Plotkin, a scientist-turned-depth psychologist and ecotherapist, notes a teaching from Native American teacher Harley Swift Deer who says early in a person's career, they complete their survival dance. They learn how to be self-reliant, secure a job, and even take social action. It is only after one completes their survival dance that they begin to establish their sacred dance (Exercise 3). The sacred dance includes a person's deeper work—the thing that calls to them and provides them with deep fulfillment (Plotkin 2003). We, the authors of this chapter believe that this chapter itself is an outcome of our sacred dance.

By leveraging courageous authenticity, we lay down a template for others to touch the depths of their own. When we allow ourselves to sink deeply into the truth of who we are—to know ourselves fully—then, we know what moves us and we recognize what moves others. We bring our soul to our work, and the wisdom from our ancestors and from our creative fire. When we can express this authentically, engaging our intuition and discernment, we invite in the development of our own personal inner-wisdom process that has the potential for more transformation,

> **Exercise 3. Self-Inquiry: What Am I in Service To?**
>
> 1. Draw a line down the middle of a piece of paper.
> 2. On the left, make a list of the five areas where you spend most of your time and energy in your work. What are you focused on currently, and what is taking the most time?
> 3. On the right, make a list of the five areas where you long to spend more of your time and energy. Are there things you would you rather be in service to? Is there something calling to you, waiting to be born into being? Write it down even if it seems out of reach.
> 4. Identify where time in your schedule can be allotted to these new areas. Have courageous conversations with mentors, partners, and champions who can support your vision to move into more of what is calling to you—for this is your Call of Self.

heart, and meaning in our global health work not only for ourselves but for those we serve. What an incentive to be in service to our true selves, so we may be a clear channel for the contributions that wish to come forward for others.

## 7 The Invitation

Courageous authenticity does not require you to adopt an entirely new way of being. It only requires you to accept this invitation:

Acknowledge and honor all aspects of yourself.
Explore and activate how you can access your own deeper ways of knowing.
Courageously reveal them to your partners and incorporate them into your shared global health vision.

The essence of your future work is already an alive force within you. Every seed of inspiration—seemingly logical or otherwise—is calling you to explore. Trust your knowledge *and* your intuition, imagination, and other ways of knowing to guide you in building deeper partnerships to co-create your unique global health vision and contribution, longing to be born into existence.

## References

Assagioli R. The act of will. Harmondsworth: Penguin Books Ltd; 1974.

Benjet C, et al. The epidemiology of traumatic event exposure worldwide: results from the World Mental Health Survey Consortium. Psychol Med. 2015;46:1–17. https://doi.org/10.1017/S0033291715001981.

Chang C. Before I Die. 2011 – Present. New Orleans, Louisiana and Worldwide.

Donovan D. U.S. officially surpasses 1 million Covid-19 deaths. 2022. https://coronavirus.jhu.edu/from-our-experts/u-s-officially-surpasses-1-million-covid-19-deaths

Plotkin B. Soulcraft: crossing into the mysteries of nature and psyche. Novato: New World Library; 2003.

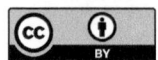

# Correction to: Nipah Outbreak Investigation in Bangladesh, 2007: A Case Study of One Health Partnership and Intersectoral Coordination

Mahmudur Rahman, Nadia Ali Rimi, Rebeca Sultana, Nusrat Homaira, Jonathan H. Epstein, and Stephen P. Luby

**Correction to:**
**Chapter 14 in: A. Stewart Ibarra, A. D. LaBeaud (eds.), *Transforming Global Health Partnerships*, Sustainable Development Goals Series,**
**https://doi.org/10.1007/978-3-031-53793-6_14**

In Chap 14, page 210, the year in the introduction part was incorrectly published as 2021 which should be 2001. The correct year 2001 is now updated in this revised version of the book.

INCORRECT:

" … back to the advent of outbreaks of Nipah (first reported in 2021) and avian influenza viruses (first reported in poultry in 2007)."

CORRECT:

" … back to the advent of outbreaks of Nipah (first reported in 2001) and avian influenza viruses (first reported in poultry in 2007)."

---

The updated version of this chapter can be found at
https://doi.org/10.1007/978-3-031-53793-6_14

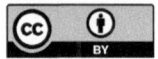

# Correction to: Building Partnerships and Confronting Challenges: Implementation of an Ebola Virus Vaccine Clinical Study During an Outbreak in the Democratic Republic of the Congo

Daniel G. Bausch, Hugo Kavunga-Membo, Rebecca F. Grais, Nathalie Imbault, Natalie Roberts, Robert Kanwagi, Deborah Watson-Jones, Jean-Jacques Muyembe Tamfum, and on behalf of the DRC-EB-001-JnJ Ebola Vaccine Study (TUJIOKOWE) Team

**Correction to:**
**Chapter 12 in: A. Stewart Ibarra, A. D. LaBeaud (eds.), *Transforming Global Health Partnerships*, Sustainable Development Goals Series,**
**https://doi.org/10.1007/978-3-031-53793-6_12**

In Chapter 12, one of the author's name was inadvertently published as "Deborah Watson" which should have been "Deborah Watson-Jones." This has now been corrected in this revised version of the book.

---

The updated version of this chapter can be found at
https://doi.org/10.1007/978-3-031-53793-6_12

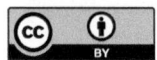

# Index